MODERN CLINICAL PSYCHIATRY

Eighth Edition

LAWRENCE C. KOLB, M.D.

Professor and Chairman, Department of Psychiatry,
College of Physicians and Surgeons, Columbia University;
Director, New York State Psychiatric Institute and
Psychiatric Service, Presbyterian Hospital of New York

W. B. SAUNDERS COMPANY — Philadelphia — London — Toronto

W. B. Saunders Company: West Washington Square
Philadelphia, Pa. 19105

12 Dyott Street
London, WCIA 1DB

833 Oxford Street
Toronto 18, Ontario

Modern Clinical Psychiatry   ISBN   0-7216-5486-X

Print No.: 9   8   7   6   5   4   3   2

Preface to the Eighth Edition

This edition of Modern Clinical Psychiatry is the first which does not bear the name of Arthur B. Noyes, the original author and the sole writer of the first four editions. His contributions to the text ended with the beginning of his long illness which terminated with his death on August 21, 1963, and yet his influence is clearly continued through this edition, particularly in his superb discussions of psychopathology; in the many illustrated case reports; and in his discussions of Psychiatry and the Law.

Those acquainted with previous editions will recognize the organizational changes with this eighth edition. They will note as well that, although the significant theoretical and phenomenological material of concern to the practice of psychiatry is retained, every chapter contains new information of importance to the practice of modern clinical psychiatry.

As before, the first chapters are devoted to a brief survey of the historical development of psychiatry and the conceptual frames of reference needed to achieve an effective comprehension of the complex and variegated array of behaviors which force the attention of the practitioners of this specialty, of medical workers in general, and of others in the mental health professions.

The major organizational change contained in this edition is the reordering and redesignation of chapters devoted to consideration of the various clinical syndromes so as to conform to the new Eighth International Classification of Disease. Such a rearrangement seemed wise in view of increasing international transactions within this and other fields of medical specialization, and because of the wider readings and the several translations of the text into languages other than English. This order has been modified when it has seemed best to assist the student in organizing his learning task. Thus, Mental Retardation follows Chapters 28 and 29, which are devoted to other conditions generally first recognized and treated during infancy, childhood, and adolescence. These three chapters, as readers of the earlier editions will note, offer a much expanded account of our knowledge of the disorders of early life. The new chapter on Special Symptoms exemplifies this expansion. This is, of course, the same period of life in which psychiatrists and others recognize the majority of individuals with personality problems derived from the various causes of retardation. As in previous editions, the content of Chapters 31 through 33 is concerned with currently used methods of treatment and management.

All bibliographies have been updated, retaining from the past only those writings of primary seminal or historical importance. Preference in the new selections has been given to outstanding review articles or other articles published in the English psychiatric literature, since these are the communicative media used by the majority of the readers of the text. The extent of the updating

iii

of this edition is evident by noting the addition of many new terms in the index. Some of the more interesting and important of these new topics are General Systems Theory, Poverty, Racism, Athlete's Neurosis, Hemodialysis, Open Heart Surgery, Organ Transplantation, Transsexualism, Behavior Disorders of Childhood and Adolescence, and Encounter Groups.

I remain much indebted to my colleagues worldwide for their continuing suggestions and critical advice. It is my particular wish to express my very deep gratitude to Professor Arthur Carr of the faculty of this university's Department of Psychiatry. Over the years he has given a continuing close reading and appraisal of the text throughout the various editions with which I have been associated. His perceptive and wise advice, too, has come unsolicited; it has added a special sensitivity and flavor, particularly to those sections concerned with the contributions of modern psychology to psychiatry. Most deserving of special appreciation are Mr. James W. Montgomery, Librarian of the New York State Psychiatric Institute, and his colleagues who have so carefully and faithfully aided me in obtaining the needed literature for review and in checking the bibliographies of this and earlier editions. To Mrs. Sara Klein Geneshier I remain warmly thankful for her able assistance in typing the updated chapters and sections for each of the successive editions.

LAWRENCE C. KOLB, M.D.

Contents

Chapter 1

"Those who fail to know the past are doomed to repeat it."

Santayana

The Beginnings of Psychiatry

Modern psychiatry is that branch of medicine which is concerned with the manifestations and treatments of the disordered functioning of personality which affect either the individual's subjective life or his relations with others as well as his capacity to adapt to life in society. Psychiatry is directed, as well, to the origins and the dynamic interactions of the personality which contribute to the development of mental disease. "Origins" include the genetic determinants, whether of chromosomal derivation or arising as the result of prenatal factors, family and social transactions, and experiential deprivations, which often underlie the specific selection of forms of behavior. "Dynamic" refers to the motivations that direct the behavior and the adaptive processes and mechanisms utilized to fulfill the requirements for maintenance of personality functioning at the biological, familial, and social levels of life. The variations of disturbance include those involving disorders of overt behavior as well as those influencing feeling, thought, and the functioning of various organ systems. Psychiatry's concern is directed to failures of personality development, expressed in certain persisting immaturities as well as in more severe disorganizations of the individual.

Since disordered behavior touches upon many aspects of life in society, the psychiatrist and psychiatry have an interest in the knowledge obtained not only from all the biological sciences which contribute information on personality growth and pathology but also from those other professions and institutions which contribute to the management and social control of those with personality disturbances. The latter include psychology, the social sciences, law, philosophy, and theology. In the former, modern psychiatry seeks for explanations in the individual's genetic inheritance. This includes predispositions, the influence of anatomical, physiological, and biochemical processes, and the determining effect upon the maturing nervous system of the recording of the individual's life experiences. The recording begins in the prenatal period and extends through childhood in the family to the later environmental and cultural pressures. To the psychiatrist, the interaction of these factors determines the personality of the individual.

Personality has been defined in a multitude of ways; some are concerned only with the outward expressions of behavior, while others consider as well man's subjective experiences. For psychiatrists, both aspects of individual experience are covered by the term "personality." Personality is perhaps best recognized as each individual's characteristically recurring patterns of behavior. These patterns, which are characteristic for the individual, are evident in response to both the sudden and the persistent stresses of life.

THE BEGINNINGS: PRIMITIVE CONCEPTS

The origins of the majority of the scientific concepts of psychiatry are, of course, rooted in the past. There are, at best, conjectures as to the manner in which disturbed behavior was viewed by prehistoric

1

man. The study of the primitive tribes of this day lends support to conjectures concerning the concepts of illness held by prehistoric men which are reflected in the myths and records of the early pages of history. Comparative studies also have provided valuable insights into the ranges of behavior of man under varying conditions. They have made evident the modifying influence of culture on the symptom expressions of psychopathology and illuminated the deficiencies in certain theoretical explanations of behavior that come from a study of man in a particular culture during a given time span.

The concepts of disease found among primitive people differ from those held by the scientific communities of today, although remnants of such primitive ideas of illness may be noted from time to time in the general populations of even the most technologically advanced societies. To primitive man, all illnesses are attributed to forces acting outside the body. Such forces are seen as supernatural; they are the evil spirits, witches, demons, gods, or magicians. These demonological explanations are particularly strong as explanations for illness affecting behavior. It is pertinent to speculate that primitive man came to such ideas from his own personal experiences and his contacts with the sick. His own dreams of return of the dead and his remembrance of their threats, demands, and affections perhaps fostered the belief in influence from beyond life. His observations of the nonsensical, impertinent, meaningless, and destructive behavior of the delirious and psychotic, his apprehensions in the face of a convulsive attack, and his efforts to explain the phantom after the loss of a limb must have fostered the concept of demonological possession as the causal means for the peculiar and frightening changes of behavior which fell upon those with whom he was close and familiar.

Primitive societies devised methods of treatment which are used even now almost exclusively in the framework of magical and religious practices. Within these methods (which often were followed by recovery of the afflicted) one may perceive the rudiments of psychotherapy.

Since like produces like to primitive man and since objects once in contact continue to have an influence even at a distance, the use of charms for their protective or healing force is frequent among such men. Charms may be viewed as homeopathic or imitative magic. Another way in which imitative magic is used constructively is in the rites of the healers who act out the experience of the person to aid him. Good examples are the healer among the Dyaks of Borneo who plays the role of the parturient woman or the medicine man who enters a state of trance before indicating the treatment. The effectiveness of such methods of treatment may have rested on the patient's identifying himself with the healer and entering into a state of death and rebirth. The therapeutic use of trance states is another widespread measure among primitive groups. In some tribes, trance states are induced by fixation on objects much as one may induce hypnotic states.

The quest of the medicine man is often to find the lost or afflicted soul, to drive out the demon, and then to return the soul to the body. Exorcism, the forcing of an evil spirit from the possessed, is brought about by many means in different groups and areas and may be easily recognized as a form of psychotherapy in which the ill person is encouraged to speak of those actions and misdeeds which have guilty connotations. The rites of self-punishment appear to have the same purpose. Other primitive ways include the use of spells and incantations with their repetitive offerings, the rituals of silence, and also the applications internally and externally of herbs and other medicines. Throughout one may recognize the primitive methods as beginning with simple cause-and-effect explanations and empirical observations, without recognition of the operation of internal forces of either a biological or a psychological nature. Nor does the medicine man direct his efforts to the individual but rather to a malignant invading force foreign to his primitive patient. The meanings and aims of primitive rites, while psychotherapeutic, hold no relationship to modern treatments which find the sources of illness within the biosocial organization and development of man.

GRECO-ROMAN ERA

References to mental disorders in the early writings of Egypt, India, China, Greece, and Rome disclose the beginnings of those major streams of thought and action which now pervade the growth of psychiatry as a science. The beginnings of the humanitarian attitude, reflected today in the area of social psychiatry, were seen as early as 860 B.C. when Greek priests supplemented incantations and exorcisms for the mentally disturbed with recommendations for kindness and suggestions for the use of physical and recreational activities.

A significant move occurred in the sixth century B.C. as the Greek healer's interest turned toward observation and experimentation; these were the first scientific steps in biological science. Alcmaeon dissected and noted the connections of the sense organs to the brain, from which he inferred that the seat of reason and the soul were located in this organ.

This early scientific movement is best observed in the writings of Hippocrates (460–375 B.C.). He initiated a classification of mental disorders into mania, melancholia, and phrenites. His descriptions of disease indicate the existence then of knowledge of epilepsy, hysteria, postpartum psychosis, and the acute brain syndromes (delirious states) which occur with infectious diseases and after hemorrhage. He flatly rejected the influence of the gods as causative of mental disease. Hippocrates influenced, as well, the social atitudes of his day. While Athenian courts recognized the rights of the mentally disturbed in civil affairs, they gave no consideration to their rights in a capital offense. Through his influence, if it could be proved that the individual on trial suffered from a condition which Hippocrates designed as paranoia, the court appointed a guardian for the accused.

Although others expanded the Hippocratic approach, undoubtedly the high point of scientific observation during the Greco-Roman period was reached in the time of the Roman physician, Galen (130–200 A.D.). Using the scientific approach, he studied the anatomy and physiology of the nervous system and postulated that the existence of symptoms did not necessarily indicate that the organ or part of the body which served as their expression was the affected part. Galen developed a theory of the rational soul as divided into external and internal parts. The former, in his system, consisted of the five senses; the functions of the latter were such things as imagination, judgment, perception, and movement. Galen concluded, as Plato thought and Aristotle denied, that the brain and not the heart was the seat of the soul.

The problem of mental disorders occupied the attention of the Greek philosophers as well. Empedocles spoke of the importance of the emotions and pointed out that love and hate were fundamental in determining changes in human behavior. His concepts were incorporated by Plato in his consideration of Eros in the personal life of man. Plato propounded the idea that a psychologic biography might be written of the individual man, commencing with his earliest years through his relations with his family members and educators, to explain his adult behavior. So, too, he conceived of a tripartite soul composed of rational, libidinous, and "spirited" portions, the latter containing various animal qualities. This concept of the soul has been likened to Freud's structural concept of the personality. Thus, one of the main streams of modern psychiatry, the psychodynamic, had its recorded beginnings in the Greco-Roman period, largely disappeared in the Dark Ages, and occasionally reëmerged in the philosophical writings of the Middle Ages. It is finally recaptured in the modern psychodynamic movement initiated by Sigmund Freud.

With the decline of the Roman Empire and throughout the Dark Ages of Western man, there occurred a revival of demonology, spiritual explanations, and tortuous exorcisms, with disagreement from only a few solitary individuals.

At times throughout the Middle Ages and even later, in Europe and in the Americas, large groups of individuals simultaneously seemed affected with psychic epidemics. The majority were poor peasants, artisans, and other impoverished members of the societies in which they lived. In the belief that they were infected by the devil, masses danced together in the streets, cried out the names of demons, publicly exposed and exorcised themselves, and told of their ecstatic visions. The study of these epidemics led to some of the earliest conceptions of social factors as causation of mental derangement—the beginning of social psychiatry.

The physician whom some describe as the first psychiatrist, Johann Weyer, worked openly against the then current beliefs of supernatural possession as the cause of mental phenomena, condemned those who blamed women of witchcraft, gave explanations of the mass psychoses, and described many as arising from symptoms of melancholia proceeding from love. He suggested that reputable physicians be called in before adjudging women as witches, as in his opinion their behavior was due to illness. Weyer, too, advised that one might find the pathogenesis of mental phenomena through developing detailed information about the sufferer. He successfully treated some accused of witchcraft by sitting alone and talking with them for long periods.

Beginning with Francis Bacon in the seventeenth century, the philosophers recognized that the functions of "mind" were of concern to the natural order of the universe. These views came to have a profound influence on medical thought. At this time the philosophic interest of Descartes and others in the "mind" and its function established a dualistic explanation of human behavior. It will be noted that in the definition of psychiatry there was no mention of the word *mind*. There need not be, however, any objection to the use of the word, provided it is employed as a collective designation for certain functional activities of the organism, particularly those of the organism as an individual personality. As a corollary to this definition of mind, the reactions of parts of the organism would be designated as physiological, while "mind" would be considered the integrated response of the organism to the complex physiological, psychological, and sociological forces that impinge upon it. The "mind," therefore, is merely one aspect—the psychological aspect—of biological functioning of the organism and not a metaphysical entity having an existence parallel to the body. The dichotomy which is implied by "mind and body" does not exist in the organism.

THE MODERN ERA

At this historical time, there again took place a revival of interest in the humanitarian care of the mentally ill. Under the leadership of Chiaruggi in Italy (1759–1820), Philippe Pinel (1745–1826) in France, Daniel Tuke (1827–1895) in England, and Dorothea Dix (1802–1887) in the United States, the shackles of patients were removed and hospital surroundings were developed for their care. Today, with the almost universal acceptance of mental illness as a medical problem in Western European and North American society, these changes continue to expand and are currently manifest in the "open hospital" movement started in England and in the new British Mental Health Act.

More or less coincident with the humanitarian reforms in treatment, there transpired the growth of medical interest in mental illnesses. Following a long series of observations by the brilliant clinicians in Europe, Emil Kraepelin (1856–1926) gave to psychiatry the first comprehensive description of what he believed were entities of mental disease. Prior to his time, psychiatric attention had been directed to the symptom, which was regarded as

the illness. Kraepelin assumed that mental disorders were definite disease entities analogous to the physical diseases and defined by etiology, symptomatology, course, and outcome. This led him to stress clinical observations and the search for physical origins for mental diseases. His system of classification was based on descriptions, symptoms, and outcome, since it was frequently impossible to make the diagnosis by laboratory examinations. Thus the classifications were not based on an understanding of etiologic factors including those of psychodynamic processes. While his system brought clarity to a mélange of psychiatric observations and thereby aided scientific study, yet, in fact, Kraepelin appears to have had limited appreciation of the inner life of his patients. His work did little to promote understanding of mental disorders, particularly the psychodynamic forces operative in them. His name, nevertheless, must be considered among those of the psy-chiatric great, as he observed with discernment and systematized the results of his observations—a necessary stage through which every science must pass.

BIBLIOGRAPHY

Ackerknecht, E. H.: A Short History of Psychiatry. 2nd revised ed. New York, Hafner Publishing Company, 1968.

Alexander, F. G., and Selesnick, S. T.: The History of Psychiatry. New York, Harper & Row, 1966.

Braceland, F. J.: Kraepelin, His system and his influence. Amer. J. Psychiat., 113:871–876, 1957.

Kiev, A. (ed.): Magic, Faith and Healing. New York, Free Press of Glencoe, 1964.

Mora, G.: On the 400th Anniversary of Johann Weyer's "De Praestigiis Daemonum." Amer. J. Psychiat., 120:417–428, 1963.

Rosen, G.: Madness in Society. Chicago, University of Chicago Press, 1966.

Schneck, J. M.: A History of Psychiatry. Springfield, Illinois, Charles C Thomas, 1960.

Zilboorg, G., and Henry, G. W.: A History of Medical Psychology. New York, W. W. Norton & Company, 1941.

Chapter 2

"Now we, like all animals, carry with us vestigial traces of our past ancestry, not least in our mental processes. To develop psychologically we must understand ourselves, and it should help us to do so if we can find ways to investigate those hidden depths in our minds from which we draw our impulses."

Sir Walter Langdon-Brown

Development of Dynamic Psychiatry

That body of knowledge which is directed to understanding the psychological influences and maturations that determine psychopathology is known as dynamic psychiatry. It rests essentially on an evolutionary basis. In its theory, behavior, no matter how abnormal, is the result of needs and drives which are built into the personality through the biological inheritance. It is complicated and modified by other needs, affects, and counter-strivings acquired in the long learning experience of family and cultural interactions that establish the foundations for man's social life. The basic maturational forces or drives are considered often to operate beyond the range of conscious awareness; that is, they are "unconscious." While dynamic psychiatry is oriented toward the understanding of motivations as determining behavior, it recognizes as well capacity to function as a central determinant in eventual adaptation. Capacity to function rests on the genetically determined anatomic-physiologic structure. Its development is influenced through experience and learning but is, in turn, influenced again by the biological and social motivations which determine aspiration and drive intensities. *Psychodynamics* is the term generally applied to the systematized knowledge and theory of human behavior and its motivations.

EVOLUTIONARY BASIS OF PSYCHODYNAMICS

It is now generally conceded that many of the symptomatic expressions of personality disorders are rooted in modes of behavior which have been manifested earlier in life; that is, they are ontogenetically determined. Through failure of maturation, which may be the consequence of either physical maldevelopment or deprivation of those experiences necessary to foster maturation of a function, evidences of immature and maladaptive behavior may persist into later life. Another type of failure in the maturational growth of the personality occurs through excessive stimulation or gratification during the sequential stages of personality development. Whether it be through deprivation or excessive gratification, the term *fixation* is applied to the process by which facets of the personality do not progress to maturity.

The recurrence of infantile and childish behavior is noted frequently in the clinic when the patient is unable to solve some emotional conflict. A simple example is that of the six-year-old who has long since learned to control his urinary functions but again wets himself with the birth of a sibling. In this instance, the child, frustrated in his need to hold the attention of his mother, "regresses" to an earlier mode of behavior when it was presumed that this need was gratified satisfactorily by the parent. Such *regressions* explain many of the bits of behavior characteristic of the severely ill.

The evolutionary orientation of modern psychodynamics stems directly from the genius of Charles Darwin and later Herbert Spencer, who influenced the great English theoretical neurologist John Hughlings Jackson (1835–1911). Jackson set forth an evolutionary theory to explain the functions of the nervous system in health and disease. In so doing, he drew from his careful clinical observations of epilepsy and other diseases of the brain. Jackson postulated that the functions of the nervous system were integrated at progressively more complex levels, mentation, the highest level of function, being subserved by the vast cell aggregations of the human cerebral cortex. He viewed the symptoms accompanying disordered brain function as representative of both the loss of more recently acquired functions of the brain and the reappearance of more primitive functions which are submerged in evolutionary growth. According to him, when a brain injury produced a permanent deficit in the functioning of the nervous system, in addition to the symptoms due to loss of function, the reëmergence of more primitive actions was also recognized by the clinician as symptoms. A classic example of the latter is the Babinski reflex, a primitive toe sign which disappears during infantile life with myelination of the corticospinal pathways to reëmerge as the result of disease to the pathways from the cortex. Jackson also indicated that the organism tends to adapt to the loss of function by a substitutive or compensatory behavior which sometimes also is viewed as a symptom by the clinician. The Jacksonian theories on evolution and dissolution of function within the nervous system inherently contain the postulate that the understanding of any behavioral disturbance is dependent upon knowledge of the progressive development of that

behavior in a given organism. While Jackson's attention was directed principally to the functions and dysfunctions at the lower levels of integration of nervous activity, he wrote briefly on higher functions and commented that the study of dreams and jokes would provide an important means of furthering understanding of the origins of psychological pathology. Jackson's works and his concepts were known well and were incorporated into the later theories of Sigmund Freud, then a promising neurologist, who established the major premises of dynamic psychiatry, and also of Adolf Meyer, the proponent of the dynamic evolutionary school of psychobiology.

HISTORICAL BASIS OF PSYCHODYNAMICS

Anton Mesmer

When Anton Mesmer (1734–1815), a Viennese outcast, stirred a furor in Paris by curing many diseases, including hysteria, by his technique of "animal magnetism," the scientific world first took cognizance of the influence of purely psychological processes on symptoms of illness. Members of the committee of the French Academy of Science, which included Benjamin Franklin on its roster of distinguished members, were impressed by the results of Mesmer's touching of his patients but duly noted the lack of evidence of animal magnetic fluids. While Mesmer's success was short-lived, his technique was picked up and used in both England and the United States. The English surgeon, James Braid (1795–1860), provided a descriptive formulation of mesmerism and introduced the term *hypnotism*. The French country physician, A. Liebault (1823–1904), learned to use hypnotism widely in his practice and was responsible for teaching the technique to Jean Martin Charcot, the renowned French neurologist. Liebault's work represents perhaps the first direct use of psychological forces in the practice of medicine

—its use in an equivalent sense with other conventional techniques for the relief of suffering of the ill.

Jean Martin Charcot

While Charcot (1825–1893) questioned the growing view that psychological forces could cause hysteria, his eminent position in French neurology brought the study of this disturbance and others directly into the stream of serious medical investigation. From his own studies, Charcot presented a report to the French Academy of Science that the phenomena of hypnotism were manifestations of abnormality and that the hypnotic state occurred only in those with hysteria. Charcot's fame and wide publications brought him numerous students, including Sigmund Freud.

Hippolyte-Marie Bernheim

Bernheim (1840–1919), professor of clinical medicine at Nancy, vigorously disagreed with Charcot's views and maintained that the phenomena observed by the latter took place only when conditions of suggestion were set up by the hypnotist. He stripped the subject of hypnosis of much of its mystery, dispelled ideas of special hypnotic powers and magnetic influences, and demonstrated that patients are also susceptible to suggestion in the waking state. Bernheim advanced the theory that hysteria was of mental origin. He was probably the first to apply the term *psychoneurosis* to hysteria and similar states. Some consider Bernheim's work to be the first effort to evolve a general understanding of behavior. From his studies came new questions pertaining to the legal responsibilities of criminals and the etiology of criminal behavior. Bernheim challenged the thought that "will" was the agent of crime and evil by advancing the belief that the mechanism of suggestion underlies the endless variety of both normal and abnormal behavior.

Pierre Janet

Another of Charcot's students at the Sâlpetrière was Pierre Janet (1859–1947), who also fostered the growth of the psychodynamic viewpoint. Contrary to his teacher, he recognized that the hysteric's fixed ideas and inner conflict with reality were neurotic and insisted on treatment by psychological means. His therapy was essentially persuasion and the use of techniques for altering the environment of the patient. Janet evolved the theory that the neuroses represent a lack of psychic tension on the part of the patient. By psychic tension, he meant an integrating force which, when abundant, held the stream of conscious activity intact. Through constitutional deficiency or as the consequence of fatigue or stress, the psychic energy became defective. Janet saw the disintegration of the stream of consciousness as the expression of psychoneuroses. He introduced the term *psychasthenia* to include reactions characterized by phobias, compulsions, and anxiety. Psychasthenia, to him, was the consequence of a general lowering of psychic energy, while hysteria represented a limited diminution of energy. Based on this concept, the idea of *dissociation* was formulated. As the result of dissociation, elements of consciousness were considered to take on an independent existence and express themselves clinically in the form of alternating personalities, fugues, anesthesias, and other hysterical expressions. The concept of dissociation has an established position in the field of abnormal psychology. Janet also introduced the idea of subconscious processes occurring independently of the mainstream of consciousness but later rejected Freud's explanation of "repression."

Sigmund Freud

Initiating his practice as a neurologist who was well acquainted with Jackson and the French school, Sigmund Freud (1856–1939) turned his attention to the psychoneuroses following his studies in Paris with Charcot. On his return to Vienna, he became associated with Josef Breuer, who was perhaps the first to recognize that neurotic symptoms had "meaning" in relation to the patient's previous life. Breuer and Freud observed that under hypnosis their patients recalled old ideas, impulses, and experiences which they had found necessary otherwise to put aside or repress. As the patient disclosed and "talked out" his emotional upheavals, his symptoms subsided. Breuer gave up this treatment, presumably concerned over the deep attachment which patients evidenced to the therapist. Freud continued alone and soon found that it was unnecessary to hypnotize the patient. He persuaded his patients to speak freely and to bring up anything that came to their minds no matter how irrelevant it might initially seem. With the use of this "free associational" technique, Freud found that he had a means of widely exploring the earlier experiences upon which the patient's mental processes and current symptoms rested. He was able to analyze the meanings of dreams, slips of the tongue, mistakes and errors in everyday life such as simple forgetting. From his careful clinical observations, he constructed a system of psychology to which he gave the name "psychoanalysis."

Freud's psychoanalytic psychology is fundamentally psychogenetic and evolutionary. It aims to discover the motivational conflicts which determine behavior whether healthy or disordered. It provides as well a concept of personality structure and development not previously advanced by other schools. His clear penetration of the relationship existing between patient and physician with the overdetermined attitudes of affection or dislike, which he termed "transference" and in which he saw the recapitulations of earlier infantile and childish relations to a parental figure, represents a monumental insight. The analyses of the transference relationship and the patient's resistance were to Freud the essential elements in his psychoanalytic therapy.

Freud also insisted that much of mental life occurs beyond the realm of awareness and is unconscious. The concept of the unconscious has been one of the great contributions to psychiatry. While some psychologists dislike the use of such a metaphorical word as "the unconscious" for those impulses, desires, and emotional responses which are inaccessible to our introspective observation, such a hypothesis is required for the explanation of many mental phenomena.

Freud's emphasis upon personality as a process developing step by step has given us a clearer understanding of personality manifestations. Many, however, do not accept Freud's concept of infantile sexuality with its uncompleted differentiation and the influence of its persistent hangovers on personality. Freud's demonstration of the importance of inner conflict with its dynamically opposed impulses is the first theoretical system to provide meaning to the genesis of neurotic and psychotic reactions and other psychological phenomena. Although some have misinterpreted Freud as referring to the generalized systems of drives and to the structural elements of the personality (the id, the ego, and the superego) as if they were entities, yet the use of such terms for certain dynamic parts or functions of the personality has simplified thinking concerning personality functioning. Freud's emphasis upon a determinism of psychic processes has led to a greater clarity in our thinking. His psychological theory revolves around the problem of the development of infantile drives into adult personality. He contended that psychopathology resulted from a failure of a smooth, scheduled progress through the successive stages of psychosexual development.

Alfred Adler

This Viennese psychiatrist (1870–1937), an early student and associate of Freud, later came to dissent from the latter's emphasis on infantile sexuality and believed that the child's resistance to domination and his drive to self-assertion, domination, and superiority were more important than the sexual drive in the development and structuring of the personality. Adler's psychological formula may be stated as follows: Because of a sense of inferiority —organic, intellectual, social, or the result of past experiences—a will to power is stimulated, resulting in compensatory reactions directed to goals of superiority. Adler included these various compensatory activities under the term *masculine protest*. He adopted this term on the assumption that the exaggerated "will to power," with its drive to prestige, superiority, and achievement, might be compared to what he believed was the reaction of women to their feminine status. He observed that in European culture, women were usually regarded as inferior, a status to which he considered they reacted by a so-called "masculine protest," that is, by trying to act like men. The will to power need not have its origin in a patent organic defect but in whatever feeling of inferiority, be it organic, sexual, economic, or social, leads to feelings of inadequacy. Adler gave his psychological movement the name *individual psychology* to indicate that each individual has its own special goals and a unique manner of attempting to achieve them. These methods mark the individual off from others and largely determine the structure of his personality. The various psychological processes by which he seeks to deny his inferiority and maintain the fiction of achievement constitute the symptoms of the neurosis. Adler's emphasis on power and prestige motivations, on cultural determinants of neurosis, and on therapy as a reëducation have been absorbed to a greater extent than is conceded by adherents to other schools of thought.

Carl G. Jung

Originating in Switzerland, Jung (1875–1961) became closely associated with Freud during the early days of the latter's development of psychoanalytic theory. In 1911 he broke with Freud over the importance of infantile and childhood levels or stages of sexuality development and the effect upon personality of trauma sustained during these developmental phases.

Like Freud, Jung assumed the existence of an unconscious, but he did not conceive of it as containing the same type of material or as acting in the same way in the production of psychopathology. Jung believed that the unconscious is made up of material derived from two sources. He called one of these sources the "personal unconscious" and the other the "collective or racial unconscious." He considered the "personal unconscious" to be more superficial than the "collective unconscious" and therefore more accessible to consciousness. He contended that the "personal unconscious" contains the individual's personal urges and thoughts that developed in his individual history, forgotten impressions, and reactions to environmental experiences. The contents of the deeper "racial or collective" unconscious, however, are not related to personal experience but consist of instinctive impulses and primitive fears, feelings, trends, and thoughts connected not with personal but with racial experience and thought. According to Jung, feelings and desires related to modes of thinking and acting that have undergone racial repression and belong to phases of past human cultural epochs belong in the "collective unconscious." To this psychological movement Jung gave the name *analytic psychology*.

Jung contributed many other concepts which have received wide acceptance. Among them was the word association test for investigating hidden regions of personality, which is discussed in a later chapter. Jung was among the first to emphasize the nature of the child's interpersonal relationships and to point out that neurotic difficulties of parents are decisive influences in the difficulties of children. Working with Bleuler, Jung applied psychoanalytic concepts to the psychoses and was the first psychiatrist to suggest a psychological approach to the study of dementia praecox (1907). He presented a penetrating analytic description of personality types, developed the extravert-introvert concept, and studied artistic creations, mythological themes, and religion and their relation to dreams, phantasies, and neuroses. He greatly stressed symbolism and religion. His critics comment upon the extent to which he combined psychological, philosophical, mystical, and metaphysical elements.

Adolph Meyer

Slightly younger than Freud but with a similar interest in the basic sciences of neurology, neuroanatomy, and pathology, and having knowledge of the foremost works of the French and British schools, Adolf Meyer (1866–1950) played a prominent role in the development of dynamic psychiatry in the United States through his pluralistic and interactional concepts of human behavior. He insisted that multiple biological, psychological, and social forces contribute to the growth and determination of personality. This approach he designated as "psychobiological." Meyer, as well as Freud, stressed the importance of early parental influences in shaping the development of the child's personality and conceived of mental disturbances as progressive habit formations.

The techniques which Meyer devised for the psychiatric examination form the basis for most of those now used in English-speaking countries. He taught that the understanding of maladaptive behavior requires a comprehensive study of the life history of the individual in which is traced the growth of personality through each unfolding stage to that of the individual's life situation. In his teaching, Meyer condemned the focus upon a single complaint or single aspect of the patient's problem or the examination of it from the standpoint of a particular system of psychiatry. He inveighed against the Kraepelinian nosology with its prognostic import and spoke of psychiatric illnesses as reaction patterns.

Meyer emphasized that each personality has its assets and liabilities. The existence of faulty habit patterns implies the potentiality for teaching healthy socialization. Psychobiology, then, is the biology of the whole personality—the whole person in the whole situation—which must be accounted for and understood in assessing the personality reactions.

The weakness of the psychobiological school rests in its failure to work through the study of intrapsychic processes and their origins in the dynamic interactions of the life of the individual. It remained for the psychoanalysts to clarify through their work these processes which nevertheless, were always clearly perceived as important in psychobiology. As the first to emphasize that psychiatry is a biological science and that its practitioners must study the actual and complete dynamic situation in which the patient lives, Meyer has left an indelible imprint on psychiatry.

One of the outgrowths of Meyer's influence was the development by Harry Stack Sullivan of the interpersonal theory of psychiatry. Sullivan emphasized and sought for a particulate analysis of the communicative interchanges between the growing infant and his parents as the means of specifying the dynamic evolution of human behavior seen as a social phenomenon. He applied his theory to the study of the patient-therapist relationship and defined there the role of the therapist as a participant observer. It was particularly Sullivan who stimulated the interdisciplinary exchanges between psychiatrists, psychoanalysts, and social scientists which have so expanded the conceptual framework and research efforts in the field of modern psychiatry, in its attempts to encompass as it does contributions from biological, psychological, and clinical sciences.

THE STUDY OF BEHAVIOR

Kraepelin's effort to classify conglomerations of human behavior into identifiable syndromes represents one of the major beginnings of the study of the source of behavior. While his system of classification has been widely criticized, all subsequent attempts at improvement or modification are essentially grounded upon his system. Nevertheless, the critical attacks upon the classifications that have been established have led to new approaches that warrant some consideration and perhaps point the way to fresh methods of studying the nuclear processes which underlie the various psychopathological reactions.

The comparative studies of behavior in many species make it possible to identify a variety of patterns of activity that are directed to maintaining the life adaptation of each individual in each species. There are those forms of activity which are directed essentially to maintaining the biological needs of the individual for food, water, oxygen, elimination of waste products, warmth, and protection against attack. These may be classified as (1) ingestive, (2) eliminative, (3) shelter-seeking, and (4) agonistic patterns of behavior, the latter being any activity resulting in contact or contest, whether it results in fighting or flight. The other forms of behavior are concerned with the procreative and social existence of species, the identifiable activities of which are (5) sexual and mating, (6) care-giving and care-taking, (7) mimetic and communicative, and (8) exploratory or investigative.

Man's behavior, in times of either health or illness, may be examined in one or all of the above contexts. He differs from other animals in several ways. First is his outstanding capacity for flexible and intricate manipulatory activity acquired through the freeing of his upper extremities from locomotion by the assumption of bipedal gait. His major adaptive power, however, rests upon the range and versatility of his communicative, social, and investigatory activities associated with the enormous growth of the human brain and its expanded capacities for storing and aggregating experiences. He is able to express through language those thought processes and affective states which accompany the arousal of his needs and the outcome of those drives motivated for their satisfaction. This, in turn, has led to the evolution of the complex symbolizations that he utilizes for communication with his fellows and the capacity to allow perpetuation of knowledge over time through their recording and passage by the cultural institutions. These progressive accretions of knowledge have provided for the solving of increasingly intricate problems.

Those disorders of behavior now recognized in man involve not only various groupings of defects in his behaviors directed to satisfying his basic biological needs, but, more important, those affecting the essentially human elements of behavior: his social relations, his ability to communicate, act, think, and feel appropriate to his maturational state and his situation.

General Systems Theory

Adolf Meyer's psychobiological theory rests upon the tenet that one must approach the study of mental illness or health by a comprehensive examination and analysis of all the numerous factors and stresses which act overtime to influence the growth and emergence of the whole personality. The psychobiological perspective embodies and outlines in a very broad way the lines of study and analysis of personality in health and disease.

The generality of this theory, that is, its failure to define the role functioning of the various scientific disciplines and techniques as they might be employed in the study of personality, has left a void. That void may well be filled today by *general systems theory*, particularly as it applies to living systems. This theory, as the author perceives it, has an organizing capacity for placing the data at hand in the hierarchy of systems which comprise or bear upon man's personality functioning. So, too, that organizational frame should provide the capacity to set the limits of these data and the definition of their relevance in terms of effecting man's own actions within his own system, as well as upon other levels of the social systems within which he lives. Furthermore, within the general systems framework of living system organizations, one can recognize the contributions of others who have offered hypotheses relating to various aspects of man's behavior.

All living systems function to maintain a steady state within by taking in inputs of matter energy so as to restore or maintain their own energy and support repair in their own structures. These systems are open—means are available for input of energy as well as its output. Their walling off in any aspect leads to a failure in functioning or death. They are complex in structure. Each contains genetic materials which provide the informational template for the development of its structures and processes from origin onward. They are composed of protoplasm, containing water, proteins, and other organic compounds. Each system contains an integrating organ (the brain: the critical subsystem which controls the entire system). The brain determines appropriate coactions between all other subsystems. Each contains other critical subsystems or maintains symbiotic or parasitic relations with other living or nonliving systems. These subordinate subsystems are integrated to form self-regulatory, developing, reproducing systems with purposes or goals.

To put it another way, living systems, including man, contain three critical subsystems. They are (1) that concerned with processing information; (2) that concerned with matter energy processing; and (3) that concerned with processing matter, energy, and information—the reproductive subsystem.

The first, the brain, receives inputs from the internal and external environment. The internal environment includes the two previously mentioned subsystems concerned with matter energy.

As for the information-processing subsystem—transformations related to immediate and continued species survival—

information input is received at various receptors and carried by channels or nets to central decoders. The various inputs are relayed to and associated with stored information (memory) gained from the past. The total input related through the associative and stored information subsystems is integrated. A decoder then directs incoding of various information to various output transducers in the subsystems, thus leading to actions appropriate to maintaining or reaffirming the steady states within the system.

In all living systems steady states are brought about by feedback mechanisms that operate on the input channels and nets to either increase or decrease the input, thus providing a method of maximizing or minimizing input or stress. Cybernetics is the study of methods of feedback control. The feedback net provides a channel from the decoder to the input receptors and channels which modulate their functioning.

Man as a living system functions through the integrated actions of various subcellular, cellular, and organ subsystems. As an individual system he relates to other single individuals and group, social, organizational, societal, or national suprasystems.

As for the decision-making processes within living systems, they are conceived of as evolving from the processing of information. In the case of behavior each system develops a "preferential hierarchy of values" from its past experiences of success or failure in the goal-seeking actions required to hold the steady state. Preferential values are acquired through experience; they constrict the decision procedures as rules to facilitate rapid adaptation to the preferred steady state—its purpose. Since each system may simultaneously have multiple purposes, inputs may direct the total system toward several incompatible actions; thus conflict ensues. Effective living systems comply with conflicting inputs by responding to the commands with higher priority values.

Behavior systems theory demands that there be one system level of reference.

Thus, if one refers to a form of abnormal behavior and proposes to use systems theory in its analyses, one will identify the level of reference of that behavior, that is, its reference as function of the individual, but also as effecting or evolving one or several of the subsystems within the individual system (psychosomatic medicine or psychophysiologic disturbance), and determine its transaction with other living systems and suprasystems (social pathology).

Systems theory holds that more complex systems evolve characteristics beyond those of the sum of their subsystems. These characteristics are emergent; they appear through novel associations in the critical informational subsystems. Thus in examining function of a living system one may not extrapolate as identical the functions and actions of its subsystems or less complex living systems. One must identify the emergent functions of the more complex system.

Studies or theories about the complex system based on observations of its subsystems which fail to reflect upon the characteristic emergent functions of the former are incomplete and cannot be used as explanatory for functioning of the total system.

Earlier, I have commented on the emergent biological characteristics of man which separate him from all other mammalian forms. These emergent characteristics have provided the source for the emergence of the species-characteristic functional behavioral process that serves as an adaptive interface between individual men and the necessary social suprasystems necessary for his survival—his personality.

The heuristic value of general systems theory for research related to personality functioning, its potential for cross systems hypotheses and experimentation, and the uncovering of new information on behavior remain to be realized. Nevertheless the psychiatrist may profitably perceive his efforts as those of a clinical scientist with background to draw upon the informational network as it relates to the operations of the organ subsystems of man, as well as being concerned with man's personality functioning in transaction with the social suprasystems necessary for his survival. From his analysis of these complex systems relations, the psychiatrist may formulate the genesis and driving forces that determine aspects of maladaptive and adaptive behavior.

Motivation: Forces and Systems

Behavior may be generally recognized as directed toward some goal, some aim that promises or provides satisfaction or a state of well-being. Behavior may be stated to be motivated, that is, activated and also selected as the appropriate means to accomplish a goal. Within the concept of motivation, questions may be asked as to the forces which lead to the activation or inhibition of a particular form of behavior and those forces which select one or another form as the appropriate one at a particular time.

BIOLOGICAL NEEDS. Each form of behavior has as its goal the satisfaction of a need. Thus, the lack of food, water, or warmth impels the individual to activity which is aimed at satisfying the bodily lack. Needs are determined by the unique biological organization of the species. It is assumed theoretically that a *drive* is induced by the establishment of a need which provides the physiological substrata for the motivation to behavior. In all species, there exist certain biologically primitive or physiological needs necessary for the survival of the individual and the species. The needs for oxygen, water, food, maintenance of body temperature, and avoidance of tissue damage exist at birth and persist throughout life. The need to copulate and to procreate the species and care for the young, while innately given with vertebrate life, is activated only after full maturation of the genital apparatus of the organism coupled with appropriate stimulation and later mating behavior with another member of the species.

In recent years it has been found that another fundamental driving force exists in both man and animals, that is, a drive to explore, or, as it has sometimes been described, innate curiosity. This exploratory drive seems, from experimental evidence, to exist without direct relevance to satisfaction of general bodily functions related to self-preservation or procreation. Even very young monkeys will press levers to open and reopen windows for prolonged periods with no other reward than to look out and observe what is on the other side. Yet the drive is capable of enhancement and may be seen as one of a chain of brain-directed activities which later are molded through experience to bring about highly skilled acts to achieve the satisfaction of a need. Thus, a monkey's activity in lever manipulation is enhanced if he is allowed as a reward to sight another monkey, enhanced beyond that produced by sight of a bowl of food or a moving toy. Furthermore, this exploratory drive to satisfy a perceptual need, in this instance mediated through the visual system, provides an additional reward. Thus, monkeys that have attempted for days to solve a mechanical problem and finally are successful then repeat the satisfying manipulations many times, apparently because of the gratification gained through mastery.

Before such animal studies were made there were innumerable observations of the exploratory efforts of infants and young children which brought forth various hypotheses about the function of exploration and play. Hendrick emphasized an "instinct to master" as an important ego drive. It would seem that work satisfaction relieves tension states induced by subcellular metabolic events which are translated into the integrated exploratory drive expressed in perceptual motor activity.

As Hamburg has written, emotional behavior serves adaptive purposes by making possible "the training of the young to cope effectively with the specific requirements of a given environment."

Exploratory behavior, associated with the protective blanket of long-continued dependence upon older members of a species, offers an unexcelled opportunity of evolutionary adaptation to a diversity of environments. It extends the chance of survival of those who live beyond infancy by increasing their adaptive potential through learning. It is not surprising that prolonged periods of both family dependence and exploratory behavior exist side by side in the widely ranging primate species, including man.

SOCIAL NEEDS. While all of the biologically primitive needs are observed early in phylogenetic growth, they are neither psychologically primitive nor simple in their mechanisms of operation. This is particularly true in man who, as a result of his long period of dependency and the influence of socially determined goals, has learned many other needs. The satisfaction of the need for food, as one examines behavior from the simple to the more complex organisms, may be found to be an increasingly complex behavioral task. The simple annelid ingests and eliminates earth, removing from it the necessary nutrients by its peculiar physiological processes. A carnivore, stirred by the need for food, must stalk his prey, capture, and eventually devour it. In this action, however, there are elements acquired through repeated experiences and even observations of other animals in hunt. Even in play, kittens hunt with the mother and may, through learning, acquire new facilities for satisfying the need for food. In the growing child, the satisfaction of the need for food passes through numerous stages of development beyond that of making the need known through crying and satisfying the need with sucking and ingesting of milk. With this behavior, there is associated contact with the mother, or food giver, who thus comes to signify a source of pleasure and security. Her care determines further associations and behavior, including all those ways in which men in various cultures eventually obtain food, prepare it, and finally eat to satisfy hunger. The many patterns of food acquisition and ingestion are learned acquisitions or derivatives of the original need for food.

While the physiological needs are innately determined, those acquired through association are learned and are the products of the unique interaction of one individual with others. The acquired needs of man then develop in particular family cultures and are determined by associations. Needs for social status, whether acquired through power or prestige and whether or not they are satisfied by the different means of birth, material wealth, creativity, conformity, or capacity to gain the confidence of others, are learned.

"INSTINCT." In the past, the term *instinct* was widely used to explain patterns of behavior innately given to the organism. It is clear that the existence of an unsatisfied need establishes in the organism a set or attitude which primes it for action in the face of an adequate excitant or stimulus in the external environment. This stimulus leads to arousal of the function and also guides or cues the response to satisfy the need—whether the response will be action or inhibition, fight or flight, leaping or stalking, speech or silence. The same stimulus may, in the terms of the behavioral scientists, have both "releasing" and "consummatory" properties. For man, the smell of food may excite hunger and also direct his steps to its presence. Often, however, there is required a series of stimuli, each necessary to determine some phase in a chain of behavior required to satisfy the need. A bee-hunting digger-wasp, for example, flies from flower to flower in search of a bee. In this phase, it is indifferent to the scent of bees, as can be determined by making available the odor of bees by having groups of them nearby but concealed. Any visual stimulus by a moving object of the correct size, whether a fly or a bee, releases the wasp's first reaction of turning toward and positioning itself, hovering to leeward of the quarry. From then on, the wasp is susceptible to bee scent. Dummy bees without scent are abandoned, but those with the right odor release the second reaction in the chain, a flash-like leap to seize the bee. The third reaction, the delivery of the sting, is dependent on a new tactile stimulus.

Many studies by animal psychologists have demonstrated the necessity for the proper maturation of the organism, its necessary exposure to the appropriate stimuli, and the influence of actual experience in determining the development of effective adaptive behavior. Likewise, the deprivation by experience at a critical stage in the maturational process may result in a continuing deficiency in the evolution of particular behavior sequences.

The accumulated evidence indicates that it is misleading and incorrect to consider "instinctive" behavior as a separate form entirely unrelated to "learned" behavior. The two types blend into each other. If by "instinct" is meant that process in the nervous system which produces innate behavior, it is again misleading, as no special portion or brain process is involved that may be specifically related to innate behavioral activity in contrast to that acquired through learning. Instinctive or innate behavior is carried out for its own sake and not for what it may produce in the future. Neither does it imply knowledge of its ends. What is desirable in the study of the behavior of man as well as animals is the eventual isolation and understanding of the various fragments of each behavioral act and also the contribution of the total bodily structure. That of the brain as the integrating organ will be found the most important.

The necessity to separate learned from innate responses in man is most significant from the standpoint of treatment. Learned processes, deficient or disordered, may perhaps be modified by learning or relearning—in other words, by psychotherapy. Those disorders dependent primarily on dysfunctions of primary organization, i.e., "innate," are unlikely to be so modified.

In psychiatry, the term *instinct* is used in a psychological sense and denotes the innate biological drives which determine motivations. They are the dynamic agents not only for the maintenance of the life of the individual, including his social adaptations, but also of the energy for creative purposes in all walks of life.

Drives, Affects and Emotion

As mentioned in the discussion of general systems theory and as may be inferred from the foregoing in man as in all living systems, there exists a continuing drive to maintain a constant internal steady state. That state is characterized by the absence of the tension aroused by a need, a lack sensed in one or several subsystems. We have indicated that in man the tension of need may result from deficiencies sensed or existing in the systems concerned with maintaining his biological integrity. Tensions may also be aroused through the need to discharge, as for example, the mounting pressure in the maturing seminal vesicles for discharge of semen, or the pressures in the rectum or bladder which lead to defecation and urination. So, too, through the long process of social learning, there evolve continuous need states with related tensions which drive to many complex social behaviors.

Even in the resting or *homeostatic state,* as it was designated by Walter B. Cannon, there exists a continuous dynamic interchange of energy and activity in all bodily systems, accompanied by a continuous barrage of information delivered from both the internal bodily and external sensory receptors. A constant quantum of such information derived from all sources establishes the steady state; variations of any sort signal the need and motivate to corrective action.

We may assume that much of the vast and continuous barrage of sensed information reaching the brain is nonmotivational and never achieves conscious attention. If it has psychological meaning, it is as a sense of general awareness of personal well-being. Also, many of the tensions of need are undoubtedly so minor, leading to immediate corrections through the reserve subsystems within the body, that they, too, are nonmotivating for behavior.

DRIVES. That critical tension exists in man is signaled mostly by a reportable subjective state which we denote in terms of threat, craving, or satiation. The drive state and its signal determine when and where the organ systems are to be activated or inhibited. In the infant, hunger or thirst, need-tensions caused by lack of food or water, establish the action of sucking which continues until the need is satisfied. So, too, the infant signals through his crying that his hunger is distressing and indicates his satisfaction on presentation of the nipple by his silence. Drive states, then, are accompanied by degrees of distress and satisfaction, and are signaled by vocalizations or other actions to the social world surrounding the infant.

AFFECT STATES. As motivating forces the drive states required to maintain the physical integrity of the organism are primitive. In man, they have been observed to operate in anencephalic infants. The tensions of the need and its later satisfaction are inferred to be distressing and satisfying, painful or pleasurable. But they are obviously experienced passively; the infant is incapable of directing actions to obtain (approach behavior) or to escape from (avoidance behavior) the circumstances arousing the need tensions. Nor has he the potential for use of actions and behaviors to decrease or increase his discomfort or comfort. As Tomkins states it, the primary function of the *drive systems* is providing motivating information concerning what systems are to be activated and deactivated and when.

In contrast, the primary function of the *affect systems* may be regarded as solely *motivational.* Furthermore it is the driving force of this system upon which the essential characteristics of man's personality evolve: his cognitive, attitudinal, decision-making, and action powers.

Affects, then, may be recognized as painful or pleasurable, warning of a need or signaling satiation. Thus, fear and rage emerge when bodily integrity is threatened, as inferred from the cries and other neuromuscular activity concerned with escape from some unpleasant stimulus or injury. Rage, fear, or anxiety are primitive affects aroused as concomitants of the reactive processes of aggression, escape, and helplessness (fight, flight, or helplessness). Other unpleasant affects (hunger, thirst, loneliness) are aroused by frustration of drive states. Satisfaction of the needs in turn is associated with a pleasurable subjective appreciation of satiation. With later growth, and particularly as the consequence of the transaction within the family, primitive pain-pleasure affects are elaborated so that in maturity one discriminates such positively motivating or attractive affects as interest, joy, affection, tenderness, love, and compassion as well as the aversive affects of fear, anxiety, guilt, shame, disgust, and hatred.

It is evident that the highly discriminative affective states which influence man's personality development arise only through the long process of family and cultural evolution. Of necessity their evolution has required the vast potential of the human brain for recording, analyzing, and synthesizing information.

Affects serve as the subjective signals warning of threat or lack of satisfaction; they also provide a feedback indicating the approach of satisfaction or satiation and the relaxation of tension. Affects may be rapidly aroused and as quickly dispelled, or they may be slow to evolve and be sustained for prolonged periods.

Affects are perceptions of the internal state of the environment and, as such, in psychoanalytic theory are designated as ego states. Affects direct the integrating and executive aspects of ego functioning; however, they also direct the development of many human behaviors which are defensive in nature and serve to disguise the existence of the underlying affect so as to lessen or deflect the associated drive state. Thus, while guilt signals a need to give up a socially prohibited act—to refrain from it if it is intended or to undertake expiatory rituals if the act has taken place—guilt may also evoke behaviors indicating its defiance, denial, or repression. Behaviors associated with affective states may indeed be used to offset and deny the existence of tension induced by other emotions, as, for example, the use of laughter, crying, or rage to modify a variety of other anxieties.

It is widely thought that the recognition of the affective states, of the variability in their relative intensities, and of the evolution of their control through the developmental process is central to the explanation of individual personality functioning and its pathological expressions. These states are discussed further under Disturbances of Affect in Chapter 6, Psychopathology.

Affects, which may be defined as feeling-tones, are pain-pleasure accompaniments of an idea or mental representation. By stimulating or facilitating some innate drive, they exercise a strongly determinative influence in giving direction both to thought associations and to overt behavior reactions. The terms *affect* and *emotion* are often used loosely as if these two aspects of mental life were the same. This is because the term *emotion* is used with many, and therefore ambiguous, meanings. Its use should probably be confined to indicate either the complex biochemical-physiological processes or functions concerned with the somatic expression of feeling or else the patterns of behavior that express affect rather than subjectively experienced feeling phenomena to which the term "affect" is more applicable.

Intelligence

In vertebrates, the modifiable and integrative aspects of behavior are greatly increased. In them appears the cerebral cortex, developed for the purpose of providing a mechanism capable of elaborating, integrating, and controlling impulses and functions more perfectly than is possible with a more elementary nervous system. In fact, evolutionary stages in development are traceable in the cerebral cortex itself, associated with a corresponding hierarchy of functions. The older part of the cortex, the archipallium or limbic system, as MacLean designates it, is concerned with self-preservative and self-procreative functions and the basic emotional response and visceral functions, in contrast to the more recently developed portion, the neopallium, essential for progressively complex discriminations and integrations characteristic of the highest psychic functions. The biological advantage of its development was that the organism obtained a more flexible capacity for adaptation.

Biological processes have evolved from conditions of simplicity and diffusiveness to complexity, differentiation, and definiteness. Similarly, an imperceptible transition has evolved from innate drive states to cognitive ability of that adaptive attribute called intelligence. Since, from a practical standpoint, the intelligence of an organism is fundamentally its psychological capacity for adapting to and making use of its environment, it is quite arbitrary to say where in the phyletic series intelligence was acquired. In fact, intelligence probably was not superimposed on earlier instinctive processes at some definite stage of evolution but was an outgrowth of them. Whether we speak of species or of individual human beings, those that possess the greatest capacity in these respects are the most intelligent.

Attention

Intelligence requires that the organism explore vast bits of information and retain them within its nervous system. Also, the information-processing organ must select from among the incoming barrage of sensory registrations recurrent ensembles of sensory inputs and recode them as recognizable percepts. It must decide which percepts have priority in terms of immediate and later adaptation, and must attend or focus on the most significant. Finally, the decision-making process requires that actions be taken or be delayed. We may deduce that over time the most

intelligent of the species have recorded a vast sum of sensory impressions. They have retained what constitutes a memory bank. They have evolved a process of rapid and clear perceptivity through the progressive differentiation of the incoming sensory inputs—their perceptivity is both acute and extensive. Also, they have evolved a number of processes which we identify as attention. *Vigilance* is one aspect of the attention processes. It may be defined as the means of scanning sensory inputs obtained from the internal and the external world to select those prepotent for survival. *Concentration* is another aspect of attention; the narrowing down of interest on one part of the perceptual input is another. Again, the attentive process may be varied to allow the alert and continuing scanning of a stream of inputs to discover similarities or discontinuities—the *associative process*. The latter is used effectively by diagnosticians, whether they be physicians or psychoanalysts scanning freely the auditory and visual signals provided by their patients, or engineers attempting to discover the source of malfunctioning of a machine.

Over a time all individuals tend to evolve certain preferences in their scanning activities, decision-making, and action-taking processes. They do so through the learning motivated by affect. Those sets, attitudes, and decisions which have been reinforced by reward-pleasure or through the relief or avoidance of distress and pain, become the preferred modes of functioning.

In the analysis of behavior we must then attend carefully to these aspects of intelligence: attention, whether it be vigilance, concentration, or association; memory as recording and recall; perception and cognition; and the acquired attitudes toward attending, decision-making, and action designated in earlier psychologies as conation.

Attitudes, Sets, and Conations

For the evolution of man's personality, the functioning unit between his inner world and the social environment in which he largely lives, the major determining force rests in his capacity to learn to control and modulate his affects. Each family and each society rewards or constrains individual members through the affection it bestows, withholds, and withdraws or the punishment it renders. Excitement, joy, and contentment are the rewarding affects. Guilt and shame, anxiety and fear, and rage are the aversive affects. The learning processes by which affect display is modulated so that others are less distressed by its emergence in behavior are the molding process for personality evolution. For man in all modern societies affect control is more significant than the motivations of the primitive drive states concerned with simple biological survival. Even the derivative of need drives is now served through the shaping of social interactions. Thus to be accepted in the human world, even activation of the craving for food in hunger demands that one receive, prepare, and consume food by customs that elaborately obscure the craving. Only under extreme conditions of prolonged starvation do the human customs derived from learned control of affect break down to reveal the immediacy of the drive states in their primitive egocentric expression.

Man's affective states, too, differentiate from the primitive pain-pleasure paradigm we ascribe to the helpless infant lying in the crib. That differentiation comes about through the long process of human socialization. From attraction, to interest, to joy in company and attentive care we identify in adults the state of love —a conative set. In the love of mature man there has evolved a series of differentiated states related to parental care: tenderness, compassion, and pity. From loss of love man suffers sadness, but he has learned its variants as depression, hatred, envy, and jealousy. From early distress and fear he has elaborated anxiety, apprehension, shame, and guilt. From the pleasure in consummation he has defined the sets pride and vanity. And from each of these affects and related attitudes his creative intelligence and capacity for leisure have provided the myriad behaviors which identify his characteristic responses in the face of stress, in the anticipation of success and failure or their aftermath, in relaxed satiation, or in distressing despondency.

But these attitudes alone do not make man either healthy or ill. Modern dynamic psychiatry and psychoanalysis have overlooked those conative sets which preoccupied the earlier psychologists. These are many of the attitudes necessary in the first place for human civilization: trust, empathy, likability, responsibility, and perseverance; playfulness, humor, curiosity, flexibility, and self-confidence.

These attitudes determine successful social adaptations. They determine adaptations in many who are crippled by the appalling limitations of the maladaptive expressions of psychopathology to be described later in this book. There is underway now in psychologic research a movement to reëxamine personality dynamics in the light of the development and role function of such attitudes in establishing a healthy balance within the individual personality. Much of the diagnostic and prognostic weakness that exists in modern psychiatric practice and psychosocial research has its origins in preoccupation with the maladaptive to the exclusion of the important ongoing and highly adaptive attitudinal sets to action.

Consciousness

A prerequisite for that degree of adapting to and making use of the environment to which we apply the term *intelligence* is that function we know as "consciousness." By this term is meant a sense of awareness of self and of the environment. Its major biological advantage is that it permits the organism to adapt itself to novel circumstances.

ORIGIN. How consciousness develops is unknown, but it seems reasonable to assume that, in common with higher functions in general, it is a specialized development of lower ones. Such an assumption is in agreement with the general evolutionary propositions. Although no conclusions as to the origin or nature of consciousness can be secured by objective observation, one may speculate that it originates in the properties of irritability of protoplasm. When protoplasm—let us assume it to be in the form of an extremely simple organism such as a protozoon—is stimulated, a response occurs. A response, however simple, implies a change, a difference. As evolution progresses and the organism becomes more complex, and as the types of stimuli and responses multiply, one can imagine that the organism becomes gradually but dimly aware that modifications are induced, that changes occur in itself. Thus, a sense of comparison arises until, finally, sensations are produced, an awareness of which constitutes the dawning of consciousness.

DEVELOPMENT. These beginnings of perceptive processes undergo evolutionary expansion from the simple to the more complex until, finally, a conceptual consciousness with ideative and affective components is reached. It seems safe to assume that its development was through an expanding process, a successive integration, which has progressed simultaneously with zoological evolution. At the psychological level is to be found the highest phase in integration in the continuity of nature. A consideration of the evolutionary process suggests that there is no sharp distinction between the conscious and the unconscious and that conscious thinking represents the most highly developed and most fully integrated process of organizing and dealing with experience.

DEGREE OF CONSCIOUSNESS. Many psychobiological activities occur without conscious awareness. It was formerly assumed that consciousness or sense of awareness was a prerequisite for all those expressions of the organism we refer to as "mental." While many of these psychic functions are manifested only under conditions of clear awareness, observation of mental processes, particularly of those occurring in states of pathology, reveals that highly significant psychic processes operate under widely varying degrees of awareness, and even in the absence of awareness.

Responsiveness alone is not indicative of conscious awareness. Reflex activities may be observed in deep states of coma, and complex behavior, including pertinent verbal communication and interpersonal exchange, may take place following a head injury or in other psychopathologic conditions without the individual's later recalling these actions. Dreaming sleep also represents a state of consciousness which differs from full awareness in which there is a capacity to relate inner perceptions when attention is directed to the immediate external environment.

Full awareness or full consciousness in man demands, then, the capacity for immediate memory and the reproduction of his actions on request with, as well, the ability to perceive the surrounding environment and relate to it in terms of immediate drives and interests. Since at times these responses are held in abeyance, consciousness must be seen as a state in which thought processes, the mediating activities of the brain, intervene between the perceptions and the motivating activities of the organism.

Most students of man's mental life agree that he is greatly influenced by unrecognized psychological forces and that much behavior originates from motives of which one is not aware in his normal waking state. Psychological motivations are undoubtedly a result usually of combinations of causes, of which those least acceptable socially and morally possess the greatest driving force and are farthest removed from consciousness, whereas those which the individual considers the most acceptable are in the forefront of consciousness and are manifest.

The Unconscious

In order to explain many mental phenomena, the features of which are not manifest, it is necessary to hypothesize the existence of a stratum of the personality referred to as the *unconscious*. It includes material that under ordinary circumstances does not enter the conscious part of the personality. For the most part, those drive states determining behavior to satisfy the physiological needs of man operate unconsciously. The diabetic favors foods containing sugar, drinks excessively, and urinates frequently because of a defect in sugar metabolism and its ultimate influence on the body's fluid balance. All this behavior is determined beyond the level of conscious awareness. The individual only knows consciously what he does or must do to remain comfortable.

Various psychological drives exist beyond conscious awareness and are manifested in such forms as dreams, amnesias, purposeful forgetting, mistakes, and split personality. There is abundant evidence that unconscious drives exercise a fundamental influence upon behavior, feelings, decisions, and interpersonal relationships. In psychopathological states, it is particularly apparent that unconscious psychic forces are powerfully active in influencing personality. Emotional forces of which the individual is unaware may be in conflict and act in such a way as to determine his behavior, even though he knows nothing about them consciously.

As will be discussed later, conscious and unconscious forces or motivations may cause the individual to pursue opposite goals. Much behavior, in fact, is a complex of conscious and unconscious motivations. It is only through active repression or through dissociation that any sharp division is produced between the "conscious" and the "unconscious." A great deal of our knowledge concerning motivations has been acquired by the psychoanalytic method of studying the unconscious through the free-association technique. Some psychiatrists raise the question whether, instead of speaking of the "unconscious," one should not emphasize "unconscious mental processes."

The Preconscious

Preconscious is a term applied to mental processes which are not conscious but possess the attribute of easy recall to consciousness. Unconscious mental processes differ in that they do not have access to consciousness except under special conditions, such as psychoanalytic therapy or the psychoses.

BIBLIOGRAPHY

Alexander, F. G., and Selesnick, S. T.: The History of Psychiatry. New York, Harper & Row, 1966.

Bailey, P.: Janet and Freud. Arch. Neurol. & Psychiat., 76:76–89, 1956.

Cannon, W. B.: Bodily Changes in Pain, Hunger, Fear and Rage. 2nd ed. New York, D. Appleton Co., 1929.

Hamburg, D. A.: Evolution of emotional responses. Evidence from recent research on nonhuman primates. Science and Psychoanalysis, 12:39–53. New York, Grune & Stratton, Inc., 1968.

Hebb, D. O.: A Textbook of Psychology. Philadelphia, W. B. Saunders Company, 1958.

Hendrick, I.: Work and the pleasure principle. Psychoanal. Quart., 12:34–329, 1943.

Hendrick, I.: The discussion of the "instinct to master." Psychoanal. Quart., 12:561–565, 1943.

Jones, E.: The Life and Work of Sigmund Freud. Vols. I–III. New York, Basic Books, 1953–1957.

Lief, A. (ed.): The Commonsense Psychiatry of Adolf Meyer. New York, McGraw-Hill Book Co., Inc., 1948.

MacLean, P. D.: Contrasting functions of limbic and neocortical systems of the brain and their relevance to psychophysiological aspects of medicine. Amer. J. Med., 25:611–626, 1958.

Meir, A. Z.: General system theory. Developments and perspectives for medicine and psychiatry. Arch. Gen. Psychiat., 21:302–310, 1969.

Miller, J. G.: Living systems. Basic concepts. Behav. Sci., 10:193–410, 1965.

Pribram, K. H.: Looking to see. Some experiments on the brain mechanism of attention in perception and its distortions. Assn. Res. Nerv. & Ment. Dis., 48:150–162, 1968.

Scott, J. P.: Animal Behavior. Chicago, The University of Chicago Press, 1958.

Sullivan, H. S.: The Interpersonal Theory of Psychiatry. (Eds., H. S. Perry and M. L. Grauvel.) New York, W. W. Norton & Co., 1953.

Taylor, J. (ed.): Selected Writings of John Hughlings Jackson. Vols. I, II. New York, Basic Books, Inc., 1958.

Tinbergen, N.: The Study of Instinct. Oxford, Clarendon Press, 1951.

Tomkins, S. S.: Affect Imagery Consciousness. 2 Vols. New York, Springer Publishing Company, Inc., 1962.

Winters, E. (ed.): The Collected Papers of Adolf Meyer. Vols. I–IV. Baltimore, Johns Hopkins Press, 1950–1952.

Chapter 3

"Now the general causes of the emotions are indubitably physiology."

William James, 1890

The Brain and Behavior

The vast bulk of the earlier neurophysiologic studies have been directed on the one hand to examination of control of various systems or organs by the central nervous system and its spinal and peripheral extensions or systems, and on the other to examination of cognitive, perceptual, and volitional performances. Increasingly over the past two decades researchers have concentrated upon the structural-functional subsystems of the brain as they relate to behavior.

Inferences drawn from the study of clinical phenomena, commencing at the turn of the twentieth century, provided the impetus for the growth of physiology of behaviors and emotions which now has direct pertinence to functions significant in the daily living of the individual members of all species. Careful analysis of sequences or patterns of activity by ethologists and students of animal psychology, and their correlation with the activity of various portions of the nervous system as demonstrated during electrical or pharmacological stimulation or after ablations, have laid the groundwork for an expanding understanding of the dynamic structural-functional relationships within the nervous system which lead to arousal and execution of integrated goal-directed behaviors. Also, the empiric clinical discoveries of the powerful actions of the phenothiazines and, later, of the various antidepressant pharmaceuticals have stimulated much study. This study has in turn added to our capacity to formulate powerful new hypotheses of concern in understanding the process of synaptic transmission, particularly as related to the subsystems of the brain concerned with drives and affects.

By far the largest proportion of the observations on behavior and its relation to brain function reported in this chapter are derived from studies in animal species. Likewise, most of the hypotheses presented in this chapter are based on observations made by those whose principal concern is the study of nonhuman species. The extent to which one may extrapolate from the physiology of nonhuman species to that of man remains an open question. Yet those basic biological functions upon which the interest of neurophysiologists has focused are common to all species, including man. Furthermore, the majority of social drives recognized as essentially human are considered their derivatives. Finally, in the past there has been notable success in applying to human organ functioning the knowledge gained by physiologists from experimentation in animals. At best the information available today on brain function as it relates to behavior provides a structure for speculation upon the relationship between that function and its abnormal expressions in psychiatric disorder. At the least it has heuristic value.

The human brain differs from that of other mammalian species in the extent to which the cerebral cortex has expanded. Upon this growth rest the extensive cognitive functions of man: his capacities for language, elaborate communications systems, retention of information in memory, exquisitely discriminative and variable affective and conative sets, and the ability to solve problems and inquire. Man retains, however, the primitive brain structures found in subhuman species. Thus, the midbrain hypothalamic systems common to all vertebrates appear to control the regulating functions concerned with those primary activities needed to sustain life: feeding, drinking, breathing, sexual activity, and thermal control. The limbic system, a paleocortical development, is conceived today to have emerged in the evolutionary process to function in connection with emotionally determined behaviors that MacLean hypothesizes are related principally to preservation of the self or the species. Thus, the human brain may be thought of as a hierarchical structure which, in effective functioning, demands the integration of each of the successively more complex systems extending from the hindbrain through the forebrain. Dysfunction at any level in the successively more complex structures and their interconnecting links, whether in the midbrain, the hypothalamus, the limbic system, or the various regions of the cortex, distorts behavior and in man may lead to symptoms impairing personality function.

In the previous chapter emotion was defined as those bodily processes and activities that are generated through threats to existence or frustration and delay in gratification of a drive state. These processes include the activation of organ systems by the involuntary nervous system as well as the associated subjective state denoted in psychiatry as an affect.

Direct attack induces the emotional states of rage or fear. Pain, hunger, and thirst, with their attendant drives and associated affects, may be regarded as primitive emotional states. Satiation of these needs—or expectation of satiation—leads to varying degrees of satisfaction or pleasure, another variety of affect with attendant emotional behavior. With the procreative drives (in man) painful and pleasurable emotional states are aroused in the seeking period, in copulatory and protective activities, and in the complexly

organized rearing of the young characteristic of the mammalian species.

For the psychiatrist the most significant behaviors are those connected with the arousal of emotion, and particularly affect, and its variable modulation and control through a wide range of socially learned behavioral sequences. The mentally ill suffer as a consequence of their defective control of socially prohibited emotional expression, or their inept learning of defenses against it. Abnormalities in social functioning are seen in the senseless rages, the grotesque posturings, and the bizarre delusional and hallucinatory experiences of the psychotic, the seemingly irrational repetitions of the compulsive, or the sensorimotor inhibitions of the hysteric. In contrast to such behaviors there is the flexible and constructive expression of emotion displayed by those more fortunate in their growth and development. Owing to his development of a verbal communicative system, man alone of all the species is capable of reporting upon the variety of subjectively perceived affective states that attend the arousal of emotional behaviors. Tenderness and love, jealousy, anxiety, sadness and lonesomeness, guilt and shame, envy and hatred—all are shadings of the primitive affects of love, fear, and rage that may be defined only through the verbal reporting of the affective state in man: emotional states at best capable of inference in other mammalian forms.

Emotional behavior, then, is a complex organismal response to a perception of threat or of satiety. Such behavior represents a response to signals or cues sensed from either the internal or the external environment. Its expression may be examined in terms of the arousing percept, the goal-directed activity, or those associated subjective states capable of study only through man's verbal communications, his fantasy, and his thought. Thus, in man, one may examine the repetitive situations in which aggressive behavior occurs; the pattern of overt expression of aggressive behavior or its covert expressions in passivity and withdrawal, or, finally, the subjective accounts of perceived rage, jealousy, envy, fear, or anxiety that represent the many manifestations of human affect when the aggressive drive is stimulated.

Each emotional response varies quantitatively. The rage response may be intense or may be shown only through minor behavioral expression. The percept that calls out one emotion may be interrupted by another more prepotent for the organism's survival. Emotional behavior results from an infinity of triggering mechanisms: unfamiliar percepts, an inner awareness of lack of strength, a perceived threat. The same cause may produce differing reactions in the same subject at differing times. Each emotional state may be capable of expression in a number of behaviors. In the same subject these expressions change as the individual becomes habituated to the stimulating condition and learns different adaptations to the arousing stimulus situation.

ANALYSIS OF BEHAVIOR

For the understanding and evaluation of behavior one must comprehend not only the range and variety of pathological patterns but also the adaptive processes which maintain performance in the homeostatic state.

For the most part the physiological analyses of central nervous system function have been concerned with behaviors considered "instinctive." As defined by Tinbergen and other ethologists, instinctive behavior exists as innate hierarchically organized nervous mechanisms susceptible to certain priming, releasing, and directing impulses coming from both *within* and *without* the organism. In turn these mechanisms evince response by coordinated actions that contribute to the maintenance of the individual and the species. Such innate behavioral mechanisms are capable of discrimination in simpler vertebrate forms, as the stickleback fish or the herring gull. In mammalian forms, however, much of behavior is thought by animal psychologists to be derived from the innate drive states and learned. While the "instinctive" drives certainly exist in man, it is unknown whether innate stereotypes of behavior still exist. Because of the overriding importance of the learning capacity and opportunity inherent in the vast growth of the cerebral hemispheres and projected through the existing social systems, the analysis which might identify simple "instinctive" activity in man has as yet escaped accomplishment.

Study of submammalian species by ethologists has shown that in any sequence, whether it be to feed and relieve hunger, to find water and quench thirst, to obtain a mate and satisfy the sexual drive, or to progress through the successive states concerned with nurturing and preparing the young for independent growth, one may find "priming" and "releasing" mechanisms. The former consist of facilitating processes which build up the potential to act. Internally, the accumulation of appropriate hormonal agents sets the attention of the neuromuscular systems. The "releasing" mechanism initiates or triggers the sequence of acts which make up a coordinated series of behaviors leading to the achievement of the necessary goal. Such releasing mechanisms may come about by either the development of a certain intensity of tissue need or the perception of some stimuli in the environment facilitating the potential of the innate releasing mechanism.

In the sequence of behaviors considered instinctive the initial actions are "appetitive" or "exploratory"; they occur through the development of internal tensions. Following the preparatory appetitive and exploratory behaviors there follow the "consummatory" actions.

During the appetitive stage of a behavioral sequence, which may be very short or of prolonged duration, extending over days, the animal appears restless and agitated. Superficially, his actions sometimes appear aimless. He seems to have reserves of energy and strength, exposed in such aggressive actions as fighting to obtain food or gain a mate. Alertness to environmental stimuli is acute, and perceptual attentiveness is magnified toward those cues subserving the prepotent organismal goal, while sensitivity to other stimuli outside that urge is diminished. Organs concerned with the need demanding eventual gratification are placed in a state of readiness for functioning.

With the realization of the external goal —food, water, a sexual mate—there takes place the consummatory act, usually a stereotyped pattern of behavior. Satisfactory consummation is followed by a state of satiation accompanied by resting behavior, lessened alertness to and interest in the environment, and, as we know from man, a subjective state of satisfaction.

As the animal grows and records experience within his nervous system, his susceptibility to response through exposure to the releasing mechanisms is enhanced. Furthermore, the external releasing perceptions for particular behavior may assume a wider range of configurations or become more differentiated through learning processes. Without consummation for prolonged periods, actions directed toward certain goals may discharge spontaneously even though presentation of the external releasing stimulus has not taken place. Thus, it is apparent that innate behaviors constitute in themselves a sequence of complexly organized actions dependent upon the internal state of each organism and each species. Furthermore, such behaviors become subject to increasingly greater modifications through experience and learning according to the extent and the peculiar organization of the nervous system of the species. The components of a behavioral sequence may vary then in their capacity for arousal, in the intensity and complexity of response of the various perceptual motor components in appetitive, consummatory, and satiated states.

It seems from the analysis of behavioral sequences that the brain, as the integrative organ of each organism, must be so organized in all animal species as to assure sensitivity to environmental and internal stimuli, to effect arousal, with increased alertness and attentiveness, as well as rest and satiation. It must contain subsystems that establish the innate drives and in some species the stereotyped behaviors which take place without previous experience and learning. In other species there exist the cortical systems upon which the multivariate discrimination of sensory experiences develops as well as the encoding denoted as "memories" and upon which are based those highly discriminated learned patterns of perception, mediation, and action. From these derive the many flexible behavioral approaches available to man to serve his appetitive and consummatory drives.

INFORMATION PROCESSING

From the analytic descriptions of goal-seeking behavior as provided by ethologists, one must conceive of brain function in terms other than those offered earlier and derived from learning, theory and simple stimulus—response physiology. As an integrating organ, the brain must continuously process information registered upon the body from the exterior as well as the interior surfaces of the body, from the internal organ systems, and from its own structure. In this integrative process the brain utilizes systems which have laid down a record over time of past sensory experience and the recorded consequences of actions taken which succeeded or failed in goal-seeking or protective behavior. It must relate the incoming registrations to each other, collate them, and compare them with previous registrations.

The brain also serves a *mnestic function*. It must attend to those registrations that signal threat to the function of the organism as a whole or to any of its subsystems, and must determine the general or local response most likely to protect and preserve function. In carrying out the integrative and executive functions of the organism, brain subsystems sustain a constant watch to sense opportunity or threat and to attend to the stimulus. In so doing conscious percepts in man emerge from memories of the past.

So, too, in relation to the needs of the other major bodily systems concerned with energy processing and reproduction, man and other species, depending upon the selective needs deriving from the systems, variously attend to differing stimuli. When hungry, vigilance is intensified to cues indicating food. In man, only when the reproductive system has evolved to maturity is the brain alerted to attend to and enhance further behavior directed toward consummation with the sexual object.

AROUSAL AND SATIATION

THE RETICULAR ACTIVATING SYSTEM

Largely through the work of Magoun and his collaborators it is now recognized that within the central gray matter of the brain stem there exist cells with rich afferent and efferent connections with the spinal cord, hypothalamus, limbic system, and various areas of the cerebral cortex. Their activation is known to facilitate or inhibit the postural tonus of muscles throughout the body, to influence endocrine and visceral functions, and to be concerned as well with states of wakefulness, orienting, and attention. Thus stimulation of the corticoparietal projections of the central reticular formations sets up the low-voltage frequencies in the electroencephalogram associated with states of attention and wakefulness. Similar behavior, with associated EEG patterns of arousal, follows stimulation in the sub and dorsal hypothalamus and the nonspecific thalamic nuclei as well as activation of the well-known specific afferent pathways in the brain stem. It appears from stimulation experiments in animals that arousal of the cortex may follow impulses reaching it from the midbrain by either of two routes: an extrathalamic route, passing through the internal capsule from the subthalamic areas, or via the cortical projections of the nonspecific thalamic nuclei. Destruction of the central

tegmental areas in animals leads to comatose behavior (high-voltage slow EEG patterns are seen in such states) even though the specific sensory pathways to the brain are intact, nor is it possible to bring about arousal even by the most intense stimulation thereafter.

That the reticular activating system is concerned with the modulations of consciousness and attention seems evident. Its activity now is known to be suppressed by general anesthetics, the barbiturates, the phenothiazines, reserpine, and other pharmacological agents. As we shall note in discussing innate alimentary, sexual, and aggressive behaviors, the electrical activity within the activating system is modified likewise by other metabolic and endocrine imbalances.

ATTENTION AND VIGILANCE

The modifications of consciousness and attention to stimulations are not only dependent upon the afferent inflow to the midbrain activating system from the spinal and central sensory neurons but are also subject to "feedback" control from the cerebral cortex. Thus, electrical stimulation of diverse points in the cingulate, orbital, and lateral frontal areas, central and paraoccipital areas, superior gyrus, and tip of the temporal lobe of the cortex leads to both augmentation and reduction of activity within the brain stem reticular system. It seems likely, then, that as facilitation of performance is brought about through cortical arousal by activity in the activating system, there occurs an inverse inhibitory corticoreticular discharge or feedback which obviates overexcitation and also dampens or inhibits sensory stimulation irrelevant to the prepotent behavioral sequence.

Little is known of the means by which the brain maintains its ability to attend selectively to one set of sensory registrations and not another. Acts of attention seem enormously different. On the one hand one may be struck by the precise visual attentiveness that must be exerted for an otherwise preoccupied man to suddenly catch a ball thrown past him by a playing child. Against this, one may conceive the narrowed attention of a microscopist as he focuses upon the tissue viewed through his scope. Then again there is the consciously determined scanning attention to a large stream of incoming registrations, such as might be given by a music critic while preparing to write his appraisal of the playing of a symphony orchestra, or that of the psychoanalyst attempting to discover a meaningful thread in scanning the sequence of the often apparently unrelated free association of his patient.

Arguing from a series of experiments, Pribram has suggested that attention derives from other than associations established by means of transcortical or cortico-cortical associations and that the brain's intrinsic processing system is other than a passive receptacle of information. He is of the belief that mnemic functions (memory) occur as active recoding and that the processing cortex regulates ongoing processes under the sensory system.

Thus from his work upon the association areas of the cerebral cortex concerned with recognition, we find it divisible into the posterior part, concerned with recognition, and the frontal part, concerned with recall. As for the latter, it is divided according to sense modality. Clinical studies and experiments over time indicate that the inferior temporal cortex functions in relation to visual recognition, the middle temporal to auditory recognition, the anterior temporal to gustation, and the posterior parietal to somesthesias. Pribram was struck with the anatomical fact that the aforementioned associative processing areas are separated by a considerable span from their related primary sensory systems. He found that one could remove the cortex between the primary cortical sensory receptive and the mnestic or associational cortex without loss of visual recognition of patterns in monkeys. What does take place is that impairment occurs in behaviors in which animals are required to process a number of visual cues

in order to complete a task. Such animals fail, even though they "track" easily. Pribram states that behavioral learning (that is, identification) is based on a progressive differentiation and not on associative abstraction. He suggests the attention required in simple visual motor tracking as used in catching a fly depends only on the functioning of the primary sensory receptive cortex. Probably corticofugal impulses from that area to subthalamic system areas direct alerting. Scanning, requiring searching, relating, and selection of a series of cues, comes about through actions of the primary intrinsic (associative) processing cortex. Here the scanning attention might be directed by corticofugal pathways to the subthalamic alerting spheres. Vigilance, the monitoring of external and internal registrations to determine their prepotency seems most likely the function of the limbic system. Cognitive factors, perhaps, are the consequence of diffuse corticocortical associational actions.

Physiologists have found that, just as the reticular activating system facilitates and inhibits sensory inputs from the spinal cord and brain stem, additional feedback control is exerted at peripheral sensory receptors outside the central nervous system, in the cochlea and retina. It is of interest that Freud predicted the existence of a *stimulus barrier* (reizschutz) to protect the organism from destructive and overwhelming stimulation. The discovery of the physiological arrangements within the nervous system preventing overactivation of sensory neurons and the excessive overload of the brain itself provides experimental support for his hypotheses.

The exigencies of life and adaptation to it have required the establishment of flexible gates excluding, reducing, or facilitating the inflow of sensory impressions from one or several sources, depending upon the immediate adaptive function demanded of the individual organism. That this protective barrier may fail to function, through maldevelopment or overload, and lead to disease is a distinct possibility. Such occurrences perhaps are exemplified in the sensory hypersensitivities noted in childhood schizophrenia, in such toxic states as delirium tremens, and in the stress reaction observed in man following prolonged battle exposure or after other catastrophes. The application of this knowledge to the clinic has suggested modulating the input of auditory stimulation to mask the pain incurred during dental procedures.

Still another characteristic of the activating system is its deactivation of the cortex on the presentation of repetitive, unvarying stimulation which may be interpreted as monotonous. Here the system functions by progressive reduction of electrocortical arousal even though the sensory input reaches the cortex. The system then is concerned with the process of habituation. Prolonged deprivation of cortical arousal now is known also to have deleterious effects, as described in Chapter 7.

BEHAVIORAL REINFORCEMENT

While the activating systems in the brain stem and thalamus are concerned principally with alerting the organism and directing its attention to external or internal cues, there exist brain systems which reinforce sequences of behavior. These systems are concerned with emotional arousal and related affect. As we mentioned in the previous chapter, the anlages of the finely differentiated affective states of man rest upon primitive feeling states of pleasure and distress—states experienced first in the helpless dependency of infancy.

As with other brain systems, cellular interconnections are now understood to be made through electrochemical events taking place at the synaptic junctions between cells. The most popular of the current hypotheses relating to affect variability centers about presumed levels of concentration of the catecholamines at the synaptic junction, the cleft, and the postsynaptic receptor site.

Thus the passage of a nerve impulse from activated neurons across the synaptic junction to other nerve cells is considered to take place by discharge into the synaptic cleft of the biogenic amine norepinephrine. That substance is thought to activate the effector site of the host synaptic neuron.

Norepinephrine is found in highest concentration in the hypothalamus but is also present elsewhere, including the limbic system. The biogenic amine serotonin has a similar distribution. Dopamine, on the other hand, is concentrated highest in the basal ganglia. It has been suggested, but not yet proved, that all three of these biogenic amines may act as chemical transmitters. Some believe that one or more of these amines may act as modulators of synaptic transmissions that depend on other substances, perhaps acetylcholine.

Synthesized from tyrosine, norepinephrine is stored in intraneuronal granules at the presynaptic endings. When discharged into the synaptic cleft it is inactivated by conversion by the enzyme catechol-O-methyltransferase or is taken up again by the cell. Released within the cell it is inactivated by mitochondrial monoamine oxidase forming metabolites. The latter enzyme may then regulate the levels of norepinephrine within the cell. Epinephrine exists only in low concentrations in the brain. Peripherally it exists almost exclusively in the adrenal medulla. Serotonin synthesis takes place from 5-hydroxytryptophan by dicarboxylation. It, too, is metabolized by monoamine oxidase to form hydroxyindolacetic acid.

Earlier inference from clinical investigations related states of anger to the state of physiological arousal produced by injections of norepinephrine, whereas fear was thought to resemble those related to states induced by both norepinephrine and epinephrine injections. In monkeys in which blood levels of these amines may be measured, release of norepinephrine takes place with presentation of familiar and threatening stimuli. On the other hand, when the threatening situation is unknown or uncertain, epinephrine rises occur in the peripheral blood. So, too, improved performance with work under stress is associated with increased norepinephrine excretion. Exposure of men to emotionally arousing feelings leads to increased excretion of both norepinephrine and epinephrine; bland film exposure is followed by diminution.

It appears that the nature of differential perception of the external cues determines differentially the relative levels of excretion of these amines within the body. So, too, in animals decrements in brain norepinephrine take place with fear, immobilization, and even after intracerebral stimulation productive of heightened emotional arousal. Also, in animals adrenocorticosteroids enhance the activity of the enzymes that convert norepinephrine to epinephrine in the adrenal.

As will be discussed in the chapter on pharmacological therapy, those agents that are considered to increase norepinephrine concentrations in the synaptic cleft are associated with relief of depressive affect with its components of impounded rage and fear. The reader is recommended to the excellent review "Biogenic Amines and Emotion," by Schildkraut and Kety.

Experienced psychiatrists are highly impressed with the powerful effects of the new pharmaceuticals in modulating and changing pathologic affect and drive. The currently given biophysical interpretations of the actions by these drugs in terms of modifications of synaptic transmission must be recognized as oversimplified. Since synaptic transmission is involved in integration of all brain and peripheral neuronal interaction, one must realize that specificity as it relates to subsystem function must involve other variables. These may arise in either qualitative or quantitative production or depredation of transmitter substances. We remain far from a chemical control of man's affective state. The above work relates only to the primitive affects aroused in protective or agonistic behaviors to be described later. Yet there is physiological evidence for a central affective system within the brain.

Olds and Milner have found that animals with permanently implanted electrodes through which they might deliver stimuli to a portion of their own basal forebrains learned shortly to re-excite this brain area repeatedly and autonomously. When the electrodes were placed properly, rats stimulated themselves as often as 8000 times per hour.

Heath and his co-workers have reported pleasurable affects in some men with similar electrode placement carried out as a treatment of schizophrenia. When the electrode was placed in sites in the posterior hypothalamus or mid-brain, self-stimulation was much less frequent. Chlorpromazine and reserpine obliterate or inhibit self-stimulation in the latter sites but not in the more potently rewarding cephalic structures. The drive for autonomous self-stimulation can be modified by increasing the intensity of needs. In rats the drive for self-stimulation is much greater when they are exposed to the shocking pain of crossing an electric grid than when they are deprived of food for a day.

This system, with its capacity to reinforce behaviors, perhaps should be contrasted with the long-known sensory system concerned with pain—an emotional state which regularly leads to withdrawal behavior. Repetitive induction of this unpleasant emotion establishes behaviors of avoidance or aversion.

CYCLIC REINFORCEMENT

Many of the drive states which serve to maintain the health of man and other species and assure their procreative activities take place on time-fixed cycles of activity. Undoubtedly the most autonomous and least conscious cyclical activity is the spontaneously recurring movement of the chest cage and diaphragm concerned with the maintenance of respiration. In man this unconsciously maintained cyclical behavior is sometimes distorted in the form of respiratory tics, grunts, bouts of hyperventilation, and breath holding, or even in the disturbances of vocalization that take place in stuttering.

Equally important to the maintenance of health—and its disruption is so symptomatic of psychiatric disorder—is the sleep-wakefulness cycle. In procreative life, the estrous cycle represents a time-recurrent event as characteristic of woman as of the female of other mammalian species. Disruptions of this cycle, too, in women are among the most telling symptoms of personality disorder.

Time-bound behavioral sequences are less evident in the life of man than in his mammalian relatives. The flexibility with which he is endowed through his capacity for learning has detached him from the rigid behavioral cycles so characteristic of many simpler species. Yet evidence exists that he remains bound to behaviors determined by the function of "biological clocks." Disruption of these rhythmic functions by conflicting learned activities invariably indicates the presence of deep-seated and serious personality disorders.

Richter's studies of cyclical behaviors in man and animals have led him to hypothesize the presence of three types of "clocks": homeostatic, central, and peripheral. The estrous cycle represents a homeostatic "clock" wherein hormonal feedback mechanisms exist between distant target organs (in this case the ovary and uterus), an endocrine gland (the pituitary), and the hypothalamus. The timing systems of the central and peripheral clocks do not appear to be homeostatic and are capable of imposing recurrent behaviors through learning. Thus, one may learn to awaken at precise times; certain pathologic behaviors recurring in patients in regular time cycles appear to be learned. The anniversary reactions, to be described in Chapter 7 in connection with bereavements, are an example. While Richter states that the homeostatic systems are somewhat irregular, the central timing systems function with high constancy over long periods. The cellular timing devices exist outside the nervous system; they cycle certain phenomena of primary physical disease

such as the regularly recurring fever of Hodgkin's disease. Such rhythms are thought to be ingrained into cellular and organ systems by the day-night and seasonal cycles which modify metabolic potentials and are modified in the evolutionary process.

Sleep-Wakefulness Behavior

For centuries the preservation of the regularly recurring sleep cycle has been recognized as imperative for the maintenance of health. Typical disruptions of the sleep cycle occur in depressive reactions and in various neurotic conditions and are represented as well by the somnambulistic trances seen most frequently in children. Less frequently met are those symptomatic eruptions of sleep which intrude upon the waking state: narcoleptic and hypersomniac attacks. The physiology of sleep has direct bearing upon the understanding of the clinical phenomenology just mentioned.

Both the sleeping and the waking states are associated with characteristic electro-encephalographic patterns. The sleeping period is associated with at least two quite distinct types of brain activity. During 80 per cent of sleeping time there occurs an electroencephalographic pattern of large-amplitude slow waves and spindle bursts. This segment of sleep time is thought to represent inhibition of activity of the cerebral cortex. The other segment of sleep is characterized by an electroencephalographic pattern of low-voltage fast activity; this is thought to be a period in which subcortical function is predominantly impaired. It is now designated as "fast," "paradoxical," or "dreaming" sleep.

In the human adult, periods of dreaming sleep recur each night at intervals of approximately 90 minutes. Associated with the electroencephalographic pattern of dreaming sleep are bursts of rapid conjugate eye movements (REM). At times of such electroencephalographic and ocular activity, the awakened sleeper almost regularly reports dreaming, in contrast to his behavior when awakened during other periods of the sleep cycle. Other significant physiological changes also take place during REM sleep. Thus, respiration is irregular, heart rate and blood pressure are elevated, skin resistance is lowered, penile erection occurs, and there is a rapid and distinctive diminution in muscle tone as shown by the electroencephalograph.

Dreaming sleep occupies as much as 50 per cent of the sleep cycle in infants, decreasing in amount with aging. Similar cycles of REM sleep have been identified in many mammalian species other than man. One may infer from the periodic sleep activity of animals that they dream in association with this distinctive physiological phase of the sleep cycle.

Whether REM sleep is of greater or less depth or whether it represents a more primitive form of the dominant sleep periods remains a matter of discussion. While it has been assumed that dreaming sleep is light, at times the arousal threshold is higher during the REM period and at other times it is barely in excess of the waking threshold. As will be described in Chapter 7, deprivation of REM sleep by awakening establishes a deficit which must be made up in subsequent sleep periods and may be associated with psychopathology.

Physiological studies have established the fact that the occurrence of the rapid low-voltage electrical activity depends upon the functioning of nuclear aggregations in the pontine reticular formations. REM records persist in mammals, including man, following decortication; they have been absent in several electroencephalographic recordings of patients with evidence of pontine damage. Even in decorticate animals, deprivation of "fast sleep" by repeated awakening leads to a pattern of sleep in which REM outbursts occur at increasingly frequent intervals. Cerebral tracts other than the ascending reticular formation are involved in the cortical driving mechanism in animals. "Fast sleep" disappears only with inter-

ruption of tracts in the ventral mesencephalon. It is of interest that there has been reported in men a syndrome of "peduncular hallucinosis" characterized by isolated visual hallucinations which occur at onset of sleep in those with lesions in the area of the ventral mesencephalon.

In the past five years much research has been done upon the effects of drugs in expressions of REM and nonREM sleep. Atropine reduces or abolishes REM sleep, whereas cholinergic agents such as eserine prolong its expression. It is of interest that atropine administered to cats just prior to the time of the expected circadian rise of 17-hydroxy steroids blocks that biological rhythmic activity. The barbiturates pentobarbital (Nembutal) and secobarbital (Seconal), glutethimide (Doriden), methyprylon (Noludar), and diphenhydramine (Benadryl) all reduce the amount of time spent in REM sleep. Of these drugs the barbiturates have the most effect. Dextroamphetamine, combined with pentobarbital, eliminates dreaming sleep. Following the withdrawal of the aforementioned drugs there occurs an increase in REM sleep in subsequent nights—a "rebound."

Particularly after the withdrawal of barbiturates and alcohol given over prolonged periods, the increased REM periods are punctuated by frightening nightmares. This is in contrast to deprivation of REM sleep by awakening; although increased REM sleep occurs on subsequent nights following interruption of REM by awakening, frightening dreaming is not usually reported.

The phenothiazines tend to change the electroencephalographic patterns of sleep toward that consistent with the state of coma. Antidepressants such as amitriptyline and imipramine decrease REM sleep activity, but over a few days of administration they expand the nonREM periods and lengthen the usual 90 minute cycles of REM expression up to 120 minutes. Their withdrawal is not followed by REM rebound.

On the other hand reserpine and d-lysergic acid diethylamide (LSD) enhance REM sleep, as does L-tryptophan.

At this time it is hypothesized that depletion of the brain catecholamines, norepinephrine and dopamine, leads to a diminution of waking and REM sleep activity, whereas decrease of the brain indole amine serotonin is correlated with reduction in nonREM sleep activity. Others state it differently: the sleep-wakefulness cycle depends upon a complex balance of these amines in the brain subcellular structures.

"Napping" sleep apparently varies greatly with the time of day. Afternoon napping is associated with an earlier appearance and greater proportion of REM sleep than is evening napping. This observation suggests a greater potential for REM sleep expression during the daytime.

ENERGIC PROCESSING

RESPIRATORY, ALIMENTARY, AND EXCRETORY BEHAVIOR. All those functions directly concerned with the intake of substances and elimination of wastes occur in organs which embryologically are outgrowths of the alimentary tract. Accordingly, in this section are considered those physiologic processes concerned with respiration, feeding, and drinking, as well as the elimination of carbon dioxide, fecal matter, and urine.

Psychopathological disturbances of respiration were described earlier. Perverted eating and drinking behaviors are common symptomatic expressions of psychiatric disorders: prolonged anorexia, specific food aversions and obsessions, compulsive eating and drinking, constipation, and various diarrheas.

While the majority of the symptomatic disturbances of alimentation are learned to gratify symbolically some psychosocial need, they are mediated through and distort the functioning of related neuronal and organic systems. Others, however, are directly expressive of disturbances in the brain subsystem concerned with alimentary self-preservation.

The arousal of the need for oxygen, food, or fluids, recognized affectively as suffocation, hunger, or thirst, is mediated through the reticular activating system. In asphyxia, either a diminution in the oxygen in the blood or an increase in the carbon dioxide (the two components of asphyxia) powerfully stimulates the bulbar respiratory center as well as the mesencephalic reticular formation. During starvation, when the blood sugar level falls, there is an increase in circulating epinephrine which effects a compensatory release of glucose from glycogen. But as this latter process runs out, with depletion of glycogen stores, epinephrine may directly activate the ascending and descending reticular system, thereby facilitating cortical arousal and motor activity. Probably similar physiological processes lead to arousal in the face of emerging thirst, although there does not now exist experimental evidence for this assumption.

The innate processes which direct feeding behavior have been located in the hypothalamus and the limbic system (visceral brain). Thus, electrical stimulation of the lateral hypothalamus elicits feeding behavior in the satiated animal; its destruction causes aphagia. A dual control of eating seems probable, as stimulation of the hypothalamic ventromedial nucleus inhibits feeding and lesions in this area lead to hyperphagia and eventual obesity. Similarly, stimulation in the closely situated paraventricular nuclei elicits polydipsia, while electrical discharges related to fluid satiation have been observed in the supraoptic neurons following injection into animals of hypertonic solutions of saline and glucose.

Although it would seem that the hypothalamus is concerned solely with specifying the direction of the drive for food or fluid, shaping of the feeding behavior in mammals has been thought to depend upon the functioning of the rhinencephalon (the cerebral archicortex or limbic system, consisting of the olfactory bulb, septum pellucidum, cingulum, fornix, and amygdala). For many years clinicians have recognized that some epileptic seizures are initiated with one or several of the subjective experiences of hunger, thirst, choking, retching, or the wish to urinate or defecate, or by chewing or other oral activity, including automatisms of eating and drinking. In addition there may occur in such attacks manifestations of rage or fright expressed in screaming, running, or attack. It is known now that such convulsive seizures are due to focal lesions in the temporal lobe involving the structures of the limbic system. This system in turn projects to the hypothalamus and central gray matter of the mesencephalon through the median forebrain bundle. MacLean has found particularly that excitation in the amygdalar projections and ventral hypothalamus leads to oral activities; others have demonstrated that stimulation of the cingulate cortex in animals may inhibit feeding behaviors and related organ functions concerned with alimentation, including secretion of gastric juices.

REPRODUCTIVE BEHAVIOR

Arousal of the sexual drive, the finding of a mate, and the consummatory acts of copulation represent only the initial sequence of sexual behavior. Parturition in man, as well as other mammals, is followed by a long series of interdependent actions between the parents and the young designed to nurture the growth and development of the young. It is now recognized that the wide variety of behaviors evolved in reproduction of different species depend increasingly, as one ascends the evolutionary series, upon learned behaviors, particularly those concerned with socialization.

The midbrain activating system is known to become progressively more sensitive to electrical stimulation as estrous behavior evolves. In the period following coitus in female rabbits, when the animal relaxes, is inactive, or may sleep, the electroencephalographic recordings have shown spindle bursting, followed by REM sleep and hypersynchrony in limbic patterns.

Electrical stimulation of the tubular structures in animals induces ovulation.

Lesions or implantations of estrogen in this area inhibit ovulation following coitus and later tend to cause atrophy of the ovary and reproductive tract. Similarly, testosterone implanted in this area in male dogs causes aspermia and testicular and prostatic atrophy. This system then responds to both neural influx and direct endocrine action as circulating gonadal hormones check pituitary gonadotropin secretion.

As for other components of the consummatory act, MacLean has found that in male monkeys penile erection and its modifications, pelvic movements, and ejaculation follow stimulation of the hippocampal projections, parts of the anterior and midline thalamic nuclei, and the hypothalamus, the septopreoptic and medial dorsal nuclei being the most sensitive areas.

Even more impressive is the enormous significance to sexual behavior in man of early experience in terms of learning patterns of socialization that lead to successful mating, copulation, and eventual child rearing. The thesis is now corroborated by a long line of experimental observations culminating in the reports of Harlow, who found that young monkeys that were isolated from a mother and contacted only an experimental wire frame for nutrition, or else were isolated from their peers, were defective in sexual approach, in the consummatory act, and in mothering behavior in adulthood. Here again the recording of experience over time is dependent upon the functioning of the cerebral cortex and allows the eventual patterning of the complex series of behaviors which determine the various phases of both procreation and child rearing. In man, particularly, each of these phases may be enhanced, distorted, or arrested through his extensive capacity for symbolizing during learning.

AGONISTIC SYSTEM

Expressions of and reactions to aggression—rage and fight, immobilization, flight, and fear—are the agonistic responses designed to protect each species from attack and also to facilitate alimentary and sexual activities.

Aggression, defined in the narrow sense of initiating attack, is a universal form of behavior in all classes of vertebrates and arthropods but rarely in lower invertebrates. In the animal kingdom fighting is common, useful, and apparently adaptive. The young of many mammalian species exhibit the beginnings of fighting behavior in their play. External and internal environment both influence the emergence of aggressivity and impulsivity. Hunger, territorial restriction, and increase in male sexual hormone increase fighting activity in various vertebrates.

Man alone resorts to violent aggressiveness with widespread maiming and killing of members of his own species. He alone has evolved exquisite means of cruelty and torture as well as equally subtle controls through social methods of inducing guilty and shameful affects and inhibiting ritualistic and expiatory behaviors. It has been said that the crowning achievement of man's evolution was the emergence of conscience—to control aggressivity. Man's aggressivity and the psychological control devices evolved for its control depend upon the vast growth of his cerebral cortex.

Perhaps because the socially feared and inappropriate aggressiveness of the psychotic has been most difficult to control, both clinical and laboratory studies of the physiological processes related to the expression of rage preceded those of other forms of behavior. As early as 1892 Goltz reported upon the astounding behavior of his decorticated dog, which had displayed strong actions of growling, barking, and biting on slight stimulation, actions expressive of the emotion of rage. Walter Cannon coined the term "sham rage" after he observed lashing of the tail, arching of the back, display of claws, biting, and panting respirations, behavior which showed the components of rage and attack, in acutely decorticated cats. A long series of arousal experiments by Bard and others demonstrated that "savage" behav-

ior in cats followed precise lesions in the ventromedial nucleus of the hypothalamus. It is now known that removal of the neocortex alone, leaving the old brain rhinencephalic structures intact, leads to the behavioral expression of placidity—the obverse of rage. Rage reactions emerge spontaneously when both new and old cortices are removed or when the amygdala and pyriform cortex are resected, but not after damage to the hippocampus. The neocortex then appears to have both a facilitatory and an inhibitory influence on aggressive behaviors characterized by rage, and in addition influences the direction and timing of such behaviors. The inhibitory influence is dependent upon the cingulate gyrus and transmitted through the amygdala to influence the ventromedial hypothalamic nuclei.

It was the introduction of prefrontal lobotomy that established the relationship of function of brain to control of emotional behaviors. As the result of the many studies of psychiatrically ill persons treated by prefrontal lobotomy, the clinical indications for the procedure have been narrowed to the presence of certain symptoms which represent the expression of rage or related aggressive states. These are assaultive and destructive behavior, suicidal acts, chronic irascibility, agitation, undue anxiety, impulsiveness, and overactivity. Other behavioral symptoms often modified by lobotomy are depression, hypochondriasis, chronic pain, and refusal to eat—symptoms that often are recognized as symbolic of inhibition of rage or hostility. Lobotomy was found to offer little in terms of the social adaptation of the psychotic patient who showed apathy and indifference. It was found as well that prefrontal cortical resections made in a posterior plane which presumably damaged the amygdala induced apathy or placidity that mitigated against the social recovery of the patient.

COGNITIVE SYSTEM

The capacity to respond with increasingly effective goal-directed behavior to variable but previously unspecified circumstances defines adaptation. That capacity, in living systems, requires that incoming information be registered and encoded, that a memory of the experience be established. On the basis of the earlier memories presentation of information resembling that registered at any early time is recognized as familiar—is perceived. So, too, the responses to past experience are recorded, including those internal events which determine emotion and affect. With each succeeding experience of goal seeking or avoidance of threat, the organism learns by comparative analysis of the effectiveness of present with previous behaviors. It thus progressively discriminates the most significant cues in percepts, evolves more skillful and economical behavioral responses, and in the more complex mammalian species progressively analyzes and solves problems concerned with increasingly variable and complex environmental situations. Memory, perception, and cognition depend upon evolution of the brain.

MEMORY. It is now assumed that a series of electrochemical processes takes place to fix in the neuronal network of the brain those records of past sensory experiences which form the basis for perception and the development of motor and cognitive behaviors necessary for adaptation and defensive purposes. Much of what is written pertaining to these processes is highly speculative. Yet the mounting information and available hypothesis have heuristic value.

Memory processing is considered to be determined through two distinct but overlapping stages. The recall of immediately experienced events is recognized as different than that of past events. Electroshock shortly after experience will eradicate recall of recent events.

Clinical studies make it evident that extensive brain damage early in life impairs the storage of information and the potential for learning. With brain damage later in life specific deficits are noted in ability to retain recent percepts, while the memories encoded from the past are retained. Such impairment of storage or retention of experiences is a prominent symptom in certain of the alcoholic psychoses as well, and characterizes the psychosis associated with the senium. Similarly, during the induction of anesthesia and after electroshock therapy, memory processing is impaired. While immediate memory of short spans is possible, the recall of long-span percepts, which involves storage, is defective.

Within the past decade it has been observed that patients treated neurosurgically for epilepsy by bilateral temporal lobe resections lose their ability to process current experience into memory. Thus, retention of any cognitive material is severely impaired and there may occur as well impairment of recall extending backward for several years (retrograde amnesia). Retention of earlier memories is unaffected. The anterior mesial surfaces of the temporal lobe are significantly concerned with the processing of perceptions to become permanent memories, but such encoding of perceptions involves as well widespread processes throughout the cerebral cortex. DeJong has placed on record one human case in which precise bilateral localized necrosis of the hippocampi led to impairment of memory recording. Animal experiments have shown that bilateral hippocampal ablation is the significant lesion responsible for impairing acquisition of avoidance learning.

It has been suggested that in the processing of sensory experiences into the electrochemical mechanisms that establish permanent coding within the brain, both specific and nonspecific sensory pathways are activated, the latter discharging into the hippocampus via the fornix. In studies in animals of the electrical activity of the hippocampus, regularly recurring high-voltage theta rhythms are generally evoked in this structure. Such rhythms become localized when a learned behavioral response takes place as the result of conditioning. Early in the conditioned learning process the electrical activity in the hippocampus precedes that in the adjacent cerebral cortex. When conditioned learning is established, the electrical activity in the cortex appears to precede that in the hippocampus. It has been suggested that these shifting electrical wave changes between hippocampus and cortex which occur in the course of learning bring about enduring biochemical changes in the cytoplasm of fast synaptic neurons and related neuroglia upon which permanent registrations depend.

Since it is now known that the processes of the astrocytic glia are intimately applied to the neurons and seem to serve as metabolic bridges between them and the circulating blood, they may be implicated in any biochemical process which determines structural change related to acquisition of memory.

The permanent recording of sensory experiences — long-term memory — would seem to require the transformation of electrical energy generated in the neurons into some permanent changes in their structure or their relationship within the net. The analogy of the genetic code information processing through the template of RNA (ribonucleic acid) has been offered as a possible explanation for the structural change in the neurons which establishes the codes for a permanent memory. Yet in order to establish with certainty the evidence that one or another neurochemical process takes place to assure permanent encoding of an electroneural impulse and thus to demonstrate that a given molecule or set of molecules, or structure or set of structures, is specifically concerned in effecting a memory trace, a number of convincing demonstrations pertaining to that molecule or structure must be assured. Thus the molecule or structure must be shown to undergo a change of state in response to the experience to be remembered. That altered state must be shown to persist as long as the memory. The disappearance of the alteration must coincide with the loss of the memory.

Today convincing evidence meeting the general criteria above does not exist to establish any protein, lipid, or other brain constituent as the substance involved in structural alteration related to memory storage.

Certainly the metabolism of RNA may relate to memory storage, as its major function is participation in the synthesis of proteins. Many are convinced that the structural changes related to storage do concern brain proteins, but point out that cellular metabolism is dynamic and not fixed, and that there are many regulatory mechanisms within the neuron and between the neuron, its processes, and its numerous synaptic functions. It has been suggested that coding then is not related to a permanently enduring state of change in the human. It occurs only when brain protein synthesis takes place above a certain critical rate. Experiments have shown that in small mammals (mice) interference with the rate of protein synthesis in the brain by such an inhibitor as the antibiotic puromycin prevents learning of new behavioral expressions and disrupts old learning as well. Flexner has suggested that the establishment of enduring memory traces depends upon the existence within the brain of a self-sustaining system for synthesis of necessary proteins. He suggests that in the evolution of the process of long-term memory the initial learning experience triggers the synthesis of one or more species of messenger ribonucleic acid (MRNA). This MRNA alters the synthetic rate of one or more proteins essential for structural change in various neurons. In turn, these proteins modify the characteristics of the synaptic network so as to variously effect the transmission of nerve impulses. Finally, the proteins or their products induce the related MRNA production to sustain a critical level of their synthesis. When the level of synthesis falls, there takes place a temporary memory failure. It is unlikely that this hypothesis alone is sufficient to explain either short-term or long-term memory.

Earlier theorists postulated memory as based upon the establishment of synaptic resistances or efficiency of reverberating electrical circuits. Probably in the future the electrochemical hypothesis will be related to the current fashionable molecular theories of memory. At any rate, at the moment the integrity of the hippocampal structures bilaterally seems necessary for the fixing of a trace event for immediate or long-term recall. Perhaps, as was discussed earlier under the subject of vigilance, this structure is concerned with the monitoring of meaningful internal and external information to determine its priority in terms of survival of the organism. High priority information is likely to be recorded. For a thorough examination of the past and present hypotheses and data relative to mnestic function, the reader is referred to Johns.

LEARNING

From both clinical and laboratory evidence there is reason to believe that the cerebral processes associated with learning in early life are fundamentally different from those which take place after maturation of the nervous system. For many years it has been known that children born blind because of corneal opacities do not develop good vision unless that defect is repaired by corneal transplant very early in life. Likewise the dreams of children born blind or deaf never contain visual or auditory images, presumably because the patterns of cerebral organization fail to evolve without early perceptual experience. The same holds true for the organization of the body percepts: children born without a limb do not experience a limb phantom as do adults who suffer amputations.

Hebb has suggested that early sensing is necessary for the establishment of perceptual functioning. Furthermore, all later learning depends upon the appropriate early experiencing which apparently stimulates the basic organization and integration of cerebral systems concerned with perception and cognition.

A long series of animal experiments now makes it clear that the organization of various sensory systems and behaviors depends upon experiencing at critical periods in the early life of each species. In the absence of the appropriate experiencing at the "critical time," the organism may be left with an enduring deficit in perception or behavior—an ego deficit, in psychoanalytic terms—a defect of personality functioning. The degree to which such deficits may be repaired by later experience is unknown.

"Imprinting," the specific emotional attachment of the young of some species to their parents, is a case in point. Discovered first in various birds, "imprinting" takes place when the young bird perceives a moving object during certain critical days following hatching. The attachment may be made to any moving object at this point in maturational development. Thus, when contact with man or some mobile inanimate object is substituted for contact with the parent, birds exposed to the substitute will thereafter follow that substitute when it is presented. From his observations on imprinting Hess points up the differences between *imprinting,* the early type of learning, and later *associational learning.* The former is dependent upon an experience that takes place at a critical period in early life. It is depressed by the prior administration of such pharmacologic agents as meprobamate or carisoprodol, and it is enhanced when painful stimuli occur with the visual percept. In contrast, later associational learning does not depend upon experience at critical periods in life, is not depressed by meprobamate, and leads to avoidance behaviors when associated with pain. In imprinting, the first percept is the most significant in the formation of the bond that leads to following behavior; in later associational learning the more recent learning has greater influence on behavior. Since this form of early learning, so important in establishing a social bond between young and their parents, may be adversely influenced by drugs which disturb electrochemical events in the brain,* we may generalize

---

* Whereas associational learning is not affected by such drugs.

and assume that the electrochemical events of learning differ in the nervous system of the immature as compared to the mature member of the species.

In the adult brain the evidence for the occurrence of electrochemical change comes from several sources. By using the Pavlovian technique of conditioning, the classic method of associational learning, it is possible to establish a blocking of the alpha rhythm of the electroencephalogram on presentation of a click as a conditional stimulus associated with eye opening that regularly acts in such a way as the unconditioned stimulus. In the initial stages of learning to respond to the click, the blocking of the alpha rhythm is generalized over the cortex; later it is localized to the occipital cortex, the projection site of the visual unconditioned stimulus. Other experiments in animals have shown that painful and pleasurable stimuli both augment the amplitude of cerebral electrical discharges and increase the distribution of afferent signals over the brain. As affective reinforcement is continued and learning occurs, the electrical discharges that were generally distributed initially are restricted to the site of projection of the unconditioned stimuli.

Learning theorists tend to distinguish between classical Pavlovian conditioning, associational learning, and instrumental conditioning. In the former an unconditioned stimulus, such as food which would lead a dog to salivate, when paired repeatedly with another signal such as a light or noise, would over a span of time bring an animal to salivate on presentation of the hitherto biologically unimportant but paired light or sound. Pavlov spoke of the latter as the conditioned stimulus and the salivation following its presentation as the conditioned response. So, too, he found it possible to pair signals with painful stimuli to produce conditioned evasive responses. Pavlov pointed out the necessity to assess the state of need or satiety of the animals he had under study. He came to know of the influence of the human experimenter upon the responsivity of his subjects and recognized that

symbols could replace physical stimuli as signals for conditioned learning. To him sensations, perceptions, and direct impressions formed the primary signals of reality for man. Words constituted the secondary signals, as abstractions of reality, that permitted generalizations. In this psychology the reflex concept is primary, but reflex here represents a behavior response with afferent, mediating central, and efferent portions. Pavlov conceived of processes of cortical excitation and inhibition, sleep and hypnosis representing inhibitory cortical states.

Instrumental learning differs from conditioned learning in the sense that the animal is rewarded when he performs a desired task. Thus an animal comes to learn that if he carries out such an action as striking a lever he will receive a food reward. So, too, he may learn to depress a lever in order to avoid a painful shock. In the course of instrumental learning, each time the correct response is given for either need reduction or escape the animal is rewarded. When he fails to carry out the desired behavior the positive reward is denied or the aversive stimulus is given. Such instrumental or operant conditioning is associated with the work of a long line of American psychologists, of whom Skinner is the best known current spokesman.

Doubt was expressed in the past that visceral responses could be "learned" through trial-and-error rewarding methods of instrumental conditioning. As DeCara reports, a long series of experiments by Neal Miller and his associates has demonstrated otherwise. Increase and decrease in heart rate, blood pressure, constriction and relaxation of the vascular bed, intestinal contraction, and rate of urinary secretions may all be influenced by such learning procedures. So, too, the learning is relieved by periodic reinforcement and extinguishes or disappears if the reinforcement is not provided. It is of interest that the same reward may be used to obtain learned visceral responses of opposing character. It seems from this experimental work that conditioning through the sympathetic nervous system may occur with a much greater degree of specificity than thought possible earlier. The work on visceral conditioning is of paramount significance in considering the operational forces concerned in the psychophysiological (psychosomatic) disorders.

While imprinting, conditioned, or instrumental learning paradigms are of importance in comprehending the evolution of adaptive and maladaptive (psychopathological) behavior on man, they have yet to explain many phenomena evident in his learning or creative conceptualizations. Thus many behaviors follow single exposures to stimulating events. Brilliant conceptualizations often appear to arise from sudden coalescence of internal associations.

Of immediate interest to the psychiatrist are the experiments of Hunt, who has found that a series of electroshocks attenuate a conditioned emotional response (CER) to a signal previously learned by rats in association with painful shocks given to their feet—but do not affect behavior learned in relation to a reward. Furthermore, amphetamine potentiates the attenuating effect of electroshock on the conditioned emotional response, while chlorpromazine given after electroshock strengthens the conditioned emotional response. So, too, learning theories relate directly to the now widely tried behavioral therapies.

In comparative psychopathology the paradigm of the CER in animals represents most closely the acute stress reactions or traumatic neuroses of men suffered immediately after threatening catastrophes—as in battle experiences in war time, or the multitude of sudden catastrophes of modern civil life. It is of interest, too, that the strength or acquired CER in animals varies in relation to the circadian rhythm. Thus if an animal is trained by an unavoidable shock at 8 A.M. daily, he will show the strongest response thereafter at the time of training and the weakest 12 hours later. So, too, this response is inhibited by adrenalectomy, or by suppression of adrenal function with methopyropine and phenothiazines.

Understanding the learning process is of paramount importance in man, since his large brain gives him a learning capacity far beyond that of other species. This capacity for learning new behaviors has made possible both the increased complexity of his intellectual creativeness and the extraordinary range of his socially maladjustive behavior and psychological defenses, described in later chapters. The gap remains great between the known physiology of behavior and the explanations it offers now of psychopathology.

While much of the investigation of these systems has been concerned with the discernment of their anatomical location and interpreted in electrophysiologic terms or in terms of neurohumoral transmission, it must be appreciated that the expanding knowledge of the ultrastructure of the cell and its intricate biochemical interchanges later may add an even more significant basis for understanding the regulatory systems of the brain and the influence of pharmacologic agents on behavior.

BIBLIOGRAPHY

Bliss, E. L., and Zwanziger, J.: Brain amines and emotional stress. J. Psychiat. Res., 4:189–198, 1966.

Cannon, W. B.: Wisdom of the Body. New York, Norton, 1939.

Collinson, J. B.: Ill-defined procedures in learning and growth. Arch. Gen. Psychiat., 19:298–299, 1968.

DeCara, S. V.: Learning in the autonomic nervous system. Sci. Amer. January 1970, pp. 31–39.

DeJong, R. N., Habash, H. H., and Olson, J. R.: "Pure" memory loss with hippocampal lesions. Trans. Amer. Neurol. Assoc., 93:31–34, 1968.

Dell, P. C.: Some basic mechanisms of the translation of bodily needs into behavior. In Wolstenholme, G. E. W., and O'Connor, C. M. (eds.): Neurological Basis of Behavior. Boston, Little, Brown & Co., 1958, pp. 187–201.

Harlow, H. F., and Harlow, M. K.: Social deprivation in monkeys. Sci. Amer., 207:136–146, 1962.

Hartmann, E.: The Biology of Dreaming. Charles C Thomas, Springfield, Illinois, 1967.

Heath, H. G.: Electrical self-stimulation of the brain in man. Amer. J. Psychiat., 120:571–577, 1963.

Hebb, D. C.: The Organization of Behavior. New York, John Wiley & Son, Inc., 1949.

Hess, E. H.: Imprinting in birds. Science, 146: 1128–1130, 1964.

Hunt, H. F.: Electro-convulsive shock and learning. Trans. N. Y. Academy. Sc., 27:923–945, 1965.

John, E. R.: Mechanisms of Memory. New York, Academic Press, 1967.

Kales, H. (ed.): Sleep. Physiology and Pathology. Philadelphia, J. B. Lippincott Company, 1968.

Levine, R. (ed.): Endocrines and the central nervous system. Assn. Res. Nerv. & Ment. Dis., 43, 1966.

Lorenz, K.: On Aggression. New York, Harcourt, Brace & World, Inc., 1966.

Luce, G. G.: Biological Rhythms in Psychiatry and Medicine. National Clearing House for Mental Health Information, National Institute of Mental Health, Public Health Service. Publ. No. 2088. Washington, D.C., U.S. Government Printing Office.

MacLean, P. D.: Contrasting functions of limbic and neocortical systems of the brain and their relevance to psychophysical aspects of medicine. Amer. J. Med., 25:611–626, 1958.

Magoun, H. W.: The Waking Brain. 2nd ed. Springfield, Illinois, Charles C Thomas, 1963.

Miller, N. E.: Chemical coding of behavior in the brain. Science, 148:328–338, 1965.

Olds, J., and Milner, P.: Positive reinforcement produced by electrical stimulation of septal area and other regions of the rat brain. J. Comp. Physiol. & Psychol., 47:419–429, 1954.

Pavlov, I. P.: Experimental Psychology and Other Essays. New York, Philosophical Library, 1959.

Pribram, K. H.: Looking to see: Some experiments on the brain mechanisms of attention in perception. Res. Publ. Asso., Nerv. & Ment. Dis., 48:150–162, 1970.

Richter, C. P.: Biological Clocks in Medicine and Psychiatry. Springfield, Illinois, Charles C Thomas, 1965.

Roizin, L.: A review of ultracellular structures and their functions with special reference to pathogenic mechanisms at a molecular level. J. Neuropath. & Exp. Neur., 19:591–621, 1960.

Scott, J. P.: Critical periods in behavioral development. Science, 138:949–958, 1962.

Schildkraut, J. J., and Kety, S. S.: Biogenic amines and emotion. Science, 156:21–30, 1967.

Stroebel, C. F.: Behavioural aspects of circadian rhythms. In Zubin, J., and Hunt, H. (eds.): Comparative Psychopathology. Animal and Human. New York, Grune and Stratton, 1967.

Tinbergen, N.: The Study of Instinct. Oxford, Clarendon Press, 1951.

Chapter 4

"We must watch the infant in his mother's arms; we must see the first images which the external world casts upon the dark mirror of his mind; the first occurrence which he witnesses; we must hear the first words which awaken the sleeping powers of thought and stand by his earliest efforts if we would understand the prejudices, the habits and the passions which rule his life."

Alexis de Tocqueville, 1855

Personality Development

Each organism undergoes a process of development of biological structure from the time of the fusion of the male and female germ cells until maturity has been reached. At any time during this maturational process, noxious factors may impair the growth of the organism, produce malformations, or limit the functioning of an organ or of the entire living being. Relative lack of appropriate foodstuffs and nutrients, including the necessary vitamins and ions, also limits bodily growth. It seems well established now that growth may be restricted as well by lack of appropriate stimulation: an experiential deficit at critical periods in maturation prevents the full unfolding of the functions of a system or organ. Thus environments in which the available diet or social stimulation is restricted or impoverished will tend to limit brain growth and personality development in the growing child. Also, lack of early experiencing may lay down a continuing vulnerability to various stresses throughout the remainder of life.

Each person, then, has an anatomical structure conforming in general to the species pattern yet unique in certain details. It is this structure and its physiological functioning which in part determines and limits the personality development. The growth of the central nervous system establishes the limits of temperament and intelligence. Temperamental variations, those capacities for range of active responsiveness to the environment, are considered both to influence the experiential effect of an environmental change and perhaps in turn to be modified by that change. That distinguishing property of the nervous system—the capacity to register, store, and integrate the experiences of the organism so as to bring about the most effective behavioral responses for adaptation—makes it possible for human personality to evolve. Thus, over time, through a prolonged series of social experiencing, more or less enduring and consistent attitudes, beliefs, desires, values, and patterns of adaptation develop which make each individual unique. The distinctive whole formed by these relatively permanent behavioral patterns and tendencies of a given individual is spoken of as *personality*.

To a limited extent, certain patterns are already laid down at birth, yet for the most part only the potentials for the development of personality components exist at that time. Whether the successive stages of the unfolding personality proceed in a wholesome manner and in a normal harmonious sequence of biopsychological and biosocial maturation through infancy, childhood, maturity, and old age, with realization of personal potentials, subjective satisfactions, and social adaptations, or whether there is an arrest or uneven growth of various personality components, depends upon complex genetic, environmental, social, and emotional factors. There is normally a *maturational sequence* in personality development, each stage developing as a logical sequel to the previous one—an emergent growth through distinctively different stages, each having its particular needs and problems. If residues of an earlier stage are carried over to later ones, they may produce malformations of the personality and become a source of psychopathology. Early experiences also continue to exert their influence on the developing personality, even though they are not available to conscious recall.

Genes cannot transmit acquired characteristics. Although the biological development of the fetus may be influenced by the intrauterine environment, there is no reason to believe that personality, as just defined, is largely influenced by prenatal life or even that it exists in the newborn infant. This statement does not deny a genetic anlage or congenital aspects of biochemistry and reactivity which create biological predispositions to the temperamental components of personality in later life. However, while extreme abnormalities in vegetative, central nervous, and endocrine systems may have a demonstrable relation to personality characteristics, there seems to be little relation between them and persistent features of the normal personality.

PERSONALITY STRUCTURE

It is convenient to think of personality as having parts or divisions which perform specific functions—in other words, as having structure. Such a concept facilitates the idea of dynamics in the functioning of the personality. However, these parts must not be considered as concrete realities or self-acting entities but as groups of forces and functions. The concept of personality structure now generally followed is that proposed by Freud, who postulated three psychic segments in the structure of the personality. While these structural divisions are hypothetical, they offer a useful classification of the system of drives. Many of the terms used in describing their dynamic interrelationships are highly figurative.

The Id   *biological need*

The *id* is a collective name for the primitive biological impulses. It represents the innate portion of the personality. The physiologically determined drives for air, food, water, and other nutrient substances, maintenance of bodily temperature and physical integrity, and procreation are thought of as id functions. Thus dependent longings, aggressive and flight tendencies, and sexuality are thought of as id drives and affects. Associated with these primitive drives are the protective aversive states of pain, distress, and rage and the cravings we denote later in life as hunger, thirst, and suffocation. The major affective states of man only unfold with development of perception and cognition; they more properly must be recognized as components of the ego. When ego functions are maldeveloped or impaired, id derivatives appear in conscious fantasies or may erupt as overt behavioral expressions.

The Ego   *social need*

The *ego,* or reality-testing self, is that part or function of the personality which establishes a relationship with the world in which we live. The ego, of course, is a group of functions for which a metaphor is employed for ease of conceptualization. The ego deals with the environment through conscious perception, thought, feeling, and action and is, therefore, the consciously controlling portion of the personality. It contains the evaluating, judging, compromising, solution-forming, and defense-creating aspects of the personality. The ego organization, concerned as it is with such important functions as perception, memory, evaluating and testing reality, synthesizing experience, and acting as intermediary between the inner and outer worlds, may be regarded as the integrative and executive agency. Its functions are to deal rationally with the requirements of reality, to adapt behavior to the environment, and to maintain harmony between the urges of the id and the demands and aspirations of the superego.

For normal development of the personality, the ego must be able to modify both the id drives and the superego's demands for acceptable conduct without extreme sacrifice of either emotional and instinctive satisfactions or of ethical ideals. In this way the ego serves as mediator and directs behavior into acceptable compromises between the blind drives of the id and the inhibitions of the superego. In contrast to the id drives, which demand immediate satisfaction and are thus stated to operate by the *pleasure principle,* ego functions are guided by the *reality principle.* Thus, the ego directs instinctual energy into channels which will, in the long run, bring the maximum pleasure and satisfaction. Its processes take place largely, but not entirely, at the conscious level. It constructively integrates impulses and thus secures mastery over them. If, through conscious control, it deals effectively with inner and outer stresses, and through reason and circumspection it deals rationally with the requirements of reality and of society, the ego is said to be strong and healthy.

The individual with well-developed and mature ego shows flexibility in handling the various stresses of life without resorting to the inflexible and repetitive defenses that distinguish neurotic or psychotic symptoms or to character defects. If the ego structure is underdeveloped or dominated by unconscious factors, it may undergo disintegrative processes and may be unable to withstand the strain of continued repression, with the result that mental symptoms or character defects appear.

Ego development takes place through the series of transactions between the growing infant and child and his parents and others who influence his growth. While the defensive functions of the ego, to be described in detail in Chapter 5, are born through resolution of conflict between the id and the evolving superego, other ego functions develop from conflict-free activities and have intrinsic generating and satisfying properties of their own. Thus, Hartman notes the development of perception, intention, object comprehension, thinking, language, and memory as autonomous functions of the ego which take place in conflict-free experiencing. One might conclude from the study of exploratory behavior in monkeys, described by Burton, that there is a primary drive state serving to satisfy a perceptual need. As is described in Chapter 2, perceptual deprivations in turn may lead to serious impairment of ego functions.

Ego functions are directed, then, to bring about psychosocial adaptation. But such adaptation requires as well the evolution of a series of interpersonal attitudes which establish for the individual a certain consistency in his relations with others—the means by which he customarily perceives them and functions in relation to them. In addition, others have expectations of his social responses—his ego identity. Erikson has described the development of the ego attitudes from the progressive identification of the growing child with aspects of parents and others immediately affecting him. Erikson has postulated specific psychosocial crises at each stage of interaction whose solution establishes an attitudinal position upon which the growing child proceeds to work through the succeeding stages in his psychosocial evolution, either relatively free of conflict or laden with conflict. Thus, infancy, with varying degrees of mutually satisfying and dissatisfying exchanges, lays the basis for varying degrees of *trust* or *mistrust* of others. The psychosocial crises of early childhood lay the basis for degrees of *personal autonomy* as against degrees of personal *shame and doubt;* later childhood brings the forerunner of *initiative* versus acceptance of *guilt;* school age, that of *industriousness* versus a *sense of inferiority;* adolescence, the crises of *identity formation* or *diffusion.*

The phases of adult life, too, bring their special crises. The young adult must work through the issue of intimacy against that of isolation, the later adult that of procreation versus self-absorption, and the mature adult that of integrity versus despair.

The primary requisite of the transactional process required for personality development is the learning of satisfying and acceptable attitudes and actions designed to control and modulate man's affects. Man's complex affective states are themselves the consequence of the long ongoing process of socialization which allows their progressive unfolding and differentiation. We recognize the syntonic affects of interest and excitement, as well as joy. In addition there are the dystonic and aversive motivating states of distress, fear, shame and guilt, disgust, anger, contempt, love, tenderness and compassion, or sadness.

These motivating and sometimes conflicting affects over time become established within the personality as prevailing mood characteristics, too: curiosity, cheerfulness, apprehensiveness, contemptuousness, or hatefulness. Again affective reaction formations may establish transient or enduring attitudes of envy, jealousy, pride, and courage.

Aside from the work of S. S. Tompkins, little attention has been paid to the dynamics of affective differentiation and its relation to ego development and personality.

But beyond the ego attitudes and affective sets described, psychopathologists are now striving to define and search for determined forces which establish conative sets, found in the mood action complexes which exist in the ego organization of those who successfully adapt to life or cope with its many enduring or sudden stresses. We mentioned in the previous chapter the balancing force of such ego assets as responsibility, perseverance, empathy, likability, humor and playfulness, flexibility, and self-confidence—the complex traits found in creative and constructive persons even though they may often be burdened with severe pathological ego defenses.

The Superego

The third hypothetical segment of the personality structure is the *superego,* that segment conceptualized as an observer and evaluator of ego functioning, comparing it with an ideal standard—an ideal derived from standards of behavior perceived over time in parents, teachers, and others significant to the growing child. The *ego ideal,* the internalized picture or image of what one desires to become and toward which the ego strives, provides the aspirational direction and demand for achievement within each personality.

The concept of the superego had its origin in Freud's analysis of psychotic delusions of being watched. He conceived then of an "observing" portion of the personality.

Around the ages of four to six the child evolves a sense of constraint in his actions as he gives in to the superior strength of the parents. He accepts the parental dictates as absolute and demanding unquestioned obedience. He is unable then to judge his acts or those of another in terms of their social meanings but only as right or wrong. Only after the child has come to share his perspectives with other children and adults in play, action, and thought does he evolve the differential perspectives that allow a less bound and more open and cooperative moral realism. Young children respond only with the narrow and rigid moralism of their homes, and particularly so when insecure. As they discover new images of morality in their play with peers or adults other than their parents, the earlier moral absolutes of the parental figures give way to a wider, more realistic appraisal of morality in general social values and goals.

The superego is derived particularly from identification with parents and their substitutes—figures of authority capable of punishing or rewarding. The prohibitions and obligations noted in these identifications are internalized and incorporated into the unconscious psychological structure of the child. Later, the injunctions and prohibitions of other authorities and of cultural influences are absorbed into the superego, the whole acting as censor. It acts as the supervisor of the ego and of inner, unconscious tendencies and, therefore, as the repressing part of the personality.

If early training has been severely punitive and shaming and unrelieved by later broadening experiences in role playing with others, the superego will contain irrational and even sadistic elements. It may threaten and punish and thereby seek to maintain its authority when the ego tends to accept impulses from the repressed part of the id. It does this by creating anxiety and by producing guilt and remorse. If the superego is severe and inflexible, the resulting fear of it will lead to a rigid, inhibited, unhappy, anxious, and often neurotic personality. Alternatively, the superego facilitates pleasurable satisfactions when ego functioning is evaluated as striving toward or achieves the ideals and goals. Thus, gratification comes from increased self-respect, personal integrity, pride in effort or accomplishment, or self-righteousness.

Balance of Segments

In the well-adjusted person, behavior simultaneously and successfully meets the demands of the id, the ego, and the superego. On the other hand, the behavior of the neurotic, the psychotic, and the pathological personality with serious and repetitive social maladjustment may be considered to result from a disturbance in the dynamic checks and balances of the id, the ego, and the superego.

PERIOD OF INFANCY

Neonatal Period

Birth brings with it a major shift in the physiological functioning of the infant. Thus, there takes place the establishment of respiration and the closure of the umbilical blood flow and the cardiac bypasses, with opening of the pulmonary circulation. With the termination of transplacental nourishment, alimentary feeding commences, with its requirement that the infant form a relationship with the mother or some mother substitute. The body surface and its active sensory receptors are exposed now to a wide variety of variable stimuli, and the homeostatic mechanisms of the central nervous system must establish means of protecting the growing infant from overwhelming excitation and must also assure water balance, nourishment, oxygenation, and temperature regulation. The period of physiological shift and adaptation to the extrauterine environment is one of inconstant and irregular physiological regulation and extends for two to eight weeks after birth.

At first the neonate's respirations are shallow, irregular, and noisy, but later they become steady and deep. Sucking is uncertain, and, while the infant may ingest well, regurgitation is frequent. Initially he loses weight. Urination and defecation occur spontaneously, but his sweat glands will not function for the first month after birth.

Much time is spent in variable stages of sleep, with periods of deep sleep associated with easy respiration, light sleep associated with irregular breathing and bodily restlessness, or stages of drowsiness when the eyes are alternately closed and open. Up to 50 per cent of the sleep of the newborn is associated with the characteristic low-voltage fast-wave electroencephalograph identified in the adult as stage I "fast" or dreaming sleep. The infant, too, shows during this stage increased eye and bodily movements, irregular respiration, and absence of muscle tone.

When awake the neonate appears alert

and active, crying, or inactive. Awake and crying he gives vent to the signal which establishes and sustains the needed relationship with his mother, providing not only nourishment through nursing but also those bodily contacts which stimulate particularly the kinesthetic and tactile systems. There exists, then, between infant and mother a new extrauterine biological relationship.

While awake and alert the infant also at times initiates contact with the external environment other than his mother through the early functioning of his distance receptors—his eyes and ears. The infant responds to most sudden and intense stimuli such as noise, pressure, or jars with a *startle reaction* under all conditions except when vigorously crying. The response to less intense stimuli depends on the infant's initial state; activity is increased when the infant is inactive and is reduced when he is active (except during periods of vigorous nursing or crying). Similarly, the heart rate accelerates if it is slow initially and decelerates if it is rapid initially (law of initial values).

The responsiveness of individual infants is highly variable, however, indicating temperamental predispositions even in the neonatal state. These predispositions, in turn, influence the pattern of mutual interaction with the mother. In some infants the startle response is vigorous, while in others it is slight. Infants are dissimilar even in their response to soothing contact.

Bridger has found that there is a discrepancy between many neonates' behavior and the responsiveness of the autonomic nervous system to various stresses. From his observations he has postulated that those infants who show little behavioral response to stressing stimuli but respond strongly in terms of such indicators of autonomic activity as increased heart rate may later show autonomic hyperactivity and predisposition to psychosomatic disease. The evidence suggests that in the early developmental stage the autonomic nervous system has a lower threshold for reaction than the musculoskeletal system. Thus, with intense soothing stimulation neither system responds to stress, but if that stimulation is lessened autonomic responses appear without musculoskeletal reactions.

While the physiological needs of the human infant are innately determined, their satisfaction both in the prenatal period and for a prolonged period after birth is dependent entirely upon maternal care-giving. The ongoing dependent relationship of the infant establishes from the very beginning of extra-uterine life the association with others from which derive the forces that mold his personality and his eventual capacities for social adaptation.

Maternal Dependency

"Object relations," that is, relations with others, are no longer considered to exist only after a year or so of life. They are initiated with the first acts of mothering which are centered on satisfying the infant's needs for food and warmth. The mother must provide constant attention to maintain the child's comfort through avoiding the irritations caused by wet and dirty clothing or exposure to other damaging forces around him. Maternal care is directed to much more than satisfying the "oral" needs of the infant, who, in turn, must be envisaged as sensing in the early days not only just through the oral mucosa and perioral musculature but also by means of the general tactile-kinesthetic sensory systems which are known to be myelinated at the time of birth. The early interactions between most mothers and infants extend beyond satisfying these basic physiological needs, since the infant is stimulated by the play of the mother, by the fondling he receives, and also by the attempt to gain from him by facial gestures and vocal signs some indications of response. As early as three or four months the infant responds differently to people; he is in contact with those upon whom his life depends.

In the first several weeks of life, the responses to the immediate discomforts of the infant dominate his behavior. He demands, through crying, immediate help in relief of his tensions, whether they are induced through external discomfort or from internal unrest. In this stage as well, the earliest indications of a smile have been noticed—a slight upward inflection of the mouth taking place usually just after feeding and during periods of alert inactivity, drowsiness, or irregular sleep. Soon the response of the facial musculature can be elicited by high-pitched sounds, particularly by the mother or nurse. A fuller smile is evident by the third week; this, in turn, generates in the mothering one efforts to reproduce it through rocking, cuddling, or cooing at the baby. Thus, the smiling response is reinforced in the infant and further intensifies the mutually gratifying, stimulating, and nourishing mother-child relationship. This crying and smiling are the infant's earliest indication of the affects of distress and joy or pleasure.

The infant may be described as directed by the "pleasure principle," unable to delay his demands. Until he is several years old, he will not be able to delay the urgency of his need for relief and to accept delay in response for some future gain or greater satisfaction of desires in terms of the perceived problems and goals and the problems of others—that is, to be guided by the "reality principle." The persistence into later life of emotional states characterized by dependency and the immediacy and urgency of demands, with absence of responsibility for or consideration of others and associated with stages of rage when the need is not met, may be identified then as *infantile*.

The early mothering process, if warm and consistent, lays the groundwork for a continuing sense of satisfaction, security, and trust in others, while its absence, as Erikson suggests, may establish the early roots of mistrust and insecurity. These are the origins of ego attitudes significant for carrying the infant through later stages of growth.

It may be surmised as well that the intermittent contacts with the mother, alternating with states of discomfort and comfort, establish those varying sensory experiences that set down the infant's slowly growing discriminations of self from another, the basis for a sense of space, and also the rhythms that establish time as a modality.

The descriptions given before of the transactions between growing infant and mother as providing the sensory experiences and thus the basic percepts making for personality emphasize the current interest in the precise study of development. There has been amassed an impressive body of evidence from studies of both child development and animal psychology to demonstrate the major significance of healthy development of the early mother-child relationship. Thus, infants deprived of the stimulation of mothering, even though good care of bodily functions is assured, appear weak and listless, cry much more than others, and become apathetic. Odd grimaces and gestures appear. These phenomena disappear if the mother rejoins the infant within the first three months of life but are more obvious and severe when maternal deprivation takes place during the second half of the first year.

Critical Periods

Equally important is the discovery of critical experiential periods needed for the formation of the primary social bonds that are basic for later social relations and for learning. Critical periods for establishing the early social bond in mammals and birds are timed in development by the appearance of behavioral mechanisms which maintain or prevent contact and thus perhaps are related to internal processes associated with emotional arousal. From animal studies it has been inferred that the establishment of the important dependent relationship comes about through the presence of the mother, whether her behavior may be judged as gratifying or thwarting, as rewarding or punishing. The essential feature is her presence to the infant as an object arousing emotion. Scott goes so far as to say that the process of socialization is accelerated by the arousal of any strong emotion related to contact, whether it be hunger, fear, pain, or loneliness.

The primary bond between mother and child appears as well to be a form of attachment that takes place irrespective of learning through contact gained in the feeding process. Thus, "imprinting" in birds is immediately related to the muscular effort made to follow an object during a critical period and can be reduced in intensity if ducklings are given the muscle relaxants meprobamate or carisoprodol. Harlow has shown, too, that young monkeys isolated at birth and supplied with dummy mothers prefer a dummy with a cloth-covered surface without a nipple to a wire-framed dummy with a feeding nipple. Monkeys raised on such dummy monkeys become, as adults, uniformly poor mothers in turn, neglecting and punishing their young.

These observations open to question many of the basic assumptions of psychoanalysis regarding the early developmental period.

Oral Stage

The period of infancy is described in psychoanalytic terms as the *oral stage*, which is conceived of as progressing from an essentially "receptive" to an "aggressive" phase. Prior to birth, the infant is fed through the maternal blood stream and has never experienced the satisfying pleasure provided by the gratification of an instinctual need. With birth, however, a biological need for food arises and he receives satisfaction through sucking. Not only is the discomfort from hunger relieved by the sucking, but, as other and more complex tensions arise, the infant turns to the most available substitute as a source of security and satisfaction and therefore sucks his thumb. The mouth becomes, accordingly, the part of the body in which interests, sensations, and activities are centered and through which gratification is secured. The second phase (from about eight to eighteen months of age) of the oral stage is that in which the pleasure of biting is added to that of sucking, and when one may hypothesize that aggressive drives appear.

AUTOEROTISM. It is conceivable that the oral satisfaction secured from nursing may be the first primitive manifestation of what through many subsequent stages of development will ultimately become adult heterosexuality. At this stage, however, the pleasure seeking is related to the mouth and contains no discernible relation to the genitals as in the adult.

Because of its pleasure-giving potentiality at this stage of psychosexual development, the mouth is spoken of as an erogenous zone. Satisfactions secured from such pleasure-giving zones are called *autoerotic*. Too little or inconsistent "psychological mothering" is apt to promote autoerotism in the form of prolonged or excessive thumb-sucking, constipation, or early and excessive masturbation. On the other hand, consistent and healthy emotional satisfactions in the child's relationships to his parents shorten the autoerotic period of development and promote a natural sublimation of the instinctive drives—a wholesome progress in the successive stages of these aspects of personality development and differentiation.

ELIMINATIVE INTERACTION. Coincident with the stage of increasing motor skills, the interaction between the child and mother centers over the effort to have the child learn to control his eliminative activities; it is bladder and bowel centered.

The manner in which the mother attempts to instruct her child in these first efforts at personal autonomy determines the development of later personality traits. If, for example, urinary or bowel control is attempted before physiological maturation with myelination of the necessary pathways in the spinal cord has made the child capable of recognizing, announcing, or controlling his need to eliminate, or before the child can walk to the toilet or manipulate his clothing, and if the child is punished for his failures, rage or fear will be directed toward the controlling parent. The child then centers his attention on the power struggle between himself and the parent. He may respond with fear of the parent and gradually evolve a pattern of cleanliness, orderliness, submissiveness, and punctuality sometimes referred to as the *anal character*. Or again, his subjective response may be one of rage with the evolving defiant reactions of dirtiness, obstinacy, and unreliability. Most frequently the response to the usual mothering process is vacillating.

From the experiences in this period of interaction, the beginnings of the capacities for self-control, personal independence, and a sense of autonomy and pride may be envisaged. With them arise the learned affects of shame and disgust which are incorporated in response to the parents' attitudes toward the child's excretory functions and are communicated to him through various means. Shame must be recognized as an important infantile emotion, learned by early training—a feeling of being exposed, looked at, and being the object of disgust. Too much shaming may lead to defiant shamelessness as a character trait.

In using the term *infantile sexuality*, Freud never attributed to infants and children the complex pattern of adult sexuality. If the restricted, even figurative, use of the term sexuality is borne in mind, one may, following the terminology of Freud, trace an orderly step-by-step development of the psychosexual aspect of personality from its earliest expression to the mature, heterosexual, socially approved mating upon which the family is founded.

As mentioned in the foregoing discussion, the initial manifestations of *aggression* may be thought of as taking place during the oral stage of psychosexual development. Even at a very tender age, the nursling is not a passive recipient of his mother's milk. On the contrary, the milk is secured by a surprisingly vigorous activity. According to this point of view,

aggression makes its first appearance in infantile personality traits characterized by energy, application, and determination and is of a constructive nature. Others suggest that the arousal of aggression arises relatively later in personality development and only as a reaction to frustration, particularly to the frustrations which the child inevitably feels that he suffers at the hands of parents during the process of being brought up. Undoubtedly, there are many occasions in the child's life for developing resentments and aggressive impulses against a frustrating parent.

ORAL PERSONALITY. If the individual, far beyond the age when the mouth should have ceased to be a focus of satisfaction, continues to be mouth-centered, he is said to be of an oral type of personality. His characteristics are dependency, egocentricity, demanding and taking but not giving, and preoccupation with mouthing as well as ingestive and alimentary fantasies and satisfaction.

Body Ego or Image

BODY PERCEPTS. By the third or fourth month, the maturing infant shows by his responses to others that he perceives the world about him. He perceives smiles and returns them; he is beginning to learn to express emotion through gestures. By the sixth month, the child is capable of binocular vision and appreciates vision at a distance. Also, coördinated activity is possible between several parts of the body; earlier, the eyes turned toward sound, and now so does the body. At the same time, hand and arm movements are well coördinated; and the hand brings objects to the mouth easily. This is the beginning of the infant's exploration of his own body, first with the mouth and then with the hand. These perceptions, largely tactile and kinesthetic sensations in the early months, establish for him the integrated percept of his physical wholeness. They function at a level below conscious awareness to position the body in space, to manipulate objects it may control, and to provide knowledge of the body surface. That percepts of body parts exist is strikingly demonstrated after the loss of a limb in an adult, when the hallucinated "phantom" of the lost arm or leg causes a continuing sensation of its presence.

EARLY SENSORY EXPERIENCES. Early perception by the infant of the body members is necessary for the evolution of these body percepts. If the infant or growing child fails in this experience, either because of congenital absence of a body part or because the limb is lost before the child is five years old, the sensory projection of a limb as a phantom never occurs.

The importance of early infantile sensory experiences in effecting the functioning growth of various integrative systems in the brain is established by other clinical and experimental observations. The most convincing illustration has to do with the permanent defects in vision which occur in children with congenital cataracts but intact retinas and visual apparatus who fail to have the corneal defect repaired by implanting of a healthy transparent cornea before five years of age. Such children are unable to develop adequate vision, while others with earlier transplants go through long periods of learning before they can perceive accurately and recognize formed images. Artificial blinding of infant chimpanzees with later uncovering of the eyes has duplicated these findings.

Such clinical observations indicate once more the importance of critical periods in infancy for experiencing certain sensations and establishing the neural patterns required for later functional maturation of various sensory systems. Much more knowledge is needed of the critical periods of growth in various systems, of the nature of deficits caused by infantile sensory deprivations, and of the capacity and means for correcting the functional impairments. Undoubtedly, this information will influence our appreciation of the etiology of many personality problems as well as the treatment of such defects.

BODY CONCEPT. It must be recalled that the child not only develops bodily perceptions over time which are modified gradually and extended in the course of growth so as to conform with the current body structure, but also takes unto himself the attitudes of others toward his body and its parts. He may develop a satisfying body concept, or he may come to view his body and its parts as unpleasant, dirty, shameful, or disgusting, by which he reflects the interaction between himself, the parental figures, and, later, other significant persons. The clinician will find it useful to distinguish *body percepts* from *body concepts*. Theoretically both are included within the well-known term *body image*. Body image is that perception of the body by the ego. The body ego contains percepts, concepts, and affects related to the body. The child's concept of his body will form a nuclear structure of his later personality and will, to a large part, determine his capacity to adapt successfully to the stresses of illness, trauma, and physical changes.

Motility

As the child develops, the focus of maternal attention gradually shifts from the giving of food to assisting the child to develop his maturing capacity for motility, the manipulation of objects with his hands, and later walking and speaking. The general motility of the child appears to arise from an autonomous drive. The patterning of motor activity and its successive and more intricate mastery in various actions, play, and games is in itself satisfying and induces pleasurable affects. Likewise, restriction of motor activity induces conflict, with the arousal of rage. Commencing at about the age of 10 months, the infant engages in two different types of motor activity. There are those which seem to serve no other purpose than the experience of movement, such as crawling, running, jumping, and whirling; many of these activities are rhythmic and circular. The second type are those motor activities undertaken to manipulate objects; these activities are often autonomous and appear driven. It is through his motor activities that the child expresses his impulsive urge to action, an urge which must later be controlled for effective social participation. Activity is used in the service of aggression and sexuality and as a means of communication through imitation, gesture, and posture. It is associated with a range of affective stages including joy, rage, anxiety, and depression.

Motility, too, is the means by which the ego gains competence and security in its executive and synthetic functions. The carrying out and trying of intentions in action—the accomplishment of a successful series of operant behaviors that are processed as such by the rewarded ego—assist in establishment of sound concepts of reality about self functioning as well as the outer world. Also, they support the establishment of the ego sets of autonomy, initiative, and competence.

It is not surprising that patterns of disturbed motility frequently present as symptoms of personality disturbance in adults. Thus, one finds the tics and other compulsive activities, and the motor inhibitions of the hysteric, the grimacing and posturing of the schizophrenic, and the waxy flexibility of the catatonic.

PERIOD OF CHILDHOOD

For purposes of descriptive analysis and study it is useful to distinguish between various periods of growth. Yet these distinctions are arbitrary, and it must be kept in mind that stages of maturation gradually melt one into another; there are no real distinctions. Childhood is here conceived as beginning with the capacity to speak—some time between the end of the first year and during the second year of life. Of course, it runs coincidently with those processes of maturation concerned with increasing motility of the child, his growing capacity for elimination and control of excrements, but also marks a major shift in his interpersonal relations as he now grows beyond signaling by

means of cries or those early gestures learned in later infancy.

Since the earliest experiences of the child occur in the family setting, his perceptions and interpretations of these experiences will determine his attitudes toward and evaluations of later, even adult, experiences that contain some apparent similarities. Such a *transference* of an attitude derived from some personal relationship in the family to others in the larger world will exert either favorable or unfavorable influences on his relations with others and thus upon his ability to reach his ultimate social goals. Persistent attitudes of resentment or hostility that are built into the personality structure through the early experiences may form the repetitive responses of the neurotic in later life and may become the focus upon which paralyzing reaction-formations are built.

For example, if a young child sees a comforting and protecting mother repeatedly hurt or made to cry by a cruel father, he may acquire a lasting hatred for the father and later transfer this attitude to all men who resemble him in some way. Again, if the mother is vacillating in her care, sometimes comforting and at other times cruel, the child will be unable to make the clear discriminations from which unambivalent attitudes of love and hatred would emerge.

A major determinant in personality development is the unconscious modeling of the growing child upon the parents, spoken of as *identification*. The child identifies with the perceived aspects of the behavior of the parent; included are those which arouse tension or pleasure, the overrated body parts, and actions and capacities which, in the child's growing fantasies, probably give the parent the strength and power he wishes for himself. If the parents are emotionally mature persons, the adaptive process of identification promotes healthy growth.

The widening ability of the child to care for himself now brings him greater relationship with the father and other siblings in the family; his social development extends beyond that of the primary relationship with the mother. With this period of expanding social contact there evolves the necessity to share. In these experiences with others, the associated emotions of jealousy, rage, envy, and guilt develop. His greater activity provides him the opportunity to exercise his exploratory tendencies, his curiosity, and his initiative at solving simple problems. Differences are discerned between the sexes, and the foundations for eventual sexual identification are laid down. The striving for the first place in affection and acquisition, from the mother against the father and in a struggle with brothers and sisters, establishes competitive rivalries that stimulate those wish-fulfilling dreams and fantasies of overwhelming strength and reward or, later, the fear of retaliation, of harm and attack from others.

With the striving initiative of the child and the arousal of the emotions of jealous rage and anger, there also emerges the superego, the *conscience*. In the face of his struggles the child is curbed by one or both parents, and in turn develops both feelings of hatefulness and those adaptations of escape from retaliatory attack that may be retained in some form to adulthood—sulking, withdrawal, and finally the internalization of the prohibitions against his expressions of anger.

For psychoanalysis, this period represents the *phallic stage*. Attention has already been called to the theory that at about one year of age the source of pleasure shifts from the oral to the anal region. Similarly, at about three years of age there appears another stage in the development of pleasurable interest with a shift of source from the anal to the genital region. This phase continues until about the seventh year. With the advent of this phase, there is a concern with the difference between sexes and the size, presence, or absence of the phallic organs. There is a predominance of genital sensations, and masturbation may become a source of psychosexual pleasure. The interest is not a sexual one in the adult sense of the term. The boy merely comes

to realize that his penis is important and devotes narcissistic attention to it. The girl may become aware that she has no penis and believes she had one but lost it, with the result that she develops feelings of inferiority and jealousy. The oral, anal, and phallic stages of libido development are often spoken of as the pregenital stages.

OEDIPUS COMPLEX. Continuous throughout the phallic stage up to the fifth or sixth year there exists a period of attraction to the parent of the opposite sex accompanied by jealousy and rivalrous hostility toward the parent of the same sex. To this situation between father, mother, and child, Freud gave the term *Oedipus complex*. Various anthropologists reject the universality of the Oedipus complex. That it is, however, a basically correct psychological feature of our own culture is generally accepted. Some suggest that the Oedipus reaction is determined by the behavior of the parents, not of the child. It is certainly frequently true that fathers are more severe with their sons and more indulgent with their daughters. That mothers frequently reverse this relationship is constantly observed by psychiatrists. In either case, the rivalry and hostility associated with the Oedipus reaction would follow quite naturally. Others regard the oedipal period as a convenient and expressive metaphorical term for designating the phase of personality development in which the child feels and expresses hostility against one of the parents because of the frustrations experienced.

Normally, this potentially pathogenic relation is resolved by the mechanisms of identification in which the boy identifies with his father and incorporates his father's goals and standards into his own pattern of behavior. Likewise the girl identifies with her mother, advances toward a healthy emotional maturation, and finds gratification and security in a feminine role.

From clinical observation, it is frequently recognized that when the Oedipus complex is inadequately resolved, the in-

dividual may introject some of the qualities of the parent of the opposite sex, with
the result that the development of "normal" relationships with persons of the
opposite sex is precluded. Familiar examples are the adult son who lives with a
widowed mother and is oblivious to the
charm of women of his own age, or the
young man who falls in love with a much
older woman who in some way resembles
his mother. Psychoanalytically it is said
that such fixation occurs at the homosexual stage of personality development.

Socialization Period

Later childhood, that period from six
or seven to twelve, is one in which the
child's socialization is relegated to others
outside the family in our Western culture.
The influence of teachers as authority
figures outside the home, of older and
younger playmates, and of other relatives
and friends provides important opportunities for new identifications and discriminations which allay, modify, or intensify
the patterns of behavioral reactions
established in the family and also offer
opportunities for the acquisition of new
skills and roles. The child is eager to do
things; he has the opportunity to learn
habits of industry. Yet, if he fails to gain
the patterns and otherwise measure up to
his peers in school and on the playground,
a sense of inferiority is instilled. His play
activities provide him the opportunity for
gaining pleasure in mastering tasks and,
for some, that of prestige in accomplishment. Through socialized play he has the
opportunity to learn mastery of his glee
in triumph and his frustration and rage
in failure. Group play activities allow the
gradual growth and pleasure in the companionship of others, in sharing their
problems. The era carries with it as well
the learning of other patterns of group
behavior, those of teasing, disparage-
ment, and ostracism. If the juvenile suffers
as a consequence of group actions, his
responses may seem to deepen the already

existing personality reactions to frustrations at home.

At this time in the child's life, his
sexual curiosity is limited; this is the
latency period of psychoanalytic psychosexual development. While sex interests
and activities do not disappear, there are
no such marked and significant psychosexual changes as are seen in both the
preceding and the following periods. The
child does, however, identify more
strongly than before with the parent of
the same sex and begins more differentiation along masculine or feminine lines.
Therefore at this time it is important that
there be close association with a parent
or some other satisfactory person of the
same sex with whom the child may identify in establishing masculinity or femininity. This period is notably one of training in the customs and attitudes of society.
There is a progressive development of
the ego as a result of growth on the one
hand and of education and experience
on the other. It is a period during which
ideals are formed. The child is exposed
to more complex social pressures; also
environmental opportunities play an important part in directing individual
interests and capacities. In the latter part
of the latency period, a quest for status
becomes a strong motivating force. It is,
too, the period when inner control of
aggressive-destructive impulses should be
attained.

PERIOD OF ADOLESCENCE

With increasing group relations, the juvenile often develops an intense interest
in one other child, usually of the same
sex. This interest extends to consideration
of the feelings and sensitivities of the
friend. It represents the first efforts at
those intimate contacts which occur in
adulthood. This interest in the friend
extends to satisfying his wishes as well
as being moved by and interested in his
successes and failures. Groups of juveniles
get together and the roles of leader and
supporter are learned. These social inter-

actions provide satisfaction and security for the growing youngster.

Adolescence proper sets in with puberty, with its rapid physiological development of the sex organs. The maturation of sexual and reproductive capacities stimulates genital and heterosexual interests and activities in the genital stage of psychosexual development. Sexuality is no longer diffused throughout the body as in the pregenital phases of personality development but becomes focalized on the genital organs. The sexual area, however, is only one aspect of the personality in which there is an inherent drive toward maturation.

The growing adolescent is now preoccupied with how he appears to others and how he perceives himself. He is in search of a *personal identity,* a sense of self. Since the adolescent stands midway between personal independence and continued dependence on the parents, many acts of emancipatory behavior occur. For example, the effort to establish a sexual identification leads the boy to seek reinforcement with men or other older boys who are idealized, while the girl finds similar sources for her growing femininity. Overaggressive and competitive attitudes, exhibitionistic poses, or cynical and antisocial actions may represent these struggles for a masculine independence from authority at home. Usually there is a searching out of members of the other sex, with courting as a preparation for eventual intimacy and mating. These adolescent interests break up the more juvenile friendships and call upon the adolescent to relive the separation experiences of early life and also the emotions of sadness and jealous hatefulness engendered in the Oedipal conflict. Concomitant with his sexual drive, the adolescent develops a fantasy life filled with fulfillment of his desires, yet finds himself in conflict between the latter and the prohibitions of his family and society.

The adolescent must commit himself eventually to a choice of intimacy with another and must make, as well, an occupational decision, and he must couple this with a persistent and energetic competitive drive. Without such commitment the adolescent is exposed to a sense of personal isolation, or else he becomes preoccupied with a multiplicity of sexual relations of varying kinds or becomes involved in self-effacing attachments to others. He may attempt to maintain the illusion of youth, refusing to believe that the passage of time will affect his choices or his ability to find opportunities in industry and to acquire skills. Fear of and oversensitivity to competitive activity may develop. Some adolescents choose a *negative identity* founded in the presumed strengths and fascinations of the most undesirable and dangerous figures offered for identification.

Since the crises to which the adolescent is exposed are so varied and so critical, it is not surprising that personality disturbances are common in this period.

ADULTHOOD AND MATURITY

While chronological age may be recognized legally as an indication of responsible maturity, it is no guarantee of the emotional growth of the individual. The mature adult is one who has developed a clear personal identity, demonstrated by the ability to form an intimate, satisfying, and loving relationship with a mature member of the opposite sex and to take on the responsibilities of rearing children. He is able both to assume personal responsibilities when necessary and to accept the decisions of those with competent authority for the general good. He independently pursues his own goals, with recognition of his limitations and with willingness to seek advice from others when indicated, and is able to maintain and enjoy his personal relations with others, making due allowances for their deficits with an understanding tolerance. The healthy adult is one who is absorbed and satisfied in achievement relative to his family, vocation, and avocations rather than in personal self-assertions. He functions well at home and at work in terms of developing gratifying relations with others as well as in being generally free of symptoms of illness.

Problems of Maturity

In all periods of adult life, the conflicts that occur recapitulate those of earlier life. For the young adult, these struggles center largely over the necessity for decisions relative to the selection of a mate and a vocation. In each instance the young adult may find himself in conflict between his personal drives and estimates of capacity and opportunity and those expressed by his parents or their representatives. Anxieties that develop in arriving at these decisions may adversely affect both marital and vocational life. Undue dependence upon the parents, if marriage occurs, will deprive the marital partner of the tenderness and attentiveness required to establish a satisfying and growth-promoting home. Attitudes of unusual defiance or submissiveness, originating in the relations to parents and teachers, are likely to be transferred to those in authority in the vocational world. In turn, these may lead either to derogatory attitudes toward the defiant young adult or to failure of associates to recognize potentialities of the submissive person that might lead to advancement. The birth of children often revives the sibling rivalries of earlier years in one or both parents, with reappearance of inappropriate hostilities or resurgence of infantile demands.

In middle adulthood, with advancement to senior positions, the rearousal of sibling rivalries leads to paralyzing anxieties over envy and hostility suspected in peers, or to overbearing attitudes of revenge for their assumed earlier punitiveness. Failure to be advanced also can bring forth hostilities and resentments that can lead to sulky withdrawal, depression, or accusations of favoritism or influence. With menopause, women experience the conflicts centered on waning sexuality

and inability to bear children. Later life poses again the problems of increasing dependence with surrender of personal responsibility owing to increasing physical weakness or relinquishment of positions of power and prestige, with consequent recurrence of drives of rivalry. The older person must also face the anxieties consequent upon impending death.

Separation and Death

One of the major emotional problems of the elderly, but one to which men are exposed throughout all periods of life, is separation from those whom one loves and upon whom one is dependent. Mourning, the period of grief that follows loss through death or an important separation, or even the loss of a body part as from amputation, must be regarded as a process of anxiety with restitution and reëstablishment of the personality in the face of the loss. During mourning the intensity of grief leads to both physiological and psychological disturbances which are evidenced in withdrawal from others and preoccupation with the loss. The process of mourning is the psychological effort to maintain the lost object by fantasy reviewing of the experiences, meanings, and emotional significance of the relationship and the eventual taking in of certain qualities derived from the association.

Older people frequently suffer this process and may defend themselves against it by adopting attitudes of personal omnipotence and pride in self-sufficiency, or they may be recurrently overcome by overt anxiety and other defenses against it.

For the infant and child, death of a person upon whom they are dependent leads to profound emotional disturbances, as Spitz, Bowlby, and others have demonstrated.

The growing child's appreciation of death is not that of the adult, however; until the age of five or thereabouts death is perceived as a departure, a further existence under other conditions, without finality, to which the separated child responds by asking for the lost person. The child at this time interprets the loss frequently as a malignant, premeditated act to which he responds with the emotions of both sadness and rage. He is taught to repress these emotions. Later, between five and ten, children tend to personify death as someone who carries others off, a fearful person. It is only after this age that death is recognized as a universal process with final dissolution of life.

Deaths in the family through suicide or illness, or threats of suicide, may be perceived by the young child as hateful or manipulative acts and may in turn lead to retaliatory fantasies, which form the basis for later suicidal thoughts and acts that have revenge as their motive.

Thus mourning and separation anxiety must be recognized as regular emotional responses to a loss, with a recognizable course of development and resolutions. Mourning for adults runs a course of six to twelve months; it is to be differentiated from depression.

FACTORS INFLUENCING EMOTIONAL RESPONSE

Family Constellation

While the *only child* may develop well and has often been reported to be superior to others in terms of health, physique, intelligence, and facility at school, his emotional position in the family exposes him to the full intensity of any emotional disturbances that may exist in the parents. As an only child, he may represent the parents' single effort to appear as sexually mature adults and thus he represents a denial of interested and wanted parenthood. The parents' exploitative drives are channeled into the only child, and their over-solicitude leads to an excessive protection, which further isolates him from his peers. He is deprived of the learning experiences of living and sharing with siblings; frequently he has fantasies of brothers and sisters. With others of his own age he may be shy and awkward, thus becoming the victim of teasing and rejection; this induces either further withdrawal or over-compensatory efforts to gain attention and prestige. Such efforts may be expressed in exhibitionistic activities, boastfulness, or bribery of others if the means exist. His isolation often leads to the persistence of childish dependency on others, which impairs his capacity for adult relations.

The *adopted child,* particularly when adopted outside the parental family, also is exposed to developmental difficulties that lead to a high incidence of personality disorder in later life. Thus, the adopted child may perpetuate intrapsychically a split in his parental object relations, since in reality he has two sets of parents and maintains one as "bad" and the other as "good." Also, one or both of the adoptive parents may be disturbed by unconscious guilt, which is then projected onto the heredity or conception of the adopted child. Adopted children frequently have wish-fulfilling fantasies that their real mothers will reclaim them. Their ambivalence toward their adoptive parents often is difficult to resolve, as they tend to perceive these parents as inadequate and support their conflict with fantasied satisfactions in the relationship with the lost parents. Such fantasies maintain and generate their frequent desires to come to know and find their real parents. Furthermore, the adoptive status is often used by the new parents as a means of shaming the child and controlling his behavior, thus magnifying a sense of being unwanted and unloved. Adopted children exposed to such family transactions more often appear to be aggressive and to indulge in sexual "acting out" in adolescence and later life.

The *institutionalized child* is often exposed as well to an environment unfavorable to emotional maturation. Deprived of a close, continuing, and warm emotional contact with an interested mother substitute and later a paternal figure, the child reared in an institution lacks the personal stimulation and the opportunity for the growth of affection and trust that permits development later of the capacity for successful relations and identifications with others. Thus impairment occurs in the maturation of both ego and superego functions. It has been found that such children show a greater frequency of problem behavior characterized by lack of control, anxiety, and aggression, and an affective impoverishment. Specifically, they are more restless, overactive, and limited in concentration, others have temper tantrums and may be impudent, cruel, and destructive. More frequently they show impairment of speech and mental activities which resemble retardation and lead to difficulty in school.

Twins, both identical and nonidentical, as well as those born in other multiple sibships, have special problems in personality growth. The maternal attitude toward twins is sometimes one of shame and rejection followed later by efforts to explore and differentiate the siblings as a means for the mother to direct appropriately her responses to one or other of the children. The care of twins demands much of the mother; each receives less attention than the single child. Yet this drives the pair together and establishes the matrix which makes it difficult for them to establish independent self-identities. Their constant closeness interferes with their independent learning of social functions. Twins develop more intense rivalry problems to which they may adapt by attaching themselves to one or the other parent or, more commonly, by assuming similar desires and thereby repressing their individual drives. The strong jealousy for the parents generated in the relationship intensifies hostile drives toward the other twin which, in turn, require compensatory efforts at repressions that again bring the twins together. While these pressures are not inevitable, they occur frequently in twin development and make the individual both insecure in his own identity and extremely vulnerable to the loss of his sibling on whom he is usually excessively dependent.

ORDINAL POSITION AND FAMILY SIZE. Both the quantity and quality of interaction between the growing infant or child and his parents will be influenced by the maternal drive and affective satisfaction of the parents and by the time available to them from their other goal strivings. Thus large families will tend to decrease the amount of parental contact for those most recently born. On the other hand peer transactions tend to increase and may therefore make up for the relative degree of deprivation of maternal and paternal interactions. First born children usually arouse and obtain the greatest degree of maternal and paternal interest and joy. They obtain the most attention, because there is less competition for parental time. As the new and shared object hopefully expressive of parental aspirations, the first born's hold on both parents exceeds that of the later born siblings. As one might predict, studies of those who have achieved most in terms of creative effort demonstrate a preponderance of first born children. Yet a child in this position is highly vulnerable, too. When his physique or his early or later development disappoint or deviate from the parental expectations, he often suffers severe rejection and may become overloaded with distress, anguish, guilt, or shame, which in turn stimulates the development of pathological defenses.

So, too, the youngest child may generate a greater maternal interest and attention as a way of recapturing or retaining the satisfactions of the mother's earlier years. Spoiling or overprotection are more likely here than for the oldest; maternal attitudes are conducive to maintenance of oral dependent characteristics.

Infinite variations exist for highly variable personality development in the many differing transactions stimulated between parents and children of moderate and large-sized families. At the same time, extended kinships or friendships offer many alternative modes for identification for the growing child. In the attempt to understand the individual personality, the diagnostician must seek to identify all the significant relations and the nature and result of their transactions with the child or adult who has become his concern.

BIBLIOGRAPHY

Adler, A.: Individual Psychology. London, Routledge, 1946.

Bridger, W. H., and Birns, B.: Neonates' behavioral and autonomic responses to stress during soothing. Recent Advances Biol. Psych., 5:1–6, 1963.

Burlingham, D.: Twins: A Study of Three Pairs of Identical Twins. New York, International Universities Press, 1952.

Chassell, J. C.: Old wine in new bottles. Superego as a structuring of roles. In Gibson, R. W. (ed.): Cross Currents in Psychiatry and Psychoanalysis. Philadelphia, J. B. Lippincott, 1967.

Clark, L. D.: A comparative view of aggressive behavior. Amer. J. Psychiat., 119:336–341, 1962.

Clark, R. A., and Capparell, H. V.: The psychiatry of the adult only child. Amer. J. Psychother., 8:487–499, 1954.

Dubos, R., Lee, C. J., and Costello, R.: Lasting biological effects of early environmental influences. J. Exp. Med., 130:963–977, 1969.

Dyrud, J. E., and Donnelly, C.: Executive functions of the ego. Arch. Gen. Psychiat., 20:257–261, 1961.

Engel, G. L.: Psychological Development in Health and Disease. Philadelphia, W. B. Saunders Company, 1962.

Erikson, E. H.: Identity and the Life Cycle, New York Psychological Issues. New York, International Universities Press, 1959.

Erikson, E. H.: Childhood and Society. 2nd ed. New York, W. W. Norton, 1963.

Frank, L. K.: Play in personality development. Amer. J. Orthopsychiat., 25:576–590, 1955.

Freud, S.: Collected Papers. London, Hogarth Press, 1924.

Freud, S.: The Ego and the Id. Translated by J. Riviere. London, Hogarth Press, 1927.

Harlow, H. F., and Harlow, M. F.: Social deprivation in monkeys. Sci. Amer., 207:136–146, 1962.

Hartman, H.: Ego Psychology and the Problem of Adaptation. New York, International University Press, 1958.

Hooker, D.: The Prenatal Origin of Behavior. New York, Hafner Publishing Company, 1969.

Kardiner, A., Karush, A., and Ovesey, L.: A methodological study of Freudian theory. J. Nerv. & Ment. Dis., 129:11–19, 133–143, 207–221, 341–356, 1959.

Kolb, L. C.: Disturbances of the body image. In Arieti, S. (ed.): American Handbook of Psychiatry. New York, Basic Books, Inc., 1959, vol. 1, pp. 749–769.

Nagy, M. H.: The child's view of death. In Fiefel, H. (ed.): The Meaning of Death. New York, McGraw-Hill Book Co., 1959.

Provence, S., and Lipton, R. C.: Infants in Institutions. New York, International University Press, Inc., 1962.

Sandler, J.: On the concept of superego. Psychoanal. Stud. Child, 15:128–162, 1966.

Schechter, M. D., Carlson, P. V., Simmons, J. A., and Work, H. H.: Emotional problems of the adoptee. Arch. Gen. Psychiat., 10:109–118, 1964.

Scott, J. P.: Critical periods in behavioral development. Science, 138:949–958, 1962.

Stone, A. A.: Consciousness: Altered levels in blind children. Psychosom. Med., 26:14–19, 1964.

Sullivan, H. S.: The Interpersonal Theory of Psychiatry. New York, W. W. Norton & Company, 1953.

Tomkins, S. S.: Affect, Imagery and Consciousness. 2 Vols. New York, Springer Publishing Company, Inc., 1963.

Vaillant, G. E.: Theoretical hierarchy of adaptive ego mechanisms. Arch. Gen. Psychiat., 24:107–118, 1971.

Chapter 5

"During man's growth, mere individuality becomes personality: and the developed individual personality is not only the most complex type of organization known, and one which exhibits a far greater range of diversity among its members than any other single type of organization, but the highest product of evolution of which we have any knowledge."

Julian Huxley

Adaptive Processes and Mental Mechanisms

NEED FOR ADAPTIVE MECHANISMS

In the course of evolution, all species have developed various means and mechanisms to adapt to the life conditions which confront them. Some butterflies, for example, develop a protective coloring whereby they so simulate the appearance of the surface on which they rest as to escape detection by their enemies, and members of the same species adapt their coloring when the environment to which they are exposed differs from that of their original habitat. Since adaptation is the very essence of life, it is not strange that man, as the most highly developed species, has evolved not only anatomical adjustments which protect him structurally or physiologically in respect to his environment but also psychological devices which assist him in dealing with his emotional needs and stresses. These devices help to meet such needs as those for affection, personal security, personal significance, and defense against perturbing affects. By acting without conscious recognition on his part, such devices effect adaptation to inner situations and experiences that would otherwise be sorely, even intolerably, troublesome. The self-conscious personality with its intense need for a sense of

security and self-esteem evokes mechanisms of a protective nature as instinctively as self-preservation prompts the avoidance of approaching physical danger. Just as the body through its physical and biochemical processes strives to maintain a physiological equilibrium or homeostasis, so the personality through automatic and unconscious psychological processes seeks to maintain a psychological stability.

The evolution of a healthy personality requires especially the development of those behavioral processes which are necessary for adapting to life in human society. Therefore the development of the communicative and explorative or problem-solving behaviors, especially language and the thought processes, must be considered of paramount importance as human adaptive processes. These processes are acquired through learning, as are the various mental mechanisms by which the personality attempts to enhance and defend itself, to mediate between its conflicting drives, and to allay tensions. In terms of psychopathology, the definitions of disturbance will be found particularly in failures of the integrative function of the personality—its ego functions. Thus disturbances of language, perception, thought, and memory and of the capacity to delay gratifications of needs, discharge tensions, and learn the ordinary social behaviors, or the acquisition of inflexible character defenses against such tensions, provide the recognizable symptomatic expressions of the personality disorders.

LANGUAGE AND COMMUNICATION

There is strong reason to believe that man's neocortex alone evolved the structural and functional organization necessary for human speech. Judging from experimental brain stimulation, vocalization in nonhuman primates appears to be functionally organized, outside the neocortex in the areas of emotional behavior. According to Lenneberg's work, language development follows a regular maturational development even in children in whom the process is impeded owing to retardation such as in Down's syndrome (Mongolism; see Chapter 30). The acquisition of language in children is not prevented by physical impairments such as blindness or deafness, or by deprivation of rearing by deaf parents, provided that appropriate stimulation is given early in life. It has been suggested that the "critical period" for language acquisition extends from the age of two until puberty. Fluent second language acquisition is difficult after this age.

Chomsky and other linguists propose that the human brain is organized to act upon a "generative grammar" and that the varieties of grammar required to cover all languages are small. Thus, all of language is not learned. The neocortical organization of man is programed to accept language. Observations that language comprehension always develops before language expression and that language comprehension evolves in children incapable of any form of verbal expression seem to support these opinions.

While the acquisition of language as a communicative device distinguishes man from all other living species, it is often overlooked that he retains and uses other forms of communication as well. When communication is accepted as representing all those methods of influencing others which lead to a response on the part of the other, there is that continuing cognizance of nonverbal communication which is necessary for the understanding of conflict and abnormal behaviors.

To return again to the developmental history of man, the infant's original communications consist essentially of vocalizations which signal his distress and need for help. These vocalizations essentially signal emotional states. The responses from the mother set up the pattern for the growth of the later and more complex communicative systems, the smiles, pointings, and other gesturings between the two which again signal emotional reactions—signs which later may be adapted, as in the language of the deaf-mutes, for an elaborate nonverbal symbolic communicative system. The early gestures are the rudiments of the kinesthetic system wherein bodily movements and postures provide information and convey messages to others. Thus the tightstepped gluteal pressed walk and stiff posture of a young woman signifies her overconcern with the taboos of sexual behavior, while the condescendingly haughty walk of a young man—erect, head thrown back, stiff armed—tells of his effort to cover up his unspoken feeling of social inadequacy with disdainful poise.

It must be held in mind that the gestural characteristics of human communication vary not only from individual to individual but also from culture to culture. Gestures have now come under study by anthropologists, who indicate that each culture has a limited range of these communicative acts; in the United States there are said to exist approximately 30 which may be regularly recognized.

Verbal communication, language, has its beginnings between the first and second years, when the necessary neuromuscular structures are fully developed. First the child uses interjections to inform of his emotional states. Later he denotes those about him by naming, and still later designates objects with nouns. Next comes the use of verbs, and by the end of the second year simple sentences are formed. The child indicates his ability to separate himself from others clearly by using pronouns and enriches his informational activity by learning the use of adjectives and adverbs. If the child has failed to speak by the end of three and one-half years, some defect almost invariably exists in the neuro-anatomical structures concerned with speech—failure in the auditory apparatus per se leading to deafness, in the auditory nerves, or in those brain pathways and interconnections mediating the reception, cognition, and activations of speech—or else there has occurred a failure in the teaching and learning of speech, in the intercommunication processes that structure language through interplay between parent and child. Language does not evolve in nonspeaking environments, as various observations have shown.

But even with the development of verbal communication, language continues to reflect the emotional states and attitudes of the speaker in the hidden meanings of accompanying tone, inflection, volume, and gesture. Wit and humor especially, as well as various creative efforts, reflect and reveal the hidden and conflicting motivations through their nonverbal meanings. The psychiatrist must observe the discrepancies between the content of language, verbal communication, and the meanings conveyed in the nonverbal accompaniments of language, including the postures and gestures which establish the speaker's character. In these discrepancies the psychiatrist may detect evidence of conflict, the subtle expression of hidden affect, and the modes of defending against its expression. It is of utmost significance to bear in mind that there is not only verbal language but also a nonverbal organ and action language.

Communication involves relations between peoples. As has been described in Chapter 4, growth is associated with establishing successively the capacity to communicate well with one other (the mother), then with the family members, and finally with increasingly varied and complex groups of persons, in the process of which the individual assumes at one time one social role and at another time another social role.

PERCEPTION AND THOUGHT

Even more distinctive of man than language has been his unparalleled evolution of a system for problem solving which has demanded an organization of neural functions of much greater complexity than that of a simple receptor-effector relationship with the environment. In contrast to the simple organizations of a reflex-stimulus-reflex system, the interposition of the highly elaborate cellular structure of the brain establishes delay in response, storing, and retention of previous experiences and the capacity for increasingly effective discriminations in exploring the environment.

It has been said that man never contacts reality directly; he first reacts with himself and his preconceived emotions, hopes, fears, and aspirations. It is the interposition of this mediating system, the human brain, which has made possible the potential for the use of symbols. Through the progressive storing of accumulated knowledge and its transmission from one generation to another by the various cultural institutions, modern civilizations have arisen.

Beyond its communicative function, language with its purposive drives made possible for man the designation and categorization of objects and thus the ability to regroup words to form different meanings or to use the same word in different combinations to specify still further meanings. Thus in the development of language the ranges of discrimination and thought were extended far beyond that found in animal species which use only a nonverbal communicative system.

Yet, if thought is considered the means for problem solving, verbal language is not a necessary precursor. Experimental psychology has acquired a wealth of data to show that animals may solve problems and also use symbols as signs. Nor is problem solving dependent upon learning, as new insights and solutions depend upon recombinations of previous experience. The parts of the old experience used in the new solutions or conceptions nevertheless must have been explored or learned. Thus, animals reared in isolation and denied the experiences of those reared in groups prove inferior in problem-solving tests. Man's great capacity for thought as a purposive problem-solving device rests upon his greater capacity for recording past experiences, for remembering, for questioning—and therefore for making progressively precise discriminations and complex combinations. It is fixation of the past through memory which allows those comparisons with current percepts or images that establish the capacity to formulate questions, the other component of man's thought processes, which distinguish him from other species.

Perception and learning are necessary concomitants of the thinking process. Perception is not sensation; it implies the recognition of an object, an image, or a thought. Perceptions then often represent integrations of many sensations recorded in the brain as the central integrating organ. Thus perception of an orange implies the sensing of both color and form visually. The latter requires the kinesthetic sensing of the ocular muscles as they circumscribe the shape, as well as the olfactory and gustatory memories of previous contacts with the orange. Perception, then, is the act of knowing objects, images, and thoughts, by sensory experiences or by recollective thought. *Imagery* takes place when some central brain process is set in action which is similar to the process aroused on earlier occasions on sensing the object. *Concepts,* in contradistinction to percepts, are mental images of something formed by generalizations from the particulars.

The acquisition of percepts takes place only through a long process of repetitive experiencing of the object, a learning process which involves the mental processes of discrimination and generalization. The child who perceives the orange has discriminated it from other round objects and is now able to transfer this percept to other images of the orange such as pictures or models. He generalizes the percept. Yet now he again recognizes the orange image and discriminates it from the real object. In the previous chapter, reference has been made to the serious defects which occur if the growing child is prevented before the age of five from experiencing visual sensation, which lays down the patterns of arousal in the central nervous system that lead to recall and the potentiality for effective visual perception. Mention was also made of the acquisition of perception of one's body, through experiencing it in the sensing and explorations of the early growth process, as well as perception of other objects external to the body.

Early Perceptual Processes

To return once more to development, the beginnings of perceptual and conceptual processes are hypothesized to commence in the experiences associated with the early mothering of the infant. Through repeated experiences of being nursed, the infant comes to associate satisfaction or discomfort with the presence or absence of contact with the mother—either direct contact or contact with the nipple. These early percepts are diffuse, and represent the physiological responses later associated with emotion in the sense that the internal state of the infant is recorded. It is unlikely that the infant distinguishes himself from the mother—the "me" or "not me." What is perceived, then, is hunger or satiation, satisfaction, cold or warmth, and pain, but without conscious meaning.

The continuing contact with the mother leads to a discrimination of nipple and breast as distinct from the infant's self and later the percept of the mother's face, with eventual recognition of its varying expression of affect in smiling, laughing, frowning, or indifference. It is assumed that at this time the infant's brain has made the perceptual distinction between the body of the infant as separate from that of the mother and has established the fundamental basis for a personal identity.

It is conceivable that in periods of contact on feeding frustrations the infant develops an image, or hallucinates the presence, of the breast or the mother as a wish-fulfilling substitute for gratification. There is now evidence from electroencephalographic studies that there is a capacity for dream life in earliest infancy. This suggests the plausibility of this early type of imagery. In this psychoanalytic theory of thinking, failure to satisfy the need for food forces a form of substitutive mental representation, the infantile prototype of ideation. The unsatisfied need also may be thought of as leading to a heightened awareness and attention which establish the set that determines what eventually appears in consciousness.

In infancy attentiveness is short lived, yet the infant, with his limited capacity to sense, has difficulty shifting from one percept to another. He may be said to be "stimulus bound." When he is exposed to a number of objects, his incapacity to attend the multiplicity of impressions is evinced in crying or other behavior indicating tension.

With recognition through repeated experience, the infantile percepts take on meaning as the external objects, human or inanimate, repeatedly induce feeling states within him. About the fourth month of life, when he commences to grasp, external percepts are given another meaning in terms of what the infant may do to them. The early percepts are largely tactile—kinesthetic senses. At about six months of age visual perception enlarges and becomes dominant.

Conceptual Development

Piaget's direct study of the growing child provides the best source of information on the development of the early perceptual and underlying cognitive processes. Within the first 18 months of life, before any evidence of language expression, the child's sensorimotor behavior demonstrates the existence of a practical intelligence centered on a logic of action. Once he has pulled toward him a blanket on which a toy has been placed, he will then pull the blanket to reach any other object placed upon it. Further, he will generalize that action to pull a string to which an object is attached. Piaget argues that the growing child's sensorimotor experiences with objects lead him to assimilate into himself that which is repeatable and capable of generalization as a logic or scheme. These sensorimotor actions organize reality outside the child by constructing action categories which define objects, space, time, and causes. By so manipulating objects beyond himself the child comes to separate himself from the outer world. At five to seven months objects are not permanent; their withdrawal sets off indifference or screaming. By nine months the child will look for an object he has seen if it is placed behind a screen —yet then he does not search elsewhere. A few months later he will use inferences to look for it elsewhere. The object has become permanently fixed in his mind; he organizes space and time as he searches and finds objects. So, too, as in the blanket experience described earlier, he has commenced to recognize that his own actions offer a cause. By the beginning of the second year the child has an understanding of space—that a movement in one direction may be cancelled by a movement in another or that a point in space may be reached by several routes.

From a year and a half to seven or eight the sensorimotor knowledge seems to be internalized and shaped as representations or symbols, of which language is the best one. Gestures and imitations are highly important. Such development takes place in deaf and dumb as well as blind children; the latter are more delayed, however, in their symbolic development than the former, as they are impaired in their ability to explore space.

To Piaget, percepts and concepts of objects are derived from early sensorimotor experiencing. They may evolve simultaneously. The percepts may precede conceptualization by a long period; or, in the case of perspective, there occurs a divergent evolution of percept and concept. Thus not until after seven will the child commence to recognize changes in size and shape and to represent perspective in drawing—a development progressive to ten.

To Piaget the symbolic or semiotic function takes place through *operations*: the child begins by imitating in the presence of a model. Later he will carry out the imitations alone. A child may imitate the stamping or crying of an angry playmate, but later will repeat the same actions when alone—a deferred imitation. So, too, through the play of pretending, the child establishes a gestural symbol of some act such as sleeping. Not until after two and a half is the child capable of a graphic image—a way station between the symbolic play and a mental image or concept.

Imitation is the prefiguration of representation. Symbolic play and drawing form the next way station before the establishment of mental images. Symbolic play for the child assimilates reality to the self, the play representing both affective states and cognitive interests. The child may play as an object, holding himself stiff "like a skyscraper." His symbolic play may deal as well with the unconscious conflicts of the child—aggressive, sexual, and so on.

Before seven, the images are static; motion or change is difficult to reproduce. In this period of life his thinking is absolute and unidirectional. Although he may identify his left hand from his right, this will be difficult when he is asked to make the distinction before a mirror. To Piaget this suggests that imaginal reproductions require anticipation and depend on operations which make it possible for the child to understand these processes.

From seven onward to approximately twelve, the healthy child turns to concrete operations, classifying objects according to similarities and ordering them in series. His thought processes are reversible, and the child now increases his capacity to think of points of view of others. Yet he is incapable of abstract thought. His command of language symbols expands his knowledge over vast ranges of time and space. It is the communicative process in gesture, language, and play which broadens the child's perceptivity of his world—decenters it from himself to others. This conceptual decentering occurs simultaneously with the decentering of affective and social (moral) thinking. Thus while children before seven will state that the quantity of liquid being poured from one glass to a narrower or wider one is increased or decreased, after this age they note that the water poured is the same and may be returned to the original container, and they will argue that the quantity is unchanged. States are subordinated to transformations and are reversible. They relate directly to concrete objects and not yet to verbal abstracts. With the thinking abilities mentioned, the child is able to play games with other children, to learn the social rules. These are first received as absolute dictates from elders, are applied without allowances, and only later are softened as group decisions between contemporaries.

It is only in the preadolescent period that the beginnings are made in accepting and thinking in terms of abstractions—not in relation to observations or representations regarded as true. The reader is referred to the extensive observational data reported by Piaget. The important point for psychiatry is the recognition that many clinical phenomena related to communication and thought are recognizable as partial regressions to or fixations at earlier levels of conceptual development.

Registration and Stimulus Barrier

Consciousness includes not only percepts and images of current happenings and those of the past, but also the images of the possible future. There is now mounting evidence that conscious percepts and images are influenced not only by consciously available past percepts, but also those that have been *repressed*. More recently there has accumulated some data to indicate, in addition, the registration of external stimuli that go unrecognized, since they are so subliminal that no immediate conscious recording ever occurs, yet such registrations appear to influence other perceptions. Thus experiments have demonstrated that subliminal exposures of emotionally toned words such as "angry" and "happy" given simultaneously by subliminal tachistoscopic projection will modify the percept of a clearly exposed photograph of a man's face to include the subject's report of the associated subliminal affect word.

It appears, then, that of the many stimuli impinging on the human receptor system, many more register and achieve some subjective representation than may be surmised from simple examination of the thoughts or overt behaviors of the subject. Man, then, is much more receptive of his world and its impingements upon him; his senses range actively and restlessly over wide areas that fall outside the range of perception and immediate consciousness. For such "incidental registrations" to reach consciousness, it seems likely that they must be recruited to reality-attuned schemata.

Registration and perception are considered now by many researchers as distinct processes, the former highly efficient but less selective. The barriers to perception of registered stimuli depend upon their endowment with qualities significant to consciousness at a particular time. Accordingly, it may be said that the state of consciousness at a particular time determines the structure of perceptions and registrations; the "set" or "attitude" of mind selects from the vast barrage of incoming sensory registrations, both internal and external, those to which the individual attends and thereby establishes an effective barrier to perception so as to make adaptations to those most significant

to the state of the organism at the moment. Recent neurophysiological work has shown as well that stimuli may be blocked from registration centrally by "feedback" which reduces registrations at the peripheral sensory organs, again providing the organism a *stimulus barrier*. The foregoing discussion is consistent with clinical observations. As an example, many soldiers fail to recall perception of pain at the time of impact when wounded in battle, when other threats and activities preclude attendance to the pain-inducing wound.

The concept of the stimulus barrier, now supported by physiological studies, bears directly upon such issues as the sensitivity of individuals to varying degrees and kinds of sensory experiences as well as preferences in the selection of perceptual experiences. Thus, many childhood schizophrenics are hypersensitive to auditory stimuli and prefer to use the contact receptors of touch, taste, and smell rather than the distance receptors of vision and audition.

Again, it has been postulated that disruption of the stimulus barrier occurs in the acute stress reactions and other neuroses, leaving the individual pathologically hypersensitive and overreactive.

Early Fantasies

The psychoanalytic theories of the early beginnings of hallucinated wishes in the infant have been mentioned earlier. Later, waking images or fantasies, thoughts, and dreams also are considered to fulfill the function of damping the tensions of unmet needs. It has been further suggested that these fantasies evolve in relation to the growth of the child. Thus with the period of toilet training and the exposure of the child to efforts to control him, the thought processes are repetitive, oscillating between the wish to excrete and the defiance of withholding. Here one may conceive of establishing the polar thinking of "is it right" or "is it wrong," or "I am good," "I am bad," or "I shall do it" or "I shall not do it"; modes of thought which are fixed characteristically in the obsessive-compulsive mind. Later on, with the child's exposure to the emotional interplay between himself and both parents and siblings, there arise those fantasies dealing with the consequences of relations with others. "If I love father, mother will punish me," or pseudo-masochistic, "If I die, you will be sorry." Finally, the child evolves a variety of thought in which he projects himself into the future and attempts to organize his world for satisfactions to be attained at a later time. By using his past, he attempts to organize his future through thought to both avoid dangers and attain pleasures.

A distinction is made between the type of prelogical emotional thinking or fantasy of the young child, which emerges as well in states of fatigue, intoxication, or psychoses, and the dreams of adults. Designated by psychoanalysts as *primary process thinking*, it is highly charged affectively. Its images are relatively unorganized, usually visual, and/or subject to the ego defensive operations of condensation, displacement, and symbolization. In contradistinction to primary process thinking, *secondary process* thought is highly organized and logical and is related to ordered word representation or abstractions concerned with the realities of the external world.

The Uses of Fantasy

The child's capacity to separate himself from the early fantasy world described before and achieve freedom for organizational thought depends not only on his innate intellectual endowment, but also upon the preservation of his curiosity and a limitation of early fears and anxieties. The parental relationship again, through its capacities for guiding the child's exploratory behavior, protecting him from too great arousal of emotions, allows the potentiality for gaining a period of autonomous thought, free from the intrusive and disturbing fantasies of early infancy and childhood just described. Thereby his capacity for the progressive differentiations, generalizations, transfers, and recombinations that constitute new conceptualizations and underlie creative thought and productive human activity are fostered by contact with adults who desire to impart their knowledge and protect the child through their own mature behavior from behavioral sequences that lead to emotional fixations and repetitive intrusion of immature fantasies.

In the next chapter the deleterious effects on mentation due to isolation from others will be described as an etiologic factor in the disruption of personality functioning. However, it must be mentioned that the healthy individual often finds periods of limited isolation highly significant in terms of creative thinking. In such instances it may be surmised that numerous perceptions and registrations from the past are brought to preconscious and conscious states that allow their associations and recombinations for purposes of gaining new insights and solutions of formerly insoluble problems. There are on record numerous instances of sudden insights into highly important scientific discoveries which took place under such circumstances. Kekulé's conceptualization of the benzene ring is one of the best known.

Such emergent and creative thought is considered by some to take place through associative linkage between repressed primary and secondary thought processes. If such is the case, the suggestion of Noy that primary processes be considered not as an infantile side of thinking but rather as one of two ongoing and continuously developing processes of thought must receive serious consideration. To him, primary processes of thinking are used for all functions aimed at preserving self-continuity and identity, and for assimilation (as used by Piaget) of new experiences and lines of action into the life scheme. Secondary process thinking is used for encountering reality, for integration and mastery in relation to reality. The latter is subject to continuous feedback from the environment; only portions of the former are so directed. Both methods of thinking continue throughout life, and both mature through experience during the life span. For most of daily living the secondary, reality-centered thought fills consciousness. Secondary process is concerned with processing more and more information, of representing complex events by quick and effective symbols and signs—the bits of conceptual thinking. This is in contrast to the more subjectively oriented primary process concerned with assimilating feelings, ideas, memories, and values and integrating them into the self system.

The sudden emergence of a new creative act perhaps occurs at moments of reflection or withdrawal from ongoing external feedback, allowing the emergence of new insight. Thus an encounter with reality may be processed first by the logical thought activities and later dealt with in dream and fantasy. The coalescence of these several processes achieves mastery sometimes in the sudden insight. Or the emergence of a personal motivation may emerge in fantasy or dream, to be worked through by secondary process thought. These suggestions do not dismiss the continued existence of early life primary process condensations which may arise, in consciousness, in psychotic or neurotic imagery of thought, or in dream or fantasy.

Other Adaptive Processes

In the last chapter we mentioned the existence of certain ego assets as important in defining the total personality. The relative strength of such ongoing attitudes or conative sets as trust, autonomy, initiative, as well as others, is not well understood. A sense of personal responsibility, perseverance, humor, playfulness, courage, and empathy must be recognized as powerful forces in ongoing attempts at coping with both acute and enduring stresses to the individual personality.

MENTAL MECHANISMS

Through the long period of development the personality acquires various psychological techniques by which it attempts to defend itself, establish compromises between conflicting impulses, and allay inner tensions. These mediating and integrating activities, functions of the ego as described before, are internal mechanisms of control, unconsciously selected and operating automatically. The personality develops defenses designed to manage anxiety, aggressive impulses, hostilities, resentments, and frustrations. All of us make continual use of defense mechanisms. In themselves they are not necessarily pathological. Life would be unbearable without resort to rationalization and similar psychic protections. Neither is it always the goal of therapy to eliminate them. Since at times they may promote the individual's ability to live in peace with himself, it may, in fact, be a therapeutic objective to strengthen them. The type of motivating device unconsciously selected to meet emotional needs and stresses and to provide a defense against anxiety, the extent of its employment, and the degree to which it distorts the personality, dominates the behavior, and disturbs the adjustment with others determine the measure of mental health. Processes similar in kind take place, therefore, in both the "normal" and the "abnormal."

Conflict

Unfortunately, the conscious desire of the individual, the recognition he craves, and the gratification of biological impulses with which he was endowed are frequently not compatible with the conventionally sanctioned habits, attitudes, demands, and values of the larger social group of which he is a member, nor with the prohibiting and censoring forces of his personality. Conscious and unconscious forces pursue incompatible goals. A struggle exists between two powerful incompatible response-tendencies—between the attitudes, habits, and values he has absorbed from the family, school, church, and various other carriers of ethical and moral standards and traditions on the one hand, and his unconscious needs and strivings on the other.

The dilemma in which the individual is impelled by mutually incompatible mental forces and irreconcilable, competing impulses and personality needs is known as a psychic conflict. The conflict may be thought of as a clashing—an internal struggle—between different parts of the personality. According to psychoanalytical theory, many conflicts have their origin in the early struggles of infancy and childhood but through repression become inaccessible to conscious introspection. In this dynamic clashing of impulses, the individual is torn between his conflictful drives, his wishes and aversions, his loves and hostilities, his fears and longings, his urges and resistances. His satisfactions, stability, and peace of mind may be seriously disturbed because of conflict between his drives and wishes on the one hand, and the codes, traditions, beliefs, and loyalties which he has adopted from his social group on the other.

There is, as it were, a civil war within the personality. The individual is driven simultaneously toward behaviors of opposite types. The personality becomes divided against itself, and a sense of tension or inner restlessness exists. It is the task of personality, often a difficult and painful one, to establish a compromise satisfactory to its conflictful strivings. Frequently it is not successful, and as a result the individual experiences anxiety, a condition of diffuse apprehension and of heightened and persistent inner tension.

Anxiety

Conflict induces the affect of *anxiety*, considered central to the understanding of the psychodynamic processes. Anxiety is generally considered now as a state of tension signaling the potentiality of an impending disaster, a warning of danger from the pressure of unacceptable internal attitudes erupting into either consciousness or action, with the consequent responses of the individual personality or society to this eruption. To put it in another way, in the face of emerging aggressive or sexual drives, the tension of loneliness or sadness or the revelation of love or tenderness, which might expose the individual to the suffering of the affects of guilt or shame, anxiety is first felt in the context of the conflict situation.

While anxiety and *fear* have much in common in that both represent signals of danger, there are certain fundamental differences. Fear is the affective response to an actual current external danger which subsides with the elimination of the threatening situation, either by its disappearance through conquest or by escape. The danger most frequently is one to the physical integrity of the individual, whether from the threat of illness or from some external physical attack. Anxiety, on the other hand, may be thought of as the signal of an impending threat to the personality in the context of the social environment. Sullivan has provided a useful operational definition of anxiety in this context. He describes anxiety as a state of tension existing when one apprehends an unfavorable estimate by a significant person. The sufferer of anxiety is at best dimly aware of the conflict, aware only of the state of dread.

During development of personality, various mental mechanisms evolve to protect the individual from anxiety and other affects and their physiological accompaniments. These are described and illustrated in the following paragraphs. Overt anxiety and its associated physiological expressions are observed only when the defensive mental mechanisms break down as the consequence of overwhelming inner or outer threat to the personality.

Serious personality disorder exists when personality functioning is limited through repetitive and inflexible use of a limited number of immature ego defense mechanisms. Such defensive limitation may occur either through arousal of intense and ongoing anxiety as the consequence of persistent conflict within the personality, or through failures to evolve a full and unlimited range of potential psychological devices useful in warding off and protecting from impairing intensities of affective arousal.

Psychotic behavior is characterized by the use of such defenses as delusional projection, denial, fantasy, regression, symbolization, and acting out. The neurotic will more frequently utilize repression, isolation (intellectualization), reaction formation, displacement, or dissociation. For both there will be a limitation or lack of effective balance in the personality's ego adaptive attitudes.

Repression

One of the commonest of mental mechanisms developed for the purpose of dealing with the conflict, i.e., with irreconcilable desires, competing strivings, tendencies toward acts that constitute a threat to the image which we have of ourselves, is that of *repression*. By this mechanism, desires, impulses, thoughts, and strivings which would be incompatible with, or disturbing to, the individual's conscious self-requirements and motivations are excluded from the field of conscious awareness, being pushed into the unconscious. Here, through a psychological inhibition of recall, they remain inaccessible in order that they may not be recognized and give rise to unbearable anxiety. Repression acts as a defense against drives and memories that cannot be controlled by the ego. It is not produced by a deliberate and conscious effort or rejection on the part of the person in whom it operates. Rather, it is an involuntary repudiation or denial, a nonconscious process acting automatically. Experiences involving guilt, shame, or the lowering of self-esteem are particularly apt to be repressed. In repression there is an elimination from consciousness of unrecognized motives and of all ideas or memories that

might tend to arouse a painful anxiety.

Impulses which the ego cannot handle except by repression nevertheless retain their dynamic drive and tension. They continue to lead a subterranean life beneath a conventional surface, yet they are liable to manifest their influence in traits of personality, in special interests, in some system of beliefs or code of values, or in more marked form as neurotic, psychosomatic, or psychotic symptoms. Frequently repressed material may be dealt with rationally if it can be rendered accessible to the scrutiny of consciousness. It is therefore often desirable to make such recall possible. As will be pointed out later, this may be done by the technique known as free association.

Repression, then, is a primary defense against anxiety which is likely to arise when unbearable ideas and impulses threaten to enter conscious awareness. From a different point of view, one may think of repression as having been induced by anxiety rather than the reverse. In either case, the present tendency is to think of repression as the cornerstone of dynamic psychiatry. If repression is unable to prevent anxiety, then other mechanisms, such as projection or symbolization, may be called on to assist in its failing efforts. If repression breaks down the capacity for evaluating, reality may be impaired and defenses disregardful of reality may be called into action. These may, for example, permit the patient to disown an unacceptable impulse or threatening feeling of hostility by having it attributed to a source, perhaps a voice, outside himself. As we come to consider symptoms, we shall find that the patterns of defense against anxiety may be of various and even of changing forms.

By forbidding the undisguised expression of instinctive strivings and socially forbidden tendencies, repression operates to maintain ethical and social conventions, thus assisting the individual in adjusting to the mores and social institutions. Unfortunately, repression is not without disadvantages. Deep-seated drives and urges are not destroyed by repression; on the contrary, although automatically restrained, they remain unchanged in quality and intensity. These drives and urges are, in fact, unmodified in any respect save that the individual is not consciously aware of the disowned strivings. Though frustrated, they constantly seek satisfaction. To make sure, however, that the undesired awareness and expression of these strivings and wishes may not be permitted, the mind, automatically and without conscious deliberation, seeks to crush the strivings, wishes, and thoughts and to reverse their effect by the cultivation and promotion of characteristics sharply opposed in nature. These contrasting aims and efforts, ·designed to reinforce repression, lead to the formation of prejudices and of pronounced character defenses known as *reaction-formations*. These will be discussed later in the chapter. The more repressions a person has, the more prejudices and biases he develops in order to prevent the arousal of his repressed desires. Similarly, intolerance of the wrongdoings of others is often indicative of the effort required to repress similar unrecognized tendencies on his own part.

It must not be concluded from what has been said that repression is always pathological and its results undesirable. It is a mechanism which, if it operates smoothly and without undue effort, may result in a well-adjusted life. In some instances, repression and other mechanisms designed to deal with conflicts and unacceptable impulses may result in the formation of qualities of character that are estimable and yet, because of the sources from which those qualities have arisen, the psychological purposes and needs they fulfill, and the uncompromising tenacity with which they are pursued, they must be looked upon as psychopathological products. We need not be unduly concerned about the genetic source and psychodynamic function which these commendable personality traits are serving. Such desirable character traits might be characterized as representing the conversion of liabilities into assets. A

careful scrutiny often reveals the same psychological theme running through character, personality traits, and the neurosis or psychosis. This is consistent with the principle of scientific thinking —that boundaries in nature are not fixed. One is forced to the conclusion that an unbroken line of continuity exists from normal behavior through neurotic to psychotic behavior. From the standpoint of dynamic development, many personality traits serve the same psychological purpose as do neurotic symptoms. Intolerance, submissiveness, meticulousness, extreme shyness, and other traits may, like neurotic symptoms, be developed as protection against an awareness of early fear, hate, or resentment long buried in the unconsciousness.

Repression should not be confused with *suppression,* in which a conscious effort is made to dismiss repudiated strivings and undesired memories from awareness.

Conscious Control

From what has been said, it is plain that repression is a mechanism which, when employed, operates without conscious recognition. The most successful adjustment to life conditions is not possible if there are tendencies or feelings of which one is not aware so that they are therefore beyond the reach of control. The motives directing our behavior cannot be guided into desirable constructive channels unless their hidden sources are exposed to the light of full consciousness, permitting us to face all the facts and direct our promptings by the mechanism of conscious control. It enables us to replace automatic adaptations and repressions by conscious and flexible adjustments. Likewise, if we can learn to recognize and understand our mechanisms of escape and defense, we may exercise a greater measure of conscious control. Conscious control requires a realistic and efficient capacity for perceiving, deciding, and regulating— that is, a strong ego.

Identification

Identification is the most important of the psychological mechanisms for determining the growth of the ego. As mentioned in the discussion of personality development, the child takes over the attitudes and behavior patterns of his parents and others significant to him. The motivation for identification is wish-fulfillment, in that the child admires or aspires to the strength and qualities of his elders and their associates and attempts to gain for himself their patterns of success by acquiring their modes of behavior. Identification contributes also to the growth of the superego functions. Thus a son may identify with his father and mold his personality on that of his parent, following his patterns of behavior and interest and sharing his ways. This mechanism is not one of conscious deliberation nor of simple imitation.

The process of identification takes place in the family setting and is related to the child's drive to mastery, excitement in novelty, and joy in mastery. It occurs in the repeated transactions of separation from the supporting parents, first from the mother, as the child gains mobility to move away from her and to explore little by little. Later he seeks strength for other tasks in his imitative play—attempts to assimilate the actions of parents, teachers, playmates, and others. Significant identification demands continued reinforcement through constancy of the presence of persons to whom the child relates, and through the child's gaining a sense of competence and rising self-esteem from the use of the identified actions.

Successive identifications over time gradually evolve into *adult individuation* —a firm personal identity separate from the pathological identifications characteristic of psychopathology.

Early and traumatic separations from parents sometimes stimulate drives toward "parenting identities"—such as overanxious concerns for children, pets, or others.

Although identification provides a means for constructive influence on personality growth, this depends upon the personality of those to whom the child is exposed. A child may take on, as well, the socially undesirable characteristics of a parent if these appear to him to provide some special strength or merit. This occurrence is sometimes referred to as *hostile identification*. The brutality of young Germans preceding and during World War II may be interpreted as hostile identification with the actions of the Nazi storm troopers of that time. Identification is seldom complete, since the personality of the admired person is never perceived in its totality by either child or adult. Certain traits alone may be picked up and assumed.

A young male school teacher was observed by his friends to change in the sense that he developed an erect posture and spoke to them looking over his glasses with a precise and clipped speech. He had moved from one city to another to assist in teaching under an outstanding superintendent of schools. His friends were surprised, on meeting the superintendent, to note that his posture and speech were those assumed by their friend.

Identification may be wish-fulfilling in its psychological purpose. This function may, for example, be observed in the self-gratifying sense of superiority felt by the servant of a distinguished personage with whom he identifies himself, or again it may explain the self-satisfaction of the psychotic patient who believes he is Christ and who, to complete the role, wears his hair and beard in the manner in which Christ is ordinarily represented.

Through this mechanism, certain circumstances, including relationships with certain people, may be selected because they fit into specific personality needs. The exaggerated sympathy at times shown by one person for another (even though the second person may be charged with some serious legal offense) results from identification—from a certain unconscious sensing of a common quality of impulse shared with the second individual. Through this mechanism, some desire may be vicariously satisfied, any fulfillment or even a conscious recognition of which would not be knowingly permitted. The false confessions of crime of which one occasionally reads in the newspapers are the results of identification which is based on a desire to commit the offense which the confessor alleges he has committed.

The mechanism sometimes is utilized repetitively by those who have failed to establish a well-organized personality identity. As mentioned before, stable identifications require the presence over time of constant and reliable models, who provide emotional support and encouragement. *Pathological identifications* are those wherein the ego attempts to achieve a sense of power through magical efforts of symbiosis with an ideal. Thus pseudo-identifications occur that are often transient, stilted, or caricatured, and that fail to relate convincingly to others. Now referred to in psychoanalytic writings as *as if* characters, such persons strive for security by successsively attaching themselves to one person after another in whom they perceive some desired strengths. Many attempt to take on their wished-for traits. Since such identifications represent an infantile wish-fulfillment, these are usually transient and cast off when the seeker for a magical security loses or feels rejected by his current supportive image.

TRANSFERENCE. As thus far described, identification is an individual's unconscious molding of himself after the fashion of another or his feeling of a sort of effective oneness with a second person. It is more than the conscious modeling of a child after the pattern of a loved and admired parent.

In a second type of identification, more properly recognized as *transference,* the image of one person is unconsciously identified with that of another. The more recent acquaintance becomes the surrogate of the person previously known and is invested with the same attitudes and emotions with which the individual has come to surround the image of the original party. Here identification is transferred and projected on to the other. This explains some of our apparently causeless likes and dislikes of persons whom we have

unwittingly identified with other persons who had once aroused similar emotions. A person representing authority may come to be identified with a tyrannical father, and the surrogate may be regarded with the same emotions as was the original image. This is doubtless the dynamic determinant of the activity shown by some persons who constantly struggle against the regulations and institutions of society. Hostile and other negative feelings having their original source in attitudes created in early childhood may be displaced or transferred to others in later life and thereby seriously distort human relationships.

EMPATHY. Empathy is a healthy form of identification which is limited and temporary but which enables one person to feel for and with another and to understand his experiences and feelings. The empathetic individual possesses a warm capacity for projecting himself into the situations and feelings of others. This quality will be found only in those with a flexible, mature, and well-established personality.

INTROJECTION. *Introjection* is best understood as a development in an earlier phase of personality than that during which identification occurs. The child introjects or perceives pleasure-pain experiences from which there are derived "good" or "bad" images of the self. In these early experiences the child hardly discriminates between his need and the gratifying or denying source. Thus, satisfaction or frustration of the need is unrelated to its human source and taken in as part of the childish personality. Identification, on the other hand, occurs after the child has been able to differentiate himself clearly from others; it originates in well-defined perceptions of others rather than in the primitive perceptions of inner bodily sensations. Introjection is the obverse of *projection,* to be discussed later.

INCORPORATION. *Incorporation,* another psychoanalytic term, refers to a defense in which a lost or abandoned source of identification is introduced into the ego structure without transformation of the ego. It takes place with an open expression of unneutralized aggression toward the incorporated object. With incorporation, representation of the self becomes like representation of the hated object.

A young married woman was referred for treatment by her husband owing to her recent crying spells, self-denunciation and deprecation, and inability to care for her home and infant. She quickly stated that her mother was a woman who was frequently in tears, only then held her on her lap, and constantly denounced the injustices done her. The patient stated she was afraid she was like her mother and she disliked herself for these traits.

Reaction-Formation

Another important device for the establishment of character is that known as *reaction-formation*. Thus is formed a character trait that is usually the exact opposite of what would naturally follow from the expression of unfettered tendencies, a trait developed to maintain the repression of these impulses and to deny and disguise personality trends that have existed under cover. Perfectionistic and uncompromising character traits are often reaction-formations against forbidden tendencies, desires, or impulses. Often such traits unwittingly reveal troublesome aspects of the personality. The defensive character of conspicuous traits and attitudes is betrayed by the very quality of their exaggeration and at times by their inappropriateness. Such overemphasized character and personality traits may be described as constituting the first line of psychological defense. They can scarcely be called pathological unless they disturb adjustment. Feelings of rejection and hostility may be disguised by scrupulous politeness or effusive expressions of gratitude. So far as conscious intention is concerned, a reaction-formation is always honest and sincere. The overtly aggressive person, constantly demanding his rights and ready to fight at any provocation, may be defending himself against a deeply seated sense of insecurity. On the other hand, submissiveness may be a reaction-formation that serves to cover up unrecognized aggressive tendencies. A façade of excessive amiability may conceal intense hostility.

Great concern for a certain person may be a disguise for unrecognized feelings of hostility, jealousy, or even wishes for his death. Beneath devotion there may lurk a concealed wish for death—e.g., of a widowed mother for whom a spinster daughter has sacrificed herself and refused an offer of marriage in order to remain with her. Such devotion serves to appease a sense of guilt. If employed within rational limits, reaction-formation may be a desirable choice of defense against anxiety.

The unmarried sibling of an identical twin pair presented himself for treatment due to mounting anxiety over his flagrant promiscuous homosexual activity. His brother was happily married. He described his adolescent hatred of his mother for her betrayal of the family in a sordid extramarital affair and his conviction that he could obtain a trusting relationship only with another man—like his brother—indicating that no woman could be trusted. Later he revealed his close and tender relationship with his mother during early boyhood and his expressed wish for a similar feminine companion. The homosexual orientations represented a spiteful reaction-formation against the, to him, fearful wish for a woman.

Compensation

Physiological and physical compensations are phenomena which the internist and the surgeon observe daily. If a valve of the heart is incompetent, the heart muscle hypertrophies in order to compensate for the impairment in circulation that would otherwise result from the valvular defect. If, from disease or faulty habits of posture, a spinal scoliosis develops, a secondary curve, opposite in direction to the primary one, is produced above or below the former in order that the center of gravity may not be displaced. Such compensations represent attempts of organs to adjust to physiological defects and inadequacies. Similarly the organism as a whole, in distinction from its component organs, by compensating for its inadequacies and imperfections attempts to secure the recognition which it craves.

Such compensations may easily become exaggerated and are often unwittingly betrayed by behavior. The person of small stature but with aggressive and dominating traits is an example of over-compensation familiar to all. His pompous and pretentious manner may have been adopted to indicate the strength and authority which a diminutive size fails to suggest. His deportment may make the undersized person feel more comfortable and secure and help him forget his physical inadequacies.

Prestige seems to be one of the fundamental needs of the personality. Methods of enhancing our self-esteem and of covering up deficiencies are widespread and vary from the simple showing off seen daily on the playground or the pretentious display observed in Peacock Alley to the formations of delusions of grandeur. It should not be forgotten, moreover, that socially acceptable degrees of compensation and even admirable personality traits may be an expression of neurotic needs. Their neurotic origin is often betrayed by the striking degree to which they are developed.

Handicaps and limitations, as factors in the production of compensatory products, may be of a widely diversified nature, being in some instances physical, in others mental. The inferiority, too, which lies at the basis of compensatory mechanisms may be either real or fancied. In persons whose reactions in relation to reality in general and to social stimuli in particular are well integrated, the existence of a physical inferiority may provoke constructive activities which result in qualities of outstanding social usefulness. Handicaps may spur one on to greater efforts, as in the case of Wordsworth's happy warrior who "turned his necessity to glorious gain." On the other hand, diseases or deformities that thwart normal instincts or ambitions or cause the individual to stand out unpleasantly from the group may fail to promote desirable qualities of the personality but may lead to wishful thinking, unpleasant traits, or even at times to a psychotic sacrifice of reality. In whatever form manifested, the products represent the results of the personality's efforts to attain a satisfying self-esteem and sense of security. All too often, unfortunately, the mechanism leads to over-compensations which, although satisfying to the individual, are fictitious so far as social values are concerned.

A boy who was so tall, angular, and ungainly that he had always been extremely self-conscious enlisted in the Army. (It is quite probable that, without consciously realizing it, he had been prompted to enlist because the military uniform and a certain glamor connected with the military life seemed to offer hope of relief from the unpleasant sense of being different.) Here he soon became an object of raillery because of his clumsiness in attempting to execute the various drills. After having struggled in vain for adeptness, the boy was placed in the "awkward squad," where he naturally felt even more self-conscious and more painfully aware of his deficiencies. The indignity suffered by his self-esteem was too great; the need of his personality for a more satisfying recognition and for a sense of security exceeded its limited resources and he therefore constructed a fictitious substitute by developing the belief that he was a major general. He was no longer the awkward soldier, unable to compete with his associates, but their commander, directing affairs of great military importance. The compensatory delusion satisfied the recruit's emotional needs but destroyed his usefulness for the realities of military life and required his hospitalization.

Rationalization

Probably none of us realizes the extent to which the mental mechanisms operative in our everyday lives are defensive in nature. One of the commonest of these devices designed to maintain self-respect and prevent feelings of guilt is that of rationalization, a term introduced into psychiatric literature by Ernest Jones.

We prefer to believe that our behavior is the result of thoughtful deliberation, unbiased judgment, and a full awareness of all the motives prompting it. As a matter of fact, only to a minor extent is behavior the result of such conscious intellectual considerations. After we have acted in response to these unrecognized motives, we formulate presentable reasons which we believe determined our conduct, although they are really but *ex post facto* justifications. This mechanism provides rational intellectual explanations of behavior that has really been prompted by unrecognized motives. We think we can fully explain our conduct but are deceived by pseudorational explanations. Our real desires and attitudes remain concealed and disguised.

At times certain of our rationalizations contain a minor element of truth which, however, is so unduly emphasized that it serves to conceal the essential prompting motive. Those motives which are acceptable are selected and considered to be the only ones. Our thinking defends our feeling. Since we believe that our behavior ought to be determined by certain motives, rationalization through its self-deception leads us to believe that it is. In fact, several motives usually combine and are operative in originating our behavior, some of them having a distinctly ethical value. Other components are of a more selfish, emotional, or instinctive nature.

When behavior is determined by such a coalescence of motives, it will be found that the individual selects the most acceptable from the complex group to explain his behavior. The more self-centered and instinctive ones are the more dynamic, and these exercise greater influence in determining behavior, yet they are not those recognized in consciousness as determinative of it. The motives which, from an ethical standpoint, are the highest are those that dominate consciousness and are therefore offered as the real motives, although they are of less influence in determining behavior than are those components that are unrecognized.

The student may ask whether the individual is not aware that the reasons he offers for his behavior are not the actual ones and that he is therefore guilty of a falsehood. To this, one must reply that in the case of a lie one consciously knows that the reason is fictitious, whereas rationalization is so thoroughly a nonconscious mechanism that he does not recognize that motives cannot always be taken at face value. To employ rationalization in discussing his behavior does not mean that he is not honest and sincere. The self-deceptions of rationalization are usually defended with great emotional intensity, since their creation was designed to conceal a truth that would be painful to the ego.

Rationalization is a mechanism that serves a useful purpose insofar as it is conducive to psychic self-protection and comfort. It leads, however, to self-deception and its conclusions are untrustworthy guides for further conduct. Its products, which are often employed deductively as premises, are so fallacious that they may readily contribute to the formation of delusions.

A not uncommon reaction closely allied to rationalization which helps to maintain self-esteem in the face of inadequacy is the depreciation often spoken of as "sour grapes." In this defensive devaluation reaction, the individual disparages some particular goal which, inwardly at least, he would greatly like to attain but which, because of some obstacle, often personal inadequacy, he cannot reach. Depreciating that for which one is unqualified is not infrequent. It is, of course, one form of response to anxiety. Somewhat allied as a defensive mechanism is a blasé indifference in the face of circumstances that would naturally offend self-esteem.

Substitution

Substitution is a mechanism which may be employed to reduce tension resulting from frustration. Through it are secured alternative or substitutive gratifications comparable to those which would have been enjoyed had frustration not occurred. To yield satisfaction and reduce tension, the substitutive action must have certain similarities to the frustrated one. Many psychiatric symptoms represent substitutive and symbolic satisfactions.

In the effort to solve a conflict, the organism has available to itself the options of (1) continuing to strive toward the desired goal; (2) overcoming the obstacles to achievement of the goal by some aggressive drive; or (3) avoiding or fleeing from the obstacle. Among the adjustments possible in personality functioning when it is not possible to utilize aggression or avoidance is the acceptance of a substitute goal or insight. Such a potential exists when the commitment to the goal or the use of a particular adaptive technique prevents the individual from relinquishing that goal. If he is so committed, frustration and the inevitable affective response must follow, although defense against the latter may be achieved with some other mental mechanism.

Displacement

Another anxiety-reducing device which also operates by a process of substitution is displacement. By this defense mechanism, an emotional feeling is transferred from its actual object to a substitute. The feeling originally directed toward a certain person, object, or situation is transferred and attached to another person, object, or situation which becomes invested with the emotional significance originally associated with the former. In a phobia, for example, there is an unconscious transfer of fear and threat from its original hidden and internal unconscious source to another one which is external and apparently unrelated insofar as the patient is consciously aware. In the frequent handwashing observed in certain compulsive neuroses, affect is displaced from an earlier experience with which a feeling of moral uncleanness was associated to the idea of dirt, which comes to evoke the feeling value originally attached to the consciously repudiated experience. Feelings and attitudes, such as love and hate, are particularly apt to be displaced from one person to someone else, who comes to be a surrogate for the first person. A feeling of hostility toward a parent may, for example, be so intense that it cannot be consciously entertained. By shifting the hatred to someone who has a resemblance to the parent, the person may

be protected against conscious recognition of his attitude toward the parent.

In many instances, symbolism is a kind of displacement. An object becomes a symbol of the person or object which originally stimulated the feeling or impulse. Displacement enables the individual to maintain repression of dangerous or unacceptable impulses, wishes, or thoughts. The displacement of anxiety from the significant to the less significant is common. Allied to displacement is the mechanism described by Freud whereby the conscious may defend itself from material in the unconscious by treating it as a joke.

A 30-year-old housewife entered the hospital for treatment of a phobic condition which prevented her from leaving her home. Her condition was initiated after the birth of her third child, when she developed feelings of panic associated with the idea of being sexually attacked. In treatment she proved to have been very dependent since early childhood and to be seductive. She eventually revealed that in her desire to have men care for her she feared loss of sexual control to the point of becoming a prostitute. This anxiety was displaced by fear of street walking.

Restitution

The mechanism of relieving the mind of a load of guilt by restitutive acts (a making up for, or reparation) is not uncommon. Restitution arising from feelings of guilt may become the main motive in life, as exemplified by the indefatigably, almost wearisomely, benevolent person. Operating to a less extreme degree and in a less obvious manner, the restitutive reaction to unconscious guilt may play a large part in a drive toward creativeness.

Projection

This mechanism is, in many respects, a form of displacement, a means of defense which, to a limited degree, one may observe daily among his associates and which is seen to a psychotic degree in paranoia and in other paranoid psychoses. Acting as a defense against anxiety, projection is directed outward and attributes to other persons those objectionable character traits, attitudes, motives, and desires one wishes to disclaim. The mechanism enables one to remain blind to important drives in the personality, while their influence distorts one's picture of the outside world.

One constantly meets people who severely criticize in other persons the very faults which are the weak points of their own character, utterly failing to recognize the fact that they themselves possess the despised traits and motives. The material projected might be said to be an echo of the projector's own unconscious. By projection, one's own aggressive designs and id impulses are attributed to others. Through it repudiated tendencies find outlet.

Feelings of guilt which give rise to anxiety may be alleviated if one is able to cast the blame for shameful tendencies or wishes onto the outer world, leaving one's self guiltless or even victimized. One may feel less guilty, too, if someone else can be made to feel guilty. As a further defense against anxiety, one may respond with hostility and aggressive behavior toward the external object which is the focus of projection. Some treat others as projections of certain of their own unconscious trends—hate, fear, and similar feelings. Often they hold others responsible for their difficulties.

It will be noted that projection is closely associated with the mechanism of denial. This is well illustrated by the formula stated by Freud: A, unable to tolerate the anxiety aroused by his hatred of B, unconsciously changes his attitude, "I hate B," to "B hates me." Repression and projection protect the ego from being overwhelmed or disorganized by the effects of aggression, hate, or guilt.

Sometimes a striving for supremacy and security by persons who, compared with others, are actually or in imagination at a disadvantage in life may lead to projection as a defensive means. If the ego fails or becomes disorganized, other phenomena—hallucinations, ideas of reference, and delusions—often become associated with projection.

DELUSIONS AND PROJECTIONS. Material may be projected in the form either of ideas or of perceptions. In the former case, projection may lead to the formation of delusions, particularly ones of persecution.

During the World War an American soldier, in order to escape from a highly dangerous situation, shot himself in the foot. He was at first treated in an Army hospital and later transferred to the United States, where the self-inflicted wound healed but slowly. The retrospective discomfort or sense of guilt created by his cowardice and dereliction was alleviated psychologically by projection. He believed that the delay in the healing of the wound was a result of neglect on the part of the physician. The soldier felt no self-reproach since it was not he but the physician who was culpable. He was, of course, quite unaware that the attempt he later made on the life of the physician was an effort to destroy *qualities of which he was the actual possessor.*

Such a projection stimulated by a sense of guilt is at times one of the important mechanisms in the production of paranoia. By this mechanism, a patient may persuade himself that his persecutor is so unspeakably evil that he deserves death, and to inflict this, far from being a criminal act, is a laudable one.

HALLUCINATIONS AND PROJECTION. Frequently in the psychotic, the disowned aspects of the personality are projected, not in terms of ideation but in terms of perception. In such a case, the repressed mental material or unacceptable tendencies, striving, or qualities may be externalized in the form of hallucinated voices accusing the patient of practices which represent the rejected aspects.

The soldier just mentioned, in his effort to kill the physician, naturally did not destroy the sense of guilt produced by the violations of his code of mental honor, nor did his attempt to kill his physician destroy the despised defects of character. Finally, their projection led to a still greater distortion of reality in the form of hallucinations. One day, as he was walking along a city street, he heard accusing remarks that seemed to refer to him. Glancing about, he saw that the person in the direction from which the accusing voices apparently came was the driver of a passing automobile. Without warning, the former soldier shot and killed the man. Thus he killed a person who, by projection, had become the representative and incarnation of his own hated but unrecognized qualities.

IDEAS OF REFERENCE. The symptom known as *ideas of reference* arises through the operation of the mechanism of projection. The individual who utilizes this type of projective mechanism egocentrically believes that he is the object of special and ill-disposed attention by those about him. Casual remarks by others, for example, are understood as relating to him and interpreted as accusatory or vilifying.

MOTIVES OF PROJECTION. Projection is a psychological expedient which, by its defensive process, makes the individual more comfortable. It is less disturbing for him to discover an undesirable tendency in someone else than to admit consciously that he possesses it himself. Protection against disowned impulses and wishes and the anxiety which they would stimulate is secured by their paradoxical denial and reversal.

Even in the so-called normal person, the mechanism of projection may be employed for its protective function, but it readily becomes a danger to peace of mind and to the integrity of the personality. It prevents him from seeing himself as he really is and leads to excessive criticism, sarcasm, pessimism, cynicism, brooding, prejudice, intolerance, and hatred. While defensive against anxiety, it is often highly provocative in producing disturbance of human relations. It is a mechanism which may set in motion a process that leads to a vicious cycle.

The attitude of the projecting person toward those on whom the projection is focused frequently becomes one of suspicion or even of overt hostility. This attitude readily leads to one of mutual estrangement which, in turn, activates in the projector a sense of an increasingly hostile world. This feeling easily promotes misinterpretations and perhaps the formation of delusions which tend to create more problems. Thus the mechanism feeds on itself.

Symbolization

At first men communicated with each other through the use of concrete objects, but with the development of language they used words in place of objects. Gradually words were employed to represent ideas as well as objects. Similarly, objects became the symbols or substitutes for ideas, feelings, and tendencies. *Symbolization* with its meaning-carrying signs is therefore a mechanism whereby one idea or object is employed to represent some other idea or object. It is characteristic of words or objects used significantly charged with meaning. This arises from the fact that the displacement of emotional values from the object to the symbol is the essence of symbolization. Symbolization is a mechanism extensively employed in psychopathology.

We have seen that conflicting drives and ideas, or groups of associated ideas, with which painful emotions are associated may be repressed because they are distressing to the conscious personality. Such repressed material is still too active, too heavily charged emotionally, not to be constantly seeking for expression. Since they are denied direct, conscious, and frank expression, the repressed impulses and other psychic content break through and obtain expression at the conscious level in direct, undisguised form. The wish or drive, therefore, that cannot be acknowledged consciously may be dealt with or satisfied in a symbolic manner.

The resemblance between the symbol and the object symbolized is generally so slight or superficial that the conscious mind will overlook it. The individual is, therefore, quite unaware of the meaning of the symbol he has employed; indeed, he is often unaware that he has used one at all. To his conscious mind, the symbol is not a symbol; it is reality in and of itself. He therefore treats symbols as if they were real and directs his behavior in accordance with the affective value with which the symbols are invested.

In both the normal and the psychotic individual, repressed material may be expressed through symbolism. It is manifested not in forms of esthetic value, as in the case of the artist, but in forms equally symbolic, although often in disguises more difficult to read. It is frequently said that symbolism is the language of the unconscious. Appearing in the content of dreams, hallucinations, and obscure or apparently meaningless ideas, symbols express particularly those contents of the individual's inner life with which much feeling is connected.

The disguises under which such material may be manifested are numerous. Various affectations of dress, gait, speech, or manner as observed among persons who are never regarded as suffering from mental disorder are often symbolic disguises expressing products of repression.

A recently married woman was admitted to a hospital for treatment because of her unusual behavior. She stood on her head, was mute, and would communicate by using ball point pens which wrote in red ink. Later she explained her behavior as a means of expressing her anger at her husband for taking her money. She was in love with him so could not speak of her rage, yet the red ink symbolized it. Standing on her head represented both a defiant gesture and a wish for help by being found ill.

Dreams, which are products of thinking that lack the awareness and direction supplied by consciousness, involve various processes, one of the most frequent of which is symbolization. Although not all dreams contain symbolic material and not all psychiatrists agree as to the interpretation to be placed upon dream imagery, many of the images and experiences of dreams represent such products of repression as unacknowledged motives and desires.

Fixation

We know that from infancy to maturity there should be a progressive development, differentiation, and maturation in the instinctive, emotional, and other aspects of the personality. There should be a progressive development not only in the psychosexual aspects of personality, but also in methods of thinking, in meeting difficult situations and the frustration of wishes, in dealing with reality, and in the control and expression of emotions and instincts. Unfortunately, the development of some aspect of the personality may be halted at an incomplete stage of its evolution with a resulting persistence of certain incompletely matured elements. Such a personality shows a lack of harmonious integration. Its emotional organization particularly remains at an immature level, and there is a lag between biological status and emotional independence. This cessation of the process of development of the personality at a stage short of complete and uniform mature independence is known as fixation. Certain phases of development are not successfully passed through and left behind. Just as the child may continue his baby talk and his dependence on his mother beyond the period when these characteristics should have been outgrown, so phases of his personality development may be arrested at various stages. The arrest is not in the intellectual but in the emotional, dispositional aspect of personality maturation.

There are many theories concerning the origin of fixation. According to one theory, fixation is the result of experiencing such excessive satisfactions at a given level that this level can be renounced only with reluctance. According to another theory, a similar effect may be produced by excessive frustration at a given level.

An analogy from somatic pathology will illustrate the mechanism of fixation. It will be remembered that before birth the blood of the fetus passes directly from the right auricle to the left auricle through the foramen ovale, thus short-circuiting the pulmonary circulation, the activity of which is not necessary during fetal life. Sometimes the patulous condition of the foramen ovale persists after birth, with the result that the individual suffers from congenital heart disease. This passage between the auricles is normal for a certain stage of development, but if the fetal arrangement persists beyond the period of its usefulness, its existence constitutes a serious biological handicap In the same way, the persistence of tendencies and emotional attitudes which should have been relinquished prevents mature development and harmonious integration of the personality.

Regression

Attention has just been called to the fact that certain aspects of the personality may be arrested in their maturing process, with the result that a full and harmonious development never occurs. By another anxiety-evading mechanism known as *regression,* the personality may suffer loss of some of the development already attained and revert to a lower level of integration, adjustment, and expression. Thus a child who is toilet trained may again wet his bed following the birth of a sibling who now takes the maternal attention from him. He seeks by his regression to regain the gratifications of an earlier period in life. If the individual is unable to deal realistically and constructively with the various problems and frustrations of life, including those that arise from outside himself, but particularly those that arise from his inner mental life—his conflicts, instinctual drives, and emotional needs —a normal progression to successively higher levels of adjustment may be checked and he may retreat to a lower level of personality development characterized by immature patterns of thought, emotion, or behavior. An infantile or juvenile approach to the world which may have been latent for many years may be awakened by some frustrating experience or situation. Regression to the dependence of infancy or childhood allays the fears and insecurities which arise from the necessity that adult existence meet life situations and responsibilities in an independent fashion. While

adjustive in its purpose, regression is disruptive and does not promote a desirable adaptation.

The stronger the fixations which may have been established during the course of development, the more readily will frustrating and conflictive situations be evaded by regression to those fixations. Extreme forms and degrees of regression result in a serious disorganization of personality and often constitute an important element in schizophrenia. In the process of regression, the total personality, or the whole of the personality, does not regress from one developmental stage to the next lower in clearly defined stages or as a total unit. Certain aspects of the patient's feelings, thinking, and behavior may be perceived as operating at various levels within various stages concurrently. The patient may, for example, think, feel, and behave partially as an adult but at the same time may manifest infantile needs.

Following a trip abroad with some friends, an 18-year-old adopted child became withdrawn and preoccupied herself with religious matters and fantasies about her own parents. Some few days before her hospital admission she commenced to repeat whatever was said to her (echolalia). This behavior persisted for some weeks after her admission. Later she said she had suffered from other children mocking her early in life through echoing her words but learned that she could satisfy her own angry feelings to her teasers by adopting the same method.

Dissociation

Another mechanism to which the organism may resort in order to secure a measure of satisfaction when the various components of the personality are not well integrated is that of dissociation. A portion of the personality which is a source of emotional distress may be eliminated by this mechanism. In dissociation, certain aspects of activities of the personality escape from the control of the individual, become separated from normal consciousness, and, thus segregated, function as a unitary whole.

DUAL OR MULTIPLE PERSONALITIES. We are accustomed to looking upon our perceptions, ideas, emotions, memories, and wishes as all belonging to a consciousness, a personality, that cannot be divided. Ordinarily a given topic occupies one's consciousness one moment and some other topic the next moment, but it is felt that there is some connection between the two topics, that both are part of awareness, that consciousness has been continuous, and that one's mental life has not been divided. Occasionally, however, in a person in whom there is an active incompatibility between repressed elements in his mental life and the rest of his personality, the repressed components may escape from the forces that are repressing them, become separated from the usual consciousness, organize a personality of their own, as it were, and thus dictate behavior. This new or secondary personality has its own consciousness which has no recollection of the usual or primary personality and carries out acts independent of it. The consciousness possessed by this independently functioning experience was designated by Morton Prince as the co-consciousness.

The disposition and character possessed by the secondary personality may be quite different from that shown by the primary personality. This contrast should naturally be expected, since the secondary personality is made up of material that has been repressed, that is, has been rejected by the primary personality because it was not of a nature to be consciously entertained or satisfied.

Occasionally more than one body of associated repressions and affective experiences may become sufficiently organized to acquire independent activity, in which case there will be more than one secondary personality, each possessing a character and disposition different from the others and from the primary personality. To these independently acting personalities is given the term "multiple personalities."

A 28-year-old married woman was admitted to a hospital, depressed and retarded, after a suicidal attempt. Several days later she became angry and assaultive, claimed that it was "her" fault that she was depressed. She then stated that "Mary" was the depressed person; she was Cynthia. As Cynthia she reported frequently leaving home, picking up sailors and lesbians, and acting in a loose and lascivious manner. As Mary she acted as a dutiful, quiet, submissive housewife and mother, angry and depressed over her husband's poor relationship to her. Periodically she abruptly assumed the character of Cynthia and became loud, boisterous, and uninhibited. In the depressed state she accepted the dictates of her superego, repressed the rage toward her husband, and dutifully attempted to assume her responsibilities as a housewife, as Mary. When overwhelmed by rage, she expressed her rage through defiance and acted her aggressive and sexual urges as Cynthia. Only the latter dissociation recognized the former.

Somnambulism. One of the simplest forms of dissociation is that of somnambulism, in which, while the usual personality is asleep, a fragment or some aspect of the personality assumes direction, with the result that, without the awareness of his usual personality, the sleeper arises and executes some complicated act. Other examples of automatisms, or dissociations of personality in which unconscious factors temporarily gain control, act independently and dictate behavior, are automatic writing, fugues, and multiple personalities. In all these dissociated states, the organization of the repressed tendencies and desires into systems has usually been aided by daydreams. Recently it has been demonstrated that somnambulism occurs only in association with the electroencephalographic concomitants of nondreaming sleep.

Automatic Writing. In automatic writing, the usual consciousness may or may not be aware that an automatism is being executed, but in all other forms of dissociation the usual or primary personality is not aware.

Fugue. Sometimes the organized material that has broken away from usual consciousness to form the secondary personality may initiate activities that lead the patient far from the scenes and efforts of his ordinary life. Stengel defines such a flight or *fugue* state as consisting of "transitory abnormal behavior characterized by aimless wandering and more or less alteration of consciousness, usually, but not necessarily followed by amnesia." A desire for escape from some intolerable situation is usually the immediately precipitating factor in the production of the fugue. Frequently the prompting desire is escape either from justice or from domestic stress. An accompanying depressive mood is common. In fugues of short duration, the patient wanders aimlessly, is highly emotional, and when found is agitated and confused. In long fugues he travels far, appears self-possessed, and lives in every way like a normal person except that he is not where he should be. The patient may be his normal self when he emerges from his fugue, aware of his identity with full memory of his past life except for the fugue period, or he may be unaware of his identity and of his past life. Clinically most cases fall into a poorly defined psychopathic-neurotic group. Many have shown a previous tendency to lying or to hysterical features.

Resistance

This defensive mechanism produces a deep-seated opposition to the bringing of repressed (unconscious) data into awareness. Through its operation, the individual seeks to avoid memories and insights which would arouse anxiety and be painful for him to face consciously. It is also observed in psychoanalytical therapy when the psychiatrist encourages the patient to bring repressed material into awareness through free associations. It was through the difficulties and obstructions encountered in free association—the blocking, embarrassment, silences, and anxieties shown by the patient to which he gave the name resistance—that Freud built up his concept of repression. Resistances afford a clue to repressed material.

Denial

Denial is an intrapsychic defense mechanism by means of which consciously in-

tolerable thoughts, wishes, facts, and deeds are disowned by an unconscious denial of their existence. What is consciously intolerable is unconsciously rejected by a protective mechanism of nonawareness. Reality is regarded as nonexistent or is transformed so that it is no longer unpleasant or painful. The term denial used in a psychiatric sense does not include a consciously attempted endeavor to repudiate or disown as in malingering or lying.

A distinguished neurologist in his mid-40's developed headaches, over subsequent weeks incurring weakness of his left hand. He suddenly became comatose and was admitted to the hospital, where a craniotomy revealed the presence of a rapidly growing glioma in the left cerebral hemisphere. Following decompression and recovery of consciousness, he repeatedly assured his family and friends that he had had a minor cerebrovascular accident.

Sublimation

We have seen that repression is a mental mechanism designed to deal with conflicting drives and desires. If it is successful in its purpose and there are no accompanying feelings of anxiety, it facilitates a well-adjusted life. Since, however, repression is, in effect, the overcoming of one force by another, the energy in the repressed impulse is not available for constructive, consciously directed activity. It would be highly desirable, therefore, if the energy inherent in primitive or unacceptable impulses could somehow be transformed and flow with relative freedom into the conscious mind and there direct the individual's interests and activities. The mechanism by which this energy is transformed and directed to socially useful goals is known as *sublimation*. Instinctive needs and unacceptable impulses find an acceptable outlet and mode of expression when anxiety arising from the threat of these needs and impulses is channeled into patterns of social acceptability. Instead of utilizing primitive tendencies and impulses for selfish or forbidden purposes, sublimation transforms and directs them into vocational channels or into art, literature, religion, science, or other activities that promote cultural development and a richer life both for the individual and the social group. Aggressive impulses, for example, may be sublimated through sports and games or other socially accepted channels.

Rarely does the individual recognize that his activity which serves the material, mental, and cultural welfare of himself and his fellows derives its energy from impulses originally developed for biological and selfish ends. The scientist engaged in research on problems of importance to the health or welfare of the entire race does not consciously recognize that his researches are but the disguised and refined expression of a pronounced, innate drive of curiosity.

DEFENSIVE PROCESSES

We may designate as defensive processes of the ego, rather than as specific mental mechanisms, those more complexly organized ideomotor, perceptual, and cognitive ego functions in which one may discern the utilization of a variety of the previously described mental mechanisms. Among such processes are certain character formations, conversions, some fantasies, and dreams.

Certain ego-defensive processes were categorized as *complexes* in earlier psychoanalytic writings. Thus the frequently encountered excessive behavioral reaction or sudden emotional outburst in response to an apparently slight stimulus, as well as certain mannerisms, slips of speech, or forgetfulness, were seen to occur as the result of complex internal responses to an outwardly insignificant or seemingly trivial external stimulus. These reactions are linked to deeply repressed experiences that are highly charged emotionally against which the individual has erected a complex of defenses. Repression plays the major role in the evolution of such processes. Not only may taboo instinctive desires, strivings, and tendencies be repressed, but also ideas, particularly those with painful affect loading. A group of associated ideas invested with common affective accompaniments becomes associated as a complex. The affect imparts the dynamic element, as a result of which it comes to constitute a sphere of emotionally charged thought and thus exercises a strong unconscious influence on behavior. It is these complexes, attached to an organized and often equally complicated series of ego defenses, which are designated as *defensive processes*.

Character Defenses

A variety of persisting attitudes, modes of approaching or responding to others, mannerisms, and affectations which give each individual his particular character are means by which anxiety and other long-continuing affects are walled off or discharged. By such character defenses conflict between id impulses and the requirements of reality are maintained in an equilibrium which often is compatible with a more or less satisfactory, if inflexible and narrow, social adaptation. Such character formations represent the means by which the personality habitually copes with enduring states of anxiety. Often these character formations offer the symbolic means of fulfilling some perceived demand from the outside world and simultaneously provide a form of gratification for the hidden and repressed drive. Character defenses are to be contrasted with psychopathological symptoms, which erupt to contain anxiety that occurs despite character defenses. The symptom is an exaggerated expression of one or several of the ego-defensive mental mechanisms; it conspicuously impairs the social adaptation of the individual and appears as a regression in reaction to some acute stress.

Certain character traits represent sublimations of drives, whereas others are reactive. Thus unremitting striving for power or prestige may represent a reaction to the anxiety evoked by deeply repressed perceptions of inferiority, while excessive kindliness may be a defense against hidden aggressive and sadistic drives. Particular aggregations of traits are referred to as establishing the oral, anal, and urethral characters. These character formations are seen as the reactions to vicissitudes of early development and the consequence of excessive tension at that particular stage of growth, or as the consequence of relative denial of satisfaction at a later period leading to a regressive fixation.

Perfectionism represents a common character defense wherein one demands of oneself and others a higher quality of performance than situations require. Thus the insecure child who seeks affection from his parents by complying with their demands for high performance characteristically must excel to allay his anxiety in later life. Perfectionism as a character defense offers a means of sustaining a satisfying self-image as well as a way of life that avoids self-disparagement. Again it appears to offer the means of continually satisfying the need for affectionate appreciation by others. The symptom of compulsiveness, on the other hand, fends off unacceptable feelings and impulses. It must be kept in mind that character formations occur with symptomatic expressions which may or may not have common psychodynamic roots.

Conversion

Conversion is a psychological process in which one finds utilized the mechanisms of repression, identification, displacement, denial, and symbolization. Thus a conflict inducing a painful affect is converted to an inhibition of some motor or sensory functions and in so doing neutralizes the affect discharge. With the paralysis or sensory disturbance the conflict is denied, the affect repressed, and yet the inhibition of function symbolizes the repressed wish and the need for its inhibition. It appears as well that those utilizing conversion often select the symptoms on the basis of identification.

Fantasy

Earlier, fantasy has been discussed as an ego-adaptive process, one important for mental health and creative thinking. Fantasy may also be defensive. If, however, the gratifications of reality are insufficient, thinking may not be controlled by the demands of reality but may serve as a regressive or substitute satisfaction. Such musing is known as fantasy. Fantasy provides the illusion of a fulfillment of wishes which cannot be satisfied, either because of the frustrations of reality or because the individual's standards of behavior forbid actual gratification of strivings and wishes. Often these strivings and wishes are of such a character that direct reflection on them would scarcely be permitted. Fantasy is a defensive or tension-relieving mechanism offering either solace and an illusionary release from unsatisfying reality or an imaginary satisfaction of wishes, any actual gratification of which has been forbidden by repression. In Freud's words: "The pleasure-principle triumphs over the reality-principle." By the former, he meant the unconscious processes that strive toward the immediate gaining of affective pleasure. By the latter, he meant the conscious tendency of the individual in his attempt to satisfy his pleasure to consider such practical necessities as the outer world imposes and, if necessary, to postpone the satisfaction of these pleasures. Because so seductive and so satisfying in itself, fantasy may replace necessary reality thinking or effective action and serve as a substitute for effort directed at adjustment to the actualities of life. Fantasy has much in common with dreams, differing chiefly in being more coherent and in occurring during waking hours.

Fantasy is not an isolated function but an integrated synthesis of idea, conation, feeling, interpretation, and memory in which instinctive and affective elements predominate and largely direct it. By disregarding reality and providing a substitute satisfaction, it aids in resolving conflicts and in preventing the development of anxiety. In extreme cases it tends to enlist the aid of delusions and hallucinations; wishes, particularly those that remain unsatisfied and beyond full conscious awareness, are projected and come back realized. In many cases, at least, fantasy may be regarded as a defense against anxiety. The psychotic patient may live simultaneously in two unrelated worlds—one of fantasy and one of reality.

One patient in his fantasy world owned the United States Treasury and its contents; he built and controlled the hospital in which he lived but had just lost the key to it. Almost daily he would hand his physician an order for a billion dollars, at the same time begging for some tobacco and that he be given parole of the grounds.

This coexistence of the consciousness of fantasy and the consciousness of reality is made possible by the mechanism of rationalization and its production of what is known as a "logic-tight compartment." Related ideas exist in each compartment, undisturbed by those in the other, each group pursuing its course segregated from those which are incompatible by a barrier through which no reasoning or argument can force a passage. "Logic-tight" and "affective-tight" compartments produced by rationalization are not confined to the psychotic but may be seen among those who are considered of sound mental health. In such cases, the compartments assure an affective segregation of incompatible strivings and emotional material.

Dreams

Dreams, like fantasy and conversion formation, combine and expose many of the defense mechanisms, as Freud so beautifully showed in the study of dreams. In dreams one may find condensations, displacements, symbolizations, regressions, and other ego mechanisms. The mental representations of dreams are a form of sleeping fantasy or imagery commonly considered to represent a means by which the ego attempts to resolve problems, protect against unpleasant affects, and offer wish-fulfilling gratifications. The analysis of the psychic content of dreams is an established technique in psychoanalytic therapy and is described in Chapter 31.

The recently discovered fact that dreaming sleep represents a distinctive aspect of the sleep cycle characterized by a number of associated physiological concomitants has provoked many new explanations for sleep and dreaming sleep, regarding their physiology, their function, and their relation to healthy and disturbed psychological processes. The physiology of sleep is discussed in detail in Chapter 3.

BIBLIOGRAPHY

Birdwhistell, R. L.: Kinesis and Context. Essay on Body Motion Communication. Philadelphia, University of Pennsylvania Press, 1970.

Brody, M. W.: Introjection, identification and incorporation. Int. J. Psychoanal., 45:57–63, 1964.

Fenichel, B.: The Psychoanalytic Theory of the Neuroses. New York, W. W. Norton & Company, 1946.

Fisher, C.: Psychoanalytic implications of recent research on sleep and dreaming. J. Amer. Psychoanal. Assn., 13:197–270, 1965.

Freud, A.: The Ego and the Mechanisms of Defense. (Translated by C. M. Baines.) London, Hogarth Press, 1927.

Freud, S.: A General Introduction to Psychoanalysis. New York, Garden City Publishing Company, 1938.

Hollender, M. H.: Perfectionism. Compr. Psychiat., 6:94–103, 1965.

Klein, G.: Perceptions, Motives and Personality. New York, Alfred A. Knopf, 1970.

Lenneberg, E. H.: Biological Foundations of Language. New York, John Wiley & Sons, Inc., 1967.

Noy, P.: A revision of the psychoanalytic theory of the primary process. Int. J. Psychoanal., 50:155–178, 1969.

Piaget, J., and Inhilder, B.: The Psychology of the Child. New York, Basic Books, Inc., 1969.

Rapaport, D.: The Organization and Pathology of Thought. New York, Columbia University Press, 1951.

Rioch, D. M., and Weinstein, E. H. (eds.): Disorders of Communication. Baltimore, Williams & Wilkins Company, 1964.

Ross, N.: The "As If" Concept. J. Amer. Psychoanal. Assn., 15:59–82, 1967.

Ruesch, W.: Disturbed Communication. New York, W. W. Norton & Company, 1957.

Schechter, D. E.: Identification and individuation. J. Amer. Psychoanal. Assn., 16:48–80, 1968.

Scheflen, A. E.: The significance of posture in communications systems. Psychiatry, 27:316–331, 1964.

Vaillant, G. E.: Theoretical hierarchy of adaptive ego mechanisms. Arch. Gen. Psychiat., 24:107–118, 1971.

Chapter 6

Psychopathology

Psychopathology, the definition of abnormal personality functioning, has evolved from the recognition of easily discernible and gross disturbances of human behavior in terms of action, thought, and consciousness to an expanding awareness of the variations in the individual's total reaction pattern—his personality. The gross symptomatic expressions of disturbed behavior were known centuries ago; their occurence in more or less persistent and recognizable groupings led to the Kraepelinian elaboration of the various categories of psychotic behavior which still constitute the matrix for the syndromes now recognized in modern clinical diagnostic nomenclature. Further studies of abnormal behavior have established the various forms of the psychoneuroses, the mental deficiencies, and personality disorders of both adult and early life.

The so-called abnormal is but an exaggerated or unbalanced expression of the normal. It seems most fruitful to look upon most manifestations of psychopathology not as the result of expression of some "disease" but as a mode of behavior or of living which is the logical, although socially maladjusted, outcome of the particular individual's original endowment, of the molding influence of the home, of traumatic experiences which modified personality development, of the stresses and problems springing from within his emotional and instinctive life, of his inability to meet these strains, of the type of self-defensive reactions habitually utilized for minimizing anxiety, and of any bodily ailments which impair the integrity or efficiency of his biological organism. Mental disorders should, therefore, be regarded as patterns of human reaction set in motion by stress. The tendency to look on those who manifest nervous or mental symptoms as being different in their organization from the so-called normal is erroneous.

Just as mechanical objects if subjected to stress beyond the limits of their elasticity suffer distortion, so the personality if subjected to anxiety-producing stresses beyond the limits of its capacity for adaptation may suffer disorganization in both overt and symbolic behavior. Doubtless everyone, however healthy his adaptation appears to be, has particular psychological spheres which are vulnerable to stress. If his experiences touch these areas and the degree of their anxiety-producing nature exceeds his ability to deal with their stresses by healthy adaptive methods, he will be compelled to deal with them by neurotic or psychotic ones. Through repeated or cumulative stress, the individual's "normal" defenses no longer suffice and his adaptive capacity is exhausted. Stress alone, however, should not be considered the precipitating factor in mental disorder. It must be a particular stress for a particular person and, perhaps, at a particular time.

Criteria of Mental Illness

Definitions of mental health, or absence of illness, though more general are useful in assessing the presence and extent of illness. In addition they have made more precise a series of personality assets which define capacities for readaptation in the face of stress or recovery from illness. The World Health Organization speaks of health in broad terms as "the presence of physical and emotional well being." To the psychiatrist, the healthy adult shows behavior which confirms an awareness of self or personal identity coupled with a life purpose, a sense of personal autonomy, and willingness to perceive reality and cope with its vicissitudes. The healthy adult has a capacity to invest in others, to understand their needs, to achieve a mutually satisfying heterosexual relationship, to be active and productive with evidence of persistence and endurance in pursuing tasks to their accomplishment, to respond flexibly in the face of stress, to receive pleasure from a variety of sources, and to accept his limitations realistically.

In the field of mental health, as elsewhere, there are no fixed boundaries. Perhaps the criteria of mental illness are largely the degree to which behavior becomes undesirably substitutive and symbolic and the extent to which problems are dealt with in a neurotic manner rather than by rational decision. The presence of character fixations, with their limitations on self-actualization, the appearance of symptoms, the loss or impairment of preexisting functions, the recurrence of regressive behavior, and the distortion or impoverishment of affects provide the clinical evidence of illness.

Like more narrowly biological phenomena, such as fever, inflammation, and other morbid processes, mental disorders are defensive, protective, and reparative in purpose, but as they deal largely with the affective and psychosocial aspects of the organism, the adaptive ends they serve are those of personal situations. The symptomatology of the personality disorder represents either the individual's attempt to effect an adjustment to the interplay of psychological, social, and physiological forces impinging upon him or his failure in that effort. Again, the symptoms may represent an attempt to hide the truth from one's self, to retreat from difficult situations, to deal with anxiety, or to shut out the stresses of life. The result then is that one employs substitutive methods of adjustment that lead away from reality, which is sacrificed to attain emotional comfort, maintain self-respect, or provide satisfaction in the easiest way. The comforts and compensations, however, are highly egotistic and often do a disservice or are objectionable to the social group.

Abnormal Development

Although each person has his own particular characteristics which distinguish him from all others, certain general types of personality have been defined as disordered. For the most part the groupings are descriptive; a better understanding of the dynamics of personality development in each instance represents one of the areas in which study is greatly needed.

The task of the physician and psychiatrist in clinical practice is to define the psychopathology of the patient and then attempt to understand the genesis of the abnormality. As has been pointed out, the personality of the patient determines largely the manner in which he will respond to stress and thereby the specific definitions of the symptomatic expressions of his illness. In the study of the patient, the type of personality organization that the patient has acquired must be defined as well as the symptomatic psychopathology which he brings with him. This chapter therefore commences with a description of the commonly accepted types of personality disorder and then proceeds to decribe the recognized symptomatic expressions of psychopathology. The types of personality disorder are the cyclothymic, hypomanic, melancholic, schizoid, compulsive, hysterical, and passive-aggressive personality structures.

DISORDERS OF PERSONALITY

Cyclothymic Personality

Kahlbaum introduced the term *cyclothymia* to designate the predisposition of the individual to alternating moods of cheerfulness, vivacity, and mild depression; cyclothymia also indicates the tempo of the personality, i.e., whether it is lively or retarded. While oscillations are not uncommon, mood and tempo continue to harmonize and the different components of the personality in their reactions and expressions function as a unit. Kretschmer characterized as *cycloid* those people who are subject to cyclic variations of mood, tending to swing between exhilaration and depression, but not to pathological extremes. As might be expected, the cycloids or cyclothymes are predisposed to the development of manic-depressive or affective psychoses. Christopher Smart (1722-1771), the English poet who on at least one occasion developed what was undoubtedly a manic-depressive psychosis, said of himself, "I have a greater compass both of mirth and melancholy than another."

Polar variants of the cyclothymic are the hypomanic and melancholic personalities.

Hypomanic Personality

The hypomanics are outgoing, cheerful enjoyers of life. They are free from internal inhibitions, many being vivacious and sprightly and showing a sustained buoyant, confident, aggressive, optimistic, perhaps exhilarated reaction. They are usually energetic, gregarious, pleasure-loving, unstable, given to fleeting enthusiasms and easily swayed by new impressions. Some are blustering, domineering, argumentative, and hypercritical. Their judgment often appears superficial and they have a ready excuse for their failures. The hypomanic cannot subordinate himself, resents frustrations and disappointments, and is usually adept at talking himself out of difficulties. The hypomanic woman is often a chatterbox.

Melancholic Personality

Those cyclothymics at the melancholic pole are often kindly, quiet, sympathetic, good-tempered people, lacking in strained eccentricity but tending to be easily depressed. They feel but little of the normal joy of living and are inclined to be lonely and solemn, to be gloomy, submissive, pessimistic, and self-depreciatory. They are prone to express regrets and feelings of inadequacy and hopelessness. They are often meticulous, perfectionistic, overconscientious, preoccupied with work; they feel responsibility keenly, and are easily discouraged under new conditions. They are fearful of disapproval, tend to suffer in silence and perhaps to cry easily, although usually not in the presence of others. A tendency to hesitation, indecision, and caution betrays an inherent feeling of insecurity. A few are irritable and paranoid. Many psychiatrists feel that the melancholic temperament develops as a reaction formation against aggression.

Paranoid Personality

Suspicious, stubborn, secretive, obstinate, and resentful of discipline, the paranoid individual is lonely, insecure, unhappy, and brooding. When his wishes are not met he tends to become sullen, morose, irritable, or threatening. He is strikingly sensitive concerning the attitudes of others, usually exaggerates their behavior, and misinterprets it as directed by wishes to harm him. Lacking in a sense of humor, he is often perceived by others as sarcastic, derogatory, querulous, embittered, or resentful. When his points of view or actions are questioned, he responds with arguments and with aggressive and uncompromising positions. Moreover, he belittles and criticizes others. His interpersonal relations characteristically demonstrate a "chip on the shoulder."

His insecurity is often disguised by an intense drive for achievement which may impel him to strive for goals beyond his innate capacity.

While often highly efficient because of his striving, meticulousness, and precision —compulsive features—his interpersonal competence is impaired by his envy and

jealousy of others. In positions of authority his behavior is often tyrannical.

Schizoid Personality

The schizoid (Bleuler) or schizothymic
(Kretschmer) personality is marked by
incongruities of the feeling-life coupled,
characteristically, with a poorly socialized
personality. In the schizoid personality
the feeling-life lacks the resonance and
responsiveness that characterize the cyclothymic. Its contrasting affective poles are
sensitiveness on the one hand and dullness
or coldness on the other. The sensitive
schizoid feels lonely, imperfectly understood, and isolated. Timid, shy, self-
conscious, often self-dissatisfied, perhaps
stubborn, secretive, and suspicious, he is
wounded constantly.

In childhood, he is often teased by his
playmates who look upon him as "queer."
In school or college, he rarely takes part
in rough-and-tumble games but strives for
a sense of security through superiority in
school work. Silent and unsociable, his
love of books is often a substitute for
human companionship. He chooses subjects of an abstract, perhaps philosophical,
nature rather than those of a concrete,
objective type. He may be imaginative and
idealistic, perhaps with vague schemes for
bettering humanity. Many schizoids of this
group attempt art or poetry. Some are
successful in transmuting their daydreams
into cultural values.

Many of these sensitive persons suffer
from a sense of isolation. What their
thoughts may be is often unknown, even
to friends, since others are rarely admitted
into their confidence. Many have feelings
of inferiority and of discomfort in interpersonal relations and are aloof to the
opposite sex. In speaking of the sensitive
schizoids, Kretschmer comments that they
close the shutters of their houses in order
to lead a dream life. Many have a genuine
love of nature, while those who have had
cultural opportunities often show a rare
esthetic taste, gentle manners, and an
uncommon avoidance of the coarse or
vulgar.

Frequently, they are ambitious, conscientious, meticulous, and perfectionistic.
The overconscientiousness of the schizoid
tends, however, to exert a paralyzing effect
on initiative or variation, with the result
that he often performs his duties in a
stereotyped, almost ritualistic manner.
Some schizoids are overscrupulous, and by
making a virtue of their repression become
ascetics or prudes. To a certain number
of these frail, sensitive individuals, the
harsh realities and frustrating experiences
of life become too painful and they retreat
into a world of fantasy.

Many schizoids, while retaining an
imaginative attitude toward life and its
experiences, lack the finer sensibilities
just described. The most attractive members of this second group are kindly and
honest, but they are also emotionally dull,
taciturn, unsociable, and given to rites
and cults. Because of a lack of spontaneity, they appear to be indifferent, indolent, colorless persons. The less attractive
members are often cold, reserved, callous
individuals, frequently jealous of those
more happily adjusted. Some shrink un-
happily away into themselves and become
preoccupied with unwholesome ruminations. In adolescence they are usually
willful, disobedient, headstrong, moody,
passively stubborn, ill-tempered, easily
offended, and resentful of advice, supervision, or correction. Such a schizoid may
be described as a "lone wolf" who prefers
to get along without strong ties to other
people. Often his early relationships
within the family are disturbed and
unsatisfying.

The self-confidence which sometimes
characterizes these unfeeling, distrustful
individuals will be found to be of compensatory origin and to arise from a sense
of insecurity which, in turn, stimulates
defensive attitudes and reactions that
tend to increase and complicate the problems of adjustment. They have to show
the world how tough they are lest they
betray their shyness, diffidence, and sense
of insecurity.

The mistrustful schizoid who expects
and detects disapproval and insult may

feel safer to endure in silence with self-restraint and sullenness, retaliating, as it were, in daydreams, fancying how he may punish and destroy his alleged adversaries. In less marked types, the dearth of esthetic sensitiveness may be shown by a neglect of personal appearance, home, and family, or by a lack of tact and other evidences of social sensibilities and amenities. A rigid moral idealism expressed in inflexible rules of conduct and associated with a self-satisfied intolerance is not rare.

Actually but few schizoids belong to the purely sensitive or to the purely unfeeling type. In the majority of them we find characteristics from both groups. Often, to our surprise, we find a sensitive and tender nature hidden beneath a cold and unresponsive exterior. Similarly one must not conclude that the schizoid type always exists in pure form. Often it is not clearly differentiated from the cyclothymic type, in whom there is a sliding scale between the cyclothymic and the schizoid.

Bleuler preferred the term *syntonic* to Kretschmer's *cycloid* to describe a personality tendency opposed in characteristics to the schizoid. The syntonic person is in vital contact with his environment, is emotionally lively and responsive, and his affects are versatile in expression and appropriate to the occasion. Syntonic characteristics reach their greatest development in harmoniously adjusted persons, whereas schizoid elements reach their maximum development in the schizophrenic psychoses.

Obsessive-Compulsive Personality

Individuals of an obsessive or compulsive nature are those whose superego functions are severe. They tend to be punctilious, rigid, fastidious, formal, meticulous, may be in constant doubt what to do, and have to go over things again and again. They are overinhibited, perfectionistic, self-doubting, and are unable to carry on their work if under pressure. They lack a normal capacity for relaxation. They show a tendency to literal obedience, have an exaggerated sense of duty, are harrassed by their responsibilities and scrupulosities, and cannot make decisions. If circumstances require a decision, regret is expressed for the choice which is made. The person of compulsive character is stubborn in his convictions and manifests a tendency to hair-splitting. In contrast to the suggestible, demonstrative, extroverted personality of the hysteric, he is likely to be of a day-dreaming, introverted, self-centered type. The compliance and "correct" behavior of the compulsive personality are frequently a defense against hostile impulses.

If the individual is relatively free from anxiety, the existence in the personality of a certain degree of obsessive-compulsive drive and persistence adds a desirable quality. Compulsive personality traits are within the range of normal personality variants—as distinguished from symptoms of a compulsion neurosis, which are pathological exaggeration of these variants. Such traits impart a desire to succeed; the compulsive person, too, is a hard worker. A degree of compulsiveness adds to strength of character. The difference between a compulsive personality and a compulsive neurosis is therefore one of degree, of the amount of anxiety present and of the extent to which the personality habitually defends itself against chronic anxieties by ritualistic devices. Frequently the traits are safeguards against hostile impulses, unconscious aggression, and accompanying guilt. The chronic tension of the compulsive personality may as a result of stress lead to an obsessive-compulsive neurosis.

Hysterical Personality

More clearly defined for women than for men, this type of personality makeup is recognized by the traits of vanity, self-indulgence, and self-centered attitudes associated with histrionic behavior, dramatization, or exhibitionism. Affectively the hysterical personality is labile, emotionally capricious, and prone to emotional outbursts. Sexual behavior in women of this type is provocative and coquettish, with erotization of nonsexual relations. In actuality there often exists sexual fear with frigidity in women who have a pronounced masculine protest. The provocative attention-getting behavior appears to overlie a driving dependent need, demanding in quality. There is reason to consider that many women of this type have been spoiled and overprotected in earlier years.

Thus the hysterical woman is actively engaged in the social world yet responds to frustrations in reality badly. Possible attainment of the wish-fulfilling fantasies arouses excessive excitability. Her active fantasy life is filled with distortions of the environment into sensual and sexual preoccupations which exaggerate her excitement and lead to tension due to the inner inhibitions against this drive. Her self-presentation is that of the child-woman.

Such women are fearful of their sexual drives, yet seek through seductive behavior to achieve security and power vicariously through the passionate engagement of a man to themselves. Secretly they are competitive—against men as a means of conquering them and against women as a method of exclusion. Their seductive behavior to men then covers both an aggressive element and a wish for a dependent childish relationship. Often they complain of shyness yet appear highly competent in actual social life, as they are lively and engaging. They avoid and are uncomfortable with the exact and precise. At home with their families their behavior is frequently regressive and thought of as childish and helpless. Some women of this type have been brought up closely attached to the mother yet also stimulated and treated seductively by the father, who, as they approach adulthood, then condemns their budding sexuality.

Another group of women have essentially similar personality traits but expressed in more blatant forms, with the competitiveness and dependency needs insistent. These women demonstrate an exaggerated exhibitionism, sometimes coupled with lying and deceitful behavior or play-acting to attract attention or avoid shame. Here the affective responses may appear shallow or fraudulent. Their personal contacts, initially strong and idolatrous, usually dissipate, when their hopes are not fulfilled, into bitterness, isolation, and depression. These women with less well-structured personalities come from more inconsistent and disorganized families where there is often evidence of a greater degree of maternal deprivation due to illness or egocentricity. Evidences of emotional immaturity are seen early in life in such childish neurotic symptoms as enuresis, thumbsucking, and fetishism and a history of an early fantasy world peopled with imaginary companions to offset an actual isolation. They have seen themselves as isolated, alone, or different.

The "Don Juan" character represents this personality type in men. Again there is the histrionic display. The drive for sexual conquest and exhibitionism often rests upon a hidden feeling of masculine inadequacy and is coupled with the need to deceive, outwit, and conquer. The Don Juan makes evident through the repetition of his conquests the lack of satisfaction in each successful affair.

Passive-Aggressive Personality

The passive-aggressive personality is thought to result from failure to attain a mature emotional development of the personality manifested in one of three ways.

PASSIVE-DEPENDENT TYPE. In this type there is a frank expression of an absence of mature self-confidence and self-reliance. The individual is overwhelmed by feelings of helplessness and indecision. He is irresponsible and childish and may cling to others as a dependent child does to a supporting parent. He requires approval and assurance. The clinical picture may include anxiety manifestations. The passive-dependent husband may depend on his wife for all major decisions. Individuals of this type shun overt expression of aggression and withdraw from any situation likely to arouse hostility. They are passive, timid, and fearful. The underlying hostility, covered by a rigid shell of timidity and passivity, is entirely unconscious.

PASSIVE-AGGRESSIVE TYPE.   In this type the personality contains a considerable element of aggression, doubtless largely defensive in origin, expressed by passive measures, such as sullenness, stubbornness, procrastination, inefficiency, and passive obstructions. Some persons of this type complain and are dissatisfied. They usually work poorly with others and may have a demoralizing effect on a group. Some have been fearful of or have shown a covert hostility to their fathers, who have been dominant, rigid, unapproachable, demanding, and difficult to please.

AGGRESSIVE TYPE.   In this type, the outstanding manifestation is a persistent reaction to frustration with such immature measures as irritability, temper tantrums, and even destructive behavior. Sometimes there is resentment of pathological degree. Many persons of this type are hostile, provocative, antagonistic, competitive, and ambitious. They manifest a "chip-on-the-shoulder" attitude. They may be sharp and biting and aggressively resistant. They demand special attention and assume unwarranted authority. Frequently they attempt to lure those in authority into long argumentative discussion. Grandiose fantasies are common. Earlier in their lives these persons have been openly hostile to their fathers. A deep dependency can be discovered below the surface. The aggressiveness here originates in a reaction formation.

Explosive Personality

Individuals of this type of personality are characterized by the explosive intensity of their emotions in reaction to relatively slight external stimuli. Between their outbursts they are usually outgoing and friendly, happy, and likable. Their relationship to other persons, however, is constantly subject to fluctuating emotional attitudes because of strong and poorly controlled hostility, guilt, and anxiety. Their emotional tension is usually at a rather high pitch and may suddenly and unexpectedly burst out in uncontrolled anger or other disproportionate emotional display. At these times such persons may shout, bluster, threaten, or even become destructive and assaultive. In some, the excitability may be manifested in outbursts of despair, sulky irritability, or obstinate inaccessibility. Suicidal attempts in response to frustration or as an effort to relieve a situation regarded as intolerable are frequent. Jealousy and quarrels with those of the opposite sex are common. Far from being the desired evidence of vigor and strength of personality, the outbursts of the excitable are often poorly concealed attempts to disguise an inherent weakness. Such reactions, characterized by fluctuating emotional attitudes, unstable and explosive feelings, and undependable judgment, are to be regarded as expressions of an immaturity of personality and probably may not be distinguishable from the passive-aggressive personality type.

Inadequate Personality

In spite of average educational and other opportunities and of normal intelligence as measured by psychometric tests, individuals of inadequate personality type fail in emotional, economic, occupational, and social adjustments. They are often good-natured and easygoing but are inept, ineffective, and unconcerned. Their judgment is defective; they lack ambition and initiative and may be dreamy and seem to lack physical and emotional stamina. When it is clear that effort would be rewarded, they lack sufficient perseverance to achieve the results already in sight. They can neither work nor wait for deferred pleasure or reward. As a result, they are improvident and shiftless. Many of the ne'er-do-wells belong in this group.

Other Types

From certain clinical studies of patients with both organic brain syndromes and other psychotic processes, a "denial personality" reaction has been described. Those so classified have been persons who explicitly deny the presence of their illness or its symptoms, even if so grossly apparent as a limb paralysis caused by a brain lesion. They tend to be highly conventional in their behavior, perfectionistic, prestige-oriented, and limited in empathy as well as in introspective capacity. Their traits and their responses on the appropriate psychological tests are similar to the "authoritarian personality" identified by Adorno and his colleagues. Attempts have been made to suggest that those with this constellation of personality traits, when psychiatrically ill, respond more effectively to treatment with physiological therapies such as electroshock than to the psychotherapeutic approach. As yet, this conclusion remains unwarranted.

Important, too, for the clinical practice of psychiatry is the understanding of such personality traits as resignation, tranquillity, apathy, boredom, or gloating, traits that tend to defeat attempts to intervene therapeutically in spite of the existence of gross malfunctioning of the personality. The psychoanalytic literature contains what is known of the existing psychodynamic understandings of such traits. The bibliography of this chapter records the more recent references.

SYMPTOMS AS PSYCHOBIO-LOGICAL REACTIONS

Origin and Function of Symptoms

Symptoms are the results of many forces, some of them from without but more of them from within the patient. Symptoms, therefore, even though they may be bizarre and therefore baffling to our understanding, have a cause and meaning.

Some symptoms, such as impairment of memory in senile dementia, or confusion in a toxic state, are the results of physiological disturbances of neuron activity involved in the process of thinking. As such they represent a loss of function.

Neurotic symptoms, however, in contrast to those due to impairment or loss of physiological or biochemical dysfunction, are manifestations of psychological processes of which the patient is little aware. These symptoms represent defenses or substitutions to cope with some impairment of psychosocial functioning.

To discover the meaning of those unusual personality manifestations that are called symptoms and the functions they perform in the life history of the patient, one must ascertain the needs and meaningful factors or situations that led to their production. It should be remembered that the pathological psychiatric formations termed symptoms represent the patient's attempt, in the face of great difficulties, to maintain his existence in the best possible way. Symptoms, too, may be not only an expression of a mental illness but also an attempt by the patient to fight the illness. Regression, for example, with its withdrawal to an earlier developmental level, may be not only a symptom of mental illness but also an attempt to deal on that level with tasks consonant with his reduced ability.

The method of approach to an understanding of mental disorder is to correlate the symptoms with the current physical and emotional status of the patient, with his life history, and with forces which have played a part in molding his personality. The psychiatrist attempts to interpret symptoms not only in their relationship to past experiences but also in terms of the known dynamics of behavior.

DISORDERS OF MOTOR ASPECTS OF BEHAVIOR

While the isolation of any aspect of the mind is purely artificial, yet the disturbances to be considered here lie in the field which the psychologists designate as *conation,* action tendency, or impulse toward action. This includes an implication of affect and desire. Conversely, all affects have conative elements and impulses. Conation is the intention-set or striving aspect of the personality. It represents the purposive activity of the personality but lacks the degree of consciousness which has usually been associated with the idea of will or volition.

Attitude

Certain other terms dealing with the action sphere of the personality may be briefly mentioned. By attitude is meant a continuing set or predisposition to react in a characteristic feeling or manner. Attitudes are determined largely by one's feeling state and may be consciously or unconsciously acquired. They may become ingrained in the character structure of the personality and influence personality functioning. A bitter feeling, for example, may affect memory, judgment, and reasoning.

Disposition

By disposition is meant the sum of one's tendencies or inclinations as determined by the affective and conative components of the personality.

Assertion

Assertion may be defined as a deep-seated drive or pattern of the personality to react in a definitely forceful way. The term assertion carries a certain implication of will to overt action, in contrast to aggression, with its implication of hostility, as explained before.

DISTURBANCE OF ACTIVITY

Increased Activity

Disturbances of activity may conveniently be classified as overactivity (typically seen in mania), underactivity (depression), and dysactivity (schizoid and paranoic). An increase in pressure of occupation is known as increased *psychomotor* activity. Such activity is purposeful but no objective is attained, as the goal of the activity is constantly changing. The patient is very busy but his activities are not productive. A new activity is undertaken before there has been opportunity to complete the task already begun. This celerity is often shared by all conative aspects of the individual so that the stream of thought is characterized by a flight of ideas.

Decreased Activity

A distinct slowing up of conative expression occurs in decreased psychomotor activity or *psychomotor retardation*. Typically there is a prolonged delay before initiating the intended activity and, once begun, it is executed slowly and as if with painful effort. In extreme cases, the patient is mute and motionless and does not spontaneously undertake any activity. As in increased psychomotor activity, the other conative aspects of behavior may participate in the disturbance, with the result that a retardation of the stream of thought is often associated.

Repetitious Activities

In certain mental diseases, especially in the compulsive reactions and schizophrenia, it may be found that, when an activity has been initiated, there is a tendency to repeat it in the same manner for an indefinite period. This persistent and constant repetition of certain activities is known as *stereotypy* and may be of position, movement of body, or speech. A constantly maintained immobility of position is known as *catalepsy*. A cataleptic form of immobility frequently seen in schizophrenia and probably to be regarded as the expression of a high degree of suggestibility is *cerea flexibilitas,* or *waxy flexibility*. This is so called from the fact that the joints of the patient's extremities may be flexed or extended with a wax-like rigidity, continuing to retain the position imposed as do the limbs of a jointed doll. The extremities may thus be placed and maintained in an uncomfortable position for a much longer period than would be permitted by a normal person. Stereotyped movements, known as *mannerisms,* are common as well in schizophrenia. These may be in the form of grimaces, repeated gestures, peculiarities of gait, or numerous other types. Sometimes a complicated series of movements may be repeated and constitute a fairly definite ritual. The same rather meaningless word, phrase, or sentence may be repeated. Such a reiteration in which no coherent thought is expressed is known as *verbigeration.* Stereotypies have a definite psychological meaning, the symbolic significance in each case being peculiar to the individual and determined by his complexes or other affective experiences. After a time, their repetition may become a matter of habit, in which case the original affective value is largely lost.

Automatic Behavior

A phenomenological but not psychological counterpart of negativism is observed in *command automatism,* in which suggestions or requests from without are compulsively or automatically followed. Automatic obedience may also assume the form of repeating words or phrases uttered in the presence of the patient (*echolalia*), or it may be exhibited by the imitation of movements noted in others (*echopraxia*). Echolalia and echopraxia sometimes represent regressions to childish forms of "mocking" behavior or mimicry in which hostility and resentment are expressed under the guise of compliance. Mimicry is seen as one of the evolving sensorimotor activities in childhood, moving from simple imitation to take on significant meanings in terms of interpersonal relations.

Negativism

Negativism is a psychological defense reaction characterized by opposition and resistance to what is suggested. It may be manifested by behavior which is the opposite of what would ordinarily be called for in a given situation. It is frequently expressed in such forms as mutism, refusal of food, noncompliance with requests, and resistance to efforts to care for the patient. Psychodynamically the negativistic act provides gratification by the acting out of hostile, revengeful feelings toward significant persons—acts which the sufferer has learned are specifically anxiety provoking to the other and lead through the latter's evident concern to an expression of interest in the negativistic person.

Compulsions

A morbid and often an irresistible urge to perform an apparently unreasonable act repetitiously is known as a *compulsion.* The obligatory act may be of a simple nature, such as touching an object twice, or walking on cracks in the sidewalk, or it may be complex and constitute more or less of a ritual. A compulsion may be regarded as the result of an obsession —an obsession in action. Such acts are so closely linked with obsession that the combination is often referred to as the compulsive-obsessive syndrome. The acts are not meaningless, but, through the operation of the mechanisms of displacement, substitution, and symbolism, serve as defenses against anxiety. A common form of compulsion is hand-washing. Frequently the basic force behind this is guilt over masturbation, the repetitious act serving through the mechanisms of displacement and symbolism as an anxiety-relieving measure. Many people whom no one thinks of as suffering from mental disease have various obsessive-compulsive habits which serve as defense reactions for keeping anxiety, feelings of guilt, and unacceptable instinctual drives at a minimum. Among such habits of personality traits are tendencies to exaggerate the importance of carefulness and details and to stress cleanliness and orderliness. Various perfectionistic strivings and a rigid adherence to routine are obvious.

Violence

As discussed in previous chapters, aggressive behavior must be recognized in vertebrates as facilitative to species survival through its functions in protection from attack and in support of the ingestive and procreative drives. Violence as practiced by man—in wars, assassination, murder, assaults, rape, cruelty in mutilating others and the self, and suicide—is an expression of aggressivity unique to his species.

Such expressions of violence may be regarded as pathological when they are expressive of a deficit in development or an impairment of function of the superego. In some, deficiency in brain growth leading to mental retardation may determine inability to absorb the family and cultural values which lead to internalization of control of rage. In others severe emotional deprivation in early life owing to parental loss, neglect, or hatred may impair the process of identification and internalization of values necessary to constitute superego control and ego ideals. In still others parental discipline or that provided in schools or other institutions may be so brutal and hateful as to establish identification with the aggressor, thus allowing acting out of similar violence to others later in life. In the instance of some emotionally deprived children thirsting for support, frustration leads to reaction formations with denial of internalized social values. Such children—and adolescents and adults—reared to produce these formations may evolve a repertoire of shrewd and devious expressions of cruelty and destructiveness as a means of revenge and testing of others. Still others, raised in seemingly healthy and socially conscious and law-abiding families, express violent or destructive behavior in a narrowly defined form owing to superego lacunae derived from some subtle expression of condoning behavior of parents or other persons in authority.

Socially sanctioned violent or destructive acts ordered and allowed by public authority in wartime may not be considered as psychopathologic. Nor should violent acts aroused in protection of self in the political interactions of various groups be so construed. Regarding both these categories of violent actions, certain individuals predisposed to violence through impairment of superego formations often indulge their individual psychopathology in overdetermined ways during wartime or in revolutionary periods.

Persistent and continued expressions of cruel, destructive, or other violent behavior on the part of an individual require a social accomplice. Sado-masochistic matches between individuals are common.

Among adults impairment of superego control with impulsive acting out of violence in murder or assault is commonly associated with impairment of brain function by poisons or other damage. Thus murder and assault are more frequently committed by the alcoholic than by others. The hallucinogens also act to impair brain function and related superego control. Brain damage from any cause may so act as to predispose to lack of impulse control when the individual is aroused to rage. Psychiatrists have found that perpetrators of unmotivated murders (those without preconceived planning) are more likely to show electroencephalographic evidence of brain damage than are the perpetrators of premeditated murders. In the instance of mass murders, there usually exists a paranoid personality development in which increasing frustration leads suddenly to revengeful acting out against a humanity conceived of as unsympathetic. The act is demonstrative, too, of the megalomaniac wish fulfillment of the murderer.

Studies in the past of patients hospitalized for psychiatric illness have shown that those discharged are less likely to be detained for criminal action, including violence, than the population at large.

Suicide

For practicing psychiatrists, self-directed acts of violence constitute a major challenge in prevention and treatment.

Suicide, suicidal attempts, and suicidal ideation are generally considered evidence of psychopathology, although this is not necessarily so. Transient thoughts of death and dying are universal, and thoughts of self-destruction are frequent. Obsessive preoccupation with suicidal ruminations, however, is pathological.

Although suicide has many precipitating events and motivating forces, all persons with suicidal ideation have an intense underlying sense of deprivation of affection and love, a deep sense of personal rejection. The suicidal attempt is motivated by the wish for revenge, by hopelessness, or by wish-fulfilling fantasies of reunion. Perhaps the most commonly recognized motive is the wish to instill guilt in the significant person who is perceived as abandoning; in this case, suicide is a means of control and revenge. Similar motives exist in those groups of patients who indulge in repeated acts of wrist-cutting or *self-mutilation*—often carried out with a seeming delicacy. Overwhelmed by an acute sense of despairing loneliness following an actual or fantasied abandonment, the patient impulsively acts out his revenge, often in a fugue-like condition, upon his body as an object entirely owned. Stengel has emphasized that those who make unsuccessful suicidal attempts and those who threaten suicide manage to give warning of their distress in such a way as to prevent success and also to influence favorably their important interpersonal relation.

Fantasies precede suicidal acts. Fantasies of identification and reunion in death with a loved person are frequently the motive for the "anniversary" suicide—an attempt that takes place on the anniversary of death of the wished-for person. Sometimes there is a regressive wish for reunion ·with the mother, a wish to live once more in an ideal state of passivity and infantile gratification. Another fantasy is of rebirth, of recommencing life in a more satisfying manner. This fantasy is said to be usual in periods of recovery following depressions or acute schizophrenic episodes. With splitting of the self-image into "good" or "bad" parts, the wish to destroy the maligned part of the self may, in periods of great tension, lead to an impulsive attempt at its elimination. This fantasy often precedes self-mutilative acts as well, particularly in the schizophrenic, who sometimes makes horrifying efforts to remove an organ or body part conceived of as the source of evil. Finally there are the fantasies of escape into death from the hopelessness arising in the course of psychotic or other illness or even from the stringencies of living. There remain some presumed suicidal attempts, particularly in patients with delirium, that represent a desperate effort to escape fearfully imminent illusory or hallucinatory threats.

Suicidal threats are pervasive in society as a means of interpersonal domination and control. They are used to induce both heterosexual and homosexual love relationships, including marriage, to prevent dissolution of such relations, to force parental acquiescence to the desires of children or vice versa, to obtain favored treatment, and to avoid certain varieties of required service (such as military service) to friends and country.

Unsuccessful suicidal attempts are estimated to occur from five to fifty times as frequently as successful suicides. The suicide rate varies between countries and cultures and is inversely proportionate to the homicide rate.

Suicide is significantly more frequent in discharged mental hospital patients in the *six* months immediately following their release. In Japan and Austria the annual rate of successful suicides equals approximately 23 per 100,000. The United States rate of around 10 per 100,000 ranks in the middle of the listing of countries; suicide is the tenth leading cause of death in this country. In urban suicides, the majority suffer affective psychosis or are alcoholic.

Suicide is rare in the very young; it occurs with increasing frequency as adolescence advances. Among adolescents in the United States it constitutes the second largest cause of death. It is more frequent among the aged, in men, and among the single, isolated, divorced, and widowed. At least a third of those who have attempted suicide unsuccessfully are without psychopathology, but the vast majority of this group give evidence of recent serious socio-economic distress.

It would appear that in the United States less than one third of those who successfully commit suicide have been seen by a psychiatrist, and perhaps not more than half have consulted a physician.

For the psychiatrist, the significant judgment has to do with the recognition that there is a high risk of suicide attempts in those patients who admit to suicidal ruminations. A history of successful suicide in other family members has been found to be statistically related to successful suicide. Clinical experience indicates that suicidal attempts are more common in patients who have been brought up in families in which they were coerced by suicidal threats or made to feel guilty by their parents by being told they were responsible for impending death. It may be surmised that such family transactions lead to impairment of superego development which allows the acting out of suicidal impulses. In psychotherapy such patients may be expected to threaten the psychiatrist. On the other hand, it has been found that the risk of successful suicide is low in those who have made a previous attempt.

Most of those who commit suicide suffer as well from self-derogatory attitudes, profound feelings of hopelessness and helplessness, and a sense of rejection prior to the act. Suicide and suicidal attempts are unrelated to particular forms of psychopathology, although they are most frequent among those with depressive reactions.

DISORDERS OF PERCEPTION

Illusions

It will be remembered that the various end-organs or receptors are so constructed as to analyze the environmental energy and select certain kinds which are transformed in the receptor and give rise to a nervous impulse. On arrival in the appropriate area in the brain, this impulse produces a visual, auditory, or other sensory image, the interpretation and meaning of which will depend upon one's previous experiences and interpretations.

One of the ways in which the mental life of the individual may express emotional or striving elements that touch it with particular significance is through a perceptual misinterpretation of such sensory images. The elements which are particularly likely to lead to misinterpretations of these images are intense affective states, ardent wishes, or urgent drives and impulses. Repressed elements are especially apt to be highly dynamic and produce misinterpretations that reflect some affect or express some wish or drive. A patient with a deep feeling of guilt, for example, may interpret the rustling of leaves as reproaching voices. Such a perceptual misinterpretation is known as an *illusion*.

The illusion has the same psychological function as a hallucination, but less reality distortion is involved. The nature of illusions is especially likely to be determined by the prevailing trend of the patient's emotional state and needs. Strained expectation or fear predisposes to illusional interpretations. In mental health, but particularly in mental disorder, the emotional life imbues and tends to influence perceptual experience according to the needs of the personality. In confused toxic states, caused either by ingested poisons or by infection, perceptions may be misinterpreted because the sensory stimuli and impressions are not properly transmitted and integrated in the brain. Such illusions usually possess less psychological significance than do those occurring in fully clear consciousness.

Hallucinations

In an illusion, an image symbol of a real object is formed, but for psychological reasons it is misinterpreted. Hallucinations are generally regarded arbitrarily as perceptions which occur when there is no impulse created by the stimulation of a receptor. Whether the absence of sensory receptor activity actually occurs remains undetermined, since the casual observer has no means of verifying this assumption. The word *hallucination* was introduced by Esquirol (1772–1840), a pupil of Philippe Pinel (1745–1826). He defined it in accordance with its present meaning as a perception without object and clearly differentiated it from illusion.

Although lacking a basis of reality in the sense that the percept is not aroused by a current stimulus in the periphery, hallucinations constitute an actual part of the patient's mental life. They should be looked upon as mental products which, arising from within and therefore not related to any external stimulus, possess an idiosyncratic certainty which, however, may not attain the vividness that is usually associated with impressions derived from the external world.

The content of the hallucinations usually suggests their dynamic significance. They represent a breakthrough of preconscious or unconscious material into consciousness in the form of sensory images in response to psychological situations and needs. Anxiety often plays an important part in their genesis. These hallucinated images which the patient accepts as reality represent the projection onto the outer world of such psychological needs and situations as wishfulfillment, enhancement of self-esteem, criticism, censure, a sense of guilt, self-punishment, the satisfaction of repressed and rejected impulses, or the desire for a more satisfying reality. The dreams of normal persons are prototypes of the mental patient's hallucinations. Sometimes in case of internal conflict there is hallucinatory expression of the internal debate; some of the hallucinations express approbation or commendation, while others express insults and antagonism. It will be seen, therefore, that *hallucinations are never symptomatic of a given morbid condition.*

The way in which escape from a harsh and unsatisfying reality may be secured through hallucinatory perceptual experiences is illustrated in the actions of a woman whose natural biological tendencies had been frustrated and who, because of personality inadequacies, had found economic and social adjustments too great a burden. One day as she was sitting on the bank of the Potomac River, preoccupied with her problems and dreaming of some means of satisfactory escape from them, she heard the voice of a former lover who had ceased his attentions as her personality limitations had become more apparent. In this thwarted and distressing state of affairs, she received from the old admirer a message pointing the way to an enchanting fulfillment of her fondest hopes. Although she could not see him, the patient heard the lover direct her to jump into the water, from which he promised to rescue her and row her to Norfolk, whence they would sail to Egypt, there to occupy a beautiful castle. So convinced by the vividness of the message that reality was ignored, the woman threw herself into the water, where she would have perished except for some chance passers. A correct appreciation of her experience would have been too painful and disillusioning, and so she continued to believe in the reality of these autogenous perceptions.

In the mentally healthy person the majority of perceptions produced by casual stimuli from the environment are ignored. The content of perceptions in hallucinations is so intimately subjective that in their acute phases, at least, they cannot be ignored and therefore not only absorb the attention but require that reality be made to harmonize with them. As a result, the functional capacity of the ego for testing any reality that does not harmonize with the hallucinations is usually suspended.

In so-called anticipatory illusions and hallucinations, a person in a tense emotional state, say of fear, intently expects to see or hear the object which has excited the emotion. The result is that the perception momentarily expected in vivid clearness appears, but in a projected, hallucinatory, or illusional form.

Sometimes various gradations between normal representation and hallucinations may occur, with the result that the patient is uncertain whether his mental experience has been of a perceptual (unreal) nature or whether it has been merely a thought.

Hallucinations may occur in diseases associated with toxic or organic states. Although in these cases there is perhaps an irritation of the association centers connected with the special sense hallucinated, the nature of the material hallucinated is doubtless influenced by the psychological experiences of the patient.

Psychological material may be projected in the image symbols of any of the senses, although the images are characteristically of that sense best fitted to symbolize the particular material seeking expression. Feelings of guilt, for example, may best be expressed in spoken language, and so the patient hears accusing voices. Such accusing voices represent the projection of the critical voice of the super-ego. Fear of some aspect of the personality may well be symbolized by the sight of terrifying objects, and so the patient sees frightful animals. One patient with an experience which he looked upon as one of moral contamination complained of a constant odor of carbolic acid. To him this chemical had always represented a purifying agent, and its hallucination was well adapted to symbolize his desire for a feeling of moral purification.

Hallucinations are more marked during the early and acute stages of a psychotic reaction. This is to be expected, since it is the period when repression is failing and the solution of the conflict is proving unsuccessful. Hallucinations with clearness of consciousness are of much more serious prognostic import than those occurring with clouding of consciousness. Hallucinations occur less frequently when the patient is occupied with reality than when attention slackens or he begins to daydream. They are often associated with delusions, to which they add support or corroboration. At times, they seem to be the concrete symbolic expression of delusional ideas.

The occurrence of hallucinatory experience is not synonymous with that of mental disorder. *Hypnagogic hallucinations* take place in healthy persons in that period between sleeping and waking. Hallucinations and illusions may be induced in the healthy in periods of prolonged isolation or under the influence of certain pharmacologic agents such as mescaline or *d*-lysergic acid diethylamide-25. Hallucinations induced by such agents are seldom formed, are usually lacking in ideational content, and are experienced as outside or beyond the self of the subject. In these respects they differ from the usual hallucinations of the psychotic person, who fails to distinguish his experience from reality and as beyond himself. Otherwise these experiences are *ego dystonic*. Again they occasionally occur as transient phenomena and in a benign sense in familiar situations in which the perceiver is experiencing a special need for foods, fluids, or some other unrequited physiological need.

HALLUCINATIONS OF HEARING. As already indicated, hallucinations of hearing are the most frequent form of perceptual disturbance. Sometimes the hallucinations are in the form of various noises, but most often they consist of words arranged in more or less complete sentences. Usually these sentences are remarks concerning the patient or addressed to him. The patient may converse or quarrel with the "voices." He may locate them as coming from any part of his body or from a distance. Sometimes the remarks are of a pleasant nature but usually they are unpleasant, derogatory, obscene, or in the nature of accusations. These unpleasant remarks represent the projection of disowned personality aspects or desires which may not be allowed into the consciousness in undisguised form. Hallucinations conveying a command are often convincing and compelling. They may therefore lead to direct and dangerous action. Considerations of reality are of little weight in comparison to their influence.

Auditory hallucinatory experiences often are associated with movement of the laryngeal musculature, suggesting that the patient is uttering subvocally the words which he perceives in his hallucination just as a child does as he learns to read silently.

HALLUCINATIONS OF SIGHT. These are not rare but are much less frequent than auditory hallucinations. They occur most typically in the deliria of acute infectious diseases or of toxic psychoses. In each of these states the visual hallucinations are apt to be accompanied by some clouding of consciousness. In general, visual hallucinations are confined to acute, reversible organic brain disorders. Visual hallucinations more frequently excite fear in the patient than do auditory ones, since they produce a greater distortion of reality. One of the most frequent mental disorders accompanied by visual images is delirium tremens, in which the images tend to be terrifying.

Most commonly, unformed visual hallucinations occur with disease of the occipital cortex, while formed hallucinations, sometimes consisting of complex scenes, result from disease of the temporoparietal cortex. Recently it has been suggested that formed visual hallucinations are more often associated with excitation or lesions of the dominant hemisphere. There are exceptions to these general observations; for example, various drugs may produce either type. Visual hallucinatory experiences have been induced not only by such agents as mescaline but also by amphetamine, atropine, and similar agents used in the treatment of parkinsonism.

HALLUCINATIONS OF OLFACTION. Hallucinations of smell are not uncommon in schizophrenic states and with lesions of the temporal lobe. Olfactory hallucinations are usually of an unpleasant or even of a strongly objectionable character.

Their repulsive nature is not surprising, since they are particularly apt to represent feelings of guilt.

HALLUCINATIONS OF TASTE. True gustatory hallucinations are uncommon but at times are associated with hallucinations of smell. Illusions of taste are much more frequent.

TACTILE HALLUCINATIONS. Hallucinations of touch occur principally in toxic states, such as delirium tremens, and in cocaine addiction. Hallucinated sexual sensations are observed in schizophrenia and are often associated with grotesque delusions concerning bodily organs.

KINESTHETIC HALLUCINATIONS. The *phantom phenomenon,* that is, the hallucinatory perception of an amputated limb or of a limb denervated peripherally or through spinal cord transection, represents the most common form of kinesthetic hallucinatory experience. Such phantoms may change shape or size, or they may move. Distortions of the body image most frequently noted in schizophrenia or toxic states, particularly those induced by such drugs as mescaline, psilocybin, or *d*-LSD-25, also largely fall into this category of hallucinatory experience.

DISORDERS OF THINKING

The joining of ideas one to another by imagining, conceiving, inferring, and other processes, and the formation of new ideas by these processes, constitute a function we know as thinking. This may be looked upon as a form of internal or implicit behavior. Thought is the most highly organized of psychobiological integrations. In considering this function from the standpoint of psychiatry, attention should be directed to the production of thought, the progression of thought, and the content of thought. It should be remembered, too, that thought takes place on several levels, ranging from the fully conscious, dealing perhaps with highly abstract topics, to that on a primitive, emotional level.

DISORDERS IN FORM OF THOUGHT

As just indicated, thinking is a form of behavior which implies the existence of stimulus and response, the latter serving some psychologic purpose. In mental health, the stimuli for thought come from various sources, including unconscious and affective ones, but thinking is corrected by reason and logic. Such thought is known as rational or realistic. It appears to be directed by, and to take place in, conscious awareness. In daydreaming, thinking is guided not only by realistic considerations but to a considerable extent by egocentric wishes and instinctual needs. In mental disorder, and particularly in schizophrenia, thinking may be directed even more by unconscious factors and become of the type first designated by Bleuler as *autistic* and later as *dereistic*. In dereistic thinking (in contrast to realistic thinking), complexes, drives, and other affective and conative motivations are given free rein and operate without conscious regard for reality. As a result, associations of ideas are no longer logical.

DISORDERS IN PROGRESSION OF THOUGHT

The rate and manner of associative activity cannot, of course, be learned except through the patient's stream of talk. It is a familiar observation that, as one's thoughts are expressed in language, there is a pertinent association or linkage of each idea with the one that has preceded —that one's thinking moves in a logical progression toward a more or less definite end. This progression of thought is often known as the "stream of thought" or "stream of talk." Normally, there is a logical and coherent sequence of related ideas passing uninterruptedly and without digression from an initial idea to a goal idea.

Flight of Ideas

In certain mental disorders, there occurs a disturbance in the progression of thought characterized by an increased associative activity, a rapid digression from one idea to another. Ideas follow in quick succession but do not progress toward the goal idea, which is therefore never reached. This disturbance of the stream of thought in which the thinking processes appear to run too quickly and in which no idea is completed is known as *flight of ideas.* Flight of ideas is associated with an accelerated inner drive and distractability, as a result of which the patient is unable to sustain his attention and direct it toward a goal idea. Observation will usually disclose an associated relation between the thought and a prompting stimulus springing from either an external or an internal source. Frequently a word similar in sound, but not at all so in significance, calls up the new thought. This is known as *clang association* and may lead to a senseless rhyme.

One patient with a rapid flow of thought, when asked if he were sad, replied, "Yes, you have to be quiet to be sad. Everything having to do with 's' is quiet—on the q.t.—sit, sob, sigh, sin, sorrow, surcease, sought, sand, sweet mother's love, and salvation. This is my first case—I am kind of a bum lawyer or liar—too damned honest to be a lawyer, so had to be a liar."

Retardation

As already seen, the flow of thought in flight of ideas is abnormally rapid. In retardation, on the other hand, the initiation and movement of thought are slow. Often the patient will state that his thoughts come slowly or that he has difficulty in thinking. It will be noted that he speaks slowly and usually in a low tone. Retardation is most frequently observed in the depressive phases of the affective psychoses but may be noted in schizophrenia.

Perseveration

By perseveration is meant an abnormally persistent repetition or continuance in expression of an idea. This clinging to a thought may be observed at times in aphasia, catatonia, and in those with senile dementia.

Circumstantiality

Another disturbance in the flow of thought is that known as circumstantiality. In this disturbance, the patient finally reaches his ideational objective, but only after many unnecessary and trivial details have led him into tiresome digressions. Circumstantiality occurs largely among persons who do not form sharply defined concepts or are unable to distinguish essentials from nonessentials. In mental disorder, therefore, it is frequently observed among the feeble-minded, epileptics, and cases of moderately advanced senile mental disorder.

Incoherence

Sometimes the progression of thinking is so disorderly that one idea runs into another without logical consecution, and speech is not bound by any law. The result is a disorganization of syntactical structure with a lapse into disjointed phrases or even into parts of sentences and it is known as incoherence.

One schizophrenic patient, when asked how long she had been in the hospital, answered, "Oh, three weeks—since different statements are made—because it is hot—Mr. Smith is a cheap guy—French —how goes about it?"

In incoherence there is a tendency for ideas to arise from a confusion of complexes, viz., repressed material highly charged affectively. As might be expected, incoherence occurs particularly in schizophrenia, a disease in which the thinking is characteristically dominated by complexes. Much of the thinking of the schizo-phrenic is described as scattered, which simply means that the thinking is a little less disorderly than in incoherence.

Blocking

Another disturbance in the flow of thought is that known as blocking. In this disorder, sometimes known as thought deprivation or thought obstruction, both expression and progression of thought suddenly cease. To a degree it may be considered as having a prototype in the sudden inhibition of the train of thought sometimes occurring when one is overcome by some strong affect, such as anger or terror. After a time, the apparent obstruction seems to be removed, and the flow of thought is resumed. This interruption of the progression of thought is probably caused by the activity of a dominant complex with its associated unpleasant affect. At first the blocking may be caused by some definite thought, or rather by the disagreeable affect attached to it, but it quickly becomes general so that nothing more is initiated. Blocking to a severe degree seems to be confined to schizophrenia.

DISORDERS OF CONTENT OF THOUGHT

Trends and Overdetermined Ideas

There is a tendency for the associative evolution of ideas, and therefore for thought content, to be determined more by affective factors than by logical reasoning. Ideas having the strongest feeling tones tend to dominate. It is because of this fact that thought content may exhibit a trend, viz., a propensity to center around a special topic. When an idea comes to have an extreme feeling-tone connected with it, it is spoken of as an *overdetermined* or *overvalued idea*.

The importance or value and the meaning attached to an idea are directly proportional to the inner need for such a belief. When an overvalued idea exists, it blinds the individual to all else so that only those observations and memories are selected which suit its purpose or confirm it. Anything which conflicts with it is denied admission into consciousness.

The whole personality, including its thinking and feeling aspects, is absorbed by the idea and placed at its disposal, so to speak, with the result that the overvalued idea becomes one of the most important determinants of behavior. Trends and overdetermined ideas, like delusions, to be discussed later, serve to satisfy some pressing inner need of the personality, such as a sense of security, defense, or self-esteem.

Delusions

Everyone is prone to develop comforting and other psychologically useful fictions to afford support and security to the personality. Apparently, mankind has always developed or adopted elaborate beliefs in an effort to satisfy inner needs. The construction of reassuring delusive beliefs as protection against anxiety and insecurity has been universally characteristic. This has been the unrecognized purpose in our fairy tales, in the folk stories of powerful persons, and in our father-image myths, beliefs, and creeds.

Sometimes the demand for the satisfaction of special inner needs of the personality may be so insistent that the claims of reality are disregarded and delusional ideas appear. Actuality is transformed to make it compatible with the emotional needs of the personality. The delusion is usually defined as a false belief. As we consider delusions and their meaning, value, and purpose, we shall see, however, that such a definition is fallaciously inadequate. It is often said that to be considered delusional, a false belief must be one that a person of similar education and experience would consider improbable or impossible and is not corrected in response to reason or logic. Even this definition is inadequate, since it ignores any

consideration of the important principle that the incorrect understanding and use of facts and evidence are in response to definite purposes and needs of the personality and that the prevailing factors which control delusional thinking are affective rather than ideative or cognitive.

How inner needs may produce misinterpretations, denial, and misuse of facts in a way to be considered delusional is illustrated in the following case report:

During World War I, a woman was notified by the War Department that her husband had been killed on a certain date and buried at a certain place in France. Several months later, she visited the Department and expressed the conviction that her husband was alive and that the body of her supposed husband was actually that of no person known to her. The military authorities presented evidence that no error had been made, but the widow remained unconvinced and demanded that the body of her alleged husband be returned to America and examined. This was done and the identification number and the location of wounds were found to correspond to the records of the War Department. Still the woman remained unconvinced. Finally the reason for the delusion appeared. Among the officer's papers collected after his death and forwarded to the widow were affectionate letters from another woman. The patient had protected herself from the painful realization that she was not first in the affections of her husband by developing the belief that the man who had been killed and whose papers had been forwarded to her was someone other than her husband.

We thus see that situations containing highly affective factors are accompanied by a lowering of the critical faculty and of the threshold of beliefs. Attempts through factual disproof to convince the patient that his beliefs are delusional are therefore rarely successful. The patient's experiences are assimilated and the picture of the external world supplied by his thinking is falsified according to his nonadjusted affective and instinctive demands. He acts as if his delusional system constituted reality—as to him it does.

As already indicated, the thinking which we characterize as delusional is quite similar in kind, although different in degree, to that in which we all indulge. Our beliefs tend to be subjectively colored, and doubtless all of us resort to certain fictions of security. Employment of wishful thinking by "normal" persons in their struggle for a realization of their hopes, and of rationalization or projection for defensive purposes, serves the same psychological ends as do the delusions of the psychotic and imperceptibly merges into them. Prejudices, likewise, often arise from intrapsychic conflict and serve as defensive measures.

From what has been said, it will be seen that delusions are attempts to deal with the special problems and stresses of one's particular life situation in which fantasy is called upon to supply what real life has denied. They differ from the beliefs of the healthy, however, in their irrational fixity, even in the face of what would be considered incontrovertible evidence to the contrary. As Macfie Campbell expressed it, "The fantasies are not woven into a structure which is compatible with a normal social adaptation."

Delusions, therefore, require an individual approach. Their trend is determined by the personality problems and needs of the patient before he became psychotic; the content will be found to reveal significant aspects of the patient's personal problems. The sources of these problems may often be found in thwarted trends and drives, frustrated hopes, feelings of inferiority, biological inadequacies, rejected qualities, teasing desires, gnawing feelings of guilt, and other situations which require a defense against anxiety. A deep-seated need for consolation, for example, may be met by self-flattering delusions.

Often the problem-solving value of the delusion and its relation to the situation by which it was produced are psychologically plain. Many times, however, the function of the delusion is far from obvious and its interpretation must remain a matter of speculation. This does not mean that the delusion is without significance or purpose. It possesses a definite adjustment value, but its source and purpose are concealed by its symbolically disguised content. When this central theme is extensively developed and conclusions are so logically deduced from the premises assumed that a coherent and connected organization of ideas is established, the patient's delusions are said to be *systematized*.

Since the psychological purposes and needs by which delusions are created fall into certain general classifications, and since well-defined mental mechanisms are employed in their creation, delusions may be classified according to certain types.

DELUSIONS OF GRANDEUR. Expansive delusions or delusions of grandeur arise from feelings of inadequacy, insecurity, or inferiority, any conscious recognition of which is prevented by the exaggerated ideative and affective components of the delusion. The content of grandiose delusions frequently suggests the nature of previous frustrations or insecurities. The patient who insists that he is God has, by the aid of his delusion, escaped from the troubles of reality which are too great a threat to his emotional security. If his distress was one of guilt, he has achieved perfection; if it was one of intolerable inferiority, he has achieved distinction; if it was one of fear, he has gained security and safety. The symbolic meaning of grandiose delusions is not greatly complicated and is fairly easily analyzed.

DELUSIONS OF SELF-ACCUSATION. Delusions of self-accusation are believed to arise because the repression of unacceptable trends and desires weakens and the superego becomes increasingly critical. In such a case, repression is not destroyed, but the threat, as it were, that consciously forbidden tendencies might be permitted expression creates in the patient a vague feeling of guilt. This sense of guilt is then rationalized in consciousness into ideas of remorse and self-accusation. Feelings of guilt may be appeased through self-punishment.

DELUSIONS OF PERSECUTION. Ideas of persecution are among the most frequent forms of delusions, occurring especially in chronic psychotic disorders. The threat of unworthy desires and of troublesome and disowned aspects of the personality is projected as hostility from the environment. Sensitive dissatisfactions with self, arising from unadjusted elements in the personality, may be projected as a dissatisfaction, and therefore as hostility, felt toward one by others.

The formation of delusions of persecution is facilitated by the mechanism of projection which easily leads to misjudgments of reality. The hostile and aggressive motives which the patient attributes to others reflect his own inclinations. High aspirations without qualities necessary for satisfying success accompanied by an inability to accept defeat may lead to brooding, distrust, suspicion, misinterpretations, resentment, and ideas of persecution, coupled perhaps with aggressiveness. Delusions of persecution permit a shifting of responsibility and otherwise serve to relieve anxiety arising from guilt.

As a further measure for averting blows to self-esteem, the patient with ideas of persecution may develop compensatory reactions in the form of an exaggerated self-assurance. It will often be found that persons who develop delusions of persecution have, since childhood, been critical, resentful, suspicious, and unhappy. Not a few of them have been lonely, brooding, and insecure, and have lacked friends with whom they could share confidences. Ready to criticize others, they have been unable to tolerate criticism themselves.

It is not uncommon to find delusions of grandeur and of persecution associated. This is not surprising, since they serve much the same purpose, one tending to supplement the other. By his delusions of grandeur, the patient psychopathologically enhances his self-esteem and magnifies his ego. In the delusions of persecution, he repudiates and rejects those aspects and tendencies which self-respect would disavow by attaching them to others. The two types collaborate to relieve anxiety.

IDEAS OF REFERENCE. Through ideas of reference, remarks or actions on the part of other persons, although in no way referring to the patient, are interpreted by him as being significantly related to himself and often as expressing accusation or depreciation. In paranoid states, ideas of reference represent a projection of the patient's own self-criticism onto the external world. In depression, feelings of guilt may stimulate ideas of reference, and these, in turn, contribute to loosely organized paranoid delusions.

DELUSIONS OF SIN, GUILT, IMPOVERISHMENT, AND ILLNESS. In depression, delusions frequently represent the ideational expression of rationalization of an affective depression. If repression weakens, material, such as wishes, memories, or ideas, which is of such a nature that it would cause emotional pain if admitted to consciousness is apt to give rise to depression. Depressive delusions often represent the rationalization of a sense of depression that has had its source in unconscious hostile tendencies felt toward persons against whom such feelings and tendencies should not be directed.

Depressive delusions are most frequently expressed in ideas concerning guilt, disease, or poverty. Ideas of guilt and of loss of self-esteem may arise when the repression of unconsciously desired, but consciously repudiated, tendencies is weakened. The patient, in his attempt to rationalize the vague feelings of wickedness rising into consciousness, formulates ideas of self-accusation based on criticisms by the superego. Unconscious hostile tendencies may be projected outward, giving rise to fear of punishment. Any psychological factor which makes the patient feel that he stands out in an undesirable or unacceptable way from the rest of his social group may lead to *delusions of guilt* and therefore of depression.

Ideas of disease have similar meanings. The illness represents punishment for unacceptable and hostile drives to another; they may originate in identifications with the hated person.

Ideas of poverty are often the ideational representation of subjective sense of loss of social value. Such ideas of poverty may accompany delusions of guilt, the idea of unworthiness being displaced to the most generally recognized symbol of value—money. Appearing at times with depressive delusions are *nihilistic ideas* expressing the patient's belief that he has no brain, that he has no feeling, that he is dead, or that other sections of reality no longer exist. Such nihilistic ideas probably have their origin in vague feelings of emotional change and in a subjective feeling of unreality and of changed personality. This subjective sense of absence and of change is rationalized into ideas of annihilation.

In *passivity feelings* or *ideas of control,* the patient may express the delusional belief that he is controlled or that people read his mind. Such feelings probably represent the denial of an impulse to yield to threatening internal needs or demands which, however, are disowned through the mechanism of projection.

Hypochondria

Although containing important affective elements of a depressive nature, the symptom hypochondria, with its exaggerated concern over physical health, may perhaps best be considered as a disturbance of ideational content. In hypochondria, the patient's attention is abnormally concentrated on his own body; he is depressed, and his thoughts are obsessively preoccupied with some organ which he is convinced is incurably diseased, although no pathological process can be demonstrated. A changed feeling of self may be present. Anxiety is displaced from unconscious mental sources to organs which thereby become the center of affective distress and preoccupation. The organ which is the focus of bodily complaint is usually one particularly subject to physiological expressions of anxiety or to the muscular tension of the anxious state. Hypochondria is more frequently manifested by persons who have shown a previous tendency to solicit affection or to evade the responsibilities of life through illness. In its milder forms, hypochondria may have its origin in a sense of insecurity which is rationalized as a threat to physical health. During the involutional period,

the changing psychological outlook on life, as well as the regressive physiological processes and the failing psychobiological security, may cause hypochondria. If hypochondriasis is consistent with the mood, it tends to disappear as the pathological mood does. If it is symbolic or inconsistent with the mood, as in schizophrenia, it indicates a serious disorder.

Obsessions

Thoughts that persistently thrust themselves into consciousness against the conscious desire of the patient are known as obsessions. Obsessions persist in the conscious mind so tenaciously that they cannot be dispelled by conscious processes and are uninfluenced by logic or reasoning. The obsessive thought is strongly charged with the emotions of guilt or depression, is unwanted, and usually plagues the individual almost constantly. The sufferer cannot understand why he is obsessed with the thought.

Obsessive ruminations are of various content. Often the constant preoccupation concerns some metaphysical question. The patient, for example, may be compelled to keep asking himself why he was born. The explanation of obsessive thought is to be found in the activity of the unconscious and of repression. As a defensive device, a guilty anxiety is displaced to an innocuous idea and the anxiety thereby decreased. The obsessive thought which is consciously distasteful may be related to what is unconsciously desired. Obsessive thoughts are closely related to compulsive acts, in which, after a distressing resistance to its performance, the patient feels impelled to perform some act which, because of its elaborate and repetitive nature, often seems almost ritualistic.

Phobias

Allied to obsessive thoughts are phobias, or fears, doubts, and indecisions. Like the obsessive idea, a phobia thrusts itself persistently into consciousness. Morbid anxiety always accompanies a phobia, in contrast to the guilt or depression of the obsessed. Among common phobias are fears of dirt, of bacteria, of cancer, or of crowds. In general, one may say that the patient's anxiety becomes detached from a specific idea, object, or situation in his daily life and is displaced to some situation in the form of a specific neurotic fear. The fear that he feels in the presence of a certain object or experience is really the displaced fear of some anxiety-producing component within his own personality. The situation about which he is phobic symbolizes or represents the incidents arousing affects of rage or shame, affects which must be prevented from coming to the surface, usually out of anxiety of rupturing an important relationship. The patient is not, of course, aware of the psychological source or significance of his fear, and while he may acknowledge that his fear is irrational, he is quite unable to regulate his life except as dictated by the phobia. He is constantly attempting to control his anxiety by avoiding the object or situation to which the anxiety has been displaced.

DISTURBANCES OF AFFECT

Affectivity penetrates and colors the whole psychic life, determining the general attitude, whether of rejection or of acceptance, in relation to any experience, promoting any tendency in harmony with it, and inhibiting any impulse not in agreement. As pointed out in an earlier chapter, the affective states provide the dynamic motivating drives. By *mood* is meant a sustained affective state of considerable duration.

Thus, affects serve as a signal or warning function for the ego and, at the same time, are the driving force which establish the psychological defenses that lead to their repression. As an example, guilty affect serves as a warning to refrain or desist from a forbidden act or to make restitutive actions if the act has been committed. If, however, guilty affect is too intense, ego functioning may bring about its repression and denial or evolve methods of control through defiance or masochistic reaction formation. Shame, too, warns against failure to perform to standards acceptable to the ego ideal or is suffered in restitution for performance of an unworthy act. As an anticipatory defense against shame, pride may evolve. The motor components of certain affects such as laughter and crying also serve as a means of reducing tension.

Affective factors may interfere with associative tendencies and prevent one from becoming aware of certain strivings or other consciously unacceptable aspects of his mental life. There seems to be reason to believe that profound disturbances of affectivity may even produce disturbances of consciousness, as in the perplexed, bewildered states of deep depression. In fact, as patients are observed while they are suffering from mental disorders and their feelings are largely determined by unconscious factors, it becomes evident that affective factors influence not only all other psychic functions but other physiological ones as well.

The role of affects for psychopathology is well summarized by Bleuler: "Just as those abnormalities which we call psychopathies are practically nothing but thymopathies (disturbances of affects) so affective influences play such a dominant role in psychopathology in general that practically everything else is merely incidental. Only the feeblemindednesses, the confusions and most delirious states are predominantly disturbances of intellect. But even these are colored by affective mechanisms, and often in both their practical and theoretical significance are determined by affective factors."[*]

Psychiatric literature strongly stresses the importance of psychogenic factors in mental disorder. Although not clearly so denoted, such dynamic etiological factors

---

[*] Naturgeschichte der Seele, Zweite Auflage, S. 185. Julius Springer, 1932.

are really affective in nature. It is not ideas themselves which are the important factors in determining the patient's mental content or his forms of behavior but the affects that are attached to his ideas. One thinks, therefore, according to the nature and intensity of his moods.

In the full evaluation of the significance of affect or feeling-tone in mental disorders, consideration must not be confined to that of pathological variations, since, directly and indirectly, affect exercises profound influence upon the thought and behavior of every individual. Not only is the thought content composed largely of affectively valued ideas, but judgment is constantly distorted and rendered unreliable by those ideas which are overvalued for emotional reasons. Associations are to a large degree directed by affective factors which facilitate those associations that tend to magnify the ego or aid in attaining some objective, while affects inhibit those associations which are unpleasant or opposed to some psychological need. If the tension of his emotional need or conflict exceeds the individual's capacity for evaluating reality, for appreciating its significance and remaining in contact with it, his experiences may be interpreted in accordance with affective needs and become hallucinatory or delusional.

By the mechanism of identification, an affect may extend or irradiate from the subject to which it was originally attached to one associated with or suggested by it. If, for example, a child came to hate a person who chanced to have some particular striking physical characteristic, then the child might always thereafter dislike persons who have a similar physical characteristic. In psychopathological states there is this constant tendency for the transfer of affects from material beyond conscious recognition to conscious thought content. In the psychoses, affective states of great intensity are often determined by unrecognized but highly dynamic factors. All affects possess conative elements; for this reason there is a delicate responsiveness of associations and behavior to affect.

Pleasurable Affects

A moderately pleasurable affect is known as *euphoria*. The euphoric patient is of an optimistic mental "set," is imbued with a subjectively pleasant feeling of well-being, and is confident and assured in attitude. Euphoria is most frequently noted in hypomanic states and in certain organic disorders such as general paresis, multiple sclerosis, and some cases of frontal lobe tumor. In *elation* an air of enjoyment and of self-confidence radiates from the patient, and his motor activity and drive are exaggerated. His circumstances may be such that unhappiness should be produced, yet everything that would normally produce that feeling is lightly brushed aside. It imparts a false sense of reality. Elation is often labile and readily shifts to irritability.

In *exaltation* there is an intense elation accompanied by an attitude of grandeur. A less frequent affective disorder is *ecstasy*. In this the mood is one of a peculiar, entrancing, peaceful rapture and tranquil sense of power. A religious feeling is an essential part of the state. The patient identifies himself with an immense cosmic power. He feels detached from outside things and on a new plane of existence, accompanied often by a feeling of having been reborn. He feels that he has attained a state beyond which there is nothing better. After having emerged from the experience, the patient retains a vivid recollection of it. Dynamically, ecstasy probably represents the achievement of the maximum of wish-fulfillment. Sometimes ecstasy occurs in persons who have had a strong sense of guilt. It has been observed in dissociative, epileptic, schizophrenic, and affective reactions.

Depression

Depression, an affective feeling-tone of sadness, is probably the commonest type of complaint in psychiatric patients. Depression may vary from a mild downheartedness or feeling of indifference to a despair beyond hope. In the milder depressive syndrome, the patient is quiet, restrained, inhibited, unhappy, pessimistic, and self-depreciative and has a feeling of lassitude, inadequacy, discouragement, and hopelessness. He is unable to make decisions and experiences difficulty with customarily easy mental activities. He is overconcerned with personal problems. Some depressed persons are petulant, querulous, and distrustful. In somewhat deeper depression, there is a constant unpleasant tension; every experience is accompanied by mental pain; the patient is impenetrably absorbed with a few topics of a melancholy nature. Conversation may be painfully difficult. He is dejected and hopeless in attitude and manner. The patient's dispirited affective attitude is projected toward his environment, which reflects his dolesome outlook. He feels rejected and unloved. He may be so preoccupied with depressive ruminations that attention, concentration, and memory are impaired.

Associated with this affect, some patients are anxious, perplexed, and complain of a feeling of unreality or of inability to think. Bodily complaints such as headache, tightness in the head, fatigue, loss of appetite, and constipation are common and occur in more than half of all cases of depression. Insomnia, especially that caused by awaking early, is the rule. Since mental content is greatly influenced by affective states, ideas of reference are frequent. Delusions are common, tending to express ideas of guilt, unworthiness, and self-accusation. Suicidal thoughts are frequently entertained. Events and pecadilloes long past receive an interpretation determined by the present mood. Initiative is lost, and replies to questions are delayed and often monosyllabic. The facial expression is one of dejection, perplexity, hopelessness, and perhaps of fear; the eyelids droop and the skin on the forehead may be furrowed, the corners of the mouth sag, and the eyes are often directed downward. In agitated depression, there are deep furrows between the eyebrows. Antagonist groups of muscles show slight imbalance, the flexors and adductors being moderately contracted, with the result that the neck, trunk, and extremities present the so-called flexion attitude of depression. All movements are executed slowly and with apparent difficulty.

Depression has its roots in unconscious guilt arising from interpersonal issues, perhaps from unconscious ambivalence and hostility with resentful and aggressive impulses directed toward persons who are the objects of an undesired obligation (a mother whose dependency prevents her daughter's desired marriage) or toward persons on whom one is dependent for security. The hostile impulses originally directed against other persons become directed against one's own self.

It should be recognized that the affect of depression may include varying degrees of sadness, guilt, and shame simultaneously—sadness because of a loss, guilt over a repressed hostile drive, and shame due to failure to live up to some personal standard. Helplessness, too, many be associated. The further study of depressions and the analysis of the prepotent affect underlying the various forms of this state will go far toward providing knowledge of those types most amenable to alleviation. It is said that states of shame are much less accessible to change than those in which guilt predominates.

Grief is to be differentiated from depression as an affect of sadness suffered from a loss of a close personal relation and unassociated with the affects of guilt or shame due to some repressed hostility toward the lost person. Grief, while leading to a withdrawal and preoccupation with the lost person, is self-limiting and seldom leads to serious impairment of usual activities, personal derogation, suicidal thoughts, or serious domestic disturbance.

Anxiety

Anxiety is a persistent feeling of dread, apprehension, and impending disaster. It is a response to threats from repressed dangerous impulses deep within the personality or to repressed feelings striving for consciousness, a warning of danger from the pressure of unacceptable internal attitudes. It differs from fear in not being referable to specific objects or events. The patient is ignorant of its source.

Most psychiatrists, in using the word "anxiety" without a qualifying adjective, mean neurotic anxiety arising from self-inaccessible sources as just described. Some speak of "normal" anxiety, meaning thereby that there is an actual danger which is realistically appraised and that the degree of anxiety is not out of proportion to the threat. Such an anxiety does not have to be managed by forcing it out of awareness by such mechanisms as repression or dissociation or by using neurotic defenses.

Anxiety is often displaced from its original, but unrecognized, source to some other situation which appears to the patient to afford reasonable grounds for apprehension, to be the excitant of his diffuse, unformulated uneasiness and painful apprehension. Sometimes the anxiety is not attached to any ideational content but is felt as a morbid fear without apparent source. Anxiety which is directly felt and expressed in this manner is known as *free-floating* anxiety. Again anxiety may be covert. In this hidden form, there are no obvious tension and painful apprehension with their physical manifestations. The various personality traits of the individual, together with the mental mechanisms which he has developed to conceal or displace his anxiety, may serve sufficiently well as defenses to prevent its overt expression. It may still, however, be the fundamental basis for the development of serious personality deviations or disorders. Anxiety is the presenting symptom in the so-called anxiety neuroses and may often be openly manifest in other neuroses. Anxiety, therefore, together with the various defensive mechanisms, such as repression, regression, conversion, and displacement, constitutes an important factor in the psychopathology of abnormal personalities, psychoneuroses, psychoses, and psychosomatic disease.

Anxiety occupies a position of great importance in psychoanalytical theory, according to which it results from the threat either of uncontrollable id forces or of self-destructive superego forces. According to this theory, anxiety is of significance in two roles: It serves not only as a signal or indicator of conflict but also as a reinforcing agent for repression, reaction-formation, and projection. In fact, the various mental mechanisms and devices which serve a defensive purpose exercise that function through their ability to reduce the strength of anxiety.

Through its effect upon the autonomic system, anxiety is particularly apt to disturb physiological functions and to find expression in psychophysiological symptoms. In acute forms, it may, through stimulation of the autonomic system, produce generalized visceral tension and therefore hyperventilation, spasm of the cardiac and pyloric portions of the stomach, intestinal irritability, hyperchlorhydria, diarrhea or constipation, palpitation, tachycardia, extrasystoles, vasomotor flushing, and respiratory distress. It may be accompanied by fainting, weakness, nausea, and tremor. Hands and face may perspire; the patient may assume a tense posture and show excessive vigilance and fidgety movements of the hands or feet; the voice may be uneven or strained and the pupils widely dilated. When anxiety is severe and overflows in this way into the muscular system, producing gross motor restlessness, the reaction of the patient is spoken of as *agitation*.

Tension is sometimes confused with the affect of anxiety. In tension, the patient has a continuing feeling of tautness, both emotionally and in his muscles. He senses a restlessness, dissatisfaction, dread, and discomforting expectancy. He presents a strained, tense expression of the facies, his fingers are tremulous, and he manifests an abrupt haste in movement. The patient may experience difficulty in concentration and complains of tightness or other unpleasant sensations in the head. Tension may arise when a person is torn between contradictory desires and strivings, by a struggle for security, and by various other situations. Its origin may be from either conscious or unconscious sources. It is a component of anxiety, expressive of a continuing inner perception of this affect accompanied by neuromuscular setting.

Panic is a pronounced state of anxiety which produces disorganization of ego functions. One of the best descriptions is that of Diethelm: "Panic is not merely a high degree of fear, but a fear based on prolonged tension, with a sudden climax which is characterized by fear, extreme insecurity, suspiciousness and a tendency to projection and disorganization." Misinterpretations are followed by projections that may assume the form of hallucinations having a threatening and accusatory content, and also may have the form of delusions of persecution. The situations giving rise to panic are ones in which some long-standing insecurity of the personality has created tension and become particularly threatening. Homosexual and, occasionally, disowned heterosexual tendencies are the most frequent factors. Because of the underlying sense of insecurity, the patient may react with self-assertion and aggressiveness and may rush about; in other cases, he may exhibit dilated pupils and the other usual sympathicotonic manifestations of great anxiety, yet remain immobile because he does not dare move. He often has difficulty in thinking and at times has a sense and appearance of bewilderment. Suicide is not uncommon in panic states.

Inadequate Affect

Emotional dulling or detachment in the form of indifference or *apathy* is a frequent form of affective disturbance and is characterized by an inadequate sensitiveness to those experiences which normally give rise to pleasure or pain. The facies shows an emptiness of expression. Patients suffering from this affective impoverishment show a lack of drive and interest in those matters which have previously appealed to them. There is an indifference to esthetic and other finer sentiments. Such qualities as gratitude, sympathy, hope, anticipation, grief, regret, pride, or shame no longer appear to form part of the patient's subjective experience. This absence of emotional responsiveness may cause the patient to seem out of touch with reality. Apathy may be regarded as a protective, defensive reaction, perhaps against painful perceptions.

Inappropriateness of Affect

Disharmony of affect is a common emotional disturbance, particularly noted in schizophrenia. The patient smiles when the social situation suggests a serious mien as appropriate. He laughs or cries out of context to the interpersonal milieu and apparently in relation to his inner percepts and associations, to which the affect may be quite appropriate.

Ambivalence

Recognizing that each feature of the personality has a double aspect, each having a counterpart closely connected with it, Bleuler introduced into psychiatric thought the concept of ambivalence. In affective ambivalence, contradictory feeling attitudes may exist toward the same object. Both of these conflicting attitudes are faces on the same coin; while only one may be visible, the other is nevertheless present. One of the two components of ambivalence remains repressed but may give rise to anxiety and feelings of guilt. A common form of ambivalent polarity is a subtle combination of love and hate. A person caring for an invalid member of his family may, for example, have mixed feelings. One feeling may be that of love, of wanting to be helpful, but another, of which he is not conscious, may be that of annoyance and hostility. Affection is linked with a sentiment of rejection. In the confusion of hostile and affectionate impulses, there may be an intensification of conscious love in order to repress the fundamental hatred. An expression of hostility toward one to whom a person should be indebted, a parent, for example, is not consciously tolerable. The hostility, therefore, necessarily remains unconscious lest it give rise to anxiety. The ambivalent attitudes of hostility and love are accordingly developed. Often when ambivalence of feelings exists, the repressed component of the dual affective attitude will be projected; for example, repressed hatred may be experienced as hatred directed toward one's self by the other party.

Depersonalization

Depersonalization, a pervasive and distressing feeling of estrangement, known sometimes as the depersonalization syndrome, may be defined as an affective disorder in which feelings of unreality and a loss of conviction of one's own identity and of a sense of identification with and control over one's own body are the principal symptoms. The term was introduced by Dugas in 1898. The unreality symptoms are of two kinds: a feeling of changed personality and a feeling that the outside world is unreal. The patient feels that he is no longer himself, but he does not feel that he has become someone else. The condition is, therefore, not one of so-called transformation of personality. Experience loses emotional meaning and may be colored by a frightening sense of strangeness and unreality. The onset may be acute, following a severe emotional shock, or it may be of gradual onset following prolonged physical or emotional stress. It is more frequent in personalities of an intelligent, sensitive, affectionate, introverted, and imaginative type. The patient may say his feelings are "frozen," that his thoughts are strange; his thoughts and acts seem to be carried on mechanically, as if he were a machine or an automaton. People and objects appear unreal, far away, and lacking in normal color and vividness. The patient may say he feels as if he were going about in a trance or dream. He appears perplexed and bewildered because of the strangeness of unreality feelings. He has difficulty in concentrating and may complain that his brain is "dead" or has "stopped working."

Depersonalization is probably not a specific disorder but occurs in various neurotic and psychotic states such as depressions, hypochondria, obsessional states, and hysteria, and in some early schizophrenias. Apparently it may occur in some normal persons after exhaustion or shock. It is more common at puberty and in women. The reaction may be regarded psychopathologically as a form of withdrawal from reality, as a means of escape from an intolerable situation by an insecure and self-observing personality.

DISTURBANCES OF CONSCIOUSNESS

Perhaps from a descriptive standpoint the words "clearmindedness" and "awareness" best indicate what we designate as consciousness. The sensorium is clear, i.e., the functioning of the special senses is intact, and the apprehension of external stimuli presented to them is unimpaired. The individual is able to apprehend his environment as to place, time, person, and general setting, to understand questions, and to reflect upon them.

Full consciousness demands attentiveness as well as that complex function known as *apperception,* by which through active, attentive thoughts one analyzes, integrates, evaluates, and absorbs experience. W. M. Wundt (1832–1920) defined it as "the single process by means of which any psychic content is brought to clear conception." It is through apperception that new ideas are formulated and related to ones already familiar, with the result that one is able to understand or grasp new situations, events, and experiences. In *disturbances of apperception,* the patient has difficulty in understanding questions, unaccustomed situations, and experiences. Disorders of apperception occur in psychogenic diseases involving intense preoccupation and in other disturbances of attention, as well as in toxic and organic states. Faulty capacity for apperception exists, of course, in mental deficiency. The projective psychological tests (Rorschach and thematic apperception) are examinations of this function.

Among the disturbances of consciousness are those imposed by *disordered attention*. The conscious, selective reaction by which the organism examines the external world for useful data is known as attention. Successful examination requires a certain degree of vigilance and a certain tenacity. Attention is greatly influenced by conation, affect, and associations. Feeling and attitudes influence attention, not only directly but indirectly, through their effect upon associations. Fatigue, toxic states, and organic lesions strongly modify both vigilance and tenacity and so influence attention. Toxic and organic factors, by interfering also with associations, tend to lower attention. Similarly, a poverty of associations is largely responsible for defects of attention in the mentally deficient. Even a normal person who has few associations connected with an object submitted for examination will, in the absence of strongly affective factors, exhibit but little attention. The inability to hold the attention a sufficient length of time to render adequate examination possible is known as *distractibility*. In this disorder, every fleeting stimulus or an abnormal lability of affect redirects the attention, which is lacking in normal tenacity. Profound depression, on the other hand, may cause too great tenacity of attention. No stimulus or experience can divert the attention to an idea or object not related to the patient's depressive mental content or not in harmony with it. Emotional disorganization as seen in the apathetic schizophrenic may greatly diminish the degree of attention.

As indicated in an earlier chapter, consciousness may be considered to exist at varying levels of awareness of one's environment. Thus it is to be suspected that the clinical disturbances of this function roughly describe progressively serious levels of impairment. The clinician defines as successive steps in defects, from the least to the greatest impairments, states of confusion, clouding of consciousness, delirium, dream, and fugue states, to complete stupor.

Confusion

Confusion is a disturbance of consciousness characterized by bewilderment, perplexity, disorientation, disturbance of associative functions, and poverty of ideas. The face of the confused patient presents a distressed, puzzled, and, at times, surprised expression. Confusion is confined largely to conditions in which there is a diffuse impairment of brain tissue function, especially associated with toxic, infectious, or traumatic agents, although it occurs also in dissociative reactions and epileptic dream states. Most psychiatrists believe that the term confusion should not be loosely applied to those subjects, such as retarded, depressive, or perplexed schizophrenic patients, whose replies are neither prompt nor pertinent. Many consider that true confusion is found only in toxic-organic reactions. Certainly clouding of consciousness is the basic feature in the toxic-organic states.

Clouding of Consciousness

Clouding of consciousness is a disturbance in which clear-mindedness is not complete, usually because there are physical or chemical disturbances producing functional impairment of the associative apparatus of the cerebrum. The threshold of consciousness is high, and perceptions are not produced by those sensory stimuli which ordinarily result in clear perceptions. The capacity to think clearly and with customary rapidity, to perceive, respond to, and remember current stimuli is impaired. To make the patient understand a question, it may be necessary to shake him, to shout the question, and perhaps to repeat this procedure several times before he apprehends sufficiently to reply. Attention wanders, and the patient's apprehension of his environment is incomplete and inaccurate. The symptom is often seen in general hospitals in patients suffering from infectious diseases and other conditions affecting cerebral oxygenation and metabolism. Clouding of consciousness may also occur in psychogenic disturbances, such as dissociative reactions. In this case, the clouding and the subsequent amnesia for events of the clouded period may serve the purpose of excluding from awareness material which deep-seated wishes would shut out. Clouding of consciousness may be of various degrees, ranging from hebetude to somnolence, stupor, or coma.

Delirium *

Although involving much more than a disturbance of consciousness, mention should be made of the symptom-complex known as *delirium,* also designated as the *acute brain syndrome.* This syndrome, ordinarily acute in both development and course, consists of clouding of consciousness, bewilderment, restlessness, confusion, disorientation, incoherent or dreamlike thinking, illusions and hallucinations, and apprehension or fear. Its occurrence is usually associated with infections accompanied by fever, toxic states, metabolic disturbances (uremia, pellagra, pernicious anemia), cardiac decompensation, or head trauma, which impair cerebral functioning and cause cerebral insufficiency. Some persons develop delirium more readily than do others. Perhaps in some cases this tendency is caused either by an inherently greater vulnerability of the brain to toxins

or by a less resistant blood–cerebrospinal fluid barrier. On the other hand, the susceptibility may depend upon the integration and stability of the personality. Electroencephalographic changes are usually found in delirium. Generally, the greater the reduction in the level of awareness, the greater the shift toward slower-frequency ranges. The electroencephalographic changes are reversible to the extent to which the clinical delirium is reversible.

Delirium is usually more marked at night, when the ordinary background of sensory input is reduced; at times it may be limited to nighttime, the patient seeming normal during the day. The most frequent prodromal symptoms are drowsiness, restless sleep, difficulty in grasp, and impaired attention. In very mild cases, the patient may merely appear mentally dull and sluggish and not keenly aware of just what is happening to him. He may show a little "wandering" but become clear when addressed. Attention is impaired, and there is a reduction in capacity for abstract thinking. The patient usually has difficulty in performing tests requiring concentration and sustained attention, e.g., the serial subtraction of 7's from 100. As the delirium becomes more marked, the patient seems dazed, baffled, and bewildered and fails to recognize members of his family.

Important symptoms are fluctuations in grasp or perception of reality, orientation, and consciousness. Shifting degrees of awareness and of orientation should always suggest the possibility of delirium. Moments of rationality often alternate with ones of irrationality. If the clouding of consciousness has been marked, the patient, after recovery, has no recollection of what occurred during the delirium. Frequently the memory is patchy, varying with the fluctuations of consciousness that occurred during the delirious episode. Other variations in the clinical picture often coexist and are also suggestive. Comparative calmness, for example, may exist for a period, to be followed suddenly by restlessness or impulsive activity. The pa-

---

* The clinical picture of delirium is well depicted in Shakespeare's description of Falstaff's death: "For after I saw him fumble with the sheets, and play with flowers, and smile upon his finger's ends, I knew there was but one way; for his nose was sharp as a pen, and 'a babbled of green fields." Henry V, Act II, Scene iii.

tient's mood may shift rapidly or be characterized by doubt, perplexity, irritability, apprehension, fear, and even panic. Frightening dreams and fantasies may arise, and both illusions and hallucinations occur, the former being more frequent. Visual hallucinations are more frequent than auditory ones and at first are often in the form of ill-defined or shadowy figures. The content of thought and of hallucinations is more dependent upon the patient's personality problems and tendencies and his previous life experiences than upon the nature of the underlying physical process responsible for the delirium. Frequently the patient shows motor disturbance, manifested in mild cases by tremulousness in writing, but in more severe cases by picking, grasping, and groping. Activity may vary from mild restlessness to intense and uncontrollable overactivity.

Delirium rarely continues for more than a month and in infectious diseases may be of only fleeting duration. Later delirious episodes tend to resemble any previous ones, in both content and course. Following his recovery, the patient often describes his hallucinations and other delirious experiences as having been dreamlike in nature. Although the delirious syndrome occurs frequently in infectious diseases and in their febrile period, it is by no means confined to such association. Toxic-delirious reactions occur in old age in a wide variety of physical illnesses. Postoperative psychoses, more frequent in elderly patients than in younger ones, usually resemble those of toxic-exhaustive and infective states and therefore present features of delirium. Puerperal psychoses, even those that are fundamentally affective or schizophrenic in nature, often show characteristics of delirium in their onset. Delirious reactions are most frequent with excessive use of bromides and other drugs.

Dream States

Presenting a somewhat similar but more exaggerated symptom complex is the disturbance known as *dream state* or *twilight state*. Such a state does not, like delirium, arise from toxic-organic condition, but is of affective or other psychogenic origin. Consciousness is usually disturbed, in some cases being so clouded or confused that the patient is not aware of his real surroundings. Visual and auditory hallucinations occur, in response to which the patient may perform complex acts, such as running away or committing acts of violence. These dream states may last from several minutes to a few days.

When normal consciousness is regained, the patient may report that during the twilight state he felt as if he were dreaming and he has little or no recollection of events which occurred during its existence. Such dream states occur for the most part in dissociative reactions and in epilepsy. In dissociative reactions they represent escape from unpleasant reality or the gratification of frustrated wishes. In epileptic dream states the behavior is motivated by more deeply unconscious factors.

Stupor

Stupor is identified as existing when the patient is akinetic (motionless) and mute but with relative preservation of consciousness. Movement of the eyes and respiration occur. However, the eye movements generally appear purposeful. Subsequent to the stuporous state, there is often ability to recall events, although total amnesia may result. Stupor is to be differentiated from sleepiness, loss of consciousness as in coma, and organic motor paralysis.

Stupor occurs both in the toxic-organic and in the psychogenic groups of mental disorders, but the similarity of disturbance of mental processes in the two groups is more apparent than real. Stupor may occur in a diversity of physical and mental conditions, from toxic states, organic brain disease, intense apathy, profound depression, blocking, epilepsy, and dissociative reaction to overpowering fear. In neither toxic-organic stupor nor psychogenic stupor does the patient move. In toxic-organic stupor, conscious thought processes are suspended; in catatonic stupor, there is intense preoccupation of thought which is often dereistic in nature, with a loss of reality sense but no real suspension of consciousness. A sudden change from stupor to activity, often impulsive or excessive, occurs in psychogenic stupor only.

DISORDERS OF ORIENTATION

The process by which one apprehends his environment and locates himself in relation to it is known as *orientation*. If a person knows his position in reference to time, appreciates his situation as to both space and circumstances, and understands his relationship to other individuals, he is said to be oriented. If he does not recognize and locate himself in respect to any one of these matters, he is said to be disoriented in the particular sphere in which he has an inadequate grasp. The development of personality identity, which commences with the early exploration of one's body and that of the mother, as well as the exploration of space and the growing awareness of time, established through the periodic experiencing of emerging needs and their satisfaction, lays down the individual's orientation in these spheres.

Disorientation may occur in any mental disorder in which there is extensive impairment of the patient's memory, of the extent or accuracy of his perceptions, or of his attention. Disturbances of orientation are the significant symptomatology of acute cerebral insufficiency, by which are designated the organic brain syndromes (delirious states) in which the physiological functions necessary for memory, perception, and attention are impaired. Less frequently, disorientation is caused by acute conflicts, intense affective factors, distractibility, or lack of interest or attention.

DISORDERS OF MEMORY

The function by which information that has been acquired and presented to consciousness through the observations of attention is stored, later to be summoned and again presented to consciousness, is known as *memory*. For the purpose of description, it may be considered as consisting of three processes: the reception and *registration* of a mental impression; the *retention* or preservation of the previously acquired impression; the reproduction or *recall* of the impression. Memories are defined now as recent or remote. As discussed earlier, permanent registration to establish the long-term memory trace is believed to involve complex electrochemical events within the brain. Memory is purposive and tends to promote adaptation with the minimum of effort by virtue of its role in assisting the individual to profit by his experience. Largely as a result of the investigations of abnormal psychology, it is known that memory is influenced by affect, the tendency being to modify it in the interests of the emotional needs of the individual.

Forgetting, too, is purposive in that it may be regarded as the result of the organizing process of memory. Those sensory impressions which are generalized or subordinated, or have come to be conceptualized as a means of retaining larger banks of information or memory or condensed and fused to maintain an efficiently operative working memory, tend to be forgotten. It is believed that everything registered as a memory persists, barring impairment of brain structure and function. Yet many sensory impressions may not be recorded within the brain as permanent memory. Psychologically repressed memories are not forgotten; they remain available when the affective states, inducing repression, are modified. Generally, forgetting may be thought of as a function of reorganizing of memory; newly recorded experiences have the potentiality of reorganizing existing memories.

The disorders of memory are three:

abnormally pronounced memory, or *hypermnesia;* loss of memory, or *amnesia;* and falsification of memory, or *paramnesia.*

Hypermnesia

Hypermnesia is occasionally seen in mild manic states, paranoia, and catatonia. This excessive mnemonic capacity is largely limited to specific periods or to specific events and experiences that are connected with particularly strong affects. Impressions arising from emotionally colored events are registered with more than the usual intensity, with the result that the patient has a vivid recollection of details.

Amnesia

Amnesia may be produced either by organic or by psychogenic factors. In *organic amnesia,* physiological disturbances of neurons, through chemical alterations, trauma, or degenerative changes, interfere with associative processes. Organic loss of memory is caused by impairment of both registration and retention, especially the latter. In *psychogenic amnesia,* recall, for psychologic reasons, is inhibited. Strictly speaking, forgetting in psychogenic amnesia is not a passive loss of memory trace. The absence of memory is an active defense against experiences which have proved unbearably painful or anxiety producing. Psychogenic amnesia may provide escape not only from the memory of intolerable experiences but also from the consequences of an act. If anxiety is severe, a dissociative reaction may occur with a resulting fugue or flight automatism, in which the patient experiences a loss of memory of both his past experiences and his identity. By this escape, the patient's symptoms supply him, without awareness on his part, with a seeming solution for his difficulties.

Another and more frequent form of psychogenic amnesia is that for intended action. This is a result of conflict of wishes. We "forget" to perform some task or keep some appointment because the proposed act conflicts, perhaps unconsciously, with some wish or interest.

The differential diagnosis between organic and psychogenic amnesia is important. To differentiate between these two forms the psychiatrist must determine the cause. Often this is obvious, but if not readily apparent, a careful history should be secured and a searching examination of the nervous system be made before concluding that the amnesia is of psychogenic origin. Such an origin should not be accepted unless a psychological need for its occurrence is discovered.

If there has been no disturbance of consciousness and no impairment of intellectual functions, the amnesia is probably psychogenic in origin. A selective amnesia in which inconvenient events or topics are forgotten is of psychogenic origin. A sudden and complete recovery of memory is common in cases of psychogenic amnesia but does not occur if the amnesia has been caused by organic factors. Any recovery of memory which has been lost through organic causes takes place gradually and is often incomplete. A fragmentary type of amnesia with a scattered loss of memory for unrelated details of experience, as noted in general paralysis or senile dementia, is of organic origin.

Amnesia for circumscribed periods of time may be either psychogenic or organic in nature. A generalized failure of memory for both recent and remote events denotes an organic degenerative disease of the brain. A patchy amnesia with a memory for isolated events in a period of confusion is frequent in delirium. An organic amnesia may be followed or widely overlapped by a psychogenic failure of recall, especially in head injuries.

ANTEROGRADE AMNESIA. An anterograde amnesia is one that extends forward to cover a period following the apparent regaining of environmental contact. Anterograde amnesia is sometimes observed in boxers who have received a severe blow on the head. The pugilist is hit but continues boxing in an apparently normal manner. Retrospectively, however, he reports a gap in his memory extending forward from the time of the injury and covering the period to the end of the fight or even beyond.

RETROGRADE AMNESIA. In retrograde amnesia, there is a loss of memory extending back over a period prior to the time when the onset occurred. In cases of trauma to the head, there may be a retrograde amnesia reaching back over a variable period prior to the injury with its accompanying loss of consciousness. It may also follow many other forms of organic interference with cerebral function, such as suicidal attempts by hanging or gassing, or epileptic convulsions. It is often seen after treatment by electric shock.

Recovery from retrograde amnesia is chronological, those memories nearest the injury being the last to return. The amnesia in Korsakoff's psychosis is both retrograde and anterograde. Retrograde amnesia may also be of psychogenic origin and has been known to stretch back over a prolonged period. In psychogenic retrograde amnesia, an experience has been registered but is not recalled except through an association of ideas. As it is recalled in this manner, the recall is accompanied by an emotional response appropriate to the forgotten material.

As the result of precise surgical extirpations it has been found that bilateral lesions of the medial surface of the temporal lobe, particularly the hippocampi, are followed by severe memory defects, particularly in the ability of retention. Such operations are also followed by both anterograde and retrograde amnesia; early memories and technical skills remain undisturbed.

Paramnesia

Paramnesia, or falsification of memory, as well as distortions of memory, also serves as protection against intolerable anxiety. In the form known as *confabulation* the patient fills the gaps in his memory by fabrications which are without any basis of fact, although, when relating them, he accepts them as actual occurrences. These fictions change from moment to moment and may often be suggested and directed by the person to whom they are related. Paramnesia is observed occasionally in the senile psychoses but particularly in Korsakoff's syndrome.

RETROSPECTIVE FALSIFICATION. Of different psychological significance are the retrospective falsifications, or illusions of memory, created in response to affective needs. We all tend to embroider the truth in accordance with these needs or unconsciously to select those memories which suit our interests. Two persons who have intense but different emotional attitudes relative to a certain event or experience will relate quite different accounts of the circumstances. Both persons may be honest but each will remember details in harmony with his emotional needs and forget those not consistent with his affects. In paranoid psychoses, one meets with exaggerations of this tendency. The patient misinterprets an actual event, appends imaginary details to it, or even relates experiences that have little or no basis of fact. Such falsifications of memory serve the purpose of supplying supporting evidence for the patient's delusions, which, too, are products of affective needs.

Defensive distortions of recall may serve to avert threats or to enhance self-esteem. Early childhood memories reported by patients sometimes represent such distortions. Whether distorted or not, they are worthy of note as are first and repetitive dreams. It has been reported that the early memories of psychotics are more frequently of being lost, being threatened with death, or losing control. The psychoneurotic more frequently reports self-images. Memories of sickness and death in the psychotic are often those of neglect; in the neurotic, of overdependency.

"Déjà Vu"

Mention should be made of the illusion of memory known as *déjà vu*. In this phenomenon, there is a feeling of familiarity on observing something—a new scene, for example—of which there has, in fact, been no previous observation, or of having previously lived through a current experience. It arises when the present situation has an associative link with some past experience or occurrence for which the patient is amnesic.

Various explanations have been offered for the phenomenon, but it seems to occur when the forgotten experience has been the center of psychological conflict and consequent repression. Several psychodynamic explanations have been offered. For instance, there is a drive for a repetition, a second chance to solve a conflict, so that the outcome of the incident may coincide with the wish. Again, the déjà vu both symbolizes and stimulates the revival of an anxiety-producing wish or fantasy which is then defensively dealt with as unreal and projected onto the current external situation which is offered as a substitute for the past. Thus repression is maintained. It may occur in normal people, especially in young people who are given to day-dreaming. In the phenomenon of *jamais vu* there is a false feeling of unfamiliarity with situations which have actually been experienced. These phenomena may occur in schizophrenia, psychoneuroses, lesions of the temporal lobe including epilepsy, and states of fatigue or intoxication.

Functions of Psychogenic Memory Disturbances

It is apparent from what has been said that memory loss, in the absence of structural or toxic changes in the higher cortical neurons, is a selective process and not a matter of chance. It plays an important part in promoting the comfort and self-esteem of the individual.

Largely through the observations of Freud and of Brill it has been realized that slips of tongue and pen, such as use of a wrong word, of one opposite to that consciously intended, the loss or destruction of objects consciously valued, little forgettings, and various erroneous acts of everyday life that are ordinarily regarded as merely "accidental," are determined by unconscious motives. Since these apparently unmotivated errors resemble symptoms in their relation to repression, they are often spoken of as *symptomatic acts*.

DEMENTIA

In any structural disturbance or degeneration of the higher cortical neurons, such as those caused by prolonged intoxication or malnutrition, there results a permanent, irreversible loss of intellectual efficiency known as *dementia*. If of but slight degree, the impoverishment may be manifested by defective self-criticism and by impairment in capacity for fine discriminations, in decisions involving delicate moral issues, and in ability to employ abstract ideas.

As dementia progresses, there are an increasing poverty of initiative, a restriction of interests, and a blunting of concern; impressions are taken in and assimilated slowly, with difficulty, and often inexactly. There is therefore a failure to profit from experience. Aptitude and learning capacity are reduced. It becomes increasingly difficult or even impossible for the patient to understand and follow conversation. Questions are not answered or are answered only after several repetitions. Memory is defective and disorientation and confusion may exist. There is a poverty of the imagination necessary for productive thinking. The content of consciousness is reduced in both number and variety of associations, with the result that new ones are formed with difficulty, imperfectly, or even not at all. The individual's capacity for integrating his past experience with his present is reduced, and judgment becomes defective. Emotions are unstable or inadequate.

Care must be taken not to mistake for dementia the temporary inhibition of interest caused by preoccupation, or the dulling of consciousness caused by external or internal toxins. One must not mistake the acquired dementia of organic lesions for the innate oligophrenia of the feeble-minded.

The causes of dementia may be grouped as follows:

1. Atrophic changes of the brain resulting in senile dementia;
2. Vascular disorders of the brain, including arteriosclerotic dementia and hypertensive encephalopathy;
3. Inflammatory disorders of the brain, particularly syphilis and epidemic encephalitis;
4. Degenerative diseases of the brain, notably Alzheimer's disease, Pick's disease, and Huntington's chorea;
5. Deficiency diseases, including Korsakoff's psychosis, Wernicke's encephalopathy, pellagra, and pernicious anemia or vitamin B_{12} deficiency;
6. Neoplasm;
7. Trauma.

BIBLIOGRAPHY

Adorno, T., Frenkel-Brunswick, E., Levenson, D., and Sanford, R.: The Authoritarian Personality. New York, Harper, 1958.

Arlow, J. A.: The structure of the déjà vu experience. J. Amer. Psychoanal. Assn., 7:611–631, 1959.

Carluccio, C., Sours, J. A., and Kolb, L. C.: Psychodynamics of echo-reactions. Arch. Gen. Psychiat., 10:623–629, 1964.

Chapman, J., and McGhie, A.: Echopraxia in schizophrenia. Brit. J. Psychiat., 110:365–374, 1964.

Charlton, M. H.: Visual hallucinations. Psychiat. Quart., 37:489–498, 1963.

Easser, B. R., and Lesser, S. R.: Hysterical personality: a re-evaluation. Psychoanal. Quart., 24:390–405, 1965.

Forrer, G. R.: Benign auditory and visual hallucinations. Arch. Gen. Psychiat., 3:95–98, 1960.

Gould, R.: Suicide problems in children and adolescents. Amer. J. Psychother., 19:228–246, 1965.

Jacobziner, H.: Attempted suicides in adolescents by poisoning. Amer. J. Psychother., 19:247–252, 1965.

Jahoda, M.: Current Concepts of Positive Mental Health. New York, Basic Books, Inc., 1958.

Joyston-Bechel, M. P.: The clinical features and outcome of stupor. Brit. J. Psychiat., 112:967–981, 1966.

Kolb, L. C.: Disturbances of the body image. In Arieti, S. (ed.): American Handbook of Psychiatry. New York, Basic Books, Inc., Vol. 1, pp. 749–769, 1959.

Kolb, L. C.: Violence and Aggression: An Overview. In Fawcett, J. (ed.): Dynamics of Violence. Chicago, American Medical Association, 1971, pp. 7–15.

Lunn, V.: On body hallucinations. Acta Psychiat. Scand., 41:387–399, 1965.

Murphy, G. E., and Robins, E.: Social factors in suicide. J.A.M.A., 199:303–308, 1967.

Nelson, S. H., and Grunebaum, H.: A follow-up of wrist slashers. Amer. J. Psychiat., 127:1345–1349, 1971.

Prince, M.: Miss Beauchamp—the theory of the psychogenesis of multiple personality. J. Abnorm. Psychol., 15:67–135, 1920.

Ostow, M.: The syndrome of narcissistic tranquility. Int. J. Psychoanal., 48:573–583, 1967.

Resnik, H. L. P. (ed.): Suicidal Behaviors. Boston, Little, Brown & Co., 1969.

Rozan, G. H., Feldstein, S., and Jaffe, J.: "Denial personality." Reported symptoms and the clinical course of an inpatient psychiatric sample. J. Nerv. & Ment. Dis., 145:385–391, 1967.

Salzman, L.: The Obsessive Personality. New York, Science House, 1968.

Schlesinger, N. J.: The place of forgetting in memory functioning. J. Amer. Psychoanal. Assn., 18: 358–371, 1970.

Stokes, A.: On resignation. Int. J. Psychoanal., 43: 175–181, 1962.

Whitman, R. M., and Alexander, J.: On gloating. Int. J. Psychoanal., 49:732–738, 1968.

Chapter 7

Predisposing and Precipitating Factors for Mental Disorder

The Disorders of Personality Functioning

The mental disorders emerge by the interaction of a personality, predisposed on the basis of its structural anlage and dynamic evolutions with the stresses imposed upon it. In earlier chapters, both the known physiological processes and the related psychodynamic forces from which mature personality functioning develops were described. The processes and forces operate upon the human anatomical structure through genetic and constitutional determinants. Each individual personality thus carries within himself various resistances and predispositions with which to react to the ongoing stresses of his life. Stress may occur as the result of impinging and sometimes overwhelming physical forces. In most instances the major stresses of life occur within the framework of a person's own social network, arousing within him affective responses and their associated emotional responses. Failure of ego functioning, or inability to adapt internally to the stresses of living, is most commonly the precipitating factor in the sudden or acute onset of psychiatric disorder.

Although stresses threatening life, in the forms of serious or mutilating illness or the catastropic disasters of war or civil life, may overwhelm the stimulus barrier of the individual and lead to personality malfunctions, in many instances careful analysis will disclose that the affective response to rupture or loss of a significant personal relationship is an important, if not the most significant, factor.

Insidious onset of mental disorder occurs when those with impaired personality development meet, over time, the progressively demanding performances that occur as one matures socially. Fixation to behavioral patterns accepted socially in childhood and adolescence leads to recognition of maladaptation in adulthood. Inflexible personality structure may yield to overwhelming internal affect when one is confronted with the newly emerging social stresses of adult life in a new family or vocation, or with the complex nuances of existence in a cultural or ethnic group foreign to the exposures of the earlier developmental period.

Stress for man must thus be recognized as occurring as much by the affective experiences aroused from human transactions—interpersonal relations—as by changes induced internally as a consequence of disturbance of the biophysical sphere.

The symptoms and signs of mental disorders cannot be explained as simply the result of disorganization of cellular structure or physiological processes. Only those behavioral expressions directly expressive of impairment or loss of personality functioning caused by brain tissue damage—thus the memory failures which typify the syndromes consequent to brain insufficiency—may be so explained.

In each instance of impaired personality functioning, the psychiatrist attempts to define, as far as possible, both precipi-

123

tating and predisposing factors. In many, removal or alleviation of the former may relieve the symptomatic expressions of personality dysfunction.

Communication theory provides a framework for considering the interrelationship between the structural organization of man and his immediate relationship to his environment as well as the continuing influence of past social forces and experiences upon him which allow for recognizing, selecting, and patterning response and therefore determine his later behavior. The brain then functions as a central integrating and communicating system, subserving contact with the inner organ systems, past experiences, and outer world. Today, contact with the outer world is largely contact with other men. Any disturbances of the brain or other bodily tissues which influence the capacity of man to receive and perceive information from his environment and integrate it with past information will lead to defective psychosocial functioning and thereby disturb personality functioning. Any physical disturbance which upsets man's capacity to communicate with others again will lead to ineffective communication that produces disturbing feedback. The latter, in turn, induces anxiety, conflict, and personality unrest.

Thus one may recognize as etiologic factors in disrupting the communicative activity between men the effects of constitutional defects in the perceptual receptive system, such as deafness or blindness, failures of development or acquired defects in the central nervous system, or the later dysfunction of this organ due to metabolic or toxic agents. Again, failures to learn language, to understand social codes, or to speak effectively, with resultant interference with ability to recognize and integrate psychosocial signals, or separations from those who maintain stability or provide guiding signs, may be seen as contributing factors to disturbance in communication or psychosocial illness. Viewed in terms of interpersonal communication, the arguments relative to the etiology of psychiatric illness as primarily physical or psychological become meaningless. One attempts to understand the totality of the personality functioning in a communicative relationship with others and to correct or modify for more effective social adaptation any defects found, or to develop substitutive behaviors if the defect is clearly permanent.

Once the psychopathology has been ascertained, an effort is made to formulate the etiology of the symptom picture. This chapter considers the many factors in the wide range from the biogenetic to the experimental defect that may influence personality functioning adversely.

Constitution

From the standpoint of psychiatry, constitution may be looked upon as that portion of the individual's organization derived from the genotype and the prenatal and early postnatal influences, but exclusive of the learning acquired through interpersonal experiences. Representing as it does the reactive potentialities of the individual, constitution is important in determining modes of behavior which are considered basic to the personality. Constitutional factors and predispositions must, however, be regarded as highly complex and as yet poorly understood.

In the opinion of some psychiatrists, the incidence of manic-depressive psychosis is higher among pyknics, and schizophrenia is more common among the leptosomic, the athletic, and the dysplastic types.

Sheldon has offered from his extensive studies of recent years not only a statement of three basic somatotypes but also a means of defining a series of intermediate variants. His basic types, the *endomorphic,* the *mesomorphic* and the *ectomorphic,* are very similar to Kretschmer's pyknic, leptosomic, and athletic types. Thus he states that the endomorphic relates to such viscerotonic temperaments as relaxation, physical comfort, and sociability; the mesomorphic to the somatotonic characteristics of assertiveness, energy, and competitiveness; and the ectomorphic to his cerebrotonic characteristics of restraint, sensitivity, and tendency to privacy.

Although various studies seem to suggest that endomorphy is statistically related to the occurrence of the manic-depressive reactions, mesomorphy to the sociopathies, and ectomorphy to schizophrenia, the bodily constitution of adults does not achieve clinical diagnostic value.

From recognition of the long-continuing dynamic of personality evolution in the family and the local culture, one must recognize that his affectively toned perceptions and conceptions of his body, that is, his image of his body, play the major role in determinating individual psychopathological responses. Yet the variation in body build may correlate with as yet unknown biologically determined biochemical reactivity that predisposes to certain personality disorders.

Probably of major significance as related to the concept of constitution is the accumulating evidence from animal research that prenatal maternal stimulation and such postnatal experiences as extent of handling in infancy and differential group social exposures establish lifelong patterns of bodily resistance to stress in terms of adrenocortical reactivity, as well as determining to some extent the emotionality of each individual.

Heredity

Each stage of development is determined by the interaction of hereditary and environmental forces. Since the earlier stages influence the character of the development of late stages, the hereditary and environmental factors interpenetrate more and more as development proceeds until finally this interplay becomes so complex and complete that the several factors cannot be separated. Nor is there yet adequate knowledge concerning the relationship between heredity and the psychophysiological processes of development.

Before attributing a mental disorder to heredity, the psychiatrist should recall that parents frequently transmit their emotional difficulties to the next generation, not through their germ cells but through the influence of their neuroses on the child. In most cases of mental illness in a parent, one can presuppose a prolonged period of maladjustment with difficulties and inconsistencies in personal relationships which preclude the existence of a home atmosphere conducive to healthy emotional growth and future mental health. A failure to find gratification of psychological needs in one generation may also be reflected in the behavior of the next, with the result that difficulty of adaptation and social misbehavior may follow through several generations. The patient has been conditioned by his interpersonal emotional experiences with parents and siblings; his parents, in turn, were conditioned by their experiences with their parents. Neurotic patterns have been communicated from one generation to another rather than inherited. A negative and hostile relationship toward parent or sibling may carry over and transfer negative, hostile psychopathogenetic feelings toward persons who stand in a parental or sibling role. Whatever may be the contribution of heredity in relation to mental disorder, therefore, the postnatal influences and growing-up experiences are important in determining personality structure and pattern.

Up to the present time, knowledge as to a hereditary predisposition to major mental disorders is incomplete, and opinions must remain subject to revision. It must be said, however, that the investigations of Kallmann on the familial occurrence of schizophrenia and manic-depressive psychosis are suggestive. Kallmann found that schizophrenia occurs much more frequently in families which include a known and hospitalized case of schizophrenia than it does in the general population. He found that the average expectancy in any group of persons who are not characterized by blood relationship to a schizophrenia case is 0.85 per cent but that the children of one schizophrenic parent have a probability of developing the disease which is 19 times that of the general population. Kallmann reported that the morbidity rate among the children of two schizophrenic parents is about 80 times the average expectancy. Among uni-ovular twins of such parents the concordance rate—i.e., the occurrence or nonoccurrence of the disease in *both* twins—is 85.8 per cent.

Later twin studies by others using twin pairs from general population groups, rather than from schizophrenic twin pairs discovered in hospitals as in the Kallmann studies, showed an incidence rate of schizophrenia (1.1 per cent) equal to that in the general population, whereas the rate of concordance for schizophrenia was much lower in the general population samples. Yet it remained three times higher than the rate in dizygotic twins. Also, the nonschizophrenic co-twins in the monozygotic group had a four times higher incidence of psychiatric diagnosis than did the dizygotic (30 per cent compared to 7 per cent). These studies confirm Kallman's position that the genetic factor plays a significant predisposing role in schizophrenia.

Of course, the influence of inheritance in the determination of psychopathology is directly expressed in the inborn errors of metabolism which lead to cerebral maldevelopment and consequently mental retardation. While phenylpyruvic oligophrenia is the classic example of such a condition, in recent years a considerable number of defects in amino acid, lipid, and sugar metabolism have been identified. In phenylpyruvic oligophrenia, as well as in certain other of the inborn errors of metabolism, the brain maldevelopment may be avoided by modifying the diet of the growing infant.

Nor are the genetic defects determined solely by transmission of dominant or recessive genic factors. In the past decade several varieties of mental deficiency, of which Down's syndrome, or mongolism, is the most important, have been shown to be associated with improper splitting of the chromosomes during meiosis, leading to more than the usual number of chromosomes or to the distortion of certain chromosomes. The conditions described in the past two paragraphs are discussed in Chapter 30.

The complex way in which genes may affect a behavioral trait is well demonstrated from the study of human populations and their variable taste sensitivity for such bitter compounds as the thioureas. Those who are sensitive tasters of these bitter substances find more foods objectionable; therefore their behavior in selecting and enjoying a wide range of food preparations and their responses to foods differ from those of the less sensitive. This genic influence is now known to be exerted upon the salivary system; there is no evidence of any direct influence upon the central nervous system and the perceptive apparatus. Those who are less sensitive or insensitive to the bitter quality secrete saliva which rapidly oxidizes the thioureas. The genetic factor determining this trait is also linked to other glandular functions: those with nodular goiters, athyreotic cretins and their parents, and the fathers of a sample of children with mongolism are insensitive to the bitter taste of these agents.

Prevalence of Mental Disorders

Various efforts have been made in numerous areas of the world to ascertain the percentage of persons who have developed mental illness requiring treatment, have been so treated in the past, or suffer such disturbances but remain untreated. Rates of prevalence vary widely from one survey to another; this variability is dependent undoubtedly on the methods of data collection, the sensitivity to occurrence of mental illness existing in both medical and nonmedical personnel in differing states and countries, and the criteria for establishing diagnoses.

Much more agreement is discovered on examination of the prevalence rates for psychotic reactions. Thus in a survey conducted in Baltimore in 1936, the prevalence rate for all psychoses in a local district was 6.7 per 1000 and for the psychoneuroses, 4.3 per 1000. A later survey in 1957 in the same city gave rates for the psychoses as 4.3 and the psychoneuroses as 5.26 per 1000. In England, a survey of the medical practitioners showed 4.8 per cent of the population at risk had sought advice for a psychoneurotic condition within a 12-month period, while 0.4 per cent also were seen for a psychosis or some other personality disorder. In another study in a new English housing estate 22 per cent of the population at risk were estimated to have psychoneurotic symptoms but only a portion had sought medical advice. Prevalence rates of psychological disorders as given in the Midtown Study are much higher because of the inclusion of all who reported in replies to questionnaires symptoms considered to be indicative of mental disorder. Thus in the Midtown Study 81.5 per cent of respondents to a questionnaire were judged to be "less than well," but only 23.4 per cent were placed in the "impaired group," a figure which correlates reasonably with other surveys concerning individuals who seek or have received treatment for their distress.

Dohrenwend's studies have demonstrated the methodological problems of questionnaire surveys of presumed symptoms of mental disorder. General physicians will record many such symptoms as occurring as the result of physical disease. Psychiatrists who directly interview patients considered to be psychiatrically disordered on the basis of analysis of their responses to questionnaires, will find many to be less impaired or not impaired. Certain ethnic groups exhibit predetermined bias in response to certain questions. The modern questionnaire administered by other than a physician trained in psychiatry and unsupported by the findings of a physical examination overlooks many physical, psychological, and social factors which determine response rate.

Cooper et al., reporting from England, recently found the mean annual prevalence rate for psychiatric morbidity of persons visiting medical practitioners to be 60 per 1000 for males and 72 per 1000 for females—not unlike earlier findings from this country.

For generations, speculation had centered on the question of whether mental illness was increasing in the population. The major support for the argument has rested upon the increasing number of persons in the United States certified to the state mental hospitals. Thus, in the United States in 1904 there were 183.6 persons out of every 100,000 in these hospitals, whereas by 1950 this number had increased to 381. Since the introduction of modern methods of treatment, such as the psychopharmaceutical agents, and also the adoption of changes in statutes pertaining to certification, as well as the humanization of hospitals with the "open-door" policies, there has been a dramatic drop in the population of these hospitals. On the other hand, short term hospitalization in the psychiatric services of general hospitals has risen rapidly as has registration of psychiatric patients in outpatient departments and day and night hospitals.

Increase in rate of hospitalization cannot be accepted as an indication of a trend toward increase in the occurrence of mental disorders. With the provision of more adequate facilities for the care and treatment of the mentally ill, and also with a changing attitude of the general public toward revealing the existence of emotional disturbances, more individuals enter or register as patients in the various psychiatric facilities. The single area in which there appears to be a major increase in recognized illness occurs in the admissions of the elderly to hospitals. Thus, the admissions of persons suffering from cerebral arteriosclerosis or senile psychosis to the state mental hospitals are related to increased longevity and the resulting increase of persons in the upper age brackets. Even here, the increase in hospitalization in the state mental institutions, which has amounted to a six-fold increase in a 35-year period in New York State, is not necessarily evidence to support the speculation that mental illness is increasing in the population. Rather it represents a shift in the age distribution of the population with exposure of the increasingly large incidence of illness in the senium and a failure to provide alternative facilities for the care of such persons. In states where such alternative facilities have been made available, the hospitalization rates for the aged to state mental institutions have been greatly reduced.

Where mortality rates among psychiatric patients at large are examined (hospitalized and nonhospitalized), as in the Babigian and Odoroff study, their relative risk is shown to be two and one half to three times that of the comparable general population. Although the chronically ill, aged, and alcoholic contribute excessively to the risk, even with their removal this patient population has a greater risk than the comparable population.

Age

Psychoses are rare until adolescence, when their incidence rises sharply and continues to show a definite upward trend with the advance of age. This rate of increase is especially sharp at the older age levels. In the northeastern part of the United States, over 30 per cent of those admitted for the first time to public hospitals for mental diseases are 60 or more years of age. In proportion to the population, more than five times as many persons enter hospitals for mental disorders at the age of 80 as at the age of 20. As indicated, psychoses are uncommon among children. Those which occur at that age tend to be strongly influenced by situational and psychological tensions.

The critical points in development of adolescence, involution, and senility bring not only physical changes but also new psychological problems. The rapid increase of psychoses in adolescence is due to many causes. As mentioned in previous chapters, there is an incongruity between various phases of personality growth;

there is the new problem of the integration of sex into the personality pattern. There are also social and employment problems and those of emancipation from parents. The involutional period brings an increase in mental disorders, due, in part, to declining activity of the endocrine and reproductive glands and to other degenerative involutional changes, but more often to the frustrations, threats, and other problems which the patient then meets. It has been suggested that the age at which a person develops mental disorder is an index of his frustration or conflict tolerance. After the age of 60, there is a distinct increase of emotional disorders, to which insecurity is apparently a contributing factor. The increase in mental disorder at the senium is largely due to the degenerative processes which may occur in the higher cortical neurons in old age; yet in some instances it is due to the fact that the changes in psychological situations which arise at that time cannot be met successfully. Sometimes, for example, the fact that an individual has to be supported by children, or by children-in-law, or by others arouses hostile feelings which are productive of psychosomatic or neurotic symptoms. Since one-half of the population in the United States lives past the age of 65, the incidence of senile and arteriosclerotic mental disease is high. Omitting diseases of the senium, the occurrence of mental disorder reaches a peak in the 40's and then drops sharply.

Sex

More men than women are admitted to hospitals for mental disorders, the ratio among first admissions being six men to five women; however, because of the greater longevity of women, there are more women than men in public mental hospitals. As indicated earlier, more women than men with psychiatric disability contact physicians in office and clinic practice. General paresis, alcoholic psychoses, traumatic psychoses, psychoses with epilepsy, and psychoses with cerebral arteriosclerosis are more frequent in men. Manic-depressive psychoses, involutional melancholia, paranoia, and psychoses with somatic disease are more frequent in women. Schizophrenia appears to be a little more frequent in women.

Race

Although American studies that report rates of treated patients using beds in psychiatric hospitals have shown a greater utilization by Negroes, Fischer and others emphasize the dubiousness of assuming that one may draw the conclusion of greater incidence of mental disorders among blacks than whites in this country or elsewhere. Such rates are derived only from known hospitalized and treated patients; the ratios to be derived from total populations remain unavailable. Also, rates require knowledge of available facilities for treatment. What is known today is the great disparity of such facilities in urban and rural areas where large black populations reside. In the former, many blacks are recent immigrants from backward rural areas. Also, the reported rates today vary as to whether prevalence or incidence is reported. Finally, studies of the processes of psychiatric hospitalizations and other institutionalizations have disclosed that those of lower socioeconomic status are less carefully examined and thereby more rapidly entered as admissions than are those in adequately staffed and readily available facilities. For the urbanized black in the United States this factor alone inflates admission rates to city and state hospital systems. When local facilities are available for diagnosis and immediate treatment, fewer are entered.

As to forms of mental illness, here again the various studies are highly divergent. Those from urbanized populations show that rates for psychoses among blacks— schizophrenic and alcoholic—are several times higher than among whites. Psychoneuroses are reported as less frequent, but again the less advantaged socioeconomic groups tend not to have available or to use facilities where such conditions are diagnosed or treated.

Definition of variable prevalence and incidence rates of psychiatric disorders in different races must await much more study, including extensive transcultural comparisons. Today, with vast internal migrations of populations worldwide to urban areas, the problem of relating rates of mental disorders to race alone has become exceedingly complex. Immigrant populations have been more subject to psychiatric hospitalizations than have stable populations. Such populations are usually disadvantaged in terms of communication and technical skills. Health, educational, and recreational services are limited. Family life is difficult owing to overcrowding, and malnutrition is frequent.

Beyond that, interracial tension and derogation, now termed *racism,* play a significant role in impairment of stable personality development. The evidence suggests that the black minorities in largely white industrialized societies suffer most. The blacks are often as well educated as the neighboring white groups and other immigrant groups, and the derogatory attitudes of the majorities have produced discrimination in opening all aspects of society to the blacks in a greater degree. Thus they remain selectively deprived as regards social recognition, positions of prestige and power, jobs, and equal opportunity to participate in all aspects of social life.

As a result of subjection to the long-continued attitudes of slave masters or their successors with racist attitudes, there may develop in the personality of some the variety of defenses against aggression described in the previous chapter: destructive or violent behaviors, or paranoid and regressive behaviors, including escapism into drug abuse. In others, reaction formations emerge, with undue complaisance or passivity and, for men, failures in sexual identity, including homosexuality, promiscuity, or impotence. Affectively, chronic depression with hopelessness is common. Upon personalities predisposed through cultural denigration and conflict to emergence of these personality features, additional stress is more likely to produce ego disorganizaion and emergence of frank psychiatric disability.

Environment: Familial, Social, and Cultural Factors

The environment in which an individual lives is much more than a physical world; it consists of the close interpersonal interaction within the family group and the pressures imposed upon this group by the wider culture and its particular value systems, as well as the influence of socioeconomic forces depending upon the class structure of the society in which the individual and his family live. In recent years the family unit has become a subject of special study. Ackerman now differentiates eight different types of family structure in American society.

It remains to determine whether there is a specific relationship between variety of family structure to forms of psychopathology. It is maintained that the attempt to understand personality development solely in terms of the interaction of the individual with past aspects of parents or others fails to provide the structure for a comprehension of the development of the social roles which each person plays in his adult life. The social self is expressed in group actions and modified by them; it may or may not reinforce the goals and values the individual has established for the personal self.

Overt *incest* is an example of tension-reducing "acting out" in a dysfunctional family which, while maintaining the facade of the family structure, often contributes to serious psychopathology in the involved minor. Thus the incestuous relationship between a father and daughter, the type generally reported, may go on for prolonged periods unreported by a mother. The latter, usually a rejected daughter herself, has married a weak and ineffectual man whom she despises and eventually rejects. The daughter, victimized in the family, becomes the mother substitute, supporting the mother in her housework but giving in to the father whom she perceives has been turned away by her mother. In turn, the father, unrelieved in his sexual drives, sometimes seduced by the wife to incest, turns toward the daughter to maintain the family unity of importance to him. While the family unity may remain intact for considerable periods and the reporting of the act often occurs inadvertently when some outsider notes evidence of other maltreatment of children, the emotional consequences for the involved daughter as seen by psychiatrists are invariably those of guilty depression. Such daughters often have learning difficulties in school; they may become sexually promiscuous or develop psychosomatic symptoms. In their efforts to escape their guilt they deny the incestuous relationship, seek punishment through various masochistic drives, and overextend themselves to placate the mother to whom they are unconsciously hateful. When these psychological defenses are restricted the daughters often regress with psychotic behavior.

The means by which couples come together to form the future family then has bearing on understanding the etiology of mental disturbance. It appears that psychiatrically ill men and women find each other for marriage more frequently than by chance. Such matings will lead to mental illness in the children because there may be a greater potential for genetic predisposition or, more likely, because a family transactional environment is established that is conducive to development of personality aberrations.

Those who are studying families state that it is no longer possible to treat patients as individuals. There is no question that therapy of the individual without consideration for the family homeostasis often leads to its rupture, with the appearance of overt psychiatric disturbance in others than the original patient, or that treatment of the individual often founders owing to interference by other family members. On the other hand, there is much to show from individual therapy, which is fully cognizant of the dependent bonds between family members, that such pathologic bonds are seldom severed while the disturbed individual remains within the family group.

Spiegel and others, in studying the family in relation to mental illness and health, postulate that what goes on between the sick individual and his family takes place within a series of subsystems which include the individual, the family, the community, and the value systems of each. Within this transactional system the interests center more on those processes between the individual and his family which are considered pathologic in the larger community rather than on the narrower question of the interactions of the family members in relation to the pathology. Those working with the transactional method attempt to define strain as it exists in the culture, the family, and the individual and to relate each to the others. Much emphasis is placed on value systems and the conflicts which exist between those within the various units. These new working models remain to be tested as a means of adding to the effective knowledge valued in clinical practice.

That cultural factors influence the etiology and psychopathology of mental disorders is generally agreed on the basis of studies by cultural anthropologists and by psychiatrists who have worked with persons ill in different cultural groups. Within a lifetime, the clinical phenomenology of various psychotic reactions has changed. As an example, the megalomanic delusions of being Napoleon, so common in the nineteenth century, are seen no longer. Now patients who have such a need fall upon a character of this century or develop a messianic complex. In the United States the manic-depressive reactions are less prevalent than they were a quarter century ago, although they are common in the Scandinavian countries. Conversion hysteria is thought to be less common in Western culture; alcoholic psychoses are frequent in the Irish and uncommon in those of Jewish faith.

Since man learns his patterns of behavior within a family impressed with the codes of a constituted culture, it is not surprising to recognize this important source as a fluctuant factor, determining not only patterns of neurotic and psychotic illness but also their changing symptoms and frequencies over time. The demands of the social environment with its variable competitiveness, sexual repressions, and contradictory codes bring differing conflicts, individual frustrations, and dilemmas as these factors shape the adaptive capacities of the individual.

It is known that more patients per unit of population are admitted to public hospitals from urban than from rural communities. This is due, in part, to the fact that admissions vary inversely with the remoteness of the community from an institution for mental diseases. Alcoholic psychoses, general paresis, psychoses due to drugs, manic-depressive psychoses, paranoia, and psychoneuroses are more frequent in urban areas. Senile psychoses, psychoses with cerebral arteriosclerosis, involutional melancholia, and psychoses with mental deficiency occur with relatively greater frequency in rural regions. Schizophrenias occur with about equal frequency in urban and rural areas.

In Hollingshead and Redlich's studies on the influence of social class upon the occurrence of mental illness in New Haven, it was found that schizophrenia was found more frequently in families in the lowest socioeconomic classes as well as other disturbances indicative of super-ego defects. (Ninety-five per cent of persons in prison come from these classes.) On the other hand, obsessive-compulsive disorders are most common in the highest socioeconomic groups and oedipal conflicts in the middle group. Other studies have suggested, however, that the patient's social class is perhaps the consequence of the illness rather than evidence of influence of social class on its form.

One might expect that anxiety, open

and often unopposed aggression (including sexual aggression), lowered self-esteem, and limited opportunities for emotional and cognitive growth are more often the ways of life in the personality development in those reared in the lower socio-economic groups. In the higher social classes, in contrast, demands for conformity presumably lead to the expression of compulsive patterns of living.

Marital Status

Statistics show that mental disorder is more common among the single than among the married. While this may be due in part to the more stable and regular mode of life led by the married person with the accompanying sense of domestic responsibility, this is probably only a minor reason for the better mental health among married persons. It should be remembered that the marital association is one of the most important of all human associations. It provides not merely for the satisfaction of sexual urges but for various important securities, the absence or loss of which may be very disturbing to the personality. The feeling that one is desired as a marital partner, that one is appreciated and is the subject of interest and affection, contributes greatly to a sense of security. The security from loneliness, the emotional satisfaction of parenthood, and frequently, in women, the added sense of economic security add wholesome satisfactions. With marriage the individual may be compelled to adjust to a very different type of environment and to personal relationships quite foreign to those in which he was reared. Marriage and success in the responsibilities of marriage suggest great interpersonal adaptive capacities and personal esteem. The development of mental disorder before marriage naturally decreases the prospects of subsequent marriage; many whose affective and other personality limitations are so great that they are predisposed to mental disorders are never sought as partners.

Statistics show that there is a marked preponderance of mental disorder per unit of population among divorced persons. There are several reasons for the more frequent occurrence of mental disorders among this group. In many cases maladjustments representing early stages of mental disorder lead to domestic discord and divorce before the personality disturbances are sufficiently developed to be recognized as constituting mental disease. On the whole, divorced persons represent a group suffering from conflicts so unusual in both number and intensity that the high incidence of mental illness is not surprising. The same deep-seated mechanisms which tend to lead to marital discord also lead to psychosis or neurosis. It should be remembered, too, that marriage is a relationship which demands a most highly sustained adaptation. The unmarried person may have been unable to achieve the adult toughness necessary to stand the give and take of adjustment to marriage and parenthood. Perhaps she may have been unprepared for this adjustment because her parents before her had not been healthy models for identification as mates and parents. A mental illness may be precipitated by factors concerned with sexual functions such as anxiety with motherhood, pregnancy, or abortion. Parenthood often rekindles conflicts over dependency or early sibling competitiveness, arousing anxiety, rage, and aggression.

A person who has failed to reach a mature, heterosexual level but remained, even though unconsciously so, with a basic sex interest in persons of the same sex may be unable to establish an abiding harmonious partnership with one of the opposite sex. Usually there will be no physiological interference in the exercise of sex functions natural to his or her sex, but the emotional, dispositional tendency of sex expression is directed to a homosexual partner. The attempt to meet this conflict between emotionally determined and biologically determined impulses may be made by projection or other psychopathological mechanisms which eventuate in mental disorder.

Pregnancy

Mental disorder may be associated with pregnancy or the postpartum period. There are, however, no specific mental disorders related to either of these periods. Latent or repressed psychological material may, under the stress of maintaining physiological homeostasis and of the emotionally significant situation, prove too great for the patient's ego resources with the result that psychopathological reactions occur. What her pregnancy unconsciously means to the mother is of significance as is the birth of her child. Doubtless, it reanimates the patient's old attitudes toward her own mother and may revive old complexes of bodily harm or injury. Sometimes the patient expresses delusions indicating hostility for either the husband or the child, thus reflecting a conflict about married life or motherhood. Rejection of the child may be expressed by a delusion that it is dead, by abusive treatment of it, or by fear that something will happen to it.

Psychotic illness in association with pregnancy is rare; the expectancy is about 14 cases in 10,000 confinements. About 50 per cent of the mental illnesses associated with pregnancy or the postpartum period are schizophrenic, about 25 per cent are manic-depressive, and 20 per cent are psychoneurotic reactions.

The occurrence of such a reaction does not predispose to a similar reaction in a subsequent pregnancy. Almost one-half of such illnesses occur with the birth of a second or a later child, and the outlook for recovery is similar to that of the general reaction type. These disorders occur with the same frequency in the postpartum setting as they do in any other setting.

Pregnancy, too, may induce psychophysiological symptoms in the father through arousal of anxiety. Trethowan has found that as many as 10 per cent of fathers report symptoms which in many respects are similar to those of the expectant mother: nausea, morning sickness, perversion of appetite, and sometimes abdominal bloating. So, too, toothache is common and has been recognized as such in historical accounts of the *couvade syndrome:* the paternal identification with the maternal role.

Occupation and Work Load

Aside from brain syndromes due to toxic substances to which individuals may be exposed as a consequence of the occupation (lead, particularly), occupation does not determine or precipitate personality disorders.

Overwork was formerly ascribed an important place in the etiology of mental disorders. It is now generally held, however, that so far as unusual application to work constitutes exhausting effort it is a symptom of mental disorder rather than a cause. The compulsive neurotic may work excessively hard, his job serving as a means of reducing anxiety and of support. Work may be the only outlet for an otherwise creative person. It may also in some instances serve as a neurotic outlet for aggression. It may give strong ego support through success or prestige to a person besieged with feelings of inferiority. For the withdrawn person, work may be his chief means of contacting others in a nonthreatening manner. Finally, satisfying work is important for mental health. It brings such healthy gratifications as creative expression, companionship, and a feeling of accomplishment.

The mental disorder, as recognized by the patient's family, may have been preceded by unaccustomed effort, but if a complete knowledge of the motivating forces is available, we should discover that the unusual assiduity represented an attempted flight from conflicts and problems for which satisfactory and successful solutions had not been reached. It should undoubtedly be conceded that fatigue may at times weaken the controlling strength of the ego. Probably the factors in modern life productive of nervous and mental disorder lie less in overwork, in the speed and stress of work, or in the distraction of noise and the like than in dissatisfaction, insecurity, distasteful work, and lack of incentive.

Anxiety-inducing situations, such as inability to accept the authority of competent superiors or to suppress dependent longings and demands, often lead to breakdowns or failures at work in groups. The competition for advancement with the mobilization of envy, or the fear of others' envy by the dependent person who has been advanced to a position of responsibility, sometimes precipitates emotional disturbance; an example would be the case of a dependent vice-president advanced to presidency and fearful of facing the envy and loss of acceptance by his former peers. Failures to receive advancement also mobilize aggressive fears that may precipitate disorder. There is evidence that mental effort in the presence of emotional stress and tension can produce either neurotic or psychotic reactions. There is only limited justification for the pessimistic suggestion frequently made that the pace of modern life conduces to mental breakdown.

Again, retirement from an occupation is now known to produce anxiety in many. Here, with the giving up of work, stress arises from the loss of prestige and of being valued by others, and frequently from isolation from old companions.

Alcohol

The role of alcohol in the production of mental disease is complex, and, while in some respects our ideas are becoming clarified, there are still many unknown and variable factors. That there is a direct relation between the amount of alcohol drunk in a community and the incidence of psychoses classified statistically in the alcoholic group is certain, as shown by experience in the United States during the past third of a century. In 1920, immediately following the enactment of the prohibition amendment, the number of first admissions for alcoholic psychoses

to New York State hospitals for mental diseases per 100,000 of general population fell to 1.2. This rate gradually increased to 7.1 in 1941, decreased until 1945, and has again continued to rise since World War II. During the three years (1919 through 1921) of relatively successful observance of the prohibition amendment to the Constitution there were 720 first admissions with alcoholic psychoses to all hospitals for mental disease in New York State. The total of such first admissions increased to 2013 in 1929 through 1931 and reached 3132 in 1939 through 1941, since which time there has been no appreciable change per unit of population.

The more carefully the history of a patient suffering from a chronic form of mental disorder is studied, the more frequently it will be found that any associated alcoholism is either a symptom of the psychosis or another method of dealing with the same personality problems which contributed to the mental disorder rather than an essential cause of it. The role of avitaminosis in producing a psychosis in the chronic alcoholic must be borne in mind.

Physical Defects

Physical anomalies or disturbances not caused by endocrine dysfunction, yet ones which occasionally provoke resentment and other undesirable psychological reactions, particularly of a compensatory, aggressive, or other defensive nature, are genital deformities, clubbed feet, scoliosis, kyphosis, and congenital defects of vision and hearing. Cleft palate, also, tends to create a sense of inability to meet social situations and to lead to feelings of inferiority and insecurity, again expressed in derogatory attitudes to one's self and body. Children with congenital or acquired defects develop feelings about the defects partly because of the way they see other people reacting to them. If others about them react with repugnance, revulsion, or abhorrence, so too will the child regard his deformity. Adolescence is the period in which physical defects are most apt to evoke unwholesome psychological reactions. It must be said, however, that the personalities of individuals having physical defects are not always affected by such handicaps.

Physical Illnesses

Acute physical illnesses with an associated toxic state frequently lead to an acute brain syndrome with an accompanying delirious state but are rarely directly responsible for neuroses or the so-called functional psychoses. Chronic illness, however, with its handicaps, frustrations, and unhealthy methods of attempting to surmount them, is a severe stress. The patient with a physical illness is confronted with two types of problems for which he must mobilize a variety of defenses and mechanisms of adaptation: (a) problems, largely conscious, related to the realities of the pain, inability to make a living, and handicaps imposed on or by his family, and (b) problems arising from emotional needs and from the activation of hitherto repressed unconscious conflicts. These are discussed in Chapter 25 in the section on Disturbances of the Image of the Body. There will be noted a relationship between the psychological symptoms released by the ego-weakening effect of the illness and the premorbid personality of the patient. Physical illness, then, may precipitate or aggravate neurotic or psychotic trends in the personality. Thus recognition and correction of such illnesses or disabilities are of paramount importance in both prevention and treatment of the personality disorders.

General Cerebral Dysfunction

It was formerly assumed that every mental disease was due to cerebral disease and that a psychosis without disease of the brain did not exist; it was also assumed that specific brain lesions were accompanied by special mental symptoms. While in some instances of mental disorder an associated disease of the brain is known to exist, in most instances there is not, so far as our present knowledge goes, any cerebral pathology. Even when mental symptoms accompany disease of the brain, they cannot be explained by considering the location of the brain pathology alone.

Mental symptoms arising from general dysfunction of the brain are dependent to a large extent on whether the brain disorder is of an acute or chronic nature, and, if chronic, whether the involvement is diffuse or circumscribed. The resulting symptom pattern tends, therefore, to fall into one of three types: an acute organic syndrome; a chronic syndrome due to a diffuse lesion; and a chronic syndrome due to a localized lesion. The acute organic reaction is the result of temporary, reversible, diffuse impairment of brain tissue function and is characterized by a disturbance of consciousness, difficulty of apperception, somnolence, coma, and cloudy and delirious states. The disturbance of the sensorium may release hallucinations and poorly organized transient delusions.

Chronic organic brain syndromes result from relatively permanent, usually irreversible, diffuse impairment of cerebral tissue function. The chronic brain syndrome may vary in degree of progress but usually some disturbance of memory, judgment, orientation, comprehension, and affect persists permanently. Frequently the organic syndrome is colored by the patient's individual personality with its particular conscious and unconscious impulses, fears, and wishes. The causes of general brain dysfunction are trauma, infection, toxic states, metabolic disturbances, and various deprivational states.

Trauma

Trauma of the head, with lesions ranging from a diffuse but minute separation of neuron structure through edema and hemorrhage to destruction of brain tissue with subsequent scar formation, may be followed by varying defects of mentation. The clinical picture is usually at first that of an acute brain syndrome. If the impairment of brain function is persistent, the clinical picture becomes that of the chronic organic brain syndrome with a permanent impairment of mental function.

Trauma of any part of the body may be reacted to, usually after a latent period, by a traumatic neurosis.

Infections

Of all infections, syphilis still plays the most active part in causing mental disease. The most common psychosis resulting from such infection is that associated with syphilitic meningoencephalitis (general paresis), which accounts now for less than 2 per cent of all first admissions to public mental hospitals in the United States. During the past 25 years there has been a constant decrease in the relative prevalence of syphilis with a resulting decrease in general paresis. Also, the treatment for general paresis is now begun much more promptly and carried out much more efficiently.

Toxic Agents

Certain chemicals and drugs may give rise to acute brain syndromes, not infrequently in the nature of a delirium of brief duration, although occasionally a delirious state of such an origin may continue for several weeks. The agents most frequently implicated in producing mental symptoms are bromides, barbituric acid derivatives, sulfa drugs, morphine, cocaine, marijuana, thiocyanates, and lead. In the last decade there has been a pronounced increase in the number of patients treated for personality disturbances due to use of the amphetamines and the hallucinogenic agent d-lysergic acid diethylamide-25.

Endocrine Disturbances

Abnormal functionings of the endocrine glands will undoubtedly influence personality functioning through disturbing bodily functions. Such disorders, for example, may lead to changes in general efficiency of bodily functions with resulting feelings of frustration or insecurity. Occasionally neuroendocrinal dystrophies produce biological defects which make the individual conspicuous in physical appearance and lead to a disturbance in his body concept or image. The dissimilarity between the patient's concept and the change in his body induced by the endocrine disturbance contributes to self-consciousness, which favors the development of defensive and compensatory mechanisms that distort the personality and render adaptation more difficult. Certain endocrine deficiencies are known to lead to cognitive impairment. Thus cretinism is often associated with mental retardation, and hypothyroidism in midlife leads as well to impaired functioning and associated personality disturbance.

Deprivations and Deficiencies

Lack of the basic bodily needs (oxygen, nutrition and fluids, sleep, perceptual stimulation), if sufficiently great or prolonged, may lead to serious constitutional deficits if they occur in the developmental period. Later in life such deprivations act as important etiologic factors in the determinations of various brain syndromes and in precipitating or complementing the primary psychogenic disorders.

OXYGEN DEPRIVATION. Beyond all other bodily organs and tissues the brain is the most susceptible to dysfunction and structural damage as the consequence of oxygen lack. Developmental defects and later behavioral changes are a regular accompaniment of hypoxia from whatever cause. Cerebral hypoxia in the perinatal period, inferred on the basis of clinical observation and now established by experimental studies, leads to profound defects in development from which result both mental retardation and personality disorder as well as physical defects.

In later life, transient or chronic hypoxia, as the consequence of acute oxygen lack at high altitudes, asphyxia, cerebral ischemia following arteriolar spasm, infarction, or cardiovascular failure, chronic pulmonary disease such as emphysema, anemia, or poisoning by carbon monoxide and other cellular poisons, if severe, produces the symptomatology of general cerebral insufficiency (the brain syndrome).

A drop in arterial oxygen saturation to 85 per cent which persists over a period of two or three hours has been shown to lead in otherwise healthy persons to hyperpnea, fatigue, headache, and lassitude followed by difficulty in concentration and impairment of emotional control. Depending upon the personality of the individual, the oxygen-deprived individual may become over-confident and elated and demonstrate judgmental defects in interpersonal contacts expressed in undue irritability and aggressive behavior toward others, whereas others become increasingly dull and depressed. Impaired emotional control is one of the finer indices of cerebral anoxia; evidence of it occurs long before difficulties in performance of routine tasks, psychological tests, or changes in the electroencephalogram. Under ordinary conditions of stress, healthy men exposed to hypoxia at the level of 85 per cent arterial oxygen saturation lose emotional control without warning and respond with unexpected truculence to verbal challenges directed to their superego values in the sexual or aggressive areas.

Prolonged ischemic anoxia is probably the major etiologic factor in the organic brain syndromes associated with arteriosclerosis. Whether the diminution of oxygen utilization found with the senile psychosis is representative of a primary anoxic defect or is secondary to the neuronal loss found with this condition is not known.

Cerebral hypoxia occurs with the use of convulsive therapy. It is known that the structure and probably the function of the most recently developed areas of the brain are most impaired through oxygen lack; thus the frontal lobe cortex often shows pathological damage when other areas appear healthy on examination with cellular stains.

LACK OF NUTRITION. Nutritional deprivation has profound effects on personality in terms of drive states, mood, and performance. The consequences of primary nutritional deprivation may come to the attention of the physician as in the case of those starved during the great wars or those suffering from brain syndromes as the consequence of vitamin deficiencies. More frequently encountered are the secondary states of semi-starvation which occur in depressions, some schizophrenias, and anorexia nervosa.

Prenatal malnutrition caused by starvation or a limitation of the mother's diet will impair brain and bodily growth. Thus nutritionally deprived populations or the poverty stricken will produce infants and children disadvantaged as far as brain development is concerned, compared to those populations in which maternal nutrition is adequately maintained.

The studies of experimental semi-starvation in man have shown well the subjective changes which this state induces and which may complicate the primary phenomenology of any illness. In addition to the weight loss, fatigue increases steadily. There takes place an increasing preoccupation with food, including frequent simple wish-fulfilling food visions and dreams. Increasing appetite, muscle soreness, irritability, apathy, and sensitivity to noises gradually appear, with feeling of loss of drive and ability to control oneself associated with a diminution in attentiveness and ability to concentrate. The sexual drive becomes progressively weaker. Lack of interest in the attractive sex partner, disappearance of masturbation and seminal emissions, and diminution of the sperm count follow in men and amenorrhea in women. Recovery of these functions in previously healthy men semistarved on a 1600 calorie diet for 24 weeks has required a full six weeks of re-feeding.

As observed during wartime, starvation leads to personality changes; meanness, secretiveness, and suspiciousness emerge associated with social withdrawal. In the early period of starvation there are a general lowering of moral standards and a drive for other gratifications. Some wish to be cared for like children, become emotionally labile and impulsive, and develop enuresis and interest in feces and anal functions. If food deprivation continues, aggressive impulses, sucking activity, and oral interest appear to be subsequently superseded by apathy and eventually the symptoms of general cerebral insufficiency.

LACK OF VITAMINS.   Specific vitamin deficiencies are known to produce encephalopathic syndromes resulting from metabolic or organic disturbances in the cerebrum. Pellagra and Wernicke's syndrome are among the most clearly recognized of the deficiency reactions. Brain syndromes rather than disorders of psychogenic origin usually occupy the foreground in personality disturbances associated with these deficiencies, although trends that have been developed for dealing with anxiety-producing situations may be revealed.

SLEEP DEPRIVATION.   Continuous lack of sleep, as has been demonstrated by numerous studies on healthy young people, produces deterioration in personality functioning, expressed in unpleasant subjective experiences as well as changes in appearance, speech, mood, perception, and thought. Whether these changes are due solely to lack of sleep or to the associated muscular fatigue or even associated dream deprivation is not known. When a person is deprived of sleep, his prolonged attention to any task gradually diminishes and is associated with increasing restlessness, apathy, and inability to concentrate. Lapses of ongoing behavior or periods of extreme drowsiness or sleep take place in which delays or actual breaks occur in the performance of tasks, even though the

situation is perceived by the nonsleeper as requiring action and a response. He may lose his contact with the immediate situation and confuse external and internal events. Thus a dream or intrusive thought becomes attached to the outward situation, and the faulty sleeper suffers a distortion of perception. Over a period of time, lack of sleep leads to misperceptions which range from changes in the shape, size, movement, texture, or color of objects to misbelieving and misperceiving them. Such misperceptions at times appear to be hallucinations. Temporal disorientation gradually appears. Initially time seems to pass slowly, while later the sleep-deprived subject makes first occasional and then frequent errors in designating time to the point where eventually he is unshakingly deluded. His cognitive process suffers as well, as evidenced by infrequent lapses of thought or speech with limited lack of sleep; with further lack of sleep, these lapses extend to loss of the train of thought, incompletion of statements, forgetting, and eventually rambling and incoherent verbalizations, with inability to recognize errors or make corrections. Lack of sleep gives rise frequently to a bandlike sensation about the head, the "hat illusion," while there are often other subjective experiences reflecting feelings of change in the self or the body—feelings of not being oneself, of strangeness, which may be classified as depersonalization.

Associated with sleep lack, physiological depression takes place in muscle tone, body temperature, sweating, and capacity to respond to noxious stimuli. Increased pulmonary ventilation takes place as a means of removing the greater blood carbon dioxide and lactate. Some studies have demonstrated modest activation of the pituitary-adrenocortical system with disruption of its circadian rhythm, as well as a variable increase in catecholamine biosynthesis, as a result of sleep deprivation.

With increasing prolongation of sleep deprivation the electroencephalogram shows a progressive diminution in the alpha rhythm and the development of a dominant slow wave activity. Nor does opening or closing of the eyes lead to enhancement of the alpha waves. Judging from the responses of organs controlled by the autonomic nervous system, sleep deprivation is associated with a progressive decrease in responsiveness to external stimulation but at the same time a persisting tendency to greater autonomic activity.

Prolonged wakefulness then may be interpreted as leading to decreased capacity for arousal and the emergence of a variety of psychopathological behaviors. It is evident that the sleep cycle must be preserved in order to sustain healthy behavior or to prevent the secondary complications due to oxygen deprivation with insomnia in the course of pulmonary illness.

During the recovery period after prolonged sleep deprivation there is an initial increase in both slow (nondreaming) and REM (dreaming) sleep on the first night. A relative increase in REM sleep may be noted for several nights thereafter.

LACK OF DREAMS.   Dream deprivation also has been examined recently. While it is not possible today to separate the consequences of lack of sleep from lack of dreams, the effects of the latter are of significance psychologically.

In a typical night's sleep, there occur four or five periods of dreaming which account for 20 per cent of the total sleep time. In experiments performed by Dement in which the subjects were awakened briefly on four to seven consecutive nights when they were observed to show the eye movements and characteristic accompanying low-voltage, non-spindling electroencephalographic pattern noted only during dreaming, it was observed that the amount of dreaming increased during nights after dream deprivation. Also, the healthy experimental subjects became anxious and irritable and showed difficulty in concentration in performing daytime tasks during the period of nightly dream deprivation. Some were noted, as well, to develop an increase in appetite associated with weight gain during this period. Dreaming sleep may represent a physiological drive state that is significant in maintaining the psychological homeostasis of the organism.

It has been suggested that the so-called toxic effects of drugs such as the amphetamines which specifically suppress REM sleep are due to the suppression of this portion of the sleep cycle.

SENSORY DEPRIVATION.   A series of clinical investigations during the recent years gives strong support to the hypothesis that a steady state of sensory stimulation or "input" is necessary to support the usual ego functions. As early as 1819 Dupuytren described delirious reactions with hallucinatory and emotional disturbance which occurred in the period following cataract extractions when the eyes were covered. Since the experimental studies of Cameron, it has been known that one factor causing senile nocturnal delirium is the loss of vision consequent to darkness.

The factor of lonely immobilization is thought to be responsible for the states of anxiety, disturbances in time sense, and delusional and hallucinatory experiences of some patients immobilized in respirators. It has been suggested that similar symptoms associated with alcoholism are caused, in fact, by isolation and reduction in sensory input. The factor of social isolation now is thought to contribute to "brain-washing" or "thought-reform" programs used by the Chinese with their war prisoners, to the prison psychoses, to the hallucinatory states of shipwrecked and lost persons, and perhaps also to the elaborations of the chronically hospitalized and isolated psychotic.

When healthy persons with no previous experimental experience are isolated, with vision and hearing diminished by the use of patches and ear plugs and with mobility limited after several hours, they experience anxiety and a desire for external stimulation and motor activity as well as difficulty in concentration, reduction in motivation, and progressive difficulty with directed thinking. After 72 hours in a few experiments they develop delusional and visual hallucinatory experiences. Following such experiences, visual disturbances continue for some time. They are reported as fluctuations, driftings, and swirlings of objects and surfaces in the visual field, associated with difficulty in fixing objects in space on eye or head movement, with distortions of margins, and exaggeration of contrasts and colors. During the deprivational experience, the electroencephalogram shows slower rhythms and slow wave activity.

During the deprivational experience the alpha rhythm of the electroencephalogam declines and there emerges increasing slow-wave activity which parallels the progressive impairment in ego functioning. It appears from some studies that the degree of electroencephalographic change is greater after deprivation of patterned visual and auditory stimuli than after limitation alone of light and sound.

The perceptual phenomena and other ego disruptions seem less likely to occur when some meaningful stimuli are present and when the deprived subject is allowed kinesthetic and tactile stimulation through movement. Personality plays a factor in determining the characteristics of the response, with exaggeration of the usual adaptations and defenses.

It appears that sensory deprivations during early life impose permanent developmental defects which impair later learning. As far as perceptual and kinesthetic learning is concerned, the proposition seems well established for man; the clinical observations on the children who failed to evolve good visual perception after corrections of congenital corneal defects by late transplantation of the cornea are fully supported by studies of artificial blinding of growing chimpanzees.

SOCIAL ISOLATION. Social or experiential deprivation in early life may well play a major role in many of the adult personality disorders. A mass of observations reported by child psychiatrists and animal psychologists shows that capacities for exploratory behavior, control of fear and anxiety, perception of pain and rec-

ognition of threat, somatic response to stress, effective sexual and child-rearing behavior, and affectional relations are impaired by isolation of developing young from others. As yet undetermined for the growing child and the young of other species are the critical maturational periods during which appropriate experience must take place in order to allow maturation of structure and related function. There exists now a scientific void relative to such questions as the quantity of experience required to allow full evolution of function and the ultimate capacity of the growing or adult organism to repair deficiencies or develop them through later learning.

It has been suggested that autism in children is the consequence of a deprivation of tactile and kinesthetic arousal through inadequate mothering in infants who are born with a lessened capacity for arousal due to some impairment in the function of the reticular activating system. In a family where parental fondling and body stimulation are limited, such infants presumably will develop with permanent deficits in their perceptual capacities. Also, the hypothesis has been offered that the primary deficit in the schizophrenias is lack of appropriate socialization during early life, causing a permanent incapacity to evolve mature patterns of interpersonal relations.

Poverty may be thought of as a form of social isolation, too. The relative lack of personal possession of material substances in itself does not necessarily predispose to or precipitate psychiatric illness. Many human groups live under materially deprived conditions as compared to others, yet there is little evidence that the forms or frequency of mental disease differ between the groups. When poverty is interpreted as limitation of emotional support in terms of the developmental process, even many children and others brought up in affluent families are disadvantaged.

Nevertheless, materially impoverished families in racial and cultural groups are exposed to a greater degree than others to the multitude of forces predisposing to and precipitating psychiatric disability. Malnutrition will affect maternal care, brain growth in the neonate, and physical development and susceptibility to illness of the infant and child. The various deprivations described heretofore probably operate to a greater degree for those in the often crowded, dirty conditions with limited access to education and intellectual stimulation in which the impoverished live. Such social conditions limit the potential for development of positive ego assets in trust, initiative, autonomy, and responsibility; at the same time, these conditions increase the affective drives which impair impulse control, allowing for continued expressions of aggression in destructive behavior to self and others, attitudes of mistrust, suspicion, hopelessness, and despair. The balance of the personality of those reared in conditions of poverty is likely to be warped negatively and predisposed toward personality disturbance.

Interpersonal Relationships

The earliest and some of the most dynamic stresses, which perhaps can later be met only by psychopathological techniques so disturbing to the happiness and efficiency of the individual or so disrupting to his social adjustment as to be regarded as mental disorder, arise from repetitive early interpersonal relations and their stresses within the family. This is not surprising, since human relations are the sources of those powerful affects of pain, pleasure, love, hate, loneliness, sadness, guilt, jealousy, envy, security, and happiness. The arousal of certain of these affects is so impelling that the individual can neither repress nor accept them without anxiety or emotional disturbance.

Of all interpersonal relations, that with the mother is frequently the most determinative of the future mental health of the individual. A strangling, perhaps guilt-ridden, over-protection on her part may prevent the child from developing a mature, independent personality. Again, the maternal relationship may fail to give the warmth, security, and support necessary for the emotional and social growth of personality. Instead, for example, of providing a healthful emotional climate of affection, acceptance, and approval, the mother may to varying degrees reject or overprotect the child, with consequent misshaping of his developing personality. Such attitudes, which exist particularly among mothers who have been damaged emotionally by their own life experiences, are usually unconscious ones. Other attitudes, often covert or ambivalent, which may also be manifested by psychologically important persons, are hostility, aggression, dominance, sadism, and dependence. Out of such relations are established patterns of personality which are culturally so unacceptable that they are repressed and give rise to conflict and anxiety. Ambivalent attitudes, i.e., confusions of hostile and affectionate impulses, which had their origin in some childhood intrafamily relationship often continue to influence the personality pattern throughout later life and constitute unconsciously a conflictful problem which cannot be met except by psychopathological methods.

The absent father deprives sons of a figure for identification and daughters of the opportunity to socialize over time with a member of the opposite sex. A domineering, aggressive, or exploitative father may interact with a son so as to inhibit his potential for developing an assertive self-confident esteem; an overly passive father may fail to provide the admired and loved focus for a mature masculine identification.

Divorce, too, serves as an emotional crises for the growing child. The loss of one or the other parent precipitates anxiety, grief, or depression, often acted out in release of aggressively destructive behavior.

Much of adult behavior is determined to a considerable degree by events which took place in the preverbal age period or through later unresolved childhood conflicts. The *anlage* of many neuroses and of other personality difficulties and characteristics is found in the prolonged experiences of early childhood. Early tension-laden relationships with parents seem to be particularly apt to be pathogenetic. Interpersonal situations in later life awaken previous feelings and unresolved difficulties and lead to the reënactment of problems generated in prior relationships. Difficulties in these relationships are therefore both expressions and sources of personality disturbances. Not only may aggression and hostility arise out of family relationships, but many other fixed emotional reactions, such as feelings of insecurity, rejection, guilt, dependency, overprotection, and jealousy, are acquired in response to repetitive early interpersonal experiences.

Bereavement

Through the close and intimate contact of the infant and young child with the mother, there is laid down the basic sense of security and trust upon which the child is able to face separation and its attending loneliness and to seek an autonomous identity. Meeting the early dependent needs of the child through mothering lays the groundwork for a healthy personality.

GRIEF REACTION. A bereavement by separation or death is followed by a train of events which are well known. Initially the young child protests by crying or other aggressive behavior, only after some hours to pass through a phase of hopelessness and withdrawal with inactivity. This is succeeded some time later by behavior characterized by detachment, with an unwillingness to resume the relationship if the lost person reappears. While detachment may be superseded in time, repeated separations lead to an effort at personal isolation from others, motivated, perhaps, as a protection from recurrent anxiety. In older children it is clear that the first phase of anxious protest is accompanied as well by rage. Children deprived of

mothering early in childhood either suffer inordinately when separated from significant people due to paralyzing nostalgias, or later may be hungry for dependent relationships. They sometimes develop a protective, isolated defense as a form of pseudoindependence to prevent a repetition of despair and hopelessness.

For adolescents and adults the awareness of one's own impending death or that of another presents a life crisis attended by major emotional response. This awareness arouses the fundamental anxiety of life—the basic anxiety of fear of the unknown with its related deep sense of helplessness. Also, there emerge the fears of loneliness, of loss of family and friends, of loss of one's body and identity, and of loss of self control.

Within the dying individual the crisis situation arouses all the anxieties of the past and mobilizes ego adaptations and the defenses evolved to cope with them: dependency, aggression, sexuality, and identity.

Since the parent of the same sex offers the model for identification that establishes impulse control through superego formation, the ideals for aspiration, and the sexual role, it is not surprising then that statistical studies demonstrate the more frequent occurrence in adulthood of psychotic, neurotic, and psychopathic behaviors in children reared in families broken by death, divorce, separation, or abandonment. Death of the mother before the child was 10 is found to have occurred more frequently in schizophrenics than in the general population. Death of a father before the child is 10 also exceeds the expected frequency in schizophrenic and manic-depressive psychoses and in the neuroses. On the other hand, separation of parents is more frequent in the histories of psychoneurotic, sociopathic, and alcoholic patients.

Indications of impairment of healthy personality development through early parental deprivation have been found in studies of delinquency rates in adolescents. Thus both girls and boys who lose a father by parental separation or divorce are much more frequently involved in acts of delinquency. Boys who lose their father by death and girls who lose their mother by death appear as well to be detained more frequently for delinquency than their peers from intact families. In families broken by separation with loss of the parent of the same sex the opportunity for healthy identifications with its potential for internalization of impulse control is voided.

In adults *the grief reaction* may be delayed for hours or even several weeks following death or separation of the significant person. During this period the sufferer behaves as usual but may speak of feeling numb. Thereafter he or she undergoes periods of yearning and suffering associated with reminders of the deceased or lost person and accompanied by psychophysiological symptoms, most frequently gastrointestinal. Between such attacks of yearning the bereaved person is apathetic, has a sense of futility, and also may be depressed. There occur insomnia, anorexia, restlessness, and outbursts of irritability or even anger aimed at others or the self. Ruminative and over-idealized thinking about the separated person constantly recurs with thoughts that he or she is present. The reaction, common to all bereaved, continues with varying intensity, depending upon the closeness of the relationship, for periods of one to six weeks, to subside in the healthy to minimal yearning after six months. Occasional and brief periods of yearning may erupt for several years thereafter. Often these are precipitated by events or other reminders of the lost relationship. The features of the grief reaction in the healthy must be known to the psychiatrist and distinguished from the distorted and exaggerated pathological variants which bring the separated or bereaved to him.

Parker has suggested that the specific grief reaction may be identified in typical, chronic, inhibited, and delayed forms from which one should separate out the nonspecific and mixed variants. In the latter he places those responses to bereavement capable of precipitation by other stressing incidents. Symptomatically one finds here the psychosomatic, neurotic, depressive, and manic responses and alcoholic episodes.

In chronic grief the bereaved undergoes an abnormal prolongation of the reaction often associated with ideas of guilt and self-blame and sometimes expressed as evidence of partial identification, or aggressive behaviors. Others seem to inhibit certain of the expressions and substitute other features. The young and very old more commonly inhibit their sense of bereavement. Finally, there are those who appear to repress the grief reaction for weeks, months, or years, yet its past representation is shown by attitudes of identification or by behavior not unlike that in chronic grief.

Bereavement is also associated with losses other than that of death of a parent, spouse, or other significant person. The grief reaction and all other related personality disturbances may occur as the result of loss of part of one's body, as from limb amputations or mastectomy; through aging and change in appearance as a response to loss of a function such as sight, sexual function, or motility caused by paralysis or impairment consequent to arthritic processes; or from loss of one's possessions or economic status.

ANNIVERSARY REACTION. Outbreaks of anxiety or their symptomatic defensive expressions which occur regularly on specific dates often represent a symbolic reënactment of an earlier important bereavement. Such reactions sometimes inaugurate the onset of a psychosis in which the emotional upheaval is observed to coincide with the patient's reaching a parent's age at death or sometimes when one of the patient's children reaches the same age as the patient when the parent was lost. Again, one occasionally sees recurrent attacks of anxiety coinciding with the date of death of a parent. Overbearing anxiety and grief appear to precipitate the ego break which manifests itself by the effort at restitution through emergence of pathological, neurotic, or psychotic defenses.

Aggression

In recent years there has been emphasis on aggression as a factor in the psychogenic production of personality disturbances. Aggression may be defined as a goal-directed self-assertion with an associated implication of attack, of hostile, destructive intent, and attached to an affect of rage. Undoubtedly learning to control aggression is one of the major socializing functions that occurs in the family. The arousal and placation of aggression are frequent in interpersonal reactions of the family nucleus.

THEORIES OF AGGRESSION. There are two contradictory theories of aggression. The first, stemming largely from the later writings of Freud, holds that aggression is a primary, instinctual drive (more accurately a component manifestation of the death instinct described by Freud). According to this view, each individual requires a certain amount of gratification of this destructive impulse which, if not attained in one way, will be achieved in some other.

The second theory may be characterized as the "reactive" theory, in contrast to the more speculative "death-instinct" theory. According to the "reactive" theory, aggressive behavior is provoked through emotion aroused by thwarting, frustration experiences. If an individual's habitual modes of action lead most frequently to gratifications, a limited impulse to aggression will be generated, but if obstacles arise in the habitual paths to establish goals, there will be correspondingly strong instigation to ever-pressing aggressive behavior. The sequence, then, is frustration-rage-aggression, the latter aiming to remove the source of frustration and thereby clear the path to the desired goal. Thus the formation of the aggressive personality pattern is frequently established by frustrating forces applied too early, too harshly, or too intensively in the family, with the result that an unconscious aggressive and hostile attitude evolves. Such unconscious hostile impulses stimulate anxiety in those with well-developed superego which, in turn, gives rise to neurotic guilt, depression, displaced hostility, and other psychopathological clinical expressions. The fact that the child is dependent on the very persons, the parents, who are the chief frustrating agents further psychologically complicates the situation.

Mental Conflict

One of the major psychogenic factors in the production of mental disorder is the need to reconcile discordant desires and conflicting psychological needs and to deal with incompatible response tendencies. Conflicts may be of the greatest variety. Frequently the conflict is between bodily drives on the one hand and cultural values on the other. Physiological urges may be beyond the capacity of the ego to handle at the time. Conflicts at a deep level may present themselves on the surface in the form of far-removed symptoms. For example, an unwillingness to accept a feeling of hostility toward a parent may cause the patient to focus his attention upon a local manifestation, such as a difficulty in swallowing. Sometimes an apparently insignificant experience may set off a chain reaction of deeper emotional conflict within the individual, with conflicts spreading from one situation to another. Some situation, specific to the individual, may be so highly charged with symbolic content that it may touch off a major psychotic explosion. Caught in a tangle of attitudes, the unification of the personality becomes disturbed. Unless opposing impulses are blended, one is constantly prompted by contradictory drives and disconcerted by the tensions of his emotional dilemmas. Faced with highly charged emotional issues, the individual is unable to attain a working harmony in his personality. Since the most important conflicts take place at levels outside awareness, one may not apply reason, reality, and common sense to their solution.

The personality, if confronted by conflict and by the fact that the repression of forbidden wishes and of instinctual tendencies is in danger of giving way, tends to develop *anxiety*. In the sources of this anxiety, whether it be overt or hidden, are to be found many of the causes of mental disorder. The personality devices designed to serve as defenses against anxiety constitute the symptoms of the neuroses, many of the psychoses, and even personality traits, particularly those known as reaction-formations.

The ways of dealing with anxiety are various and range from those which have social value to those which disorganize the personality.

BIBLIOGRAPHY

Ackerman, N. W.: The Psychodynamics of Family Life. New York, Basic Books, Inc., 1958.

Babigian, H. M., and Odoroff, C. L.: The mortality experience of a population with psychiatric illness. Amer. J. Psychiat., *126*:470–480, 1969.

Barach, A. L.: Physiologic Therapy in Respiratory Diseases. 2nd ed. Philadelphia, J. B. Lippincott Company, 1948.

Bleuler, M.: Endokrinologische Psychiatrie. Stuttgart, George Thieme, 1954.

Bowlby, J.: Grief and mourning in infancy and early childhood. Psychoanal. Stud. Child., *15*:9–52, 1960.

De Ajuriaguerra, J. (ed.): Désafférentation expérimentale et clinique. Symposium. Bel Air II, Geneva. George & Cie, s. a. Geneva, 1964.

Fischer, J.: Negroes and Whites and rates of mental illness: Reconsideration of a myth. Psychiatry, *32*:428–446, 1969.

Gregory, I.: Anterospective data following childhood loss of a parent. Arch. Gen. Psychiat., *13*:99–109, 1965.

Hilgard, J. R., and Newman, M. F.: Anniversaries in mental illness. Psychiatry, *22*:113–121, 1959.

Hirsch, J.: Behavior genetics and individuality understood. Science, *142*:1436–1442, 1963.

Hoffer, H., and Pollin, W.: Schizophrenia in the NAS–NRC panel of 15,909 veteran twin pairs. Arch. Gen. Psychiat., *23*:469–477, 1970.

Hollingshead, A. B., and Redlich, F. C.: Social Class and Mental Illness. New York, John Wiley & Sons, 1958.

Kety, S. (ed.): Sleep and Altered States of Consciousness. Publication of the Association for Research in Nervous & Mental Diseases. Baltimore, Williams & Wilkins Company, 1961.

Kolb, L. C., Bernard, V. W., and Dohrenwend, B. B. (eds.): Urban Challenges to Psychiatry. Boston, Little Brown & Company, 1969.

Levine, S.: Maternal and environmental influences on the adrenocortical responses to stress in weaning rats. Science: *156*:258–260, 1967.

Lewis, A.: Demographic aspects of mental disorder. Proc. Royal Soc. (Biol.), *159*:202–220, 1963.

Lewis, M., and Sarrel, P. M.: Some psychological aspects of seduction, incest and rape. J. Amer. Acad. Child. Psych., *8*:606–619, 1969.

McDermott, J. F.: Divorce and its psychiatric sequelae in children. Arch. Gen. Psychiat., *23*:421–427, 1970.

Nielsen, J. M.: Mental disorder in married couples. Brit. J. Psychiat., *110*:683–697, 1964.

Parker, C. M.: Bereavement and mental illness. Brit. J. Med. Psychol., *38*:1–12, 13–26, 1965.

Pattison, E. M.: The experience of dying. Amer. J. Psychoth., *21*:32–43, 1967.

Plaut, S. M., Ader, S. M., Ader, R., Friedman, S. B., and Ritterson, H. L.: Social factors and resistance to malaria in the mouse. Psychosom. Med., *31*:536–552, 1969.

Racism: Special section. Amer. J. Psychiat., *127*:787–818, 1970.

Rubin, R. T., Kollar, E. J., Slater, G. G., and Clark, B. P.: Excretion of 17-hydroxycorticosteroids and vanillylmandelic acid during 205 hours of sleep deprivation in man. Psychosom. Med., *31*:68–79, 1969.

Schiele, J., and Brozek, B. C.: "Experimental neurosis" resulting from semistarvation in man. Psychosom. Med., *10*:31–50, 1948.

Schoenberg, B., Carr, A. C., Peretz, D., and Kutscher, A. H. (eds.): Loss and Grief: Psychological Management in Medical Practice. New York, Columbia University Press, 1970.

Schopler, E.: Early infantile autism and receptor processes. Arch. Gen. Psychiat., *13*:327–335, 1965.

Sheldon, W. H.: Atlas of Men. New York, Harper & Row, 1954.

Spiegel, J. P., and Bill, N. W.: The Family of the Psychiatric Patient. *In* Arieti, S. (ed.): American Handbook of Psychiatry. New York, Basic Books, Inc., 1959, pp. 114–149.

Trethowan, W. H.: The couvade syndrome—some further observations. J. Psychosom. Res., *12*:107–115, 1968.

Zubek, J. P., Welch, G., and Saunder, M. G.: Electroencephalographic changes during and after 14 days of perceptual deprivation. Science, *139*:490–492, 1963.

Chapter 8

Examination of the Patient

PURPOSE OF EXAMINATION

The purpose of the psychiatric examination is to discover the origin and evolution of such personality disorders as may be interfering with the happiness, satisfactions, efficiency, or social adjustment of the patient. One seeks, therefore, to secure a biographical-historical perspective of the personality, a clear psychological picture of the living person as a specific human being with his individual problems. It will be found that there is a logical continuity in any personality manifestations, whether the manifestations be those that are called normal* or those that are called abnormal. The fundamental dynamic laws of behavior and of personality development are the same for both. By securing the maximum knowledge possible concerning the personality of the patient, the forces that have determined it, and the problems of living which he has found anxiety laden, it should be possible to understand the function of the illness and the meaning of the symptoms.

All phenomena of behavior, including those of mental disorders, are natural events and should be studied like any other object of natural history investigation. This requires that an attempt be made to reconstruct the patient's behavior, to unravel the story of his neurosis or psychosis in the light of the fullest information possible concerning physical, chemical, anatomical, physiological, path-

ological, social, psychological, and educational factors and influences. It will be seen that the mental examination should be a clinical study of personality and aims at a comprehensive appraisal of the patient.

After an analysis of the concrete circumstances of the individual's life and of the complicated forces that have entered into the organization of the personality, the examiner will reformulate the patient's particular difficulties and behavior and reconstruct his inner life history. This formulation will include statements as to the significant personal relationships during various periods of the patient's life with special emphasis on the patterns laid down during childhood. The formulation should include experiences that have been important in the development and persistence of personality traits, types of conflict present, and the development of various adaptive processes and defense mechanisms. The formulation of the patient's clinical picture is in the form of probable facts and not in diagnostic labels. These facts must be orderly and intelligible. The formulation will include a discussion of the processes responsible for the behavior of the individual patient, will trace the complicated but significant sequences of cause and effect, and will, through their dynamic relationship, reconstruct past and present events and to a considerable degree predict future ones.

Although the elucidation of symptoms is important in establishing the evidence of psychopathology, they should be looked upon as surface phenomena, and one should attempt to determine the needs, feelings, and motivations manifested in

---

* Normality is, of course, a vague concept, since everyone projects his own ideal of perfection into it.

146

them. On the other hand, study of the personality will reveal certain themes or recurrent life issues or conflicts running through the individual's life history—topics or problems to which he may at times respond in the patterns known as mental illness. An examination of the patient's history usually will show that the same anxiety-relieving mechanisms, the same psychological themes which are revealed in the illness, have been active in determining his personality type and character traits long before the illness appeared, going back usually, in fact, to early life.

THE PATIENT-PHYSICIAN RELATIONSHIP

While much has been said of the importance of the history in arriving at a diagnostic formulation, it needs to be emphasized that the psychiatric interview consists of significantly more than the verbalized account by the patient of his illness and the sought-for elaboration of his developmental history by the physician. From the beginning, the patient's behavior in relation to the physician is revealing in terms of his personality functioning, and its careful observation in connection with the verbal statements made and questions applied is most important. The relationship between the patient and physician influences to a large extent his motivation to reveal the nature of his problems and their sources in his past experiences. If the physician is perceived as helpful and tolerant, the course of history taking and personal revelation will be facilitated. When the patient thinks of the physician as critical, hostile, or demanding, he will be unlikely to unburden himself and will not reveal his innermost thoughts.

The majority of patients conceive of physicians as persons with whom they discuss their physical ailments, although in Western culture today a growing number recognize the psychiatrist as someone to whom one attempts to reveal his feeling states, thought processes, and personal intimacies, generally subjects of less interest to the practicing physician.

Conventionally it is not customary for most persons to discuss openly their intimate relations and thoughts with strangers in the first meeting, nor should the interviewing psychiatrist expect such a full revelation. Much is withheld and perhaps distorted on first contact with the patient, and one should consider as abnormal too open and precise details of usually suppressed and repressed information during an initial interview.

Largely determining the patient's behavior and the attitude he exposes in his relationship to the interviewer are the patterns of behavior he has learned in his relationships with parents and other persons significant to him earlier in life. Thus, he often projects his expectations of how others respond to him to the physician and perceives him in a distorted manner other than that of the special role of a medical aid. In other words, from its inception the relationship is shaped by a transference, and such transference distortions vary considerably from person to person. The psychotic person is most likely to misperceive the physician, while the person with a neurosis respects more closely the reality role of the psychiatrist.

With the concept of role misperception or transference available to him, the interviewer should carefully notice the attitude of the patient toward him throughout the course of their contact. Does the patient deal with him openly and frankly as an ill person seeking aid? Is the patient unusually dependent, requiring magic reassurance from the beginning or soliciting support for his actions and thoughts? Is his approach one of surliness or suspicion, or is there a seductive or provocative or exhibitionistic trend in the contact? On some occasion, the patient may attempt to ingratiate or bribe the physician for special attention or, on others, openly attack him or become sarcastic, jocular, or tearful. The type of behavior and the immediate sequence of verbal interchange in which it occurs are the important correlations that the skilled physician duly notes.

From these observations, the psychiatrist should infer similar behavior on the part of the patient in the past, an interpersonal approach perhaps revealing evidence of the personality disturbance, and he should question as well in what family setting and circumstance this behavior was learned and from what early sources of identification.

An awareness and appreciation of the dynamics of the patient-physician relationship and its potentialities for transference distortions of the physician by the patient are of major value in allowing the physician to maintain a necessary objectivity and detachment. From such a position, he may remain patient, tolerant, and sufficiently free from personal anxiety so that even the most suspicious and frightened patient will sooner or later perceive him as a nonthreatening aid. To put it more concretely, the physician, knowledgeable of the transference, will not be misled by unwarranted flattery in the initial interview or later nor will he respond either with guilty defensiveness or hostile rebuff in the face of bitter criticism presented by an embittered and suspicious newcomer to his office. He will not succumb to requests for immediate reassurances or provide promises to the magic-seeking dependent person and, in the face of a seductive approach, his information of the transference will hold him aloof since he knows that the same deceptive contact, covering hostility, has been applied to others before him.

It is the function of the psychiatrist, uninvolved in the nuances of the patient's behavior, to arrange and conduct the interview in such a way that the patient, who finds himself in a strange and unaccustomed situation with an individual who often fails to meet his expectations of the role of a doctor, is relieved of as much anxiety as possible. The success of this endeavor to ease the patient's discomfort determines the potentiality of the examiner to provide the information needed to reconstruct and understand the patient's illness.

THE CONDUCT OF THE INTERVIEW

When the patient is accompanied by a family member or friend, it is preferable at all times to interview the patient first. Furthermore, the patient should be advised of the psychiatrist's wish to discuss his illness with the accompanying person. By this means the relationship with the patient is benefited. He is provided the dignity of the responsibility of presenting his history prior to conversations with others who he may feel are motivated to distort his story. To be interviewed first may, too, allay a suspicion which sometimes exists that the physician is an enemy or is submissive to the wishes of a hostile family. The accompanying family member or friend should be seen on all occasions and, if additional information is provided that the patient has failed to present, he may again be interviewed to determine his conception of the unreported events or factors. The discrepancies between the report of the patient and of any other informant should be carefully noted.

The relative usually brings with him certain fears, misapprehensions, and feelings of guilt concerning the patient's illness. His attitude, too, may vary from acceptance and understanding to intolerance. He may be protective, demanding, condemnatory, or unrealistic. Often the relative, in an attempt to be helpful, may unwittingly contribute to the patient's illness.

It is important that the initial interview be conducted under circumstances that prevent the conversation with the patient from being heard by others. This makes for fairness and also leads to further investigation, as the patient often speaks more freely at this time than subsequently. The ease of a patient and his capacities for communication depend to a considerable extent on the manner of the physician's approach. The psychiatrist must be frank and courteous, show that he is genuinely interested in the patient, and, by the implicit elements of his character, be able to command the patient's respect.

Rarely does the patient talk revealingly unless the psychiatrist shows signs of interest and understanding. The patient must be made to feel that he is being taken seriously, is being treated with dignity and as an equal, with due consideration for his opinions and statements. Also the psychiatrist must scrupulously seek to maintain the patient's self-esteem and allow him considerable initiative in relating his history.

In order that the optimum rapport and maximum information may be secured, the examiner must be flexible and the interviewing situation must be characterized by spontaneity. A patient's spontaneous account of himself will usually expose more informative material than the patient realizes. The psychiatrist will gradually seek to gain the confidence of the patient so that he will not hesitate to mention life experiences and desires which are so private that he has not mentioned them to his intimates. The patient usually feels that he is understood and his point of view appreciated if the physician permits him to tell his own story, with only an occasional tactful, courteous, and guiding question. Judicious questioning of a patient with an emotional disturbance in such a way that psychopathological mental content will become manifest is a fine art.

A physician who has placed his patient on the defensive has usually blundered in his technique and has perhaps greatly impaired his future usefulness as a counselor. This does not mean that a sense of delicacy should prevent a search sufficient to determine what is going on behind the scenes; rather, the confidence and coöperation of the patient having been gained, the questions should be put with discretion and with respect for the patient's feelings and intelligence. Care should be taken not to frame questions in such a way that they will be interpreted as accusations. Skillful questioning should enable the psychiatrist, without arousing undue anxiety, to touch upon the most intimate aspects of the patient's life and open up subjects for exploration that might otherwise remain untouched. Often the patient is not able to respond affirmatively to certain topics suggested by the questioning. However, the fact that the psychiatrist has intimated through his questioning his acquaintanceship with and availability for discussion of such problems is of utmost importance. The patient has been made aware that he has available to him a person to whom he may reveal himself at an appropriate time.

The psychiatrist will never permit himself to become involved in an argument with a patient. The beginner is apt to think that the principal object of the examination is to ascertain the existence of abnormal ideas and to forget the significance of the social circumstances under which symptoms became apparent. He is often more interested in gross disturbances of behavior or in delusional material, with the result that he overlooks deviations in affect and mood, not to mention those of the sensorium.

The patient is initially often eager to discuss his symptoms, complaints, and present illness. While it is the custom in many hospitals and clinics to record these data at a later stage in the formal documentation of the patient's history, it will be found most satisfactory to allow the patient and the relatives to discuss these matters spontaneously and initially. To insist on a presentation of material relative to the patient's family and his life history is often regarded by patient and family informant as irrelevant and irritating.

Although the diagnostic interviews with the patient and his relatives and friends are to be conducted in a flexible manner, the recording of the data for analysis or future reference is best done in accordance with a definite schema. Such a schema is followed in describing the psychiatric examination, and the information to be considered or arranged is detailed under the various headings. In examining a patient, the error is often made of following such a schematic history with its various subdivisions in an obsessive manner, drilling the patient for information on each point. Such an effort is bound to be unrewarding, as patients are usually too anxious initially to provide pertinent material and therefore will respond to a routine staccato type of questioning only by withdrawal or irritation.

There follows a schematic representation of the headings which are customarily contained in the recorded history. Under these headings are mentioned appropriate areas of life experience upon which the psychiatrist should, at some time, gain knowledge. It is just as imperative to realize what has not been mentioned and discussed in a spontaneously flowing interview and the extent and affect attached to each area as to record what has been gained. One may then question the existence of some special suppression or repression of experience or even a deprivation that has particular significance to the patient. Later these "missed" areas may be covered either through direct probing, or spontaneously, when the patient's anxiety has lessened.

THE PSYCHIATRIC HISTORY

A brief initial description of the patient's status is to be obtained which will include a statement as to his age, sex, marital status, racial background, and occupation. His address and means of direct communication with him (telephone) are also obtained.

Reason for Consultation or Commitment

With the widespread extension of psychiatric services into the areas of private practice, outpatient clinics, courts of law, welfare agencies, schools, and the general hospital, as well as the private and state institutions, a patient with a psychiatric disorder presents himself for examination under a variety of circumstances. The patient may come personally for examination or be referred to a private office or clinic by a physician or by a social

agency or school. In other instances, he may be required by a decree of court or by certification to be examined or admitted to a hospital. Under all these circumstances, a brief statement of the manner and circumstances which led to examination or treatment should be obtained. This should include a record of the referring physician or agency and the reason for requesting the examination, if this is offered or is available. In the private office or clinic, the patient often comes alone, and the account of his illness, as he sees it, and of his life history is available only through him. This may also be the circumstance when a patient is committed to a hospital.

The Problem

A clear statement of the complaints and problems of the patient should be obtained from the patient. If possible, it is best to record statements made by the patient in verbatim form.

Present Illness

A detailed account of the development of the present illness of the patient should be obtained. This account should include not only the patient's statements in regard to the symptoms he has observed but also the acute or insidious changes in character, interest, mood, and attitude toward others, as well as modifications in his dress, personal habits, and physical health. It should provide, as well, a careful description of the social circumstances in which the symptoms evolved. The psychiatrist should attempt to ascertain what relationships with others may have been significant. He should seek to learn what has taken place in the lives of these persons and in their contacts with the patient which may have had an effect upon his emotional and psychological state. The psychiatrist should ascertain whether there have been deaths, separations, conflicts, or losses suffered by the patient in relation to his parents and other members of his immediate family or to relatives or friends who are not initially identified. The interweaving of these data and the patient's emotional responses to changes in his relations with others as chronologically related to the development of his symptoms often provides major clues to the psychodynamic factors influencing the illness and its prognosis.

The relationship of symptom development to periods of stress induced by interpersonal conflict or significant loss is seldom to be obtained by direct questioning. It is necessary for the psychiatrist to define the potential temporal relationship and then elaborate the problem.

While the search for the emotional disturbance has been emphasized as one of the most important parts of the story of the present illness, the patient and the family or friends usually tell their story by describing the symptoms that preoccupy him. It is important to obtain a clear description of each symptom, when it was first noticed, whether it is episodically observed or persistently present, its severity, the circumstances that influence each symptom for better or worse, and their effect on the patient's life. His social, sexual, and vocational adaptations must be explored.

The psychiatrist should seek to ascertain what changes were first noticed in the patient's behavior and how they developed and progressed. He should secure information concerning changes in emotion and mood and when undesirable emotional and other personality attitudes were first overtly expressed, and determine whether the patient has appeared increasingly tense and anxious or displayed obsessive or compulsive symptoms. Details as to changes in work efficiency, degree of activity, conduct, attention, speech, and memory are important as indicators of illness. Inquiry should be made as to whether the patient grasps questions and new situations as quickly as formerly and whether his judgment is impaired. Specific instances are necessary. Has he mentioned peculiar experiences? Has the patient said

or done anything that suggests that he has heard imaginary voices or has had other sensory deceptions? Has he had expansive or depressive ideas, ideas of sin, unworthiness, persecution, jealousy, or infidelity? Have suicidal or homicidal tendencies existed?

All accounts of the current illness must consider the general areas of necessary biological functioning. Therefore, an exploration must be made of the changes in the patient's zest for life, his social drive, and the physiological indications of general anxiety exposed in his sleeping and eating habits, his bowel functions and his usual sexual activities and gratifications.

Equally rewarding as the previous areas of interest in the account of the present illness will be inquiries which are concerned with the patient's concept of the origins of his illness, its meaning and significance, both now and in the future, for himself and his important relations with others. Is the illness one to which he responds with overt anxiety or sadness, or does it provoke shame or guilt?

The attitude toward the illness is revealing as well. Does the patient deny its significance and seem to be gratified by his symptomatology and the effects upon those upon whom he is dependent? In other words, is there an emotional gain from the illness? In some instances, the matter of material gain demands inquiry when insurance payments or litigation may be pending.

In contrast to the gain from illness, one will wish to consider as well the urge to recover. Some understanding of this urge may be ascertained by studying the patient's response to his previous illnesses. The duration of the dependency induced by illness in the past in relation to the specific disease and his understanding of his present illness and his expectations for its outcome may give clues to his drive for improvement.

All accounts of the present illness should contain a statement as to the reason for the request for help at the particular time that it is sought. Often patients give histories of long-continuing and unchanging symptomatic disturbance without medical consultation. The precipitating event is unrelated in some cases to symptom change and, frequently, is found in some sudden change in the interpersonal life situation. An inquiry must be made of previous illnesses of the same kind, of treatment given for the current illness and any preceding attacks, and of those who provided therapy so that additional information may be obtained from them and also an estimate made of the value of the therapy. In some instances, it will be of value to explore the patient's collaboration in previous treatment regimens.

From the present illness, the psychiatrist should distinguish as far as possible the precipitating stress situations from those that predispose. For the most part, the latter will be discovered in the account of the family and personal life of the patient.

Family History

From the family history one may obtain information as to the genetic, familial, economic, and social forces to which the patient was exposed throughout his life. In addition to an account of the parents and siblings with whom the patient lived, which should provide a picture of their personalities, ills, strivings, and other defects, it is important to learn as well of the other persons who resided in or frequently visited the home. By inquiring as to the patient's impression of his parents and other family members and associates, their methods of rearing, and the social mores of their group the examiner may infer much of the familial customs, conflicts, emotional control, and opportunities for identification offered in early life. The methods of enforcing obedience used by the parents and their substitutes are particularly revealing in this aspect. A careful account of the reactions of the family and the patient to illnesses in other family members may reveal the sources of reactions to illness or patterns of symptom expression used by the patient and others. The influence of a powerful or domineering grandparent who has set certain ideals for the family or even of the offsetting factor of training by some domestic helper is worthy of note. The patient is usually able to indicate whether he or some sibling was the favored child of either parent and to comment upon his emotional reaction of pleasure, fear, envy, or jealousy relative to his position in the family as compared to that of his siblings.

Here one should note the response of the patient to events such as loss of a parent by death, divorce, or desertion. The age of the patient at the time that the separation took place is much more important to note from the psychiatric viewpoint than the age of the parent at the time of death or desertion. Whether mourning—or a sense of relief—took place should be learned, as well as the duration of this response to the loss and the response of other family members to the same event.

Specific information should be obtained as to the occurrence of mental illness, suicide, alcoholism, delinquency, or eccentricity in direct or collateral lines, and whether the patient was of legitimate birth, adopted, or a foster child.

Throughout, it will be found that information is more easily elicited by making an effort to obtain specific descriptions of action and interaction with related report of the concomitant emotional response rather than by attempting to elicit responses to questions framed in terms of adjectival descriptions of behavior.

Personal History

It is convenient to think of the personal history as a record of the maturation of the individual and thereby to divide the written report into areas concerned with infancy, childhood, adolescence, and maturity. A report only of maturational development will be inadequate; again, the able historian attempts to define the concomitant interpersonal reactions and their possible influence on the growing person.

INFANCY. Infancy poses a particular problem, since much of the available material is beyond the range of the patient's conscious memory and thereby represents hearsay or the reports available from other family members or observers. Here one wishes to learn whether the patient was a wanted or unwanted child and what expectations the parents might have held for his sex and future development. If he was born with a physical handicap or failed to conform to the family expectations and hopes, the parents' response should be a matter of interest. The nature of the birth itself and the mother's reaction to it often determine mothering attitudes for long periods thereafter and are worthy of discussion.

An account should be obtained of the ages at which sitting, walking, talking, and bowel and bladder control took place. This information provides indications of maturation of functions of the nervous system. One should determine the mother's response to delay in these events and failure of the child to live up to her beliefs in evolving such activities. Important information may be elicited here, too, relative to the patient's infantile patterns of eating, sleeping, and playing and the parents' methods of participation in such activities.

CHILDHOOD. Childhood as a developmental period offers the opportunity to review the earliest aspect of the patient's active relationship with others than himself. It is usually possible to obtain some expression as to his reported personality traits at this time of life. Was he thought of as affectionate, trusting, generous, and active, or as shy, irritable, distant, easily frightened or suspicious, selfish or aggressive? The capacity of the child for playing and sharing with others should be studied.

Here an account of the patient's earliest memories and dreams, particularly if repetitive, offers an opportunity to discern a wealth of material concerning his early inner fantasy and emotional life. Since the major interpersonal growth at this time is concerned with the issue of dependency or autonomy, the history should describe the interplay of forces toward independence or dependence. That patient's early efforts at self-expression and assertion should be sought as well as the parental attitudes and reaction to such actions. An evaluation should be made of the response to separations from the parents, such as homesickness. Particularly to be noted are the childish responses toward parental discipline and the accompanying or related emotional responses of fear, shame, or guilt. If the patient had feelings of inferiority early, their source should be sought, and if there occurred attitudes of self-compensatory grandiosity, they should be noted. The early expressions of hostility, anger, and aggression and their chief targets, as well as the methods of coping with stress (flight, fight, or immobilization) should be observed.

Sometimes, one may obtain only reports of symptomatic disturbances in childhood of maldevelopment expressed in speech disorders or stuttering, enuresis, somnambulism, nightmares, or special phobias.

Since schooling commences in childhood and offers an opportunity of defining not only the early intellectual growth but also the initial socialization over periods of time outside the family, the patient's experiences in this milieu are of particular interest. Thus, one wishes to know the age of entrance and leaving, the occurrence of grade failures or evidence of unusual ability, the child's attitudes toward his teachers and classmates, as well as indications of disturbance expressed in school phobias, truancy, or poor deportment.

Again, the historical study of childhood illnesses and injuries with their duration, complications, and residuals must be conducted, as it reveals the origin of important deficits and later character traits.

ADOLESCENCE. Adolescence holds the potential for reëxperiencing at this later period of maturation many of the stresses of the earlier periods of life as well as those uniquely characteristic of this time of the developmental phase. Thus once again, the responses to illnesses, relations to seniors and peers, and schooling as experienced in adolescence should be reviewed. The patient's adaptations and reactions to such events should be noted. Of particular importance for the inquiry into the period of adolescent behavior is the response to pubescent development. The family's preparation of the growing boy and girl for such events as seminal emissions and menstruation needs to be known as well as the adolescent's response to their occurrence. His emerging sexual interests and his reactions to those of his peers should be noted. Signs of failure to develop a clear psychosexual identity usually are evident by this life period.

Other questions of importance are those related to the reaction of mother to sexual curiosity and experimentation of early childhood; strong, persistent, dependent attachment to the parent of either sex; preparedness for and reaction to sexual differences; guilt concerning adolescent masturbation; persistence of "crushes"; heterosexual or homosexual attitude toward sex; frankness, prudishness; overt homosexuality.

Since adolescence is a period of emerging personal identity with evident struggles for autonomy and independence, the nature of the patient's adolescent friendships must be ascertained as well as his participation in or rejection by adolescent groups, his predominant sources of idealized identifications, and his complacent or defiant attitudes to authority. In this period, special capacities or talents may be discerned and ascertained.

ADULTHOOD. Since adulthood brings with it the special stresses of marriage and child rearing as well as of vocational adaptation, plus the problems of establishing effective relations with those in authority and peers, as well as of establishing adult social relations, the history should contain information pertaining particularly to these areas.

As for the sexual adaptations of the adult, the historian will include an account of the courtship, the role played by the patient and his partner, and their areas of agreement and disagreement. As the more common areas of disagreement in marriage center about the sexual relations, rearing of children, relations to in-laws, and the spending of money, detailed information will be sought in all areas. The attitudes toward contraception, emotional reactions to infidelity, illegitimate pregnancies, abortions, or impotence should be looked into. If divorce has occurred, there should be special inquiry into its sources. If the patient has failed to marry, the sources of this lack of adult experience may be looked for in the possible overfixation on a parent, homosexual drives, aversion to the opposite sex, or some physical or social disability preventing the establishment of a heterosexual relationship.

In considering the occupational adaptation and perhaps the military experiences of males, the most significant areas of inquiry are those concerned with the motivations leading to selection of a vocation, the perseverance and performance of the task, and the ongoing relations with working associates. The patient's ability to accept the direction of competent authority or his defiance of it will indicate in some measure his level of emotional maturity. His emotional response to his advancement or that of his peers is also to be carefully searched. Undue fear or envy or incapacity to adapt to envy of others should be of particular interest. Other revealing areas for study are the various occupations entered, positions held, wages received, reasons for changing, periods of idleness and the reason for same; stationary condition or progress in efficiency and in responsibilities; attitude toward work; satisfaction from work; anything in the present position that is especially difficult, threatening, or inadequate in providing satisfaction; habits of saving or spending money; whether life aims were achieved.

LATE MATURITY. The later years of life bring their special problems. Here one should examine reactions to the menopause, the emerging independence and separation from children, retirement, and death of others. Here one will wish to know of the existence of special interests and avocations, athletic or other recreations, social and community activities. The satisfactions or stresses which they produce represent important facets of the patient's personality functioning. These should be ascertained as well as the need for alcohol and other drugs to relieve tension. An account should be given of the patient's religious interest and practices as well as the satisfactions gained thereby. It is often useful to have the patient describe a typical 24-hour day. One should also inquire about his current dreams, daydreams, and plans for the future; this information gives clues to his aspirations, ideals, and hidden drives.

Personality

On the basis of the developmental history, the interviewer may arrive at estimates of the social adaptability of the patient, his general activity, and his personality traits and characteristics. These estimates may be derived both from the patient's own comments about himself and those made by his relatives and friends, as well as the inferences obtained from the personal history. These statements and inferences should be recorded as a part of the personal history, with references as to their source.

Particularly important here are the references to the prevailing mode of interpersonal relations. Have relations with others been satisfying to himself and them? If not, why not? Has his inner feeling for others seemed to have been one of hatred or of liking? Has the patient enjoyed a degree of affection and respect from others that provided emotional security and self-assurance? Since interpersonal relationships with their positive and negative feelings may be of much significance, inquiry should be made concerning any special attitudes toward parents, siblings, spouse, or others closely associated with the patient. Has filial devotion to either parent been extreme?

GENERAL ACTIVITY AND INTERESTS. Assessment should be made of the degree of initiative and of activity, the fluctuation of activity, the industry or the indolence; intense and poorly balanced devotion to special activities in work or recreation; range of interests; use of leisure; preoccupation, alertness, talkativeness, taciturnity. What have been the patient's dominant interests and activities? What satisfactions and dissatisfactions are experienced from work and environment?

EVALUATION OF PERSONALITY TRAITS AND CHARACTERISTICS. One wishes to have an opinion as to whether the patient is given to emotional fluctuations; cheerful, light-hearted, optimistic; gloomy, pessimistic, worrisome; daring or timid; overconfident or cautious; self-reliant or dependent. Does he seek support, reassurance, and approval from others? Is he demonstrative or stolid, outgoing or shut-in, frank and open or reserved and reticent, bashful or at ease in the presence of strangers, talkative or taciturn, aggressive or submissive? Has aggression been constructively or destructively expressed? Is he generous or stingy, honest or deceitful, suspicious, given to misinterpretations, easily offended, prone to feel slighted, resentful, hostile, cynical, inclined to blame others, argumentative, stubborn, envious, cruel? Is he self-conscious, self-blaming, meticulous, perfectionistic, excessively orderly, overconscientious, overscrupulous, or boastful, overbearing, resentful, arrogant, calm or irritable, preoccupied with bodily complaints? Are his opinions and habits rigid, adaptable, characterized by special prejudices? Does he accept or shrink from responsibility? Does he have feelings of inadequacy? Is he given to daydreaming? What is his attitude toward authority? Does he have a sense of humor? What are his characteristic ways of handling stresses, failures, and frustrations? What is his tendency to evade reality and what methods does he employ? With what sets of reactions and patterns of behavior does he respond to new situations? What tension-relieving devices does he habitually use? It is also helpful to ascertain the persons toward whom the patient manifests any of the special personality characteristics described.

Information concerning the patient's personality organization will be secured by ascertaining the type of interpersonal relationships which he has tended to develop, e.g., those marked by a predominance of hostility or of affection, of aggression or of submission, of projection or of incorporation, of independence or of dependence. What type of emotional disturbance has the patient most characteristically manifested when defenses have broken down, e.g., anxiety, depression, elation, rage, or others?

Expression of the patient's attitude toward himself and his body and an indication of his ideals, goals, aspirations, and the sources of his chief identifications, if obtainable, should be ascertained. In addition, there should be a statement as to his superego function with a note as to the person after whom he has modeled his conscience. Also included should be any past indication of the manner in which he placates feelings of guilt, whether, for example, by penitence, mourning, physical suffering, deprivation, or bribery.

Emotionally Disturbing Experiences

Special attention should be paid to respects in which life has not been psychologically satisfying. Was the need for affection in childhood adequately met? Were there frustrations of hopes and wishes or wounds of pride, vanity, and self-esteem? Were love and sex experiences of emotional significance? What experiences produced pent-up emotional tension or domestic, economic, or social stress? Have family or environmental entanglements been anxiety-producing? The patient should be encouraged to express freely his associations with significant life events and his feelings about them.

Either at this point or in the account of parental relations, the age of the patient at the time of death of a parent or other significant person should be noted. Furthermore, the patient's response to this loss in terms of sadness, depression, guilt, anxiety, or failure to respond emotionally, as well as the duration of the emotional response and its effect on his various activities, should be determined.

PSYCHIATRIC EXAMINATION

An examination must include a thorough physical and neurological examination together with all indicated laboratory examinations. These investigations, which must be sufficient to discover all structural, functional, somatic, and metabolic factors, need not be discussed in this textbook. It should be borne in mind that psychotic patients may utter no word of complaint even though they are suffering from serious organic illness.

General Appearance, Manner, and Attitude

One will observe how the patient enters the room and how he shakes hands. He will note the patient's facies and the various psychomotor tensions through which emotions are expressed. The initial interview affords opportunity to note any obvious physiological signs of anxiety, such as moist hands, mopping of perspiration from the forehead, restlessness, tense posture, strained voice, wide pupils, or guarded vigilance. Note should be made of any peculiarities in the patient's physical appearance, including observation of any features suggestive of the opposite sex. Attention should be paid to his dress, gait, posture, gesture, or voice as well as the care of his person and clothing. Dress often reveals much concerning personality. Note should also be made as to whether the patient is accessible, frank, evasive, self-defensive, suspicious, ingratiating, superior, disdainful, irritable, or otherwise characterized in manner and bearing and in his attitude toward the examiner and the environment. Is he assertive and aggressive, or is he meekly submissive? Is he superior and condescending in speech and manner, or is he self-depreciatory? Is he critical, sarcastic, and verbally abusive? Is he irritable and irascible? Is he opinionated or indecisive? Is he arrogant or obsequious? The patient's general reaction to examination may be significant. Does he welcome, tolerate, or refuse the interview? It will be remembered that surface attitudes are often compensatory or otherwise protective. Aggressiveness or a rugged and rough surface attitude, for example, may be a chronic defense against internal anxiety. While many of the data under this heading may be noted and recorded at the beginning of the interview, they may frequently be modified or enlarged at its conclusion.

After having noted such general observations as those indicated, the psychiatrist examines the patients in respect to the following part-functions of the personality.

Consciousness

Under this heading one notes the sensorium, or functional state of the special senses, especially as it is related to the condition of consciousness, which may be clear or clouded to varying degrees. Deeper states of impairment are confusion, stupor, and unconsciousness. If necessary, the patient is questioned to determine his orientation as to time, place, and person. It is a matter of great importance to determine whether symptoms are presented in a setting of mental clearness or one of clouding.

Affectivity and Mood

By this, the character tone of the patient's feeling-life is referred to. The psychiatrist will note the type of affect, its intensity, depth, and duration. The prevailing mood is often suggested by the patient's facial expression, muscular tensions, and bodily attitude. One usually inquires, too, of the patient as to his emotional state. The question should not be of a leading or inappropriate type. One, for example, would not, of course, impair the confidence of an obviously depressed patient by asking him if he were happy. Frequently, the inquiry, "How are your spirits?" will evoke the desired description. Discreet questions designed to bring out the patient's estimate of self may elicit not only a reply suggesting his mood but one containing other significant information. When the patient has indicated his mood, he may be asked the reason for his feelings, although the reply frequently represents the rationalization of factors not consciously recognized. In addition to the important observations as to the intensity of affect, its appropriateness, modulation, responsiveness, and oscillation, such states as euphoria, elation, exhilaration, exaltation, ecstasy, depression, gloomy irritability, and apathy or incongruity are noted. The patient who is euphoric or exhilarated will often be optimistic, self-assured, friendly, and buoyant. The depressed patient is usually quiet and restrained, often dejected and hopeless in attitude and manner. Affective states readily influence attention, concentration, memory functions, and thinking processes. Somewhat more complex states marked by disturbed affective components are fear, panic, hypochondriasis, apprehensiveness, worry, despair, chronic dissatisfaction, irritability, suspiciousness, anger, hate, and silliness.

Expressive Aspects of Behavior

In this phase of the examination, observation is made of the patient's general activity with special reference to the urges, drives, tendencies, and habit formations that determine this activity. The examiner notes both the spontaneous and the reactive behavior of the patient. Does he act in a reality-adjusted way? The physician should note whether the patient is ready for effort or whether he avoids it; whether he is overactive and energetic or whether he is slow and retarded and perhaps unable to initiate action. Is he restless, agitated, impulsive, or assaultive? What, if any, activities does he spontaneously initiate? Distinction should be made between pressure of occupation with its eager output of energy and a mere undirected restlessness. Other disturbances of activity are inability to initiate action, reduction of activity, stupor, negativism, stereotypy, catalepsy, mannerisms, tics, posturing, grimacing, silliness, automatic obedience (*flexibilitas cerea,* echopraxia), playfulness, impulsiveness, combativeness, and destructive tendencies. The apparent stupors designated under this caption do not include those caused by an extreme clouding of consciousness. Among these apparent stupors are those associated with deep depression, those resulting from negativism or resistance, and those resulting from resentment. Note should be made of any compulsive acts or ceremonials. Any evidence of a compulsive personality as shown by scrupulosity or by excessive emphasis on orderliness or cleanliness should be described.

Considerable information can often be obtained by having the patient write a simple sentence from dictation. The handwriting may show tremors, as in the paretic. In the same disease, too, various elisions are common. The manic frequently writes in bold characters, underscoring many words or adding spontaneous productions. Negativism, retardation, or pressure of activity may be demonstrated by the manner in which the patient approaches the task. Note should be made as to the patient's degree of alertness, whether he is mute, whether he eats or refuses food, and the presence of queer postures or the sustained immobility of catalepsy.

If the patient is depressed, a careful effort should be made to ascertain any possible inclinations toward suicide. Inquiry should be made as to whether the patient considers life worth living. If his response is in the negative, he may then be asked more specifically as to whether he has considered doing anything about it and what thoughts and plans he has constructed.

Note should be made concerning sex attitudes or habits observed, including flirtatiousness, hypereroticism, anaphrodisia, exhibitionism, homosexuality, and overt or covert masturbation.

Disturbances of attention, in the form of distractibility, preoccupation, excessive tenacity of attention, and absence of attention should be included in this topic.

Associations and Thought Processes

In this field of examination the examiner observes not the content of thought but the tempo of associations and the characteristics of thought processes. Note should be made of any unusual rapidity of associations, as in flight of ideas, also of any slowness in associations, as in retardation. Disorders in the logical progression of thought will be shown by the patient's associations as he talks. The examiner should therefore note such disturbances as circumstantiality, incoherence, blocking, or irrelevance. Record should be made of any distortions of thought processes, such as neologisms, word salad, perseveration, echolalia, or condensation.

Thought Content and Mental Trend

A spontaneous development of the patient's mental content should be encouraged, and the narration should be interrupted with a minimum of guiding questions. Such questions as are asked should be carefully individualized, and be pertinent to and in logical relation to content that has already been expressed.

In the investigation of this important field, an error is often made by confining it to a search for delusions. The patient's dreams, the content of his fantasies, his ambitions, fears, and identifications afford significant glimpses into his preoccupations and personal problems. The psychiatrist will note the extent to which the patient misinterprets facts and reality in his unrecognized effort to meet his emotional and personality needs. The psychiatrist should be on the watch for a trend or general theme that runs through, correlates, and tends to determine beliefs and conducts. Some patients are eager to express any beliefs that center around such a trend, while others are evasive or suspicious.

In patients who are otherwise accessible but who are reluctant to divulge such content of thought as they fear will be considered disordered, much depends on the experience of the physician and the rapport he establishes with the patient. Usually, while giving the story of his life and of his recent experiences, the patient will have divulged whether he has resorted to delusional beliefs in his efforts to deal with personality problems and difficult situations. If, up to this point, the patient has made no references to material which suggests that it may be delusional, its existence and an intimation of its nature may sometimes be secured by asking him if he has recently had any unusual, strange, or troublesome experiences. If it is suspected that he has resorted to projection as a protective device, the patient may be asked if people have been spreading lies about him or if ill-disposed people have attempted to harm him. Efforts to solve given personality needs are often met not only by projection and delusions of persecution but also by the mechanism of compensation. For this reason, inquiry may be made as to self-flattering beliefs designed to magnify the patient's estimate of self. If the patient's mood is one of depression, he may be asked if he has done anything that is wrong or if he has sinned more than other people. Escape from intolerable reality may be provided by delusional consolations.

As the patient reveals his conscious ideational content, the examiner seeks, by the type of delusion, to ascertain what is being symbolically told him, as well as the relationship of its specific content to the patient's emotional needs and why at this particular time he has had to have the protection and support of his delusion. It will frequently be observed that the conscious content of the delusion is the converse of the true meaning. Statements made by the patient are often clues to the psychological realities they conceal. Motives ascribed to others, too, may represent the patient's own wishes and urges. Grandiose delusions often give a clue to previous frustrations.

If the patient is requested to write an account of his life, he will frequently disclose a trend or express material of psychopathological significance. Mental content previously undiscovered is at times revealed in letters or other writings.

Perception

In deeply toxic and in organic states, consciousness may be so seriously disturbed that the mental processes necessary to complete perception are impossible, with the result that imperception exists. In suspected mental disorder, particularly in delirious or in strongly affective states, the examiner should scrutinize the accounts of the patient's perceptual experiences and his observed reactions to them in order to discover any indications that they are illusionary in nature. Illusional misinterpretations which are not of psychopathological origin are usually, in the face of reasonable evidence, recognized by the individual as erroneous. If, however, the illusions have arisen from a deep-seated anxiety or other personality basis, they are not amenable to reason.

The ease with which the occurrence of hallucinations is ascertained varies greatly. One looks first for auditory hallucinations, the method of inquiring for which will depend upon many factors, particularly upon the apparent integrity of the patient's personality and the extent to which he recognizes that hallucinations are mentally pathological. If the patient's evaluation of reality is considerably disturbed, he may be frankly asked if he hears voices. The subject may often be approached somewhat more indirectly by asking him if he has observed that he has been called derogatory names, or if unpleasant remarks have been directed to him. Frequently some remark of the patient affords a lead which, if pursued, will indicate whether hallucinations exist. It often happens that the patient will describe hallucinatory experiences if he is asked if he has had any "imaginations." The same inquiry may occasionally reveal delusions when the patient has some realization that his mental content is abnormal. This is not surprising, since the unitary reaction of the individual frequently uses both perception and mental content for the same purpose. Indeed, ideational and hallucinatory content are so intimately reciprocal and complementary that in a guide for mental examination they might properly be considered under the same heading.

In Chapter 6 attention was called to the fact that both hallucinations and delusions represent an inner falsification of the outside world in accordance with the needs and wishes of the personality. The psychiatrist seeks, therefore, to determine what function the patient's hallucinations are serving in his total psychological experience. When the patient denies hallucinations, a suspicion that they exist may sometimes be confirmed by the nurse, who may observe him in listening attitudes or responding to his hallucinations. Since, in disguised and projected form, the hallucinations express mental material that intimately pertains to his personality needs and problems, the patient is usually much preoccupied during his hallucinatory experience. In toxic states, the patient's behavior may suggest reactions to visual hallucinations; in other instances, an inquiry if he has had any visions may furnish information. For diagnostic purposes, it is a matter of great importance to determine whether hallucinations, irrespective of the type of sense expression, occur in a setting of clear consciousness. If consciousness is not clear, it is probable that toxic or organic pathology exists.

Memory

If, as is frequently desirable, the patient is asked, as part of the general mental examination, to give a chronological account of his life, by his success in giving dates of entering and leaving school, the places and dates of employment and the names of employers, a reasonably correct estimate of his remote memory can be determined. Special attention should be paid to whether the stated activities and dates are properly correlated. The patient's memory concerning events of somewhat less personal interest may be tested by asking him concerning local or national events known to have occurred during the patient's life and concerning which any person in the community would ordinarily have knowledge. Frequently, particularly if there is a history of head trauma, delirium, epilepsy, fugues, or other dissociative reaction, one should ascertain if there is a hiatus of memory for a circumscribed period of time.

Recent memory can easily be tested by asking the patient when he came to the hospital, from what place, by whom he was accompanied, or concerning other events in the immediate past.

If the patient shows impaired memory for recent events, note should be made of any tendency to fill the gaps of memory with pseudoreminiscences (confabulation). Sometimes alleged activities and incidents can be suggested. In paranoid psychoses, especially, it should be determined if the accounts of any incidents are elaborated with details, really fictitious but believed by the patient to be facts. In more exaggerated cases, the entire account of alleged incidents may be a retrospective falsification of memory.

Retention and recall ability may be tested by giving a series of four or five nonconsecutive numbers and asking the patient to repeat them in the same or in reverse order. Another frequent test is to give him a street address or the names of a few objects with instructions that they be remembered. After a given period, e.g., five minutes or an hour, the patient is asked to repeat what he was enjoined to remember.

Fund of Information

This will be indicated by the patient's replies to questions concerning current events, matters of common knowledge, and retention of knowledge acquired in school. The character of the questions will depend upon the opportunities the patient has had for acquiring information.

Judgment

By judgment is meant the ability to compare facts or ideas, to understand their relations, and to draw correct conclusions from them. The correctness of the patient's estimates and interpretations of external objective matters and the degree to which he recognizes the interrelation of significant factors and incidents are indexes of the quality of his judgment. Judgment is integrated in all personality functions but is particularly influenced by the patient's general grasp and by emotional factors. It might readily be extended to include the patient's estimate of his mental disorder, but his subjective judgment in this respect is so important that under the designation "insight" it is considered as a special field for examination. If objective judgment is impaired, one seeks to ascertain if the defect is caused by a toxic disturbance of the sensorium or by degenerative or inflammatory involvement of higher cortical centers, or if it is distorted by emotional influences and confined to matters conflicting with delusional trends and affective needs. In estimating the patient's judgment, an attempt is made to learn if the patient's business affairs are conducted with prudence and if his family obligations are met.

Insight

By insight one refers to the extent to which the patient is aware that he is ill, that he recognizes the nature of his illness and understands the special dynamic factors that have been operative in its production. It refers to the patient's ability to observe and understand himself—the extent of his self-knowledge. One seeks to learn the patient's estimate of the manner and extent to which personality difficulties are interfering with his social adjustment and the successful performances of his usual duties. An endeavor is made to ascertain if the patient recognizes his adaptive limitations.

The patient is asked the reasons for the psychiatric consultation. If he is in a hospital, inquiry should be made as to the cause for his admission, whether he wished to come, his need of treatment, whether he considers himself to be suffering from a mental illness or has so suffered in the past. Frequently it is well to ask him if he has noticed any change in himself or in his outlook on life, or if there has been any change in his feelings, interest, memory, or thinking. One seeks to learn whether the patient desires to be helped and to ascertain what attempts he has made to adjust himself to the situation. Many patients state that they are or have been "nervous" or have suffered from a "nervous breakdown," and yet have no actual realization that they have suffered from a mental disorder. Not a few patients, on recovering, have what might be described as a verbal insight but are quite lacking in any psychological insight, i.e., an appreciation of the presumed motives associated with the illness and the genesis of their symptoms. They are unable to reflect retrospectively on their feelings and experiences or to understand how the past interferes with present functioning. They may readily admit that they have suffered from mental disorder, yet they have little realization as to what their symptoms have been, none as to the significance of their experiences, and no recognition of the factors which were operative in the production of their mental disorder.

Absence of an understanding insight is not surprising, since there is usually great resistance to the uncovering of dynamic tendencies that have been operating beyond the sphere of awareness. The patient is not emotionally prepared to face clearly and appreciate fully the existence of conflicts or the nature of the symptoms to which his symptoms constitute a defense. He is blind to their meaning since he needs his blindness. The patient must, too, avoid realizing that he has adopted delusional beliefs or otherwise disregarded reality in order to attain his ends. Asking the patient whether he has had any imaginations will often reveal the extent of his realization of his entertainment of delusional ideas or whether he has had hallucinatory experiences. In hospitalized patients, significant information can often be secured by asking the patient why he has been detained so long in the institution.

The extent to which the patient recognizes any continuing disabilities may at times be learned by inquiring as to what he expects to do when he leaves treatment. It is often well to ask the patient what the various psychopathological phenomena discovered mean to him and why he did this or that, not that he can or will give the real explanation, but that his rationalizations may at times betray significant factors or psychological areas that require defenses. At its best, insight is usually a mixture of self-knowledge and of rationalization. The goal of psychotherapy, frequently not attained, is that the patient gain such insight into and understanding of the unconscious roots of his problems, their genesis and dynamics, that changes in the dynamic structure of his personality will be promoted. Insight alone, however, does not cure; it must be applied.

Personality Maturity

As the psychiatrist continues his study of the patient's personality through successive interviews, he makes an evaluation of the emotional and personality maturity. He will note whether the patient's interpersonal and other attitudes are appropriate to a stage of personality development consistent with his chronological age. The degree of maturity of personality may be suggested by the perspective in which he sees his life and work. The psychiatrist will observe the patient's pattern of securing satisfaction, also the roles which he unconsciously demands from others. As a confidential rapport is established, the psychiatrist will study the patient's psychosexual development since, through the intimate and pervasive role which it plays in life, it becomes an important and sensitive indication of personality development. The evaluation of the maturity of the patient is important in assessing his capacity for various types of therapeutic endeavor.

While the levels of emotional maturity have been described previously, they are noted again in the following schematic manner. *Infantile attitude* is evident when the patient expects from others infinite service and tolerance and responds with petulance when his desires are not immediately gratified. *Childish emotional maturity* is signified in those in whom the psychiatrist finds a limited degree of responsibility with the expectation that, when required, his parents or those upon whom he is dependent will assume his care or excuse his defects. Such individuals also demand a complete trust in another as the basis of any acceptable relationship. The *early adolescent stage* is epitomized in youths concerned with the problem of independence from parents by their tendency to admire and be devoted to extrafamilial figures. They may be much interested in social organizations and mystic rivalry. Here, then, are consciousness and awareness of sex. In the *late adolescent stage,* emotional drive at the adult level is for self-advancement through growth and learning. There are strivings for independence that are often challenging to parents and other adults.

Those with infantile and childish emotional fixations in their relationship to the physician have expectations that the physician must do all things for them by some magical means, or entirely through his own efforts. The patient does not commit himself to participation in the treatment. A more adult development allows the patient the capacity to work with the psychiatrist and to learn to use his own assets and make full use of his resources. It is important to recognize that the individual's emotional development may not have advanced equally in all respects or in all relationships. An individual may function at different levels of maturity in relation to members of one or the other sex, to those in authority, or to group activities.

Psychological Testing

Although intelligence is but one of many functions of a total personality, it is often desirable to determine whether a patient is feeble-minded and, if defective, the degree of deficit. Facilities should, therefore, be available for psychometric examinations. Since the conclusions reached by such an examination are of little value unless it is performed by a trained, experienced individual, no details as to the application and interpretation of psychometric tests will be given.

From such tests, not only is the subject's general intellectual ability determined but also the level of his functioning in different areas. Frequently the psychotic patient is unable to make use in an effective manner of the intelligence he basically possesses. In such a patient, therefore, the physician should not usually expect to ascertain accurately by psychometric tests his normal level of intellectual development. However, it is desirable to know how much intelligence the patient can now use, as well as any peculiarities and inconsistencies of intelligence now existing. In spite of the fact that in many psychotic states the patient is unable to demonstrate the intelligence he possesses, considerable interesting and frequently valuable information may be secured by a psychometric examination.

It should not be forgotten that high scores in psychometric tests are not incompatible with serious mental disorder; in fact, patients suffering from paranoia frequently have a high intelligence quotient. On the other hand, some mental disorders are accompanied by an impairment of the original capacity for mental functioning, the deterioration being particularly manifested by difficulties in forming new associations, in making correct associations, in retaining recent memories, and in fixing attention. Certain functions may become impaired more rapidly than others, with the result that there may be a wide variation or "scattering" in the extent of the loss when one compares mental functioning in one area as against that in others. The use of the intelligence test extends far beyond that of simply stating the intelligence quotient of the individual. Modern tests are devised to examine a wide range of functions and mental deterioration as inferred from the variations exposed in the capacities of the patient to perform in the various subjects. A brief description of the most commonly employed test of intelligence follows. The personality tests will be included as well. These examinations may be supplemented by a variety of other test devices for special functions that are available for application under appropriate circumstances by the clinical psychologist. In cases in which particular aspects of the personality deserve study, consultation with the clinical psychologist may provide advice as to methods of examination that are not described here.

The development of these tests derives from the original work of the French psychologist, Alfred Binet (1857–1911), and Simon, a psychiatrist, in 1905. Since the series of modifications of the original psychometric test are described in Chapter 28, as well as certain schedules for examining development, the only test described here is that most frequently employed in the examination of the adult and adolescent.

Wechsler Adult Intelligence Scale

In contrast to the earlier tests of intelligence, which were largely verbal, the intelligence scale constructed by David Wechsler performs its measurements on suitable verbal and performance material in such a fashion that the age of the subject is taken into consideration. This scale is an individually administered scale which consists of eleven subtests applicable to adolescents and adults. The *verbal scale* consists of six subtests which examine general information, general comprehension, digit span, arithmetic, similarities, and vocabulary. The *performance scale* includes picture arrangement, picture completion, block design, object assembly, and digit symbol. In the verbal subtests, the responses to verbal stimuli are given orally by the patient. The performance scale includes certain subtests in which manipulation by the patient is important and others in which this element operates minimally. In scoring, items of each subtest are scored separately and the sum of these items yields a raw or unweighted score for particular subtests. These scores are then weighted and converted into an IQ in accordance with the average of the individual's own age group. The test is an advance over earlier examinations, since it is standardized by actual examination of individuals in seven separate age groups ranging from 16 to 64 years. The use of the numerous subtests provides an opportunity for differentiating an individual, for studying the "scatter" pattern of individuals with various types of personality disorder. From an examination of the scatter patterns, certain diagnostic impressions are obtained, although experience has shown that much overlapping exists between the various groups. Similar tests have been developed by Wechsler for children (4 to 6½ years; 5 to 15 years).

Personality Tests or Assessments

Although a knowledge of the individual's intellectual endowment often gives the psychiatrist useful information concerning the patient, it tells practically nothing about his personality characteristics or the underlying dynamics of his behavior. Much thought has therefore been given to the development of probing techniques whereby one may investigate factors existing in the deeper levels of the personality and uncover unconscious needs and aspects which have been important in determining its structure and the individual's behavior. Such methods are known as *projective tests,* since in them the subject interprets ambiguous stimulus situations according to his own unconscious dispositions, i.e., he reads into his perceptions and fantasied creations covert personality tendencies and processes. He projects out onto the external world the pattern of his own psychological life. The subject's performance patterns and responses, being projections of himself, reveal the personality structure and its underlying dynamics. The tests can also tell much concerning the patient's assets and liabilities. The projective tests have done much to close the gap between psychoanalysis and general psychology.

Rorschach Personality Assessment

This "test," devised in 1921 by Hermann Rorschach, a Swiss psychiatrist, furnishes some information concerning the patient's intellect but is more valuable as a means of detecting fundamental personality characteristics. It indicates tendencies within the patient that may come to overt expression once the effectiveness of his defenses is diminished. In its application, the patient is shown ten cards on each of which is a complex standard "inkblot" picture with two symmetrical halves. Five of the ten cards are dark gray but with many different shadings; two are in dark gray and red; three are multicolored. The inkblots show a great variety of form, shading, and color, so chosen that they may have suggestive value for the responder. In the test procedure, the patient is asked to state what he sees in the relatively formless blot, what it looks like, what it makes him think of, or what it suggests to him.

By creating meaningful forms out of the apparently meaningless material, he unknowingly reveals fundamental traits and dominant trends in his personality. What the patient perceives becomes an expression of himself. In telling how the inkblots look to him, he tells the examiner about his own attitudes, feelings, conflicts, and significant aspects of his personality. In the apparently meaningless inkblot, the free-running fantasy of the patient discovers and reveals content that symbolizes significant and emotionally charged elements and problems of the personality. Authority figures and attitudes toward them, identifications, suppressed cravings, the quantum of aggression, conception of the life role, sexual identification, the psychosexual level, and specific anxiety-arousing factors and stresses are among the contents disclosed.

From this material, the psychologist may determine the underlying conflicts against which the patient's symptoms have been constructed as a means of defense. He acquires an idea not only of the subject's defense mechanisms and against what impulses they are operating, but also of the rigidity, flexibility, and potentiality of his personality as a whole. By this projective technique, the examiner obtains a psychological portrait of the personality and may discover pointers to underlying psychopathology. The patient's responses are scored and evaluated by means of an elaborate system in which perceptions of and associations to the blots have been correlated empirically and logically with certain personality traits. The test gives indications as to how the patient operates, i.e., anxiously, depressively, obsessionally, and so on.

The Rorschach test should yield information concerning "basic personality configurations," intellectual aspects, and emotional aspects of the personality. The psychological aspects as well as the personality strengths and adaptive tendencies of the patient are tapped by this test. The

interpretation of the test is a task that requires skill and should therefore not be undertaken by an untrained person. It affords much insight into the personality structure, although its critics say it is difficult to tell where the test results leave off and the personality of the examiner begins.

The Rorschach test is sometimes used in psychotherapy. Its value there is its shortening of the therapist's task of elucidating the patient's personality components and reaction tendencies.

Thematic Apperception Test

Another projective test is the Murray Thematic Apperception Test, which was devised by Professor Henry A. Murray of Harvard University on the theory that the need is father to the fantasy and on the well-recognized observation that pictures are significantly provocative in stimulating projective expression of the content aspects of the personality. An analysis of the content will reveal the areas around which the patient's major problems revolve. In this test, the patient is shown, one at a time, twenty pictures of persons in various rather ambiguous but dramatic situations. From his imagination, the patient makes up a story about each picture, telling how the depicted scene came about, the relation of the individuals in it, what has happened to them, how they feel about it, and what the outcome will be. The patient usually identifies himself with a character and projects an image of himself and of the significant people in his life. He imagines situations and motives that represent projections of his own predispositions, impulses, feelings, thoughts, frustrations, conflicts, and situations. The fantasies evoked reflect inner feelings and states, latent and repressed material, and covert layers of the personality. The test yields information about the patient's attitudes and opinions in respect to his parents, death, violence, sex, and the like. The stories he tells furnish clues as to his level of intelligence, the range and type of his interests, and his unconscious directional tensions. To some degree, at least, the patient's stories represent a projection and expression of his own present or past personality. Not all the elements and incidents are significant personal references, and so care must be exercised in selecting those that are relevant. The stories, like dreams, may be used as points of departure for free associations.

Bender-Gestalt Test

This is a drawing test consisting of nine geometric designs chosen by Lauretta Bender from patterns first devised by Wertheimer in his study on perception. The nine patterns are presented to the patient one at a time and he is asked to copy what he sees. A frequent modification in the administration of this test is, after a short interval, to ask the patient to recall as many patterns as he can. The organization of the drawings, the page placement, the distortions and elaborations in the form of the individual drawings, any relative differences in pattern size, and other miscellaneous factors are used by an experienced interpreter to make inferences about personality functioning. Because of its dependence on visual-motor functions, the test is often helpful in detecting organic pathology. Although it was conceived of by Bender as a "maturational" test, many workers have in recent years found it more useful as a general projective technique and assign certain symbolic meanings to individual patterns.

Draw-a-Person Test

One of the more recent but now widely used projective techniques for personality analysis is the Draw-a-Person Test. The theory upon which this test rests is the assumption that the body or the self, because of its intimate relation to the individual, serves as a natural vehicle for the expression of his needs, interests, and conflicts when projected by him into his drawing of a "person." In the application of the test, the patient is first merely asked to "draw a person." The examiner may then ask certain questions about the drawing in order to secure associations to the drawing. The patient's concept of body image with its peculiar significance to himself is therefore elicited. This self-projection, arising necessarily out of personal experience, manifests itself in the attention and emphasis in certain parts of the body or in the difficulty in handling them in the drawing. Correlations of clinical observations with analyses of material secured by this technique appear to substantiate it as a legitimate testing device. It is now used to supplement other projective techniques.

Sentence Completion Test

This test consists of giving the subject an incomplete sentence and of allowing him to complete it after his own fancy. It explores various life areas and attitudes of the patient about himself and toward others. Among the areas tapped are fears, worries, aspirations, and regrets.

Although generally designed to elicit more conscious associations than the other projective techniques, the sentence items are still sufficiently ambiguous to serve as projective stimuli to some extent.

Word Association Tests

This is a method introduced by Francis Galton but developed by Jung, having for its purpose the discovery of experiences and tendencies to which the patient is sensitive and which therefore are of psychodynamic import. It is based on the observation that if a stimulus word arouses emotional conflict, the response is delayed, distorted, or inhibited.

In the use of this test a list of words designed to touch on all the common emotional problems is read to the patient.

He is requested to respond after each word with the first thought which comes to him. Words that stimulate some sensitive topic result in a delay in responding or evoke unusual or irrelevant response words.

After the list has been called, the words may be repeated, with instructions to give after each word the same response as first given. A failure to understand the word, or its repetition before giving a response, betrays that a sensitive problem has been touched. The topics and tendencies thus disclosed may be used as subjects of discussion. The unpleasant associations also may be used as starting points for psychoanalytic free association.

Minnesota Multiphasic Personality Inventory

MMPI

Unlike the projective techniques discussed above, this test is a questionnaire of 550 items designed to provide scores on all the more important phases of personality and personality adaptation. As such, it ranges across the areas of investigation explored in the psychiatric interview. Both individual and group forms of the test are available, as well as a shortened research version. The questions are distributed into some 26 different categories. From this usage, nine clinical scales have been developed. These are hypochondriasis, depression, hysteria, psychopathic deviation, masculinity-femininity, paranoia, psychasthenia, schizophrenia, and hypomania. This questionnaire has the special feature of additional validating scales which identify the test-taking attitude of the individual and provide an index of the degree to which the subject has been guarded and evasive, or overly frank and self-critical; a "lie scale," and finally, a set of items infrequently answered in the score directions by the standardization group and thus indicative of gross eccentricity, carelessness in responding, or deliberate simulation.

Other studies, empirical in nature, have provided additional scales for social introversion, academic achievement, social

satisfaction, and social tolerance. When used, a careful study of the item analysis in conjunction with the patterning scales may yield many unexpected insights concerning the individual.

Clinical Usage of Psychological Tests

While the various techniques of personality diagnosis are of considerable assistance in determining whether the basic personality pattern is one of dependence, submissiveness, self-depreciation, ingratiation, arrogance, grandiosity, resentment, aggression, or other type, it must be recognized that the tests alone are not diagnostic procedures and that they do not form the basis for a formulation of the personality structure and its psychogenesis. The information secured through psychiatric examination, in addition to that yielded by the psychological tests, should, among other disclosures, enable the psychiatrist to acquire a diagnostic understanding of the patient's attitudes and relationships to others. As the data from the psychiatric history, the psychiatric examination, and the psychological tests are assembled and surveyed, one may discover that a meaningful pattern of the personality of the patient has been reconstructed and that its parts and features fall into place like pieces in a jig-saw puzzle. It is well to recognize that the information derived from initial interviews is seldom adequate to answer all the questions in regard to personality organization. Areas in which information is lacking and a satisfactory account may not be found for certain aspects of the personality should be noted. Here the psychological test may give information not initially available through the psychiatric history or psychiatric interview.

Examination of the Inaccessible Patient

The student often feels at a loss how to secure significant clinical data when confronted with a patient who is unable or unwilling to speak or otherwise coöperate in the mental examination. The beginner may not realize that the various stuporous states are characterized by more or less well-defined features possessing much of differential value clinically, or that the patient who fails to utter any word, as well as the one who declines to discuss certain subjects, unwittingly reveals much of psychological significance. The inaccessible states existing when the patient is first seen by the psychiatrist are usually rather acute manifestations and yield data of great value both in themselves and when considered in connection with subsequent symptoms observed at a later stage in the evolution of the mental disorder.

Since the clinical reactions of the inaccessible patient are in certain respects less well defined than in the coöperative patient, their detection and interpretation require a systematic method of study. The following plan of examination may serve as a guide to a study of personality expressions in the inaccessible patient.

GENERAL REACTION, MOVEMENT, AND POSTURE.   After having described the patient's reactions in accordance with the plan noted in the paragraph entitled General Appearance, Manner, and Attitude, the following may be noted: Nature and degree of response to greeting: Will the patient shake hands with examiner? Is there any spontaneous speech? Are questions at times followed by replies? Is there apparent effort to reply by vocalization or by whispers, lip movements, or movements of the head? Are replies confined to impersonal questions? Are there special topics that the patient refuses to discuss? If he will not speak, will the patient write when offered pencil and paper?

Does the patient appear suspicious, on his guard, preoccupied, inattentive, evasive? Is the patient ever observed talking to himself? If so, what is the accompanying emotional state?

Are bodily positions assumed voluntarily or passively? Are they natural, affected, comfortable, or constrained? Describe any sustained, unnatural postures. Does the patient resist change of posture? Are muscles found to be relaxed or tense as extremities are passively moved? Are responses to suggested or passively attempted movements characterized by negativistic resistance or by movements in the opposite direction? What does the patient do when placed in an uncomfortable position? Any spontaneous activity and its amount and rate should be noted.

Does the patient obey commands? Are reactions influenced by distraction or command? Are movements of defense evoked by painful stimuli?

What are the patient's habits as to eating and dressing? If food has been refused, is it subsequently eaten if left near the patient? Is spoon-feeding or tube-feeding necessary? Attention should be given to excretory needs.

Are the various characteristics of attitude, speech, and behavior constant, or do they vary from time to time? If variable, by what do they seem to be influenced?

FACIAL EXPRESSION AND EMOTIONAL RESPONSIVENESS.   Should the patient's facial expression be described as alert, apathetic, vacant, placid, stolid, scowling, sullen, surly, morose, discontented, angry, or apprehensive? Does his face express aversion, hatred, bewilderment, perplexity, or distress? Is there any play of facial expressions? Are there tears, smiles, or other signs of emotion? On what occasions do they appear? Does the patient appear worried, anxious, fearful? Is grimacing noted? Describe any mannerisms observed.

Is the gaze fixed? Are furtive glances observed?

Is feeling manifested when the patient's family is mentioned? Is it shown when certain topics or certain experiences are mentioned? If so, what are they?

What reaction is shown to visits of the family? Describe any striking reaction to visits from particular members of the family or to those from certain other individuals.

Examination Under Narcosis

If, because of mutism, amnesia, or difficulty in establishing rapport, one is not successful in securing significant mental material from the patient, accessibility can often be increased by narcosis technique. Various forms of barbiturates may be used for the induction of narcosis, but one of the slow-acting forms, such as sodium amytal, is most frequently employed in this type of uncovering technique. A freshly prepared 10 per cent solution of sodium amytal is injected intravenously at the rate of approximately 1 ml. per minute. The injection is continued until the patient becomes drowsy, but care must be exercised that he does does not become stuporous. Usually after the patient has received 3 to 6 grains he will begin to respond to questions. In this lowered state of consciousness, midway between being awake and being asleep, inhibitory processes are released, rapport is produced, and suppressed and conflictual material is brought into consciousness.

Drugs may also be used on the patient who is accessible in order to bring repressed material to consciousness and to find underlying conflicts. The occasion can also be used for psychotherapeutic purposes. Since overdoses of sodium amytal produce a fall of blood pressure and respiratory depression, it is wise to have appropriate respiratory stimulants available.

While accessibility is not increased in patients with organic brain damage and toxic states, the narcosis technique, as shown by Weinstein and Malitz, may be utilized diagnostically if the patient's attitude toward and recognition of illness and hospitalization are examined. Patients with brain damage explicitly deny their illness, become disoriented for place, and misidentify the examiners. Those without brain damage fail to respond in this manner.

Diagnostic Formulation

A biographical picture of the person as obtained through a psychiatric history, together with a formal mental examination made as indicated, will serve as a guide in the search for signs and symptoms of personality disturbance and usually enable the examiner to determine the character of the patient's reaction patterns. The physician, in order that he may intelligently attempt to redirect the personality functions, desires to know what the life problems are which have led to a disorganizing and asocialized method of meeting them. Diagnosis, therefore, should be based on a case analysis, a dynamic formulation which reconstructs the complex, impelling interplay of psychological forces which have served to disturb personality.

Although in most cases these psychological forces seem to be sufficient to account for the disturbed personality functionings, it must be remembered that disturbed brain functions may also alter personality performance. The psychiatrist therefore carefully considers and evaluates all the constitutional, neurological, physiological, social, psychogenic, and other factors which the life history of the patient and the physical, laboratory, and mental examinations may reveal. The object should be to obtain not a static cross section of the psychosis or neurosis, but a dynamic longitudinal section of the functioning of the personality. The aim should be both an analysis of the present situation and a reconstruction of the personality development from childhood on.

In constructing a diagnostic formulation, an effort is made to coordinate and correlate the various symptoms and behavior manifestations and to articulate them one with the other, with the result that a comprehensive, consistent, meaningful, natural-history picture of the personality is obtained, a dynamic formulation that avoids speculative assumption and makes sensible the patient's life history. It should become apparent that the patient's pattern of behavior represents a biological approach to his total life situation. As a corollary, it follows that the human being is so complex that every human reaction is always a consequence of a combination of factors.

As the previous discussion in this chapter is considered, it will perhaps be readily observed that a comprehensive psychiatric diagnosis is analogous to the diagnosis which the internist aims to construct in order that his treatment may be rationally directed. As a result of his various studies of the patient's organs and their functions, the internist makes an etiological, anatomical, and physiological diagnosis. Through the techniques of his specialty, the psychiatrist makes a comprehensive study of his patient's personality and formulates a genetic, a dynamic, and a clinical diagnosis. In his efforts to reach a *genetic diagnosis,* he searches both for any constitutional factors which may have precluded the construction of a strong and wholesomely functioning personality and for emotionally significant and anxiety-producing experiences which made successful personality functioning difficult or impossible without resorting either to reparative or to morbid measures to facilitate its functioning. These inherent limitations to personality development, its arrests in the maturational process, and the emotionally disturbing impulses and events which have been experienced, particularly in early life, establish the primary source or determinant of the mental illness or, in other words, constitute a genetic diagnosis.

Through a study of the mechanisms and techniques which the individual has unconsciously employed to manage anxiety and enhance self-esteem, it is discovered how psychological forces have operated to produce personality characteristics and how those pathological functionings of personality called symptoms have been formed; i.e., a *dynamic diagnosis* that traces the psychopathological processes and their effects is formulated.

Finally, the general pattern of reaction which has resulted from the operation of genetic and dynamic factors is noted and classified in accordance with accepted clinical nomenclature. The *clinical diagnosis* conveys to the psychiatrist useful connotations concerning the reaction syndrome, the probable course and prog-

nosis of the disorder, and often the methods of treatment that will probably prove most beneficial.

The formulation of the case may be schematized in the following way:

1. Summary of patient's problems.
   a. Behavioral disturbances, including character traits and interpersonal attitudes.
   b. Psychological disturbances, including conceptual, perceptual activities, thought, awareness, attention, et cetera.
   c. Affective disturbances.
   d. Physiological (somatic) disturbances.
2. Salient features of genetic, constitutional, familial, and environmental influences as revealed by the history and the various medical, neurological, and psychological examinations.
3. Psychodynamic explanation. Here an attempt should be made to reconstruct the origin of the various problems of the patient in terms of the interplay of the genetic and constitutional background of the individual and the impact upon the growing organism and the influences of the family life and other environmental contacts upon his emotional and psychological development. It will not be possible to provide a complete explanation of the intricate processes of the individual's life. However, where gaps are noted or explanations may not be made, a statement to this effect should be included for further reference.
4. Diagnostic classification. The classification of psychiatric disorders as provided by the American Psychiatric Association should be utilized.
5. Therapeutic formulation. A concise statement should be provided as to the form of treatment considered most effective, its availability and its source, the needs for indicated adjunctive therapies such as vocational, occupational, or recreational therapies, and the role to be played by the social worker in treatment. The de-

sirability of inpatient or outpatient treatment, the need for certification, and the need for a guardian if the individual is considered incompetent to manage his personal or financial affairs should be stated.

6. Transference relationship. The expected repetitive attitudes of the patient toward the physician should be indicated if this can be ascertained from the developmental history of the patient. If psychotherapy is recommended, an additional statement should be provided in regard to the expected countertransference responses of the treating psychiatrist toward the patient.

7. Prognostic evaluation. A statement should be made in regard to the expected modification of the patient's problems as a result of the therapy suggested above.

NOMENCLATURE AND CLASSIFICATION OF MENTAL DISORDERS

Following the practice of other branches of medicine in which pathological entities are ordinarily demonstrable, psychiatry, usually basing its attempt either on similarity of descriptive facts or on prognosis, formerly endeavored to classify personality disturbances as if these, too, were distinct entities. Unfortunately, in such an attempt one may easily err in mistaking reaction-sets for disease entities.

From a descriptive standpoint, the problem is simplified if mental disorders are divided into groups based on clinical and behavioral differences. It is more important, however, to think of a diagnostic understanding in terms of the patient's intrapsychic processes and how they reflect themselves in the patient's behavior and interpersonal relationships. It is well to avoid thinking in categories or disease entities and to seek only to present a factual digest of the origins and types of reaction. Although classifications are necessary for statistical and other purposes, there has perhaps at times been too

great a disposition in psychiatry to consider that its objective was attained when a classificatory diagnosis had been made. The principal value of classification is not in the categorizing of a disease entity but in the quick elimination of those considerations which will be least useful in understanding the patient and in directing attention to those which are likely to be relevant.

Except in organic disorders, a classificatory diagnosis is less important than a psychodynamic study of the personality. The psychiatrist should be interested in process, not in labels. He should remember that a particular pattern of behavior may stem from widely varying psychological causes, and that a diagnosis on a purely descriptive level without regard to the patient's thought content and inner life is really no diagnosis at all. Even in such disorders as general paresis, in which undoubted organic pathology exists, a study of the earlier functioning of the personality will clear up many points that cannot be explained by neurohistology. It will frequently be found, for example, that organic brain disease has permitted the release of impulses that were formerly inhibited and repressed.

Although, as just indicated, the psychiatrist should, through his study of the patient, formulate the many data he has secured into a meaningful psychobiological biography of the patient, for purposes of statistical study and for summarized identification of similarities discovered in the study of large numbers of patients, it is necessary to have classifications of the more important clinical features which persons with personality disorders manifest.

It will be observed that the general categories recognized by the official nomenclature are quite simple and correspond to recognized principles of organic or mental pathology. Approached from this frame of reference, psychiatric disorders fall into the three groups designated by the Diagnostic and Statistical Manual of Mental Disorders of the American Psychiatric Association. (1) In the first group are disorders caused by or associated with impairment of brain tissue function. The clinical picture resulting from this deterioration of function will vary according to whether the impairment is acute or chronic. (2) The second large group of disorders is that without clearly defined physical cause or structural change in the brain, but of psychogenic origin. This group is, of course, a large one since it includes the psychoneuroses, a major part of the psychotic reactions, the psychosomatic disorders, and the personality disorders. (3) This group comprises the mental deficiencies. Strictly speaking, it includes only those in which the mental defect is of familial origin, has existed since birth, and is without demonstrated brain disease or known prenatal cause. The mental deficiencies which are secondary to or the result of chronic brain disease produced by birth trauma, mongolism, or other irreversible impairment of brain function leading to a developmental defect of mentation are for statistical purposes classified among chronic brain disorders.

Since a medical nomenclature has the function of providing a list of generally approved terms for recording clinical and pathologic observations, it must be extensive so that opportunity is offered to record any pathological condition. With increase of knowledge, the nomenclature, too, must expand to include new terms that both allow recording and improve accuracy. Thus any morbid condition that is specifically described will need a specific designation in a suitable nomenclature.

Owing to their effort at completeness, nomenclatures do not serve well for statistical classifications. Statistical compilation of data is made to furnish quantitative data useful in providing answers in regard to groups of cases; the interest is not in individual occurrences. The statistical classification then is more likely to be limited to a number of categories encompassing the entire range of conditions and chosen to assist the statistical study of disease. Titles of specific disease entities are warranted in such a classification when they occur frequently or when importance as a morbid condition justifies isolation as a separate category. The construction of a statistical classification, then, particularly of international scope, involves numerous compromises between efforts at classification based on etiology, circumstances of onset, and pathology and the forms and quality of medical reporting, and the classification must be varied to suit the demands of differing vital statistics offices, governmental institutions involved in health practices, insurance agencies, et cetera.

The Committee on Nomenclature of the American Psychiatric Association engaged in a series of conferences to bring about an eighth revision of "The International Classification of Diseases, Section V on Mental Disorders" (referred to hereafter as the "International Classification"). The major differences between this classificatory system and the "Diagnostic and Statistical Manual of Mental Disorders" of the American Psychiatric Association (referred to hereafter as the "Manual") is that the latter makes a primary division between acute and chronic brain syndromes and requires no differentiation between psychotic and nonpsychotic forms of such syndromes. These are to be designated in the Manual by qualifying phrases of psychotic, neurotic, or behavioral reaction. In contrast, the eighth revision of the International Classification requires an initial classification as to whether the syndrome is or is not psychotic and does not require a specification of acute or chronic. The International Classification does not list, under Personality Disorders, the subheadings of personality pattern, personality trait, and sociopathic personality disturbance, whereas the Manual does. The heading Psychophysiologic Autonomic and Visceral Disorders in the Manual is found as Physical Disorders of Presumably Psychogenic Origin in the International Classification. Mental Deficiency becomes Mental Retardation in the latter, with subcategories in terms of both degree of defect and etiology.

In this instance the International Classification is more specific than the Manual.

The following is the classification of psychiatric disorders officially adopted by the American Psychiatric Association in the "Diagnostic and Statistical Manual of Mental Disorders" (DSM–II).

List of Mental Disorders and Their Code Numbers

DSM-II

I. MENTAL RETARDATION
Mental retardation (310-315)
310 Borderline
311 Mild
312 Moderate
313 Severe
314 Profound
315 Unspecified
The fourth-digit sub-divisions cited below should be used with each of the above categories. The associated physical condition should be specified as an additional diagnosis when known.
With Each: Following or Associated WITH
  .0 Infection or intoxication
  .1 Trauma or physical agent
  .2 Disorders of metabolism, growth or nutrition
  .3 Gross brain disease (postnatal)
  .4 Unknown prenatal influence
  .5 Chromosomal abnormality
  .6 Prematurity
  .7 Major psychiatric disorder
  .8 Psycho-social (environmental) deprivation
  .9 Other [and unspecified] condition

II. ORGANIC BRAIN SYNDROMES
(Disorders Caused by or Associated with Impairment of Brain Tissue Function) In the categories under IIA and IIB the associated physical condition should be specified when known.

II-A. PSYCHOSES ASSOCIATED WITH ORGANIC BRAIN SYNDROMES (290-294)
290 Senile and pre-senile dementia
  .0 Senile dementia
  .1 Pre-senile dementia
291 Alcoholic psychosis
  .0 Delirium tremens
  .1 Korsakoff's psychosis (alcoholic)
  .2 Other alcoholic hallucinosis
  .3 Alcohol paranoid state (alcoholic paranoia)
  .4 Acute alcohol intoxication
  .5 Alcoholic deterioration
  .6 Pathological intoxication
  .9 Other [and unspecified] alcoholic psychosis
292 Psychosis associated with intracranial infection
  .0 General paralysis
  .1 Other syphilis of central nervous system
  .2 Epidemic encephalitis
  .3 Other [and unspecified] encephalitis
  .9 Other intracranial infection
293 Psychosis associated with other cerebral condition
  .0 Cerebral arteriosclerosis
  .1 Other cerebrovascular disturbance
  .2 Epilepsy
  .3 Intracranial neoplasm
  .4 Degenerative disease of the central nervous system
  .5 Brain trauma
  .9 Other cerebral condition

294 Psychosis associated with other physical condition
.0 Endocrine disorder
.1 Metabolic or nutritional disorder
.2 Systemic infection
.3 Drug or poison intoxication (other than alcohol)
.4 Childbirth
.8 Other and undiagnosed physical condition
.9 Unspecified physical condition

II-B. NON-PSYCHOTIC ORGANIC BRAIN SYNDROMES (309)
309 Non-psychotic organic brain syndromes (mental disorders not specified as psychotic associated with physical conditions)
.0 Intracranial infection
.1 Drug, poison, or systemic intoxication
    .13 Alcohol (simple drunkenness)
    .14 Other drug, poison, or systemic intoxication
.2 Brain trauma
.3 Circulatory disturbance
.4 Epilepsy
.5 Disturbance of metabolism, growth or nutrition
.6 Senile or pre-senile brain disease
.7 Intracranial neoplasm
.8 Degenerative disease of central nervous system
.9 Other [and unspecified] physical condition
    [.91 Acute brain syndrome, not otherwise specified]
    [.92 Chronic brain syndrome, not otherwise specified]

III. PSYCHOSES NOT ATTRIBUTED TO PHYSICAL CONDITIONS LISTED PREVIOUSLY (295-298)
295 Schizophrenia
.0 Simple type
.1 Hebephrenic type
.2 Catatonic type
    .23 Catatonic type, excited
    .24 Catatonic type, withdrawn
.3 Paranoid type
.4 Acute episode
.5 Latent type
.6 Residual type
.7 Schizo-affective type
    .73 Schizo-affective type, excited
    .74 Schizo-affective type, depressed
.8 Childhood type
.90 Chronic undifferentiated type
.99 Other [and unspecified] types
296 Major affective disorders (affective psychoses)
.0 Involutional melancholia
.1 Manic-depressive illness, manic
.2 Manic-depressive illness, depressed
.3 Manic-depressive illness, circular
    .33 Manic-depressive illness, circular, manic
    .34 Manic-depressive illness, circular, depressed
.8 Other major affective disorder
297 Paranoid states
.0 Paranoia
.1 Involutional paranoid state
.9 Other paranoid state
298 Other psychoses
.0 Psychotic depressive reaction (reactive depressive psychosis)

IV. NEUROSES (300)
300 Neuroses
.0 Anxiety neurosis
.1 Hysterical neurosis

.13 Hysterical neurosis, conversion type
.14 Hysterical neurosis, dissociative type
.2 Phobic
.3 Obsessive-compulsive
.4 Depressive
.5 Neurasthenic
.6 Depersonalization
.7 Hypochondriacal
.8 Other neurosis
[.9 Unspecified neurosis]

V. PERSONALITY DISORDERS AND CERTAIN OTHER NON-PSYCHOTIC MENTAL DISORDERS (301-304)

301 Personality disorders
.0 Paranoid
.1 Cyclothymic
.2 Schizoid
.3 Explosive
.4 Obsessive-compulsive
.5 Hysterical
.6 Asthenic
.7 Antisocial
.81 Passive-aggressive personality
.82 Inadequate personality
.89 Other specified types
[.9 Unspecified personality disorder]
302 Sexual deviations
.0 Homosexuality
.1 Fetishism
.2 Pedophilia
.3 Transvestitism
.4 Exhibitionism
.5 Voyeurism
.6 Sadism
.7 Masochism
.8 Other sexual deviation
[.9 Unspecified sexual deviation]
303 Alcoholism
.0 Episodic excessive drinking
.1 Habitual excessive drinking
.2 Alcohol addiction
.9 Other [and unspecified] alcoholism
304 Drug dependence
.0 Opium, opium alkaloids and their derivatives
.1 Synthetic analgesics with morphine-like effects
.2 Barbiturates
.3 Other hypnotics and sedatives or "tranquilizers"
.4 Cocaine
.5 Cannabis sativa (hashish, marihuana)
.6 Other psycho-stimulants
.7 Hallucinogens
.8 Other dependence
[.9 Unspecified dependence]

VI. PSYCHOPHYSIOLOGIC DISORDERS (305)

305 Psychophysiologic disorders (physical disorders of presumably psychogenic origin)
.0 Skin disorder
.1 Musculoskeletal disorder
.2 Respiratory disorder
.3 Cardiovascular disorder
.4 Hemic and lymphatic disorder
.5 Gastro-intestinal disorder
.6 Genito-urinary disorder

.7 Endocrine disorder
.8 Disorder of organ of special sense
.9 Disorder of other type

VII. SPECIAL SYMPTOMS (306)

306 Special symptoms not elsewhere classified
.0 Speech disturbance
.1 Specific learning disturbance
.2 Tic
.3 Other psychomotor disorder
.4 Disorders of sleep
.5 Feeding disturbance
.6 Enuresis
.7 Encopresis
.8 Cephalalgia
.9 Other special symptom

VIII. TRANSIENT SITUATIONAL DISTURBANCES (307)

307 Transient situational disturbances
.0 Adjustment reaction of infancy
.1 Adjustment reaction of childhood
.2 Adjustment reaction of adolescence
.3 Adjustment reaction of adult life
.4 Adjustment reaction of late life

IX. BEHAVIOR DISORDERS OF CHILDHOOD AND ADOLESCENCE (308)

308 Behavior disorders of childhood and adolescence (behavior disorders of childhood)
.0 Hyperkinetic reaction
.1 Withdrawing reaction
.2 Overanxious reaction
.3 Runaway reaction
.4 Unsocialized aggressive reaction
.5 Group delinquent reaction
.9 Other reaction

X. CONDITIONS WITHOUT MANIFEST PSYCHIATRIC DISORDERS AND NON-SPECIFIC CONDITIONS (316-318)

316 Social maladjustments without manifest psychiatric disorder
.0 Marital maladjustment
.1 Social maladjustment
.2 Occupational maladjustment
.3 Dyssocial behavior
.9 Other social maladjustment
317 Non-specific conditions
318 No mental disorder

XI. NON-DIAGNOSTIC TERMS FOR ADMINISTRATIVE USE (319)

319 Non-diagnostic terms for administrative use
.0 Diagnosis deferred
.1 Boarder
.2 Experiment only
.9 Other

Diagnostic Agreement and Quantification

Studies of agreement between psychiatrists in detection and assessment of symptoms and signs of psychopathology and of diagnosis have revealed high reliability as regards the former and complexity as regards the latter. The problem as to reliability of psychiatric diagnosis, reported in earlier studies, rests largely upon the failure to apply uniform methods for collecting data in the interview process as well as a similar deficiency for quantification of the principal signs and symptoms recorded by different interviewers.

In recent years numerous rating scales, inventories, and forms have been extrapolated from study of the process of the psychiatric interview. From such forms, which enforce on their users standardization of the interview procedure, there have been developed quantitative assessments of bits of psychopathology as well as aspects of personality. A number of them now are so constructed that their analysis on a large scale may be conducted using computer technology. The latest revisions of instruments such as the Psychiatric Status Schedule developed by Spitzer and his associates allow, in addition to the detecting and recording of psychopathological signs and symptoms, subsections designed to "evaluate (1) impairment in role function; (2) impairment in efficiency and conduct of leisure time activity and daily routine (e.g., handling of money, traveling, personal hygiene); (3) impairment in interpersonal relationships (e.g., friendship patterns, visiting); (4) the use of drugs and alcohol, and illegal or other antisocial activity."

In detection and quantification of severity of psychopathology the reliability between individual psychiatrists using such methods is high. Agreement as to diagnostic classifications is high as well when psychiatrists in the United Kingdom and the United States are exposed to televised psychiatric interviews with patients interviewed in either country, excepting in certain subgroups. Thus, as Gurland and his colleagues observed, psychotic patient subgroups with marked mood disturbance and little disorganization tended to be diagnosed as schizophrenic in New York and affectively psychotic in London. Such differences in diagnostic tendency have been noted before—between psychiatrists resident in different states or attached to different institutions. Most likely the diagnostic variability represents the consequence of the differing educational exposure of psychiatrists, differences which are likely to recede as international communication and agreement increase between educational institutions.

BIBLIOGRAPHY

Carr, A. C. (ed.): Prediction of Overt Behavior Through the Use of Projective Techniques. American Lecture Series. Springfield, Illinois, Charles C Thomas, 1960.

Conference on Normal Behavior. Arch. Gen. Psychiat., *17*:257–325, 1967.

Deutsch, F., and Murphy, W. F.: The Clinical Interview. 2 vols. New York, International Universities Press, 1955.

Diagnostic and Statistical Journal of Mental Disorders, Ed. 2 (DSM-II). Washington, D.C., American Psychiatric Association, 1968.

Gill, M., Newman, R., and Redlich, F. C.: The Initial Interview in Psychiatric Practice. New York, International Universities Press, 1954, Chap. 7.

Gurland, B. J., Fleiss, J. L., Cooper, J. F., Kendell, R. E., and Simon, R.: Cross national study of diagnosis of the mental disorders. Amer. J. Psychiat., *125*:30–38, 1969.

Holsopple, J. Q., and Miale, F. R.: Sentence Completion: A Projective Method for the Study of Personality. Springfield, Illinois, Charles C Thomas, 1954.

Menninger, K. A.: The Vital Balance. New York, The Viking Press, 1963.

Murray, H. A.: Uses of the thematic apperception test. Amer. J. Psychiat., *107*:577–581, 1951.

Sandifer, M. G., Pettus, C., and Quade, D.: A study of psychiatric diagnosis. J. Nerv. & Ment. Dis., *139*:350–356, 1964.

Spitzer, R. L., Cohen, J., Fleiss, J. L., and Endicott, J.: Quantification of agreement in psychiatric diagnosis. Arch. Gen. Psychiat., *17*:83–87, 1967.

Spitzer, R. L., Endicott, J., Fleiss, J. L., and Cohen, J.: The psychiatric status schedule. A technique for evaluating psychopathology and impairment in role functioning. Arch. Gen. Psychiat., *23*:41–55, 1970.

Stevenson, I.: The Psychiatric Examination. Boston, Little, Brown & Co., 1969.

Sullivan, H. S.: The psychiatric interview. Psychiatry, *14*:361–373, 1951; *15*:127–141, 1952.

Weider, A., and Wechsler, D.: Contributions Toward Medical Psychology. New York, Ronald Press Co., 1953, Vol. II.

Weinstein, F. A., and Malitz, S.: Changes in symbolic expression with amytal sodium. Amer. J. Psychiat., *111*:198–206, 1954.

Whitehorn, J. C.: A working concept of maturity of personality. Amer. J. Psychiat., *119*:197–202, 1962.

Zubin, J., Eron, L. D., and Schomer, F.: An Experimental Approach to Projective Techniques. New York, John Wiley & Sons, 1965.

Chapter 9

Disorders Caused by or Associated with Impairment of Brain Tissue Function

In this chapter the symptom complexes now designated as brain syndromes but formerly known as toxic-delirious reactions or dementias are discussed generally. In succeeding chapters of this section on brain syndromes these are referred to in relation to their induction by specific etiologic agents. These symptom complexes are induced by a general derangement of cerebral metabolism which produces a diffuse dysfunction of brain tissue and thereby impairs those functions most expressive in man of brain action—the positive functions of awareness, retention, memory and comprehension.

Particularly for the psychiatrist practicing in general hospitals, the disorders designated as brain syndromes are among those for which consultation is most frequently requested. The diagnosis of the psychotic brain syndrome probably approximates 5 to 10 per cent in the medical departments of general hospitals; among those over 60, some report the evidence of delirium on admission to hospitals at 40 to 50 percent. In the young the highest incidence occurs in those subjected to surgical procedures associated with pain and/or emotional stress. As for those receiving anesthesia, a large proportion of children exposed to a barbiturate basal anesthetic with later nitrous oxide as inhalant so respond. In general 8 per cent of patients given anesthetics demonstrate some evidence of delirium (the acute brain syndrome).

Although they are critical conditions, indicating serious impairment of cerebral functioning, the acute brain syndromes (deliria) often go unrecognized by physicians, particularly in their earliest stages. Nursing staffs are usually much more sensitive to the presenting symptoms of the condition, and in most well-organized hospitals the behavioral evidence is well recorded in their notes. The consulting psychiatrists will frequently obtain many more data from this source than elsewhere as to the existence of the behavioral indices of the brain syndromes, both acute and chronic.

DEFINITIONS

The term *general cerebral insufficiency,* discussed as an etiologic factor in Chapter 7, probably best designates these brain syndromes since this term draws attention to the basic etiology of all such states and relates them to the more familiar concepts of medicine such as renal insufficiency, hepatic insufficiency, and cardiac insufficiency. Thus with failure of the metabolic processes there occurs a general lowering of the function of the organ or loss through death of the cellular units, or both, so that the activity of that organ is impaired. It may be recognized, then, that dysfunction of the brain caused by disturbance of the metabolic processes may evolve into permanent impairment of function if the cerebral metabolism is disrupted to such an extent as to render a sufficient number of cells dead. In other words, the condition may be reversible when the metabolic defect is insufficient to lead to cellular necrosis, or it may become permanent if the metabolic defect is sufficiently severe or prolonged.

The designations of *acute brain syndrome* or *delirium* are associated customarily with the reversible picture of cerebral insufficiency, while the designations of *chronic brain syndrome* or *dementia* are associated with persisting damage to brain tissue. As one may surmise, it is possible to have symptomatic expressions of both states simultaneously. When symptoms occur which are consequent to both ongoing metabolic disturbance and the effects of permanent damage to brain cells, it is customary to speak of the *organic syndrome*.

The terms *acute* and *chronic* are hardly useful, since it is possible to produce a widespread irreversible necrosis of cerebral cells—e.g., after a blow on the head—which will give the picture of delirium but end with a persistent defect later to be termed dementia. On the other hand, some types of cerebral insufficiency such as those associated with prolonged illnesses, e.g., pernicious anemia, may develop slowly and last for weeks or months and yet be largely reversible when the proper treatment is provided.

In addition to the symptoms directly expressive of impairment of functioning of brain tissue and identifiable as the psychotic manifestations of this impairment, early loss of functioning induces various neurotic or other behavioral defenses in those so predisposed. We identify then the psychotic symptoms and nonpsychotic reactions to cerebral insufficiency. In the following chapters concerned with the brain syndromes, both psychotic and nonpsychotic expressions will be considered.

Pathophysiology

While it is probably correct to state that the brain derives most of its energy from those cerebral oxidative processes which require glucose as the major substrate, there is reason to believe that this statement is not completely accurate. There is some evidence to suggest that some brain function can take place at times in spite of inadequate glucose supply. For the operation and maintenance of proper cerebral oxidative processes there must be available also adequate quantities of oxygen and the necessary enzyme systems. Recent studies have demonstrated an active amino acid and protein metabolism in the brain in which the glutamic acid cycle may act as a maintenance mechanism controlling carbohydrate metabolism. There is good evidence to show that ammonia, which is known now to be produced in the brain, has a toxic effect on the function of the nervous system in certain quantities. Ammonia, apparently, is removable through the glutamic acid–glutamine system. Therefore, the syndrome of cerebral insufficiency may be expected to occur in circumstances wherein there is a lack of oxygen or glucose, an interruption of actions by toxic means, or a deficiency in the enzyme systems related to carbohydrate metabolism and those of certain of the amino acids, or in the presence of excessive amounts of ammonia owing either to excessive absorption or production or to ineffective removal from the brain itself.

In association with the progressive impairment of cerebral functions, there occurs a slowing of the brain waves. It appears that the degree of slowing is more significant in giving evidence of cerebral insufficiency than is the absolute frequency of the wave forms. Therefore, it is possible to have an electroencephalogram show a frequency generally considered to be within normal range in an individual whose premorbid frequency was 11 to 12 per second. A slowing to 8 to 9 per second will occur in such a person during a moderate delirium, yet both values would be considered within the accepted normal range for the adult population. As an aid in following the course of a case of cerebral insufficiency, the electroencephalogram may be most useful when successive recordings taken over time are examined. On the other hand, the single electroencephalogram has considerable limitations as a diagnostic method to establish the existence of cerebral insufficiency. Since the normal frequency count for the individual is seldom known beforehand, a slowing of frequency may not be surmised.

A much wider understanding is needed of the complex biochemical activities underlying the normal metabolic activity of the cerebral cortex, of the disruption of normal metabolism by toxic substances of chemical or microbial origin or by trauma, and of the various substrates and their related enzyme systems and interactions involved in carrying out the specific functions of particular components of cells. As we come to know more of the necessary substrates for the brain's metabolic activity and the associated enzyme systems and metabolites, it is possible that the effects of the various toxic substances upon the metabolic cycles and activities within different parts of the cortex will become understandable. This knowledge may lead to more rational therapy for the delirious reactions.

Symptomatology

Under the heading of Delirium and Dementia, the symptoms of cerebral insufficiency have been described in Chapter 6. The characteristic symptoms of the delirium usually associated with the acute brain syndromes are fearfulness, clouding of consciousness with bewilderment, restlessness, confusion, disorientation, and impairment in thinking, sometimes with delusions and hallucinations. Thus the acute brain syndrome differs from the so-called functional psychosis in the marked impairment of cognitive functions. It must be emphasized that the recognition of the cerebral insufficiency should not wait until the full appearance of the previously mentioned symptoms. Long before gross cognitive disorganization takes place the acute observer will note failures in cognition. In the earliest stages, in which the condition might be likened to the mild intoxication experienced by many persons when drinking, there is a blurring or haziness of perception so that the sufferer notices a limitation in the accuracy of identification and apperception of sensations. He has difficulty in focusing attention on important percepts and in screening out interfering percepts. Again, one with incipient delirium will note a difficulty in thinking clearly and coherently; he may complain of inability to bring forward desired memories and associations. In the milder stages of the delirious process, such difficulties can sometimes be overcome by heightened attention and effort on the part of the affected person. Unless complained about, they may be quite inapparent to the clinical observer, who may note only some vagueness, uncertainty, and hesitancy on the part of the patient.

At a further level of impairment of consciousness, the affected person has difficulty performing correctly in spite of personal effort, and there now is evidence of confusion and bewilderment. In addition to hesitation in responses to questions, it is possible to expose defects in memory, retention, and recall. The heightened effort is sometimes revealed by the knitted brow and a tendency to glance up and around when asked simple questions. At this level of impairment, the patient usually has some difficulty in dealing with abstract concepts; the earliest expression may be in disturbance of time orientation, initially expressed in giving days of the week and later expanding to confusion concerning the month and the year. Furthermore, an examiner will note problems in retention of instructions, grasping their meaning, and carrying out directions. The patient may complain of inability to read as he cannot retain what has been put before him. At a still later stage of cerebral insufficiency, orientation as to place fails, and misidentification of perceptions with a development of illusions is noticeable. At this time, language difficulties appear, and there develops a defect in a coherent train of expression. Eventually there takes place a deterioration in motor activity with problems in personal writing, eating, and grooming, and finally, incontinence of urine and feces may take place. In the later stage of delirium, complete disorientation exists, with delusory and hallucinatory experiences and severe impairment of motor control. Grasping and groping movements may occur. Delirium of this degree represents a *critical impairment* of cerebral function and should be recognized as diagnostically serious for life if it proceeds without arrest. The final stages of progressive cerebral insufficiency are stupor and coma.

It may be seen that impairment of cerebral functioning leads to progressive loss of the more differentiated and elaborated cognitive functions and a reappearance of more primitive activity. To put it in other terms, there exists a progressive impairment of ego functions of the individual, with interference in the ability to integrate new and current stimuli with the impressed patterns of older experience and bring them to proper thought and action.

The clinical expressions of cerebral insufficiency vary, depending on the nature of the past experience and the variety of ego defenses available to the ill individual as well as the type of support he receives from his environment. Some delirious patients experience much anxiety due to their frightening thoughts and fantasies; these individuals will present, in addition to the evidences of ego disruption and cognitive impairment, the physiological expressions of anxiety. Others, due to their personality makeup, are able to minimize their concern over the progressive impairment of their faculties through such methods as withdrawal, denial, sleep, or a confiding relationship with their attendant. Some utilize the staff of the hospital for support and present denial with an unusual façade of coöperativeness, humor, and pleasantry, while those few individuals with limited ego development react to cerebral insufficiency with gross anxiety, panic, and periods of hallucinatory

and delusional presentation. The individual prone to depressive responses to frustrations in the past may react to impairment of his mental faculties by an affective withdrawal of the same kind. Others respond with shame when they are unable to maintain their ordinary standards of performance. Yet others may act out aggressive and sexual impulses and respond to these with guilt. Such individuals may have suicidal drives.

One of the important characteristics of the delirious state is the variability in the symptoms over short periods of time. Even in one day the evidences of impaired cerebral functioning are often much greater at one time than another. Frequently the most serious disturbances are seen at night, when the patient has available to him fewer sensory cues to aid his orientation in the absence of other persons and when there is lack of light. Thus his disability is aggravated by isolation and deprivation of sensory stimuli as well as by the associated mounting anxiety.

Differential Diagnosis

It is most important to distinguish the acute organic brain syndromes with the delirious state from other psychiatric disturbances. In view of its threat to both life and future cerebral functioning, it is imperative to arrive at early recognition and immediate treatment. Schizophrenic reactions are confused frequently, but usually they may be distinguished by the patient's clear orientation and ability to retain and recall past events, thus demonstrating an effective memory. In acute schizophrenic excitement, in which the patient has been heavily sedated, the diagnosis may be difficult. However, a brief period of observation usually leads to clarification. Depressive psychoses with retardation in thought again do not lead to disturbances of orientation or mentation. In patients with hysterical amnesia, the memory defects are usually either too gross or spotty, with great clarity in certain areas. Amnesia for personal identity is not found in delirium. In all the functional psychoses and neuroses, the electroencephalogram will not show the slowing of frequency as in the acute brain syndromes.

BIBLIOGRAPHY

Eichler, M.: Psychological changes associated with induced hyperammonemia. Science, *144*:886–889, 1964.

Engel, G. L., and Romano, J.: Delirium: A syndrome of cerebral insufficiency. J. Chronic Dis., *9*:260–277, 1959.

Lipowski, Z. J.: Delirium. Clouding of consciousness and confusion. J. Nerv. & Ment. Dis., *145:* 227–255, 1967.

Wohlrabe, J. C., and Pitts, F. N.: Delirium and complex electrolyte disturbances. Dis. Nerv. Syst., *26:*44–47, 1965.

Chapter 10

"He who is of a calm and happy nature will hardly feel the pressure of age."

Plato

Senile and Presenile Psychoses

Through man's increasingly successful control of his environment, and particularly his progress against the inroads of infectious diseases and nutritional deficiencies, he has in this century vastly extended his longevity. Yet as a result many more men are exposed to the impairing processes of aging, of which progressive neuronal degeneration undoubtedly is the most distressing. Both cognitive deterioration and the emotional reactions to this and to other losses contribute more heavily each year to the total of psychiatric disabilities.

In 1900, 1 in 25 living persons was over the age of 65; in 1950 this ratio had changed to 1 in 13. The total population of the United States doubled between those years, but the number of persons of 65 years or over almost quadrupled and is said to be increasing at the rate of 1000 per day. This has naturally been reflected in the number of aged people who develop mental disorders.

Estimates made by Lassan et al. indicate the total morbidity risk for the senile psychoses (up to 80 years of age) to be approximately 0.6 per cent for men and 0.8 per cent for women. In New York state, the average standardized rate of first admissions to mental hospitals with senile psychoses per 100,000 population over 45 reached 41.3 per cent in 1950. Before 1935 such admission represented only 8 to 10 per cent of all first admissions; now the figure is above 15 per cent.

Aging

A gradual wearing down of energy, a decline in responsiveness, a waning of initiative and of creative imagination, a narrowing of interests, an increase in egocentricity, and a certain warping of personality must be looked upon as a normal involutional process operating with the passage of time. With advancing age, there is a progressive loss of physical and mental resources, a loss that tends to arouse feelings of helplessness. These feelings serve to create anxiety that the individual tries to overcome by mechanisms that he has long employed in making his adjustments. More specifically, with aging, the ability to respond to stimulation is retarded. Learning in unfamiliar contexts is more difficult than for younger persons and responses to tests of intelligence which involve time limits are poorer.

Beginning in the 40's, there takes place in healthy persons a decline in hearing and vision. Older persons have a particular deficit in their ability to adapt visually to darkness and to distinguish various intensities of light. Color vision is impaired in that the yellowing of the lens filters out shorter wave lengths and thus retinal sensitivity to blue light is reduced. The loss of nerve cells in the inner ear causes a reduction in hearing, a loss which appears to affect background noises that are vital to understanding. Thus it has been suggested that the elderly do not need, as often has been thought, "peace and quiet" but rather more light and sound. At age 60, the majority of persons have suffered a 50 per cent loss of their taste buds. Perception in the gustatory field is thus also reduced.

At least a third of those over 60 years of age also develop an abnormal electroencephalogram. The abnormality consists of focal slow waves, usually maximal over the anterior temporal area. While more often noted on the left side, it is unrelated to cerebral dominance as demonstrated by handedness. This abnormality starts in the middle years, when 20 per cent of the population show it.

The stress of increasing physical and mental limitations, loneliness resulting from the loss of friends and relatives, and perhaps rejection by children produce an anxiety that may evoke various protective mechanisms. Among the most frequently encountered responses are the depressive and hypochondriacal. Busse considers that the aging person tolerates more easily the loss of love relations and prestige than the onset of physical disabilities, particularly those disabilities which limit his mobility or disturb his communicative processes with others.

Depressive episodes increase in frequency and depth in the advanced years of life. In contrast with the psychodynamic constellations that induce depression in the young and middle-aged—that is, the guilty inward-turning of hostile impulses—the depression of the elderly is more frequently the consequence of loss of self-esteem through impairment of functioning, associated with feelings of personal derogation, shame, or helplessness.

Other personality reactions are a turning to and perhaps embellishment of the past, a paranoid projection, or a self-assertiveness to the point of being domineering. Other elderly persons, through feelings of insecurity or inadequacy, become ill-natured and contentious or regress to a dependent state. Both biological and sociopsychological factors contribute, therefore, to the personality changes of old age.

From these mild senescent mental changes, there is a sliding scale to the extreme impoverishment of mental resources that characterizes senile dementia. The dividing line may be a matter of individual opinion. Often the patient with senile dementia is one who has not felt secure and whose pattern of living has long been constricted. The person of cheerful disposition who maintains contact with the outside world, has been well adjusted in previous years, and has built up emotional and intellectual resources may well escape the dementia of senility. The person who develops senile dementia has often been characterized by rigid and static habits. Persons who have always had difficulty in adjusting to the demands of life are prone to react to the inevitable retirement from business and professional posts of honor, to deaths of friends and relatives, and the loosening of family and social ties that accompany old age by the development of mental symptoms.

The more immature and maladjusted, too, have been the adaptations of earlier life, the smaller is the stress required in old age to produce disorganized or disturbed behavior. That social activities and a wholesome variety of mental occupation may retard mental senility has long been recognized. In one of his dialogues, Cicero said, "Old men retain their intellects well enough if they keep their minds active and fully employed." It will therefore be seen that, although of great importance, organic disease of the brain is often not the only factor in the development of senile psychoses. It is increasingly recognized that frequently they result from the interaction of organic and psychological factors.

Pathology

It has been estimated that the brain of the healthy young adult contains over 12 million neurons and that in the latter half of life several thousand die daily. There is a progressive loss of brain size and weight; at age 75 the brain weight is approximately 55 per cent that of the healthy young adult.

The gross pathology of the brain in senile dementia is typically characterized by cerebral atrophy, but frequently this is not easily demonstrated. If atrophy is apparent, it will be greatest in the frontal lobes, where wide sulci and narrowed gyri may give the brain a wrinkled appearance. In extreme cases, the ventricles are widened and the ependyma presents granular excrescences. On section, the gray matter may be less atrophied than the white.

One of the most significant histopathological changes, if demonstrable, is the reduction in the number of cells. The pathologic process involving the nerve cells is usually one of shrinkage, but necrobiosis is seen as well. Another characteristic change is the intraneuronal neurofibrillary condensation and distortions. But the most striking feature of senile dementia is the presence throughout of "senile plaques," small areas of tissue degeneration, roundish in shape and consisting of a granular or filamentous detritus. They are scattered throughout the cortex, but the frontal lobes and Ammon's horn are sites of predilection. Electron microscopy has shown such plaques to contain a core of extracellular amyloid fibers, large dendrites and axons containing excesses of neurofibrils, dense and altered mitochondria, and lipofuscin bodies. Studies of the plaques have shown them to have a largely polyamide structure but with small amounts of carbohydrates. The amino acids in the structure are glutamic acid, glycine, leucine, and alanine. Sulfur and phosphorus are also found in the plaques, more so in those with cores.

Recent studies demonstrate lower concentrations of homovanillic acid in the brains (putamen and caudate nucleus) of those dying of senility, particularly dementia, than in the brains of others. Gottfries et al. argue from these findings that there must exist a diminution of release from dopaminergic nerve endings, and suggest that disturbance of this system is specific to senile dementia. They argue that senile dementia is thus not a variant of aging but a specific disease.

Since these pathologic changes are not invariably related to the severity of the clinical expressions of senile dementia, pathologists have disagreed as to their pertinence to the disturbance. The interrelationship of the clinical and pathologic states has been more certainly established by recent studies; however, such a correlation is not crucial in view of the dynamic psychologic defensive and adaptative processes which, varying from individual to individual, are responsible for personality vagaries in the face of stress.

Mental Symptoms

The transition from usual old age to senile dementia is ordinarily gradual, and any decision as to when the imaginary line is passed must often be an arbitrary one. A dislike of change, a reduction in ambition and activity, a tendency to become constricted and self-centered in interests, an increased difficulty in comprehension, an increase in time and effort necessary for the performance of familiar duties, an increasing difficulty in adapting to new circumstances, a lessened sympathy for new ideas and views, and a tendency to reminiscence and repetition are scarcely signs of senile dementia, yet they pass imperceptibly into mental destitution and personality regression. Many elderly people have little capacity to express warm and spontaneous feelings toward others.

As mentioned earlier, during relatively early stages and before mental impairment is advanced, periods of reactive depression following some specific event are common. Physical illness or severe emotional disturbance may quicken mental deterioration. Rarely are the symptoms of waning mental capacity sufficiently marked to warrant the diagnosis of senile dementia until after 60 years of age. The decreased impressionability, impaired registration, and declining interest in environment and in present affairs predispose to the loss of memory for recent events that often serves as the earliest clinical criterion for the diagnosis. Limitation of ideas and impairment of capacity for abstract thought usually appear early, as may also an indifference to the ceremonies and courtesies of social life. The patient resents what he considers interference by younger persons and may complain that he is neglected. Some show a hostile but anxious and fearful dependence. Natural affections become blunted and may turn to hatred.

A certain tendency to isolation occurs. This tendency to self-isolation and to hostility toward some living person is most frequent if some close member of the family has been lost. Altruistic sentiments are usually lost early, while egoistic, selfish ones are intensified and, like the instinctive ones, may be crudely manifested. Irritability, either as an expression of egocentric trends or a defensive reaction to the impairment of memory, is common. Exaggerated sexual activities or sexual indecencies may be exhibited, in which case they usually represent not merely a weakening of inhibitions but a defensive effort at psychological compensation for the waning of a fundamental function. Some senile dementia patients become careless in habits of toilet and dress; pride of appearance is forgotten. At times there is a tendency to be distrustful, prying, and suspicious. Hoarding and delusions of theft, of poisoning, of poverty, or of not being wanted are common.

Exaggerations and caricatures of the previous personality betray its earlier tendencies. Anxiety, irritability, timidity, and other personality changes frequently seen in senility are not attributable solely to changes in the brain. Many of them are caused by the fact that the individual has been shoved into a position that frustrates his wishes and deprives him of his usefulness and of his status as an autonomous person. A failure to find the satisfactions necessary to replace those the elderly person had when he felt needed, important, and productive tends to lead to regressive changes.

Psychodynamically the pathology of the patient with senile dementia may be understood as a series of ontogenetically related ego regressions. Thus, as the patient becomes aware of the gradual impairment of his capacities, there is at first an intensification of already existing character defenses—he "grows more like himself." As the character defenses fail to protect from anxiety, then depressive, persecutory, and hypochondriacal symptoms emerge as means by which the personality defends against fears of death and impending loss of functions and satisfactions. The senile patient undergoing a protracted course is much less likely to manifest depression; the anxiety over loss of functions or death is projected and demonstrated in his paranoid accusations. Later, with further progression of the illness, withdrawal occurs; the hypochondriacal preoccupation with his bowels and constipation or other organ discomfort demonstrates introjection of the fear. These symptomatic expressions of ego regression are not specific for senile dementia; they may be seen in other progressive brain syndromes as well as in deteriorating schizophrenia. These symptoms are brought into play with the continuing loss of gratification and represent as well the weakening functional capacity of the brain to deal with emotional arousal.

More constant and more characteristic are the evidences of progressive *impairment of cognitive functions* due to the ongoing cerebral degeneration. Accompanying, or even preceding, the amnesia is a tendency to reminiscence, the theme being characteristically personal. As memory for recent life sinks further away from recollection, the limits of recall are forced back further and further until the patient, with the loss of his ability to assimilate new ideas and experiences, comes to live in the distant past, often in the period of his childhood. The patient may speak of parents or grandparents as still living, and persons are often misidentified. Any recollection for the simplest events of recent life may be lost. This retention of memory for remote events and loss for recent ones seem reasonable in view of the theory that the hypothetical neuronal circuit patterns responsible for memories become more strongly established with time. The longer, then, the pattern has been established, the more strongly does memory resist degenerative states such as those of senility.

Orientation becomes defective, and in his confusion the patient may wander away and become lost. Judgment becomes impaired; the personal hazards of traffic or other situations are not recognized. Frequently the patient forgets where he has placed articles and accuses other persons of having stolen them. He may leave the gas jet burning and is careless with matches and fire. He may become the victim of unscrupulous persons, particularly if their technique involves an appeal to the patient's vanity, in matters of either competence or sex.

Many are restless at night and either wander about the house or engage in some aimless, perhaps destructive, activity in a confused manner. This nocturnal delirium is due apparently to the limitations of vision in darkness. Those with senile states become disoriented within an hour when placed in darkened rooms due to failure to retain their spatial location; they then become anxious and more confused.

During the day, on the other hand, the patient may sleep much of the time. Hoarding of articles of no value is common, quantities of worthless objects being carried in the patient's pockets or jealously guarded in some cherished hiding place. The *aged recluse,* living alone or with a close relative or associate, often may be recognized as one afflicted with senile dementia. The majority of those who have come to public notice seem to have been seclusive from early life, and perhaps of schizoid or compulsive personality. Often thought to be poverty stricken, living in a house of shambles and uninterested in ordinary pleasures, the recluse is discovered at his death or following an accident to have hoarded and accumulated large sums of money. Many are victims of crimes of violence when their hoardings become a matter of knowledge; others provide a

menace because of demented carelessness with fire and explosive hazards or because of an ill-kept collection of many dogs, cats, and other animals.

Physical Symptoms

Physically, the patient usually exhibits conspicuous signs of senility. The skin is often thin, atrophic, and wrinkled. In advanced forms the special senses lose in acuity, weight is lost, and the muscles are wasted; the gait becomes unsteady and shuffling, the voice harsh, and the speech slow. The handwriting becomes tremulous, while tremors of head and hands are common. Coexisting sclerosis of the cerebral arteries frequently gives rise to headache, dizziness, and the episodic and focal disturbances incident to vascular accidents.

Clinical Types

Different clinical types, such as simple deterioration, delirious and confused, depressed and agitated, paranoid and presenile types, are described, but there is frequently so much overlapping that the assignment to any particular group is an arbitrary matter.

SIMPLE DETERIORATION. This is the most frequent form of senile psychosis; it is characterized largely by progressive memory defect, at first for recent events but later for remote ones, a narrowing of interests, loss of initiative, sluggishness of thought, apathy, irritability, and nocturnal restlessness. Contact with the environment becomes less and less, and a vegetative, mildly stuporous state may finally develop.

A talented artist was referred by his wife, who became anxious and mildly depressed when his first symptoms emerged. In many respects he was very fortunate. At the age of 65 he had achieved a national, if not international, reputation as an illustrator. His talents were such that he had devised a special process used to produce color covers and prints. His illustrations were sought by the many periodicals. He was employed for his talents as an artist to do some of the highest grade illustrations in the commercial art world.

Recognition of his work gained him election to one of the distinguished clubs of artists in the city.

There had been some beginning failure in his memory. He complained of some difficulty in the use of his hands and arms, a clumsiness and lack of precision that did not exist before. When first seen, he advised that his father had become senile before his death and had had a slowly progressive course of increasing mental impairment, which the patient feared for himself, abhorring the thought. He was accompanied on his first visit by his wife, who had been his model. They had been married thirty years and had two daughters, both married.

She declared that about the house he had become critical and querulous. He seemed to avoid going out to meet his artist friends. Furthermore, in contrast to his usual self-assurance at his work he seemed anxious and upset when requested to take on a new contract. His concern over his abilities, his doubts, and even refusal of work reflected in his relations with his wife. Over the succeeding months it was learned that she had been nagging him. He complained that she had commenced to drink and did not seem as interested in the care of the house. Also, he said his daughters were hounding him. Although he was able to talk most interestingly of his past work and life, it was clear that he had difficulty in recalling his earlier visits with his physician, when they occurred, or what had been discussed. The course was slowly progressive. As time went on, the tension and near panic he felt over inability to perform, on the recognition of his slowly progressive impairment of perception and skill, accompanied by much anxiety in meeting his business and social acquaintances, continued to increase.

The therapeutic efforts were devoted to discussion of the events of the recent past, prescribing medication (Thorazine) which most effectively damped his mounting anxiety, explanation of the probable course of his illness to his wife, and the ways in which she could respond most helpfully. She had to know that he could not be held responsible, that the course would be progressive, that he would become increasingly unable to care for himself, even to the point of being unable to understand where he was, to dress, or to maintain his cleanliness. She was assured that her feelings of frustration and anger were justified, and that their control required that she be relieved at times and get away. Hospitalization was discussed. Contrary to the positions of many who have had intense attachments and perhaps live in less spacious rooms—theirs were by no means spacious—she wished to maintain the patient at home.

The failure in his mental functioning proceeded slowly. Periods of disorientation were first noticed at night when he arose to go to the bathroom. Some six years after onset he became seriously disturbed, had the delusion that men were attempting to kill him and hallucinated voices. By increasing the dose of Thorazine and reducing

other medication, this acute and overtly psychotic paranoid reaction subsided and hospitalization was avoided, but only through the warm and understanding attendance of his wife and his daughters in her relief.

The periods of anxiety and panic with breaks went on for another year or so, to be succeeded by increasing apathy and disinterest. He could no longer tell his wife of the difference between Picasso and Braque. He tried to draw, attempting to improve old sketches, but without creativity. He would talk to her of planning a Christmas card, but would forget that his daughters were married. His death, in a local general hospital, occurred quickly from cardiac arrest seven years after he was first seen.

DELIRIUM AND CONFUSION. The nature of the delirious and confused type is indicated by its name. The onset of this delirious and confused reaction is comparatively acute and may accompany a variety of physical illnesses. Among them are alkalosis, anoxia, hypoglycemia, and urinary infection. An incautious use of bromides, morphine, barbiturates, or other drugs may precipitate an attack. The reaction may be associated with dehydration occurring in fever or following a surgical operation (such as prostatectomy) requiring general anesthesia. Less frequently it may be caused by vitamin deficiency. In milder cases the patient is perplexed, disoriented, and perhaps inaccessible. Insomnia is marked, and hallucinations are frequent. In more severe cases, the patient is restless, resistant, and noisy and may exhaust himself. Strictly speaking, such a reversible process is not a part of senile dementia but represents a reaction to which the elderly person is particularly prone. Some senile subjects, however, present a chronic confusional state. Such a person may present a bewildered expression, move about in a vague and aimless fashion, and be only dimly aware of his whereabouts.

DEPRESSION AND AGITATION. The depressed and agitated type presents not merely the memory loss and intellectual impoverishment of senile dementia but also a marked egocentricity, persistent agitation and melancholic, hypochondriacal, and nihilistic delusions.

PARANOIA. The paranoid type is distinguished by the conspicuousness of delusions, most frequently of a persecutory nature. Sometimes helplessness is used as an effective means of securing and wielding power. Many paranoid senile individuals are irritable, quarrelsome, hostile, and demanding. Complaints of bad treatment are nearly always expressed. This type of behavior usually occurs in persons whose life personality pattern has been characterized by dissatisfaction, projection, and other defensive mechanisms. As its physical substratum suffers the degenerative changes of senility, the personality is no longer able to cope with its problems, its former defensive and compensatory mechanisms are exaggerated, and delusional beliefs falsify reality to protect the personality and maintain its self-esteem. Memory loss may be absent or comparatively insignificant for a long time. As memory defect appears, delusional extension and further defensive emotional reaction may take place in an attempt to repair the additional psychobiological defect. Similarly, as judgment fails the delusions become more absurd, partly because beliefs are no longer subject to any critical scrutiny, and partly because the damaged personality requires more fantastic beliefs for its support. Hallucinations and illusions occur more frequently than in any other type of senile psychosis. Consciousness is not disturbed, and orientation usually remains unimpaired. Of the various types of senile psychosis already mentioned, the paranoid form stands out most clearly as a special type. Transitions and admixtures of the various types described are common.

The following case history abstract is illustrative of simple senile dementia with an admixture of paranoid features—a not uncommon association.

H. S. was admitted to a public hospital for mental disorders when 72 years of age. When 6 years old she sustained a fracture of the hip. Four years later an operation was performed in an effort to correct the deformity and disability. It was necessary to strap her to the bed for 6 months following the operation. The functional results of this operation were disappointing, and the patient was always self-conscious concerning the considerable degree of disability that persisted. She always felt that people did not wish to mingle with her because of this infirmity and did not seem comfortable in the presence of others. It is quite possible that the few paranoid features accompanying the patient's senile dementia may have had their origin in this defensive characteristic.

Five years before the patient's admission her adopted son, with whom she resided, noted that she was becoming forgetful, especially concerning her usual household duties and recent incidents. She hoarded articles and sometimes said that someone had stolen them. She remembered events of her childhood quite well and at times was somewhat boresome in her accounts of early experiences. Her adopted son noted that she became increasingly neglectful of her personal appearance. For many months prior to her admission she would not bathe unless reminded to do so. Recently she often went to bed without removing either clothing or shoes. At times she put on her clothing inside out. For four years prior to admission she seemed to find it difficult to prepare meals at accustomed times.

On many occasions she completed the preparation of the midday meal at 8 a.m. and insisted that the family should eat at that time. In preparing coffee she often put sugar instead of coffee in the coffee pot but failed to recognize her error. In a few instances she wished to pay bills that she had already paid. She was restless at night but often slept during the day. The patient became increasingly confused in surroundings with which she had formerly been quite familiar. Often, when crossing the street, she paid no attention to approaching automobiles. At times she wandered away from home.

There were periods during which she constantly packed and unpacked her clothing. During recent months she had often failed to recognize friends. She became increasingly suspicious, and said that neighbors were talking about her, spoke of them in extremely derogatory terms, maintained that her son lied to her and had tried to poison her, and that her neighbors had threatened to kill her. She claimed that her son and an elderly woman who had been employed to give her protective care had been secretly married. She complained that everyone was trying to control her activities and threatened to commit suicide if not permitted to do as she wished.

When the patient was brought to the mental hospital, she rose to meet the admitting physician, shook his hand, asked him where he was and if there was anything she could do for him. She knew her name but could not give her address or other identifying data. She claimed that her son, who had really been extremely devoted to her, had ejected her in order to secure possession of her house, which was located "down the hill." After her admission, affectless and placid, she sat in a rocking chair all day, paying little or no heed to her environment. Her existence had become but little above a vegetative level.

PRESBYOPHRENIA. The presbyophrenic type is characterized largely by a defect of retention with confabulation. It is doubtful if it should be accorded a special classification. Probably it should be regarded as a somewhat precocious form of senile dementia exhibiting certain clinical symptoms. It occurs rather more frequently in women than in men. Usually it will be found that the pre-morbid personality was characterized by cheerfulness, energetic activity, a certain vivaciousness, and a good adjustability. The previous personality is fairly well retained, and the patient continues to manifest a warm emotional response but with a tendency to be suggestible and to vacillate between friendliness and irritability. Most presbyophrenic patients are talkative, apparently alert individuals who, however, when addressed, are found to be quite out of touch with their environment. Impressibility and retention are defective, and memory is greatly impaired. Without the slightest realization of his memory fault, the patient supplies the deficiencies with confabulations, often accepting with good humor and amplifying as facts the fabrications that are suggested to him. His absurd contradictions and repetitions pass unnoticed by him.

Many presbyophrenic patients are constantly busy with a restless, unproductive, even destructive, activity. With a certain amiable eagerness, as if occupied with his usual vocation, the patient intently disarranges or destroys his bed. The fabrication and memory disturbances are suggestive of the Korsakoff syndrome, but the age of the patient, the gradual onset, complacent loquacity, progressive deterioration, and absence of neurotic symptoms serve to differentiate presbyophrenia from Korsakoff's psychosis.

Prognosis and Course

The prognosis of advanced senile dementia is manifestly hopeless. No well-defined remissions are to be expected, although in the depressed and excited types subsidence of symptoms may occur. The course is progressive; the patient gradually becomes more demented, although life may continue for 10 years or even longer before death supervenes. Not a few mental disorders in the aged are, however, precipitated by situational problems such as isolation, exhaustion, and toxic and nutritional factors. Many of these are quite amenable to appropriate management.

Diagnosis

In well-developed simple senile dementia, the age of the patient, the progressive egocentricity, and the characteristic memory loss, particularly for recent events, make the diagnosis easy. In the paranoid form, the memory loss and evidences of dementia may be comparatively slight. Since these senile paranoids have usually had a life pattern of a defensive, paranoid type, the matter of deciding when this exaggerated pattern crosses the psychotic line may be one of arbitrary decision to be determined largely by social criteria and by the interpretation and values accorded to reality. When arteriosclerotic changes in the brain, rather than the histological ones of senility, are the basis for such paranoid psychoses, the patient usually suffers from easy mental fatigability, dizziness, or slight confusion, suggestive of changes in the smaller vessels of the cerebrum. Some depressed and agitated types of symptoms suggest involutional melancholia, but it must be noted that depressive symptoms are more common in arteriosclerotic brain disease. The differentiation must be based largely on the age of the patient and particularly on the presence or absence of deterioration.

Differentiation from arteriosclerotic psychoses is discussed in Chapter 11.

A restricted diet in the aged may lead to avitaminosis suggestive of senile psychosis. Toxic psychoses are frequently mistaken for senile dementia. It should be remembered that, in the aged, mental disturbance may be caused by uremia, anemia, decompensated heart disease, or pulmonary disease rather than by senile dementia. The differentiation of presbyophrenia from Korsakoff's disease has already been mentioned.

Treatment

The discussion in the early part of the chapter has already suggested the importance of prophylactic factors in the prevention of the senile psychoses. It is therefore highly desirable that the aged person maintain a feeling of emotional security and a sense of dignity. One will accordingly attempt to see that the old person's needs for affection, for a feeling of belonging, for achievement, and for recognition and approval are met. Equally important are the maintenance of his nutrition and careful management of his health with early treatment of any illness.

The milder form of senile dementia should be cared for in the home. It is there that the patient's roots are deeply imbedded. Unless circumstances are such that either the safety of the patient or that of the family is endangered, it is well to attempt to care for him in the usual and familiar environment. The patient is ordinarily happier there than in the unaccustomed and rather rigid routine of an institution, where the habits of a lifetime have to be reconstructed. It is true, however, that the patient's inability to recognize his failing physical and mental vigor may present a serious problem to his family. In not a few cases, too, hospital care becomes necessary because of nocturnal restlessness, disturbing response to paranoid delusions, marked irritability, assaultiveness, sexual play with children, exhibitionism, or ill-considered plans for marriage. Impaired judgment in business affairs may make the appointment of a legal guardian necessary. Care must often be exercised to prevent the confused patient from setting fire to clothing or furniture, to prevent wandering from home or falling with resulting fracture of the neck of the femur. It is particularly important

to maintain the visual orientation of the senile patient at night. This may be done by providing adequate night lighting, available if he awakens. During the day, the presence of familiar objects also supports his orientation. Also, hearing impairment should be corrected, even if minor, by the appropriate audiophonic prostheses.

Psychotherapy wherein the physician or his agent plays a supportive role is often useful in the earlier stages of the illness to sustain the patient's increased dependency needs. Advice to the family on the need to provide avenues of gratification is important as well as advice on changing the home environment so as to ease the burden of the deficits of the elderly. As mentioned earlier, adequate lighting, stimulating associations, and avoidance of overprotection and social isolation are significant in the care of the majority of the elderly. The indications for insight and dynamic therapies are unclear, but such methods have been reported helpful in limited trials with some patients in this reaction group. The goals should probably be restricted to understanding and modification of pathologic defenses related to the immediate conflict situations.

If appetite has been poor or diet restricted it is advisable to prescribe ascorbic acid, thiamine chloride, niacin, and glutamic acid. Preparations are now available in which glutamic acid is supplied in its utilizable form, monosodium L-glutamate. Vitamins are frequently of value in confused and delirious senile states. In the depressive forms, electroshock therapy can often be used safely and with great success.

For insomnia, a mild hypnotic is advisable. Barbiturates often are tolerated poorly. A phenothiazine before bedtime may prove most effective. Pentylenetetrazol (Metrazol) may be given to stimulate mental processes and memory.

In the depressed form, trials should be made with the antidepressant agents. It should be kept in mind that the elderly are often unusually sensitive to these agents. Hypotension and urinary retention are common complications in their administration. When the antidepressants fail, electroshock is indicated. For restlessness, irritability, confusion, or delirium, chlorpromazine or another phenothiazine should be prescribed.

ALZHEIMER'S DISEASE

In 1906, Alois Alzheimer (1864–1915) described the case of a woman who had died at age 51 following a rather rapidly progressing dementia and whose brain tissue showed the development of tangled, threadlike structures occupying much or all of the body of many cortical ganglion cells. These agglomerated neurofibrils are stained black with silver stains. This degenerative change may involve even one-fourth of the ganglion cells. It is now known that they are not limited to this disease but may be observed in senile dementia and even in the brain in normal senium. There are accompanying diffuse gliosis and an abnormal amount of fatty pigment in the nerve cells. Another histopathological change that practically always exists is the presence of senile plaques with their amorphous and homogeneous core. Plaques are most frequent in the frontal cortex and in the cornu Ammonis. In Alzheimer's disease the cortical degeneration is diffuse and involves the outer layers of the cortex, especially those of the frontal and temporal lobes.

Recent electron microscopic and histochemical studies have shown that the characteristic neurofibrillary tangles are composed of large numbers of closely packed hollow neurofilaments which have displaced cytoplasmic organelles. Within the senile plaques are cores of amyloid fibrils in extracellular positions. Neighboring enlarged dendrites and axons contain excesses of neurofibrils and electron-dense altered mitochondria. Lipofuscin bodies and astrocytic processes make up the other constituents of the plaque. The brain in Alzheimer's disease contains increased amounts of acid polysaccharide and reduced amounts of an unknown neutral polysaccharide, perhaps glycogen. Conflicting accounts are now given regarding lessened amounts of brain lipid and cerebroside.

Whether these new findings offer answers to the riddle of Alzheimer's disease is unclear. Are they, too, as enigmatically related to presenile disturbances as the senile plaques and neurofibrillary changes? As R. Richter has commented, "One wonders whether the black freckles in the cortex of the brain signify more than the senile freckles in the skin."

Symptoms

The onset of Alzheimer's disease is usually between 50 and 60 years of age, although earlier appearances have been reported. The disease begins insidiously, with a reduction of spontaneity, progressive intellectual deterioration, and alterations in behavior. There is no characteristic pattern in either the intellectual impairment or the behavioral disturbances. Disorientation, memory impairment, defects in calculation and general information, emotional lability, and decrease in concreteness in thinking are present in varying degrees and combinations. Pronunciation is difficult, spoken language is comprehended poorly, and errors are made in reading and writing. The patient makes mistakes in the routine details of his everyday life, words are forgotten, and speech disorders are common. A not infrequent disturbance is a preservation of speech in the form of logoclonia. In advanced stages of the disease, speech becomes an incoherent jargon without sentence formation. Prolonged periods of restless overactivity, anxiety, and depression may occur. Agnosia, apraxia, and temporary hemiplegic or paraplegic weakness may exist. Syncopal and epileptic attacks are common. A Parkinson-like difficulty in gait is often seen. Facial paresis and hypertonicity of muscles are frequent, and in late stages there may be contractures of the extremities. At this stage the patient becomes extremely demented, is entirely out of touch with his environment, and becomes reduced to a mere vegetative existence. The usual duration of the disease is five to ten years, but the course may be characterized by remissions.

The following is a rather typical clinical history of a patient suffering from this disorder.

W. M. was admitted to the hospital at the age of 52. The patient's early life, including medical history, does not appear to have been significant. The onset of his mental disorder was so insidious that his wife was able to give only an approximate date. About five or six years before his admission, he began to show less affection toward his family. His wife added that at about the same time "he grew lazy and his interests gradually dulled. He had a habit of just sitting around the house. For years he has not mentioned the payment of the interest on his mortgage or his taxes." About three years before admission his wife noticed that he could not tell time correctly and that he would make errors in writing a check. "He would set out for the store to buy feed for his cows and forget to do so. One time he wanted to walk to his father's place, thinking that it was just down the road, whereas it was a matter of 60 miles. He grew confused, and on one occasion he stopped the car in the middle of an intersection. He would put on his trousers backward and his overalls inside out. Sometimes, when a dish of food was put on the table for the whole family, he would eat the entire amount himself."

The preadmission history is obviously that of an insidiously developing and progressive dementia. On admission the patient appeared to be older than he actually was. He was completely disoriented for time and place. He did not know whether his home was in Pennsylvania or New Jersey. On the day of admission he said he was 34 years of age; on the following day he gave his age as 25 and a few weeks later, as 80. He was careless and untidy in dress and wandered about the ward in a confused and bewildered manner, often mistaking the nurse for his wife.

General hyperreflexia was noted, but there were no other neurological abnormalities. Prior to his death his extremities showed spasticity. The patient became incontinent of urine; he gradually grew weaker and even more demented. Nearly two and one-half years after admission, he suffered a rather typical epileptic seizure. Shortly thereafter he became comatose and died nine days later.

At autopsy the brain weighed 1250 gm. A coronal section through the frontal lobes showed pronounced cortical atrophy, with enlargement of the sulci. The island of Reil was also atrophic. On microscopic examination, a marked cortical atrophy was found; there was also a decrease in the amount of subcortical white matter. In some convolutions the white matter was reduced to a narrow band. The subcortex showed moderate general demyelination. Sections through the plane of the substantia nigra showed this to be depigmented. A section further caudad showed the posterior horns of the ventricles to be considerably enlarged at the expense of the white matter. Stained sections showed a focal and general loss of ganglion cells, the presence of ghost cells, severe degenerative changes in the cells that remained, and a uniform gliosis. Special silver stains demonstrated numerous senile plaques and neurofibrillary degeneration of many ganglion cells. These showed thickening and agglutination of the neurofibrils, their displacement to the periphery of the cells, and their bizarre arrangement within the cells.

Diagnosis and Treatment

When there is a history of slowly progressive impairment in cognitive function taking place in the late 40's or 50's, Alzheimer's or Pick's disease should be considered. Serial psychological tests are helpful in indicating the progressive nature of the condition. Air encephalograms show ventricular dilation and increased cortical markings. The clinical differentiation from Pick's disease, described below, is most doubtful.

Since the etiology remains obscure, treatment should be directed to maintaining the general health of the patient and protecting him from the vagaries of his increasing impairment while supporting his dependent needs and increasing demands. Metrazol and ribonucleic acid have been prescribed to assist memory functions. Their value is uncertain.

PICK'S DISEASE

This uncommon chronic brain syndrome, first described by Pick of Prague in 1892, is characterized pathologically by atrophy and gliosis in the associative areas. The motor, sensory, and projection areas are relatively unchanged. Several reports of multiple cases in one family suggest that the disease may be a heredodegenerative disorder, but it does not show any simple mendelian pattern. The involvement is of cortical areas which are relatively younger phylogenetically, areas which are concerned with higher associative functions.

The mechanisms of speech and of thinking are therefore especially impaired. It has been suggested that the disease is a premature and localized neuronic aging. The frontal lobe may look as if a constricting band had been applied to it. The clinical symptomatology is the result of a combination of the diffuse and focal processes. The majority of cases have been in persons between the ages of 45 and 60 years, the youngest being 31.

Local areas of the brain, particularly the frontal and temporal lobes, may be severely atrophied, and the total weight of the brain may be reduced to less than 1000 gm. (the average normal male Caucasian brain weighs 1340 gm.). The whole depth of the cortex may be involved. Microscopically the lesions are found to be degenerative and not inflammatory. Usually there is distortion in the arrangement of the cytoarchitectural layers of the atrophic convolutions. Chromatolysis of the nerve cells is marked, there is a progressive disappearance of the chromatic substance, the nucleus becomes pale and is displaced to the periphery, and the granulations are lost. Ballooned cells, not found in Alzheimer's disease, are regularly seen in Pick's disease. The loss of ganglion cells becomes marked, and many of those remaining are swollen and show argentophilic granules. There is hypertrophy of the neuroglia, and the microglia presents a swollen appearance, with relatively numerous fatty granules. Senile plaques and Alzheimer fibrillary changes frequently found in senile dementia and Alzheimer's disease are rarely found. The white matter atrophies early. Changes in the basal ganglia are regularly found in Alzheimer's disease but are rare in Pick's disease.

The affliction occurs twice as frequently in women as in men. Among the earliest symptoms are lack of spontaneity, loss of memory, difficulty in thinking and concentration, and a blunting of emotions. The patient becomes taciturn, indifferent, and bewildered and is unable to deal with new situations. The memory for the execution of normal, concrete tasks is relatively well preserved, but the capacity for abstract behavior is more seriously impaired. Dementia is usually well established within a year. Some patients show a euphoric contentment, while others are irritable, depressed, and suspicious. Common focal symptoms include apraxia, alexia, agraphia, or aphasia until such time as their characteristics are obscured by general dementia. The patient may have difficulty in naming objects, although he may remember their use and properties. A rather important characteristic of these aphasias is that they are of gradual rather than of sudden onset and the spontaneous logorrhea often found in aphasia due to vascular disease is not present. Echolalia and stereotyped reactions are not infrequent. The pupils, other reflexes, and spinal fluid are not disturbed.

As the disease progresses, the patient becomes asthenic, is confined to bed, and scarcely moves. Dementia becomes extreme, sphincter incontinence develops, the capacity for speech practically disappears, and cachexia becomes marked. The patient usually dies in from four to six years of some intercurrent infection.

Diagnosis

Clinical differentiation of the disease from Alzheimer's disease is extremely difficult. Many clinicians believe that this differentiation can be made only on postmortem examination of the brain. The age period, slowly progressive course, and intellectual impairment are similar in both diseases. Convulsions, facial paresis, and muscular rigidity, common in Alzheimer's disease, are rare in Pick's disease. Aphasic disturbances with perseveration and logoclonia are frequent in Alzheimer's disease but rare in Pick's. Motor impulsiveness and aggression are more common in Alzheimer's. Indifference is common in Pick's disease and anxiety in Alzheimer's disease. Defects of memory seem to occur earlier in Alzheimer's disease, and in late stages memory may be practically obliterated, whereas some retention of it continues in Pick's disease. Delusions, hallucinations, and confabulations, rather frequent in the former disease, are not common in Pick's disease. Hyperactivity is common in Alzheimer's disease; in Pick's disease the patient tends to be underactive. Many believe that deterioration of emotional factors, and especially of habit, progresses more rapidly in Pick's than in Alzheimer's disease. In the former, neurological signs are more frequently focal than in the latter. Finally, Pick's disease occurs much less frequently than does Alzheimer's.

Cerebral arteriosclerosis can usually be differentiated by the antecedent history of headache, dizziness, apoplectic phenomena, and other evidences of vascular disease.

BIBLIOGRAPHY

Busse, E. W., and Pfeiffer, E.: Behavior and Adaption in Late Life. Boston, Little, Brown and Company, 1969.

Corsellis, J. A. N.: Maudsley Monographs No. 9., Mental Illness and the Aging Brain. London, Oxford University Press, 1962.

Gillespie, W. H.: Some regressive phenomena in old age. Brit. J. Med. Psychol., 36:203–209, 1963.

Gottfries, C. G., Gottfries, I., and Roos, B. E.: The investigation of homovanillic acid in the human brain and its correlation to senile dementia. Brit. J. Psychiat., 115:563–574, 1969.

Granick, B. A., and Zeman, F. D.: The aged recluse —an exploratory study with particular reference to community responsibility. J. Chron. Dis., 12: 639–653, 1960.

Larsson, T., Sjögren, T., and Jacobson, G.: Senile Dementia. Copenhagen, Munksgaard, 1963.

Nikado, T., Austin, J., True, B. L., Hutchinson, J., Rinehart, R., Stuckenbrok, H. and Miles, B.: Isolation and preliminary characterization of Alzheimer plaques from presenile and senile dementia. Trans. Amer. Neurol. Assoc., 95:47–50, 1970.

Post, F.: The Clinical Psychiatry of Late Life. 1st ed. Oxford, Pergamon Press, 1965.

Shanas, E., Townsend, P., Wedderburn, D., Fris, H., Melholj, P., and Trethowan, J.: The Social Condition of the Aged. New York, Atherton Press, 1968.

Simon, H.: Physical and socio-psychologic stress in the geriatric mentally ill. Comprehensive Psych., 11:242–247, 1970.

Sjögren, T., et al.: Morbus Alzheimer and morbus Pick: A genetic, clinical and pathoanatomical study. Acta Psychiatrica et Neurologica, Supplement 83. Copenhagen, Munksgaard, 1952.

Stengel, E.: A study on the symptomatology and differential diagnosis of Alzheimer's disease and Pick's disease. J. Ment. Sci., 89:1–20, 1943.

Symposium: The Presenile Dementias. Trans. Amer. Neurol. Assoc., 90:9–23, 1964.

Chapter 11

"It is not a divinity but the mystery of arteriosclerosis that shapes the earthly endings of most lives."

Walter Alvarez

Brain Syndromes Associated with Cerebral Arteriosclerosis and Other Cerebrovascular Disturbances

The circulatory disturbance causing the major frequency of psychosis owing to impairment of cerebral functioning is characterized by *narrowing* or *obliteration of the lumen*. Atherosclerosis, more commonly called arteriosclerosis, is an occlusive disease that affects the nutrient vessels of the brain, heart, or kidney, and by progressively choking off the flow of blood leads to functional alteration and even to disability or death. When the term arteriosclerosis is used in this chapter, it should be borne in mind that the real nature of the pathological vascular process is an atherosclerosis with its distinctive morphological feature of stainable lipid within the atheromatous lesions.

The Dynamics of Cerebral Circulation

Through the use of angiography, surgical explorations, and more recent anatomical studies there has emerged a greatly expanded appreciation of the vascular supply of the brain, particularly as it depends upon the functional integrity of the major extracerebral arteries and their capacity for expanding anastomotic connections.

In man, the internal carotid artery is the major arterial supply to the brain. Yet extensive anastomoses exist between the branches of this vessel and those of the external carotid. The vertebral artery provides a significant contribution to this circulation as well. These anastomotic changes, the *rete mirabile,* are known now to expand widely when, through occlusive disease such as atherosclerosis, the main channels of the internal carotid system are narrowed. Impingement upon the lumen of the great vessels of the arch of the aorta or at the bifurcation of the common carotid through atheromatous plaques, thrombosis, or other constricting lesions may critically influence the blood supply to the brain and produce periodic ischemic crises which impair brain activity and personality functioning just as decisively as focal ischemic crises due to reduction of blood flow by the terminal cerebral arterioles.

In man each hemisphere is supplied by the ipsilateral carotid artery while the cerebral structures contained in the posterior fossa of the skull receive their blood from the basilar artery.

It appears that the circle of Willis, that anastomotic link at the base of the brain between the carotid and basilar arteries, customarily brings up little interchange of blood between the two arterial supplies. In emergencies with sudden occlusion of one of the major arterial channels to the brain, it provides an immediately available anastomotic channel. Thus, it is known that in young persons ligation of one of the internal carotid arteries does not reduce the total circulation of the brain. However, in the elderly, in whom component vessels of the circle of Willis may be partially occluded by an atheromatous plaque and be incapable of full dilatation, the same procedure reduces cerebral blood flow and produces extensive signs of impairment of brain function.

While the cerebral cortex has an extensive capillary supply varying from 1000 capillaries per millimeter of cross section in the gray and 300 in the white matter, to its minute vascularity is much less than that of the heart. Occlusion of blood flow for two minutes in any area leads to cellular ischemia and necrosis.

Cerebral blood flow and cellular oxygenation are held steady in health through the many homeostatic mechanisms which control cardiac output, maintenance of blood pressure, and pulmonary ventilation as well as the special receptors that influence the flow to the head, such as the carotid sinus. Constriction and vasodilation of these blood vessels are mediated by the intrinsic nervous supply of the carotid and vertebral plexi. Thus the sympathetic vasoconstrictors derive from the superior cervical ganglion while the fibers subserving vascular dilatation enter the plexi via the branches of the greater superficial petrosal nerve.

Humoral influences, too, are known to produce narrowing or widening of the brain arterioles. Dilatation occurs with high blood carbon dioxide tensions and constriction follows increase in blood oxygen tension. In pharmacological experiments in which the arterial blood pressure is raised 20 per cent with intravenous injection of norepinephrine, the cerebral vessels constrict with lowering of blood flow, while epinephrine injection brings prescribed for the elderly patient with arteriosclerosis, has little effect on brain vascularity, nor does nicotinic acid, which brings about dilatation of the external carotid system without modifying cerebral blood flow. While histamine dilates the cerebral vessels, its associated effect of lowering blood pressure also obviates change in that blood flow.

Pathophysiology

While in aged healthy men cerebral blood flow approximates that of younger persons, a gradually progressive decline in the cerebral circulation has been found in the majority of studies involving those from the fourth and fifth decade of life onward. With progressive arteriosclerosis there occurs a significant diminution in cerebral circulation associated in some instances with increase in vascular resistance to values twice those noted in healthy persons. With the resulting hypoxia there follow disturbances in cellular metabolism and eventual death of cells. Although it is true that some individuals with cerebral arteriosclerosis associated with markedly diminished general cerebral blood flow appear to show good personality and cerebral function and to withstand well sudden additional lowering of that flow, it must be kept in mind that the presently used techniques of measuring flow do not determine levels in localized subcortical areas but rather present quantitative changes only in the circulation of the brain as a whole.

The part played by age in the genesis of atherosclerosis has been discussed at great length by pathologists. Although it is now generally agreed that atherosclerosis is not a necessary result of age, it is indirectly related to the aging process. With the progressive lengthening of the life span during the present century, there has been a great increase in the number of persons suffering from arteriosclerosis. There is perhaps no better evidence of this fact than the striking increase in the number of admissions to public mental hospitals of persons suffering from mental disorders incident to this disease.

With the progressive diminution in caliber of the relatively narrow vessels of the brain, the flow of blood is slowly throttled and the nutrition of the parenchyma affected. Ganglion cells gradually deteriorate and areas of atrophy develop around the constricted arterioles. Hemorrhage or thrombosis and embolism with infarction may occur. Thrombosis is much more frequent and probably accounts for 85 per cent of vascular accidents.

While there are many case histories which suggest that those with cerebral arteriosclerosis are subject to episodic attacks of transient ischemia due to localized vasoconstrictions, the evidence for such spasms is inconclusive. An equally plausible explanation is the occurrence of transitory periods of hypotension which reduce oxygenation in an area supplied by a critically narrowed arteriole.

Symptoms

The age of onset of the arteriosclerotic psychoses varies widely, but in general it is between 50 and 65. Prodromal symptoms in the form of fatigue, headache, dizziness, diminution of capacity for prolonged concentration, drowsiness in the afternoon or evening, and an insidious impairment of physical and mental abilities are common. Frequently latent character features are revealed or previous trends become pathologically exaggerated. Any apparent change in character in a person over 50 should suggest the possibility of cerebral arteriosclerosis if syphilitic meningoencephalitis is excluded.

In somewhat more than half of the cases, a sudden attack of confusion is the first obvious mental symptom. Episodes of confusion or of excitement or, particularly, of their combined association constitute a frequent symptom of the arteriosclerotic syndrome. During such episodes, there are clouding of consciousness, incoherence, and restlessness, sometimes extreme. Recurrent episodes of this type, as well as transitory attacks of hemiparesis, hemianopia, or aphasia, should suggest the presence of occlusive atheromata in the major extracerebral arteries.

In other cases the onset is insidious and represents what has been descriptively characterized as "a slow dying at the top."

Among such symptoms are easy mental fatigability, a lessening of initiative, an impairment of attention, emotional instability with outbursts of weeping or laughter, and perhaps a tendency to depression. Some patients are irritable, aggressive, meddlesome, quarrelsome, obstinate, jealous, and paranoid. Finer sentiments, such as affection, may be destroyed. Some patients become garrulous. Memory is impaired to varying degrees. At first it may consist merely of difficulty in recollecting names, but later it may become general. The facies may become increasingly immobile and inanimate. Nocturnal attacks of bewilderment, of delirious, anxious states, or of violence may occur. As the illness progresses, the arteriosclerotic patient becomes neglectful of his personal appearance, his clothing may not be clean, and he may fail to bathe. Delusions may be expressed and are particularly apt to be of a persecutory nature, although ideas of ruin and hypochondriacal delusions are not uncommon. The patient may be distressed by ideas of jealousy concerning his wife or other members of his family. His ideational content, like other expressions of his psychosis, is influenced largely by former types of mental mechanisms and other patterns of personality expression. Occasionally a patient is noted who expresses ideas of grandeur representing a compensation for failing sexual capacity. As in senile dementia, defective judgment and decreased inhibition may result in sexual indiscretions or offenses.

Characterological changes representing alterations in adaptive mechanisms and personality defenses may occur. Defenses against feelings of dependency may, for example, be replaced by acceptance of these needs. Hostile impulses that were previously suppressed may be released. Premorbid defensive drives, such as for perfectionism, may be relaxed.

Among persons with more advanced cerebrovascular disease are those subject to "the little strokes." Such individuals may become intermittently psychotic or subject to periods of delirium. Vertical headaches that are worse in the morning, giddiness, short periods of confusion, fleeting loss of power in arm or leg, or momentary aphasias or apraxias usually give warning of subsequent more serious focal lesions. Station becomes insecure, its base wide, the gait uncertain, and the steps short and spastic. Pupillary inequalities are not uncommon, although recent studies have shown that there is no close relationship between retinal atherosclerosis and sclerosis of the small arteries supplying the brain. Coarse tremors may appear, and the patient may finally experience much difficulty in feeding himself.

Cardiovascular disease in the form of cardiac hypertrophy, coronary sclerosis, or chronic valvular disease is common. Numerous paralytic lesions appear—evidence of focal destruction of nervous tissue by occlusion or by rupture of a vessel of considerable size. Upper motor neuron paralyses and various aphasias and apraxias are most frequent. Paraphasia, or confusion of words, may occur.

Deterioration and dementia are hastened by these focal lesions, especially by those that result in serious speech disturbances. Certain intellectual functions may be much impaired while others remain comparatively intact. Epileptiform attacks, either jacksonian or general, may take place, caused, some believe, by temporary anemia or edema.

Patients with cerebral arteriosclerosis are peculiarly apt, on the occasion of a mild infection, to suffer from episodes characterized by confusion, disorientation, misidentification of persons, anxiety, fear reaction, suspiciousness, and delusional trends.

In contrast to the dementing senile patient, the arteriosclerotic patient, at least in the early stages of his deterioration, recognizes that there is a decline in the quickness and accuracy of his mental functions. He often feels keenly his difficulty in finding a word, his weakness of memory, and the diminution of physical and mental capacity.

The following abstract of a patient's clinical record illustrates some of the more frequent symptoms resulting from the physiological disturbances of brain function through arteriosclerotic changes.

W. B., aged 66, a bookkeeper by occupation, was admitted to the hospital when he suddenly suffered from an attack of vertigo and severe headache lasting for about 20 minutes. He then resumed his daily tasks although he felt weak and tired. On the following day, "for no reason that he can explain, as he claims he was not dizzy," his brother reported, "he just lost his balance and fell downstairs." He was then referred to the hospital for study and diagnosis.

The patient's brother added that 18 months previous to this episode the patient first showed a change in behavior. He talked much less and "would often sit and look at absolutely nothing for long periods. For the past year he had been saying rather peculiar things. He became silly, flighty, and confused." While in the general hospital to which he had been admitted, he was constantly worrying over loss of his money, although there was no basis for such a belief. The brother described the patient's behavior in the general hospital as follows: "He was very confused. He would remain in bed, and instead of getting out of the side of the bed, he would crawl over its foot to get out."

Upon arrival at the hospital, the peripheral and retinal arteries were found sclerotic. He said he had come from the B. General Hospital and had never heard of the Ab. Hospital. When asked the dates when be became ill, he maintained that he had not been ill. He gave his age, his birth year, and the current year correctly, but when asked the present date he replied, "The New York Giants won the first game, Brooklyn won the second game, and the third game was going home when I went." A month after admission he conversed freely and usually rationally with other patients and showed concern about the condition of the feeble ones. He continued, however, to manifest difficulty in concentration, in apperception, and in memory for recent events. He was then fully oriented as to time and place and recognized that his memory was impaired. He remarked to his physician, "I don't know. If I have to keep on this way, maybe the good Lord ought to take me." Four months after admission he was described as having periods of memory loss. Although the United States was then intently preoccupied with World War II, he took no interest in the world situation and important events. At times he showed difficulty in choosing the proper word and occasionally became quite irritated at himself for having this difficulty. Although he had completed three years of college, he was unable to answer simple mathematical questions and failed in an attempt to subtract from 100 by using 7 as the subtrahend and the successive differences as the minuend. Under the simple routine of hospital life and freedom from responsibility, the patient improved. Five and a half years after admission he was described as discussing his business affairs intelligently and as showing an interest in hospital activities and as being well informed on current events. Three years later there developed periods of 24 hours' duration during which he became excited, screamed at anyone who approached him, and often became quite threatening, although he never did violence to them. At such times he was somewhat confused.

Prognosis

The course is not always uninterruptedly progressive. It frequently happens that a patient, particularly if he has cardiac and general vascular disease also, is seen in a confused, perhaps excited, state, so that he appears to be quite demented. After rest and several days or a few weeks of the simple regimen of hospital life, the patient may become clearly conscious and apparently recover from the acute symptoms.

With early recognition by appropriate arteriography of cerebral insufficiency due to occluding atheromata of the extracranial arteries supplying the brain, it is now possible by means of appropriate surgical endarterectomy or angioplasty to alleviate immediate symptoms and also maintain improvement over long periods of time in two-thirds to three-fourths of those so treated.

There is constant danger, however, that an apoplectic stroke or another confused episode may occur at any time. Many patients, nevertheless, retain considerable, although impaired, capacity for several years before dementia or physical helplessness removes them from the scene of activity. In many cases death is hastened by general arteriosclerosis associated with cardiorenal disease.

Those who suffer transient attacks of cerebral ischemia before the age of 65 have a significantly poorer outlook for life than those whose symptoms present after this age. Later complications and death are due to both cardiac and cerebrovascular disturbances. The co-existence of hypertension does not seem to modify the mortality rates.

Diagnosis

In the early differential diagnosis of cerebral insufficiency due to atherosclerosis, it is of great clinical importance to distinguish between the type due to atheromata in the major extracerebral vessels and that due to intracerebral occlusive arteriolar disease. In most instances of the former condition, there occur transient episodes of cerebral ischemia which present as bouts of minimal dysfunction in mentation or weakness to apoplectiform hemiparetic attacks. Such symptoms last momentarily or for days. One of the few signs suggestive of extracranial arterial occlusion on physical examination is the presence of murmurs detectable over the great vessels, although the absence of murmurs is without significance. With incomplete occlusion of the internal carotid, systolic murmurs may be heard in the neck at the angle of the jaw; with partial occlusion of the vertebral arteries they may be heard in the supraclavicular region. With partial occlusion of the great vessels in the chest, murmurs may be heard at the base of the neck or in the supraclavicular region, and the pulses in the arms and neck vessels are diminished or absent. Arteriography is, of course, diagnostic and may be done with low risk of complications.

The mental disorder from which the differentiation of arteriosclerotic psychosis is most frequently required is senile dementia. Since the two forms of deterioration are often associated and the manifestations of both are about equally prominent, differentiation may be difficult or impossible. Arteriosclerotic psychosis occurs somewhat more frequently in men than in women, while senile dementia occurs more frequently in women. Arteriosclerosis usually arises earlier in life than senile atrophy. Usually there is less intellectual impairment in arteriosclerosis. Headache, dizziness, or apoplectic phenomena occur in about half of the cases of arteriosclerotic psychosis. Fainting attacks, convulsive seizures, or attacks of cardiac dysfunction likewise suggest an arteriosclerotic origin. Sudden attacks of confusion often occur in arteriosclerotic psychoses.

In arteriosclerosis the intellectual impairment is lacunar; there is good preservation of the personality and the course is fluctuating. In senile dementia there is first a defect in recent memory, then disorientation going on to progressive dementia. Signs of coronary disease, of retinal arteriosclerosis, and of kidney involvement, with associated changes in the urine and an increase in the blood nonprotein nitrogen level, suggest cerebral arteriosclerosis.

Perhaps one of the most significant and also most frequently overlooked factors in the differential diagnosis of the arteriosclerotic brain syndrome is that of the complicating depressive reaction or the depressive reaction of aging. The latter diagnosis is made much more frequently in England than in the United States. Obviously the recognition of these depressive states is highly important in that now impressive therapeutic measures may be initiated. Awareness of declining faculties establishes for the individual with the symptoms of either arteriosclerosis or aging that sense of loss with depressive affect and/or anxiety, limited drive and interest in activities and friends, and sense of hopelessness and helplessness which characterize these states. Suicidal ideation may be noted and in those so predisposed a depressive episode or a manic-depressive illness may erupt with self-reproaches, nihilistic and somatic delusions, and reduction in psychomotor activity. The correct diagnosis of these affective states, either primary or secondary to the arteriosclerotic condition, provides the indication for often gratifying antidepressant therapy.

Finally, acute brain syndromes (delirious states) due to drug intoxications, infarctions, or states of malnutrition must be discriminated from the sudden episodes of cerebral ischemia so common with cerebral arteriosclerosis. Here, the clues are most likely to be given by the history of drug administration, excessive use of alcohol, recent illness, or poor feeding habits.

Treatment

Since our knowledge concerning the causes of cerebral arteriosclerosis is so limited, little can be done to prevent its development. In any case, a carefully regulated mode of life is a fundamental requirement in treatment. Although neither heavy manual labor nor mental tasks involving burdensome responsibilities or emotional stress should be permitted, an agreeable occupation of simple type should be continued as long as possible, due attention being paid to recreation and physical rest. It should be borne in mind that suicide is not rare in arteriosclerotic depressions. The arteriosclerotic patient will be wise to refrain from alcohol. Any inadequacies of nutrition should be improved, and attention should be directed to any associated cardiorenal or other pathologic condition. The value of low-cholesterol low-fat diets, estrogens, heparin, choline, or inositol as a means of influencing the presumed disturbed lipid metabolism remains controversial. Hydrotherapy in mild forms, carefully supervised, may be employed, but measures that are too long or too vigorous may be harmful.

Chlorpromazine has been helpful with some patients in reducing nocturnal insomnia and restlessness, confusion, excitement, and aggressive, destructive behavior, but care must be taken in the case of the arteriosclerotic patient because of the possibility of a hypotensive reaction following administration of the drug. For this reason, oral administration is preferred, commencing with small doses (10 mg. three times daily) and gradually increasing the amount. The use of other sedatives often may be discontinued. The dosage needed and tolerated is highly variable. Psychotherapy should not be forgotten in the anxious patient. Barbiturates will sometimes aggravate the confusion associated with cerebral arteriosclerosis and hypertensive encephalopathy. The dizziness, headache, insomnia, confusion, and delirious confusion occurring in these disorders are often relieved by the administration of aminophylline in doses of 4 grains each four times a day.

Pentylenetetrazol (Metrazol) given orally in doses ranging from 4.5 to 12 gm. over prolonged periods is credited by some with improving the sense of well-being and relieving the general symptoms of debility.

The therapeutic value of vasorelaxant agents acting on smooth muscle of the vessel walls is unclear. Isoxsuprine (20 mg. by mouth three times daily) has been tried with reported success in relieving headaches and reducing symptoms suggestive of recurrent cerebral ischemic attacks. This pharmacologic agent with nylidrin also stimulates the myocardium and increases cardiac output without producing general vasodilation.

Surgical treatment with endarterectomy or angioplasty is indicated in instances of occlusive disease of the extracranial cerebrovascular supply, particularly in early and incomplete obstructions. With thrombosis superimposed on atheromata, lesions of the innominate, subclavian, and common carotid are almost always amenable to such treatment, but operability is more difficult when the common carotid or vertebral arteries are involved. When both carotids are stenosed but the clinical symptoms may be ascribed to major disease in one of the two vessels, effective intravascular surgery may provide relief for periods of three to five years before contralateral stenosis or occlusion occurs.

Psychoses Following Major Vascular Surgery

Postoperative psychoses are common in patients who have undergone open heart surgery. In the earlier studies psychotic reactions were noted in 30 to 40 per cent of patients treated by cardiotomy. Fewer responses are now seen. These reactions are characterized by anxiety, disorientation, transient disturbances of perceptions with illusions, visual and auditory hallucinations, and paranoid delusions. Sometimes they are accompanied by episodic attacks of hyperventilation or auras. As such they confuse the evaluation of the postoperative state and impede surgical recovery. Some patients, so affected, have attempted suicide; others, through their agitation, have pulled out or upset tubes or other measures of support needed for their postoperative maintenance

Both physiologic and psychologic factors are important as etiologic agents. Some patients have had previous cerebrovascular accidents or disease. Others undergo cardiac fibrillation or become hypotensive in the postoperative period. Those patients who tend to deny anxiety preoperatively are more prone to this response. Their isolation in intensive care units, with the often associated sensory and sleep deprivation to which they are then exposed, is believed to lead to a breakdown of this ego defense with emergence of diffuse anxiety. Its incidence may be diminished by preoperative discussion of the fear and anxiety expected in relation to such operations, the patient's previous surgical and traumatic experiences, and any overdetermined responses or expectations. So, too, postoperative stress may be minimized and psychologic support enhanced by assuring regular sleep and the presence of reassuring social stimulation.

BIBLIOGRAPHY

DeBakey, M. E., Crawford, E. S., Morris, G. C., and Cooley, D. A.: Arterial reconstructive operations for cerebrovascular insufficiency due to extracranial arterial occlusive disease. J. Cardiov. Surg., 3:12–35, 1962.

Ehrentheil, O. F.: Differential diagnosis of organic dementias and affective disorders in aged patients. Geriatrics, 12:426–432, 1957.

Goldner, J. C., Whisnant, J. P., and Taylor, W. F.: Long term prognosis of transient cerebral ischemic attacks. Trans. Am. Neurol. Assoc., 94:20–24, 1969.

Gurdjian, E. S., Darmody, W. R., and Thomas, L. M.: Recurrent strokes due to occlusive disease of extracranial cerebral vessels. Trans. Amer. Neurol. Assoc., 94:11–14, 1969.

Heller, S. S., Frank, K. A., Malin, J. R., and Korn-feld, D. S.: Psychiatric complications of open heart surgery: a re-examination. New England J. Med., *283:*1015–1020, 1970.

Kety, S. S.: The cerebral circulation. Chap. LXXI, Sec. 1, Vol. 3, pp. 1751–1760. *In* Handbook of Physiology. Washington, D.C.: American Physiological Society, 1960.

Layne, O. L., and Yudofsky, S. C.: Postoperative psychosis in cardiotomy patients. New England J. Med., *284:*518–520, 1971.

Roth, M.: Some diagnostic and aetiological aspects of confusional states in the elderly. Gerontologia Clinica, *1:*83–95, 1959.

Simonson, E., and McGavack, T. H. (eds.): Cerebral Ischemia. Springfield, Illinois, Charles C Thomas, 1964.

Sours, J. A.: Neuropsychiatric findings in internal carotid artery occlusive disease with cerebrovascular damage. Psychiat. Quart., *38:*405–423, 1964.

Whittier, J. R.: Vasorelaxant drugs and cerebrovascular disease. Angiology, *15:*82–87, 1964.

Chapter 12

"In the bottle, discontent seeks for comfort, cowardice for courage, and bashfulness for confidence."

Samuel Johnson (1709–1784)

Alcoholic Psychoses and Alcoholism

Alcoholism and the disturbances of metabolism often associated with it may lead to both acute and chronic brain syndromes. A discussion of both of these syndromes is included in this chapter, as well as that of various other aspects of indulgence in alcohol.

The subject of the use and effect of alcoholic liquors, whether considered from sociological, physiological, or psychiatric points of view, still provokes much discussion and wide divergence of opinion. Unfortunately, moralistic implications have retarded the development of a scientific understanding and rational management of alcoholism.

Those psychoses which occur as the most conspicuous complications of addiction to alcohol represent the most frequently encountered states of cerebral insufficiency caused by toxic or metabolic disorders. Thus successful diagnostic and therapeutic management demands modern medical understanding. Yet these disorders are invariably encountered in those whose behavior is characterized by continual or episodic excessive imbibition of alcohol.

Since the earliest recorded times in the history of man, he has indulged in consumption of alcohol for euphoric purposes, to celebrate various festivities, to solemnize religious rituals, to grace social functions, and to provide surcease from his immediate or continuing emotional stress. The widespread use of alcohol seems to have commenced with the beginnings of the western industrial societies, although the consequences of its continual abuse were known many centuries earlier. Since the occurrence of the psychoses is inextricably linked to alcoholism per se, both are considered in this chapter.

Prevalence

It is estimated that there are about four and one-half million persons in the United States on whose lives drinking has an adverse effect in one way or another, also that at least 12,000 alcoholics die each year from chronic alcoholism. Five out of six alcoholics are men between the ages of 30 and 55—the most productive years. Of these admitted for the first time to public mental hospitals in the United States in 1960, 14.6 per cent were alcoholics, an 18 per cent increase over 1950. Such hospital admissions rank now only behind those for schizophrenia and mental diseases of old age.

Those alcoholics admitted to hospital with psychoses or seriously impairing behavioral disturbances form only a small minority of the total who suffer from alcoholism in all parts of the world. The prevalence of alcoholism varies, apparently in relation to social and cultural factors. In France, where a high proportion of the adult population derives its income from the production and sale of alcoholic beverage, there are much acceptance of wine drinking and little public expression of drunkenness. High rates of alcoholism and its complications exist among the Irish and Irish Americans, low rates among Orthodox Jews and Asians.

These variations in appearance of alcoholism seem related to usage and acceptability of drinking within the ethnic and cultural groups.

Those psychotic reactions secondary to alcoholism occur at a mean age in the forties. They are the consequence of drinking habits initiated many years beforehand. Usually one discovers that the alcoholic commences his habituation in social drinking, in which he both enjoys relief from the usual stresses of his life and learns that his inner tensions can be alleviated by the intake of alcoholic drink. Over time he relies increasingly upon drinking as a means of reduction of anxiety.

Later his bouts of drinking are associated with amnesic episodes in which he does not seem to lose consciousness but has little or no later recollection of his actions or of events that took place, even though to others the amount of alcohol he imbibed seems small. This is sometimes spoken of as a prodromal phase of alcoholism. As a habitual drinker he has limited ability to control his intake. Once he commences to drink, he continues until he is comatose, unable to coordinate his actions for imbibition, or nauseated and vomiting. At this time in his course he may periodically discontinue drinking. However, once accepting another drink his compulsivity reasserts itself. Criticized by his family, friends, and employers who recognize his instability in action and thought, he offers various excuses, yet may indulge himself in surreptitious drinking, hiding his habit from others. Personal care declines, attention is blunted, and he neglects his work, family and social relations. It is here that he may develop vitamin deficiencies through neglect of his regular eating, or, in the state of addiction, a withdrawal syndrome with psychotic or epileptiform convulsions.

Vehicular Accidents and Alcohol

In modern societies with their great dependence on high velocity transportation, acute or chronic alcohol intoxication—and through it impairment of perception, judgment, reaction time, and quality of response—contributes excessively to accidents. Blood alcohol levels of over 0.10 per cent have been found in large numbers of persons killed in auto accidents. Impairment of functioning as a driver occurs in many others at much lower concentrations of blood alcohol. Blood alcohol levels of 80 mg. per 100 ml. impair dark adaptation. Also, at this level various investigations have demonstrated that car drivers show impaired judgment in passing other vehicles, in approaching caution lights, in interpretation of multiple sensory inputs, and in maintaining attentiveness when driving for long periods. Studies have shown that the risk of incurring an automobile accident increases appreciably when the blood alcohol level enters the range of 50 to 100 mg. per 100 ml. At the latter level the probability of an accident is ten times more than that for a sober driver. In private aviation, 35 per cent of fatalities occur in drinking pilots. In one general hospital, 20 per cent of hospital admissions for home accidents were associated with intoxication.

Alcoholism and Personality Disturbance

Alcohol addiction is symptomatic of personality disturbance. Underneath the expressions of chronic intoxication with alcohol, and in spite of the conviction of most alcoholics that they would be quite normal if they ceased drinking, psychologically well-adapted personalities are seldom found during periods of sobriety. Some two-thirds of chronic alcoholics fall outside the ordinary classifications of the psychoses and psychoneuroses. The vast majority have character traits of the inadequate, passive-aggressive personalities. A lesser number are rigidly organized, compulsive individuals or dependent individuals with depressive affect and certain paranoidal personalities. The remainder of the addicted present the character traits and symptomatic expressions of the major psychoses, particularly paranoid and "pseudoneurotic" schizophrenia and the manic-depressive reactions, as well as the psychoneuroses and the antisocial personality disturbances.

Studies of chronically alcoholic men, the "skid row" alcoholics, have disclosed that they demonstrate as much or more psychopathology as do groups of psychotic hospitalized patients, particularly in such behavioral indices as bizarre appearance and behavior, speech disorganization, social isolation, and disoriented memory. These chronically habituated alcoholics are the most conspicuous for their evidence of addiction, but they must also be recognized as predisposed to it through the existence of prior severe personality disorders.

Psychogenesis of Alcoholism

Continuing studies of the families and relatives of alcoholics reaffirm that experience of early parental loss through death, separation, or divorce is more common in the alcoholic than in others. Deprivation of both parents with subsequent institutional or foster home care for the children has been noted as significant in some series of studies. Large families with older fathers and predominantly male members generate more alcoholics in some countries. An earlier initiation of excessive drinking seems more likely in those who experienced parental loss than in those without such a loss. Alcoholism is more common among men than women. So, too, the recognition of its existence as a series habituation or addiction takes place at a mean age almost a decade earlier in men than women. Many married women commence their drinking in middle age as their role of mother and wife is challenged in the departure from the home of their children—the challenge of the "empty nest."

When one examines the families and relatives of alcoholics in relation to risk of associated psychiatric illness, it appears that primary affective disorders are discovered in a considerable proportion of the female alcoholics—in whom this term is used to mean a disorder present before excessive drinking occurred. A personality disorder, usually sociopathy, is the primary diagnosis most frequently made in the males. Yet the morbid risk for affective disorder and alcoholism is greater, as Winokor and his colleagues have found, in relatives of both males and females, with a greater risk for alcoholism among male relatives and for affective disorders in female relatives. The affective disorder found in this series of relatives was usually depression alone: "unipolar depression."

Thus, genetics, constitution, and the child's emotional experiences in its family transactions all contribute to the predisposition to alcoholism. Cultural influences reinforce the family patterns, establishing the predilection for alcohol abuse as the means of gaining relief from anxiety and depression. Later experiences of deprivation of emotional support may act, and sometimes act repetitively, as precipitants to bouts of drinking or return to alcohol in those who have given up the habit.

Often the family histories demonstrate that the future alcoholic was mothered by an overindulgent and overprotective parent who encouraged his infantile oral demands from the early periods of life so that eventually they were too excessive to be met. The outbursts of rage at frustrations of demands are met by such mothers with redoubled efforts which, in turn, intensify the infantile demands and dependency. The maternal overprotection often is brought about by conflict resulting from a remote, cold, or brutalized relationship with the marital partner or by his or her regular or intermittent absence due to a variety of causes. The conflicts with father and siblings are heightened for children reared in this way. In other families from which alcoholics emerge, the paternal attitudes also are alternately severe and overindulgent; bewildered by such inconsistency, the child evolves into a passive-dependent adult who is either unable to express his needs and is thereby frustrated and filled with guilt and resentment due to the restrained and internalized hostilities, or else is subject to periodic outbursts of aggressions when released from his inhibitions. Social and sexual identity are inadequately established as the parental roles are confused. Since the growing child is protected from environmental demands through parental ambivalence and conflict, ego functions fail to evolve well.

Alcohol is discovered as a release from the painful internalized emotions because the parents are permissive toward drinking. Alcoholism in some form is much more common in the parents, siblings, and marital partner than in the population at large. It is this open indulgence in alcohol in the family or in the adolescent society of the future addict which allows the superego defect that permits its repeated use. Secondarily there evolves the psychological and pharmacological dependency on a substitute which at first offers euphoria but which later, as ego frustrations mount, offers little more than relief from unbearable tensions.

The psychopathologic conditions leading to alcoholism vary with the individual alcoholic. Thus it appears in many instances that the addictive drinker may have been psychologically traumatized very early in life and his personality remained fixated at an early, oral stage of development. Again, alcoholism may occur in persons who, through the absence of a desirable identification figure, never developed a stabilizing superego. Lacking in responsibility and ego strength, they are closely allied to the character neurotic. Sometimes the periodic drinker seems by his alcoholic bout to be seeking for relief from an overly strict superego. In some instances there are unconscious homosexual identifications and tendencies. If his drinking continues and the alcoholic pattern becomes established, the disregard of reality which it brings about begins to operate and serves as a further but undesirable defense.

Physiological Effects

While alcohol affects all cells of the body, its most marked effect is on the cells of the brain and is therefore manifested in behavior. Since alcohol does not require prior digestion, it may be absorbed directly into the blood. The rate of absorption is much more rapid than its elimination, with the result that with heavy indulgence a considerable concentration may occur. While there is an individual tolerance, it is generally accepted that a person showing a concentration of 150 mg. or more of alcohol in 100 ml. of blood, or its equivalent in urine, saliva, or breath, should be considered intoxicated. In the opinion of the National Safety Council Committee on Tests for Intoxication, this concentration so impairs judgment and performance in driving an automobile as to render the operation of a car unsafe.

Only a small proportion of the imbibed alcohol is excreted from the lungs, kidneys, and skin (2 to 10 per cent). The remainder is metabolized in the liver by a diphosphopyridine nucleotide–dependent enzyme to acetaldehyde. The second stage of oxidation of alcohol is from acetaldehyde to acetic acid. This occurs not only in the liver but in other organs as well. (With the use of disulfiram, combustion of acetaldehyde is inhibited and acetaldehyde may reach toxic levels.) Finally, acetic acid is oxidized to carbon dioxide and water.

The presumed stimulating tendencies of the drug, in terms of behavior, are due to loss of inhibition through impairment of the ordinarily acting ego-superego controls. Thus it reduces avoidance of behaviors generally inducing fear or anxiety. It also has specific analgesic effects.

Carpenter states that alcohol effects complex thought processes by impairing inductive reasoning. Yet no change or even slight improvement takes place in deductive tasks. The release of inhibition consequent to moderate use of alcohol is the major behavioral effect of alcohol conducive to the feeling of well being, social ease, and sometimes increased capacity for creative work and effective drive. Such release of inhibition, leading to creative thought, probably results from the emergence of primary thought and its reorganization and integration with secondary thought processes. Such effects do not occur with heavy intoxication when impairment of all perceptual, cognitive, and judgmental activities takes place. Alcohol tends to be sedating and to induce sleep, but even here its actions vary in moderate doses, depending upon the individual. Some become aggressive and noisy.

In the chronic alcoholic, Johnson, Burdick, and Smith have found that long latencies exist for sleep onset. Sleep itself occurs with frequent awakenings and bodily movements, and numerous shifts from one sleep stage to another, with marked diminution of stage 4 (slow wave sleep). These researchers suggest that the deficiency in slow wave sleep may be related to a disturbance in brain serotonin and norepinephrine metabolism.

Sexual drive is usually increased in the inhibited. But in the male, although the potential for erection may present, that for ejaculation and orgasm is often reduced.

So, too, alcohol tends to stimulate the appetite in small doses. Although its persistent use leads to a chronic gastritis with associated degrees of anorexia, it is nutritive, producing 71 calories per gram. In large doses it increases the vitamin requirements of the body, perhaps because of the additional caloric intake. This, in addition to his failure to maintain a regular and nourishing diet, may be a reason for the predilection of the chronic alcoholic to suffer so frequently from such psychoses as delirium tremens and Korsakoff's syndrome.

Ethanol also tends to produce a hypoglycemia in fasting healthy persons, alcoholics, thyrotoxics, and decompensated diabetics. Fasted nondiabetic obese persons are refractory to the induction of hypoglycemia by alcohol.

Administration of alcohol leads to a reduction in the blood of a norepinephrine-like substance that is elevated in association with anxiety, a cholinergic-like substance that is elevated with arousal of tension, and a substance regularly found in association with resentment. Alcoholics consistently were found to have greater amounts of the "resentment substance" than others, and alcohol was more effective in reducing the action of all the substances in the blood of alcoholics.

Since alcohol reduces his anxiety, tension, and resentment, the alcoholic seeks its use more and more frequently. His addiction is manifested not only by this persistent use but also by the effects of its withdrawal. These results may be moderate, such as increased anxiety, a craving for alcohol, weakness, tremor, and perspiration, but may be serious and include anorexia, nausea, vomiting, fever, tachycardia, convulsions, hallucinations, and delirium tremens.

Although alcohol has long been known to be a depressant to brain function, its method of action is still uncertain. It is thought that it may interfere with synaptic transmission. The effect of alcohol on the brain is from above downward. Higher cortical functions such as judgment, memory, learning, self-criticism, and environmental awareness suffer first. With depression of higher functions, lower parts of the brain are released from higher control. Thus the excitement frequently seen in an intoxicated person is doubtless a release phenomenon resulting from a depression of the highest brain functions. With the ingestion of excessively large amounts of alcohol, this gradually descending depressive effect may extend to the entire brain and inhibit not only the supramedullary areas but even the medulla with its respiratory, cardiac, and vasomotor centers.

Alcoholism and Crime

It was formerly stated that alcoholism was directly responsible for a large, perhaps a major, part of crime. There is now an increasing tendency to consider that alcohol and criminalism are caused by similar social and psychological factors. Emotional instability and other expressions of a poorly integrated personality characterize both the recidivous criminal offender and the alcohol addict. The relation of alcohol to crime is more frequently one of a common cause rather than of cause and effect. It should be added, however, that the drinking of alcohol tends to be accompanied by a release of sexual and aggressive impulses.

Alcoholism and Psychoses

The relation between alcohol and the so-called alcoholic psychoses is not as simple as was formerly assumed. In many instances alcohol serves merely to release a reaction that is primarily psychogenic with factors intrinsic in the personality. In other cases there is such an interplay of psychogenic and metabolic factors that the picture becomes complex. In Korsakoff's syndrome and in chronic alcoholic deterioration, the psychosis is not, as was formerly believed, caused by the toxic effects of the alcohol itself but by thiamine deficiency. Even in this, the structure of the personality influences the picture. It is important to remember, too, that alcoholism may be a symptom—sometimes the most obvious symptom—of another personality disorder such as depressive psychosis, schizophrenia, or paresis.

PATHOLOGICAL INTOXICATION

Occasionally an individual of unstable personality may, on partaking of alcohol, suffer from a transitory mental state much more striking in the nature and severity of the symptoms than ordinary drunkenness, and known as pathological intoxication. The onset is dramatically sudden. Consciousness is impaired, and the patient is confused and disoriented and suffers from illusions, hallucinations of sight, and transitory delusions. Activity is exaggerated, impulsive, and aggressive, even to the point of destructiveness. The emotional disturbances are profound and may consist of rage, anxiety, or depression, perhaps with suicidal attempt. The disorder lasts from a few minutes to a day or more and is usually followed by a prolonged sleep, after which there is an amnesia for the episode.

There is an increasing tendency to consider that such episodes with their disturbances of consciousness and perhaps crimes of violence are really instances of psychomotor epilepsy released by alcohol in persons predisposed to such seizures.

The behavior observed in "pathological intoxication" is in many ways illustrated by the following case:

N. W., aged 28, was seen in jail while awaiting trial on a charge of drunkenness and disorderly conduct. The patient's father had committed suicide as he was about to be sent to a hospital for mental diseases. The patient himself was described as being a friendly but quick-tempered and restless individual whose marriage had terminated in early divorce. He was said never to have been particularly alcoholic, but one July 4 he celebrated the holiday by drinking two bottles of beer and a glass of wine. Soon afterward he attempted to fling himself down an 80-foot embankment and was so greatly excited that he was taken to the police station for the night. The next morning he had no recollection of the affair. Ten months later the patient called late one afternoon to see friends who invited him to sample what they considered choice varieties of whiskey and gin. He accepted their invitation and drank somewhat more heavily than usual. Soon after leaving the home of his friends he was observed by a police officer to be acting strangely. As the officer spoke to him he attacked him. While the officer was calling for help, the patient disappeared. About 15 minutes later two women were startled to see a strange man thrust his head through a closed window of their living room and shout, "Help! Murder!" It was the patient, who then ran on to another house where he rang the doorbell insistently. As the occupant answered the summons he again screamed, "Murder!" and ran to the street once more, where he broke the windshields and headlights of several parked automobiles and tore out the seats and pulled parts from other cars. At this point he was seized and taken to the police station where, on awakening the following morning, he had no recollection of his experiences of the previous night.

ACUTE ALCOHOLISM AND ALCOHOL WITHDRAWAL STATES

In the majority of instances, bouts of acute alcoholism may be terminated by withdrawal to a supportive, nonstimulating environment, with provision to insure adequate sleep and rest. In such circumstances, bodily processes quickly metabolize the excessive alcohol.

Much more complicated as regards therapeutic management are the acute withdrawal syndromes which erupt when long-continuing drinking bouts are terminated. After a few days of drinking, abstinence may result in tremulousness, nausea, and vomiting. If the individual resumes drinking and then abstains once more, as the signs of acute intoxication subside, convulsive seizures or delirium with hallucinations may appear. The latter occurs only when the drinking bout has lasted several weeks.

Alkalosis regularly follows in the early stages of withdrawal, and other electrolytic disturbances, including hypomagnesemia, are frequent. For proper management, blood electrolyte studies should be performed. If deficiencies are noted in the fluid and electrolyte balances, they may then be corrected with administration of appropriate intravenous fluids.

Chlordiazepoxide, given in 50 mg. dosage by mouth at six hour intervals, provides both rapid relief of symptoms and the greatest preventive potential against later convulsions or delirium tremens. Seizures occur more often and later in the course of treatment in chlorpromazine-treated groups.

Barbiturates are rarely indicated in the treatment of withdrawal state convulsions. If severe or persistent, diphenylhydantoin in doses of 100 mg. four times daily should be first administered. The use of steroids, large amounts of glucose, or gastric lavage has been discontinued, as they may adversely affect fluid and electrolyte balance. On the other hand, prescription of vitamin B complex is desirable.

DELIRIUM TREMENS

This is an acute psychosis that may develop in the chronic alcoholic following an unusually severe or prolonged debauch.

The term *delirium tremens* was first used by Thomas Sutton in 1813 in what is regarded as the classic description of this disease. The nature of the factors that operate in its production is uncertain. While it was long considered an acute psychosis developed during drinking, it is now generally thought to be a withdrawal syndrome precipitated in the chronic alcoholic suddenly deprived of alcohol. Delirium has been produced in the experimental laboratory by the sudden withdrawal of alcohol in those consuming 12 oz. or more of the agent for 48 or more days. The withdrawal may be associated not only with delirium and sometimes with convulsions but also with abnormalities in the encephalogram. On the other hand, disorder may arise from metabolic disturbances, including faulty carbohydrate metabolism, impairment of the detoxicating function of the liver, disturbed protein metabolism, acidosis, suboxidation of the brain, disturbed water balance, and various nutritional deficiencies, particularly of vitamin B, which the alcoholic usually takes in insufficient amounts and may not be able to absorb.

Delirium tremens is rare in a person under 30 years of age, or after less than three or four years of chronic alcoholism. The delirium is usually preceded by an aversion for food, restlessness, irritability, and disturbed sleep in which terrifying dreams occur. Occasional illusions and hallucinations are soon followed by more frequent ones, usually of a fleeting, terrifying nature. Figures on the wallpaper become menacing animate objects; inkspots become insects which the patient attempts to seize and destroy. The visual hallucinations are often of objects that appear to be moving, and are particularly apt to represent loathsome animals of fantastic shapes which terrify the patient and from which he may struggle to escape. These imaginary animals may be of diminutive size. At times hallucinations can be suggested; the patient, for example, may be handed an imaginary thread which, in response to instructions, he will carefully wind about his finger. Tactile hallucinations, probably associated with peripheral neuritis, are not infrequent. The patient feels as well as sees the insects on his skin. Olfactory hallucinations may occur. The patient may exclaim with terror that gas is being pumped into his room. While visual hallucinations are most numerous, auditory ones are not infrequently added.

As indicated, the mood is usually one of irritability, fear, apprehension, and even of terror. Occasionally, however, it is one of euphoria, amusement, good-natured silliness, or grim humor accompanied by the narration of preposterous confabulations.

Consciousness is clouded, and the patient may be greatly confused with disorientation for time and place. Speech is often incoherent. Persons about the patient may be misidentified. Attention is fleeting and impressions are retained but a moment. At times the delirium is of an occupational type. The motor restlessness is marked. The patient repeatedly gets out of bed to attend to some detail of his supposed occupation or to seize some imaginary object. Sleep is usually impossible.

On physical examination, the conjunctivae and face are ordinarily found to be congested. The pupils are dilated and often react slowly. A coarse tremor is an almost constant accompaniment. It is increased by muscular tension, such as extension of the fingers. The tongue is tremulous, as are also the muscles of the lips and face in well-developed cases. The pulse is rapid and often irregular and weak. The temperature is elevated and in some cases may be high. The skin is moist, the face often showing marked perspiration. The tendon reflexes are usually increased, although occasionally they are absent because of neuropathy. The nerve trunks and muscles may be painful to pressure. Albuminuria exists in about half the cases.

Differential Diagnosis

Delirium tremens is to be differentiated from other forms of alcoholic hallucinosis as well as brain syndromes. Among the latter, and particularly pertinent to the group of alcoholic patients, is the delirious state associated with *acute hepatic insufficiency* and referred to sometimes as *impending hepatic coma.* Alcoholic cirrhosis of the liver is the most common cause of the condition, although it may occur with other illnesses which lead to severe disturbance of the brain parenchyma. The importance of its discrimination rests upon the necessity of prescribing quite differing therapy; that for delirium tremens may lead to a fatal outcome in the patient with impending hepatic coma.

While both conditions may follow a period of heavy drinking, delirium tremens more often has its onset after cessation of drinking. The patient with delirium tremens is consciously responsive unless sedated, often aggressive and destructive, and his hallucinatory experiences are generally visual. The patient with impending hepatic coma more often is dull and lethargic, with diminution of psychomotor activity, and seldom has vividly formed visual hallucinations. Perhaps the most characteristic differential point is the irregular, "flapping" tremor which presents itself on extension of the arms in hepatic insufficiency. Speech is more often slowed, slurred, or monotonous, with perseveration, and a mask-like facial expression may be seen. Both flexor muscle tonus and tendon reflexes are increased.

Those with impending hepatic coma usually subside into stupor with little indication of anxiety or fear, and there is more likely to be hypersomnia than the insomnia of the individual with delirium tremens. Hyperphagia exists with liver disorder, in contrast to the anorexia of the delirium tremens.

Also, the general medical examination in hepatic coma often shows evidence of jaundice, gross hepatomegaly, and fetor hepaticus, with elevation of the blood ammonia; these findings are absent in delirium tremens.

The electroencephalogram has been useful in the diagnosis of hepatic insufficiency in that a "triphasic wave" may be found in approximately 25 per cent of cases. Furthermore, a provocative dose of oral ammonium chloride (0.05 grain per kilogram of body weight) leads to an increase in EEG abnormality within 30 to 60 minutes in this condition.

Acute pancreatitis, another complication common in the chronic alcoholic, may also be associated with a hallucinatory psychosis that must be differentiated from delirium tremens. Here the symptom of severe abdominal pain with abdominal tenderness, vomiting, tachycardia, leukocytosis, and particularly an elevated serum amylase level (over 300 Somogyi units) should establish the primary diagnosis.

Pathology

Changes both of a degenerative and of an inflammatory nature may occur. The brain is usually edematous. There are more or less liquefactive degeneration of nerve cells and an increase of glia with some round-cell infiltration. There is degeneration of myelin sheaths, especially in the cerebellum. Punctate hemorrhages occur and there is a mild degree of leptomeningitis.

Prognosis and Course

Delirium tremens usually runs an acute course, terminating in from three to ten days. Convalescence is frequently preceded by a prolonged sleep following which consciousness becomes clear and the hallucinations disappear, although brief periods of delirium may occasionally recur at night for a short time. The prognosis depends largely upon the presence or absence of coexisting disease. The existence of myocardial degeneration, which is not uncommon in such chronic alcoholic patients, makes the prognosis much less favorable. The mortality in the type of case that reaches a hospital averages from 5 to 15 per cent, the two most frequent causes of death being heart failure and pneumonia. Occasionally, instead of terminating in death or recovery within the

usual period, the psychosis may merge into a Korsakoff's psychosis.

Treatment

It has been customary to withdraw alcohol at once, but this practice is questionable. It is of great importance that care be taken to conserve the strength of a patient suffering from delirium tremens. The patient should be placed in bed immediately. As he is usually fearful he should be constantly supervised and reassured concerning his fears and hallucinations. Many a patient has died from exhaustion while struggling under mechanical restraint or from the depressing effect of sedative drugs. Restraint should therefore never be employed. Chlordiazepoxide should be prescribed orally in doses of 50 mg. every six hours. Any fluid or electrolyte imbalance or deficiency should be corrected by administration of appropriate parenteral infusion. Cardiac stimulation by means of caffeine is usually to be recommended. Other sedation should be avoided. Morphine should never be given. Thiamine chloride (50 to 100 mg.) and nicotinic acid (10 mg.) should be given immediately and repeated three times daily. These vitamins may be added to the infusions for intravenous use.

In those patients in whom delirium and marked tremor exist, the possibility of magnesium deficiency must be considered. With evidence of depression of the serum magnesium (normal 2.0 milliequivalents per liter), magnesium sulfate in a 5 per cent sterile solution may be given in doses up to 2.0 gm. four times daily for three days and then 1.0 gm. per day for an additional two or three days.

The patient has usually eaten little or nothing for several days. Since his gastrointestinal tract suffers from catarrhal inflammation because of his long indulgence in alcohol, he has little appetite and may even be nauseated. It is, however, exceedingly important that he receive an abundant, soft diet, particularly of carbohydrates. If possible, it should contain from 3000 to 4000 calories a day and should be rich in vitamins. The administration of the entire vitamin B complex is especially advisable as a preventive of Wernicke's syndrome or encephalopathy from nicotinic acid deficiency.

In contrast to the above treatment, alcoholic patients with the deliria of *impending hepatic coma* must be placed on a protein-free diet and fed with fruit juices and dextrose. Tranquilizers, sedatives, and methionine are to be avoided, while tetracycline, 1 to 2 gm. daily, and infusions of sodium glutamate (25 to 100 gm. daily in glucose solution) and L-arginine may be given to lower the blood ammonia. Recently continuous plasma and whole blood transfusions have proved effective in relieving such conditions.

KORSAKOFF'S PSYCHOSIS

Sometimes it will be noted in what, except for the absence of the usual critical sleep, appeared to be an ordinary case of delirium tremens that the hallucinations and acute delirium disappear but the clinical picture merges into one characterized by amnesia, disorientation for time and place, and a falsification of memory, associated with the symptoms and signs of peripheral neuropathy. At other times the syndrome develops in the chronic alcoholic who has not suffered from a preceding delirium tremens but has indulged excessively in alcohol for several years. This syndrome was described in 1887 by the Russian psychiatrist, Sergei Korsakoff. Because of its frequent association with chronic alcoholism, Korsakoff's psychosis has long been classified among the alcoholic psychoses. Strictly speaking, this syndrome should be classified elsewhere.

Etiology and Pathology

The condition is but one of several syndromes that result from vitamin B deficiency, a form of deficiency to which the chronic alcoholic, with his impaired gas-

trointestinal absorption, his diet largely limited to vitamin-free alcohol, and his increased vitamin requirement resulting from the high caloric effect of alcohol, is especially prone. Vitamin B deficiency may, of course, exist under various circumstances. Although a deficiency of other vitamin B constituents doubtless contributes to these syndromes, thiamine and niacin deficiencies are particularly responsible for them. The variations in these syndromes depend largely upon the parts of the nervous system in which the neuronal degeneration is localized. If this degeneration is largely in the cerebrum and the peripheral nerves, Korsakoff's syndrome results. If the degenerative changes occur in the long peripheral nerves of the alcoholic, the result is known as "alcoholic neuritis." If the greatest deficiency is in niacin and the degeneration is marked in the cerebrum, less in the spinal cord, and least in the peripheral nerves, the vitamin deficiency encephalopathy assumes the form of pellagra. If the brain stem is the site of the degenerative process, the syndrome is that of Wernicke's disease. Frequently these syndromes are not sharply defined but merge one into another, the pattern depending upon the vitamin in which the deficiency is greatest and upon the sites and extent of the degeneration. For example, symptoms of Korsakoff's psychosis and Wernicke's disease or of Wernicke's disease and pellagra may be associated. In fact, in nutritional encephalopathy it is possible in the same individual to see delirium tremens, Korsakoff's psychosis, niacin deficiency encephalopathy, and the Wernicke syndrome.

The nutritional encephalopathy is probably caused by the fact that in the absence of ample quanities of thiamine and nicotinic acid there is an impaired oxidation of pyruvic acid during the breakdown of glucose.

The histopathology of Korsakoff's psychosis consists of diffuse parenchymatous changes. Among these changes are axonal alterations, a deposition of excessive amounts of normal lipochrome pigment in the nerve cells, glia, microglia, and around the blood vessels in the prefrontal and motor cortex, and acute chromatolytic changes in the larger nerve cells in these areas, especially in the Betz cells.

Symptoms

The most conspicuous symptoms have already been indicated. Superficially, consciousness may appear clear and the seriousness of the mental disorder may not be apparent. On questioning the patient, however, one is often surprised to discover the extent of mental impairment. Although possessing a relatively good grasp of what is in sight, he is disoriented as to that which is beyond immediate observation and dependent on memory. At first the memory loss is most marked for events occurring since the onset of the disease, but later the memory for remote events is lost also. The amnesia is anterograde, and frequently the patient cannot recall what has just been said to him. He usually presents a superficial cheerfulness and often evades inquiries by jocularities. In his confabulation the patient relates fictitious memories which superficially conceal the actual amnesia. The pseudo-reminiscences, which usually vary from day to day, can often be suggested and guided by leading questions, with the result that the patient will narrate whatever fictitious reminiscence is proposed. Presumably the patient's confabulations serve as a defense against anxiety by concealing from him his defective functioning. The patient characteristically presents a jovial mood and often misidentifies people about him. Disorientation, especially as to time, usually exists. The polyneuropathy, which is sometimes absent, is most marked in the legs, with pain, tenderness over the nerve trunks, absent knee jerks, and, in severe cases, foot drop and wrist drop. The disease is relatively more frequent in women.

Course and Prognosis

Many cases clear up after six or eight weeks, with approximate restoration to mental health. If the process is not fully reversible, the disease continues for several months, with a gradual improvement but without complete return of memory. In some cases there are a permanent impairment of efficiency and a certain degree of intellectual, emotional, and esthetic deterioration. The neuropathy usually improves rather rapidly and often completely disappears. A Korsakoff-like amnesia with confabulations serving to fill in the losses of memory may occur in uremia, after brain trauma, in general paresis, and in other organic and toxic diseases of the brain—conditions in which the pathogenesis does not seem related to dietary deficiency. If irreversible changes have not already occurred, the active symptoms may rapidly disappear. Insight is not usually regained.

Treatment

The first step in treatment is the discontinuance of the use of alcohol. To correct the deficiency of vitamin B_1, 20 to 50 gm. of thiamine chloride may be given daily for a few days, to be followed by 20 gm. of powdered brewers' yeast in iced milk three times a day. Milk, fruit, eggs, meat, and other foods rich in vitamin B complex should be liberally provided. It is probably advisable to administer ascorbic acid also. If irreversible structural changes have already taken place, the symptoms are not affected by vitamins. As in other mental disorders associated with chronic alcoholism, daily doses of insulin are often advisable. When acute neuropathy exists, rest in bed is desirable. Care should be exercised to prevent permanent foot drop. As soon as pain and tenderness in the legs have disappeared, massage and electricity are of value. The patient should then be encouraged to move his feet.

ACUTE HALLUCINOSIS

Since excessive indulgence in alcohol is the occasion of the symptom complex to be considered, it has usually been classified as an alcoholic psychosis. The present tendency is to look upon it as a psychogenic reaction liberated by alcoholic excess rather than as a purely toxic expression. It seems reasonably safe to state that the clinical characteristics are determined by personality factors. Some cases lead one to believe that the disorder is a schizophrenic reaction released by alcohol. However, recent clinical studies have disclosed that the majority of individuals with this syndrome are cyclothymic or extroverted individuals, with a family and developmental history quite unlike that of the schizophrenic. Cases diagnosed as chronic alcoholic hallucinosis ultimately become obvious paranoid schizophrenic reactions.

From the histories of cases of prolonged inebriation with onset shortly after withdrawal of alcohol or restriction of intake, it appears likely that this acute condition represents a type of alcoholic abstinence syndrome, perhaps occurring in individuals with a constitutional predominance for auditory imagery or with some disturbance of the seventh nerve and the auditory pathways within the central nervous system predisposing to tinnitus, with subsequent auditory illusions or hallucinations. Thus tinnitus is reportedly found in a high proportion of patients with auditory hallucinations. Furthermore, in those with unilateral tinnitus, the hallucinatory experience customarily is ipsilateral. Pure alcoholic hallucinosis occurs much less commonly than does delirium tremens or hallucinatory states with both visual and auditory hallucinations.

Symptoms

As in the case of delirium tremens, acute alcoholic hallucinosis develops only after the prolonged and excessive use of alcohol, although usually it is precipitated by increased indulgence. Descriptively the reaction may be summarized as one of auditory hallucinosis occurring in a clear sensorium accompanied affectively by marked fear. In the majority of cases, the hallucinations are usually accusatory, or threatening, or both. The voices are particularly apt to accuse the patient of homosexual practices and to call him indecent names. In women, as in men, the hallucinations are frequently accusatory and of sexual content. The voices, however, accuse the patient of heterosexual offenses rather than of homosexual ones as in men. The hallucinated voices often refer to the patient in the third person and threaten him with such expressions as, "Now shoot him"; "Let's cut him up tonight." The patient may hear the firing of pistols or other sounds suggesting a threat of attack. Not infrequently, in the case of the operator of some mechanical equipment, the hallucinations appear at first to come from his machine and to be synchronous with the rhythmical sound of its operation. In a few the vocal hallucinations are benign and may or may not affect the behavior of the patient. Olfactory hallucinations are not infrequently associated. Illusions of sight are not uncommon. Visual hallucinations may be intermingled to a slight extent but are rarely present in a typical case.

The patient's ideational content and his behavior are determined by the acceptance of his hallucinations as reality. Ideas of reference and misinterpretations are common. A delusional system is rapidly acquired, while additions and elaborations are quickly introduced. The patient may appeal to the police for protection or arm himself in self-defense.

In contrast to its disturbance in delirium tremens, consciousness remains clear in alcoholic hallucinosis and the patient continues to be oriented, projecting his hallucinations into a real environment. In another respect, too, acute hallucinosis differs from delirium tremens: After recovery there is no amnesia for events occurring during its course.

The disturbance in mood is usually pronounced, being characteristically one of fear and apprehension. Terror-stricken by the threats of his imaginary pursuers, or reduced to despair by the accusing voices and his panic state, the patient may attempt to end his own life. The fear may at times be accompanied by anger or depression. Not infrequently there is an element of irritability, while during the temporary cessation of the hallucinations the characteristic alcoholic humor may be manifested.

Course

Recovery from alcoholic hallucinosis usually occurs in five days to a month. Recurrences are common if the patient again indulges excessively in alcohol. Unlike delirium tremens, alcoholic hallucinosis is never followed by the Korsakoff syndrome. Occasionally the hallucinatory episode continues beyond the usual period and merges into a manifest schizophrenia.

Psychological Factors

Mention has already been made of the fact that acute hallucinosis is not always an uncolored alcoholic psychosis. There seems reason to believe that if a certain type of personality takes large quantities of alcohol over a considerable period of time, a psychogenic reaction of an acute schizophrenic nature may be liberated. The frequent history of unsuccessful heterosexual adjustment in the patient with alcoholic hallucinosis and the homosexual character of the hallucinations suggest that in some cases, at least, unrecognized homosexual tendencies may be the psychopathogenic factor which has both prompted the use of alcohol and determined the nature of the hallucinations. As to the psychogenic determination of the mood in alcoholic hallucinosis, one may speculatively suggest that the unconscious sense of threat to the personality in the biologically destructive and socially prohibited homosexual impulse is greater than the feeling of guilt which this repressed impulse sometimes arouses; hence the mood is usually one of fear rather

than of depression. From the standpoint of self-respect, too, fear is psychologically preferable to shame. If the sense of guilt is relatively strong, then the patient exhibits the depression occasionally seen in the disease.

Treatment

The treatment consists in placing the patient under such supervision that he may neither commit an indiscreet act nor do harm to himself. All alcohol must, of course, be withdrawn. The continuous bath assists in calming fear and anxiety. Chlorpromazine or related tranquilizing agents are useful for this purpose. The administration of food is not so difficult as in delirium tremens, but it should be given regularly and in abundance. It is well to give large amounts of orange juice, also vitamin B complex.

ALCOHOLIC PARANOIA

Clinically it is convenient to describe alcoholic paranoia, although its recognition as a true alcoholic psychosis is scarcely warrantable. Here, too, there may be a common factor—the repressed homosexual impulse—beneath both the alcoholism and the psychosis. Usually the patient has never established a wholesome, mature heterosexual relationship. In the prepsychotic life of the patient, we often find the same incomplete developments, fixations, traits of personality, and psychopathological processes as in other paranoid psychoses. In alcoholic paranoia, the use of alcohol, prompted by these tendencies, weakens repression and causes the vicious psychopathological circle of homosexual conflict, alcoholic indulgence, and paranoid delusion to continue without interruption. Psychologically the conditions were favorable for the development of a psychosis before the use of alcohol became excessive. In some cases one might almost say that a latent psychosis already existed and that the alcohol did no more than hasten its appearance. The previous personality pattern has been characterized by stubbornness, suspiciousness, resentment, projection, and other defensive mechanisms. The history of the patient usually shows that he has accepted discipline poorly and that he has preferred the society of men.

Symptoms

This clinical manifestation is typically characterized by delusions of jealousy and infidelity. At first the patient is irritable, fault-finding, and distrustful. To these unpleasant defensive characteristics are later added accusations of marital infidelity, as evidence of which are cited the most insignificant and absurd arguments. With his jealousy motivated by unrecognized sense of guilt and fear based on the odious trends and impulses of his own personality, the suspicious husband devises numerous schemes to entrap his wife and her supposed paramour.

A noncommissioned officer in the Army, whose enlistment had perhaps been prompted by an unrecognized homosexual interest, argued that he could not be the father of the child to which his wife had given birth inasmuch as it was born 279 instead of 280 days following marital relations with her. As evidence that the family physician was the father of the child, he cited the fact that on one occasion the doctor had not submitted his bill promptly. On several occasions, he threatened the life of the physician and finally actually attempted to shoot him.

Because of their incompletely developed and poorly integrated personalities, these patients are peculiarly inadequate for the sustained demands for social adaptation which marriage brings. By imputing to the wife, too, the interest which they fundamentally feel for other men, they secure an alleviation of anxiety. The ideas which follow are psychologically protective but adjustively disruptive. At times, with the increased use of intoxicants, impotence, produced by the toxic action of the alcohol on the central nervous system, increases the patient's sense of in-security and incompetence, the prevention of any recognition of which requires a further development of ideas of infidelity.

Prognosis

The prognosis in the alcoholic paranoid state is not good. With the decrease in demands for adjustment that follows removal to a hospital, the patient may improve and no longer entertain his delusional ideas. At other times, having observed that the expression of his ideas has resulted in a deprivation of his liberty, he may dissimulate and maintain that he now recognizes he was in error and that he no longer doubts the fidelity of his wife. At any rate, after the return to the old situation, the former delusions and threatening behavior usually soon reappear.

OTHER ENCEPHALOPATHIES

Wernicke's encephalopathy, resulting from a deficiency in vitamin B, may be associated with alcoholic addiction or with other conditions in which this deficiency exists. It will be discussed in Chapter 17, Brain Syndromes Associated with Endocrine, Metabolic, and Nutritional Disturbances.

The chronic alcoholic may also develop a *nicotinic acid deficiency encephalopathy,* in which are seen typical pellagra-like symptoms with clouded consciousness, parkinsonian-like rigidities, and sucking and grasping reflexes. Improvement follows treatment with a high calorie, high vitamin diet and administration of nicotinic acid or nicotinamide.

Marchiafava's disease, with signs of aphasia, agnosia, and apraxia, is related to long-continued excessive use of cheap red wine. Pathologically there are found degenerative changes in the corpus callosum and multiple cortical and subcortical areas of encephalomalacias. Cerebellar ataxia may also develop in chronic alcoholics.

ALCOHOLIC DETERIORATION

A considerable number of persons who consume large amounts of alcohol over a prolonged period ultimately suffer a certain disintegration of personality, the change ranging from an impairment of emotional stability and control to a noticeable dementia. The principal organic damage that alcohol inflicts upon the human nervous system probably is caused by avitaminosis rather than by primary toxic injury itself. From the standpoint of anatomical pathology there is, in the more severe cases, a progressive, chronic parenchymatous nervous degeneration, sometimes affecting a considerable part of the neuraxis. As previously indicated, so-called alcoholic dementia is caused by progressive atrophy of the cortex of the frontal lobes.

Symptoms

One of the earliest mental symptoms of the abuse of alcohol is an increased tendency to act impulsively in accordance with primitive instinctive forces and the momentary affectivity. The alcoholic patient develops resentment, hostility, and feelings of guilt. Although, at least for a considerable period, a capacity for ethical sentiments remains, these are not sustained or applied, with the result that ethical purposes and strivings suffer, will is weakened, perseverance of endeavor is lost, and the patient becomes untruthful and unreliable. His tendency to deceive and to gloss over whatever is discreditable in behavior or character is but a part of a fundamental inability to face the facts of reality and of his own situation. He blames others for his failure and represents himself as abused and as the victim of circumstances for which he is in no way responsible, while at the same time he exaggerates his own achievements.

Affection is lost and ambition disappears. The confirmed alcoholic becomes careless as to his personal appearance and neglectful of his family. With an increasing egocentricity, his former sense of social or other responsibility disappears, or rather is avoided by the process of evasively treating it facetiously and superficially. Usually the patient's mood is one of unwarranted euphoria and carefree good humor, but a word of implied reproval may evoke a violent and profane outburst of irritability. A word of commiseration calls forth a ready tear, but, with a hearty slap on the back, his tears promptly give way to a cheerful laugh. With his friends, the alcoholic may be a congenial and welcome companion who enters enthusiastically into their pleasures, but at home he may be brutal, surly, and without shame. In nearly every instance, the patient's sex life is poorly adjusted, this failure in some instances serving as a cause of the alcoholism and in others representing a result. Not infrequently, this maladjustment operates to continue the vicious circle. A defensive attitude is assumed toward those who are not alcoholic in their habits, and the patient is touchy, irritable, and critical in the presence of those who he believes do not approve his excesses. There is an increasing poverty of ideas, with a growing incapacity for sustained attention and for more delicate discriminations. After a time, memory becomes impaired, and the insidious dementia finally becomes extreme. One patient, a physician, whose practice had been ruined by his habits, had abused his children and accused his wife of neglect and infidelity; he was unable to remember how long he had been in the hospital or give the name of his ward physician who had seen him daily for months. Psychometric examinations performed on alcoholic patients indicate that impairment of the mental functioning of various abilities precedes any clinical evidence of brain lesion.

Course and Outcome

If the use of alcohol is discontinued as soon as any early character changes are noted, there may be a nearly complete restoration to former mental health which, however, must always remain precarious, since the alcoholic was never well-adjusted to life. Moreover, the alcoholic, in spite of his protests to the contrary, rarely is motivated to give up his addiction because alcohol provides the easiest way of escape from the difficulties which his inadequately integrated personality has precipitated. Deterioration of personality is permanent, and any actual dementia is, of course, quite irremediable.

Treatment

Unfortunately, alcoholism has been regarded as a moral problem, with the result that the complex contributing factors have not received the scientific attention they have merited, and attention to therapy has not been commensurate with the extent of the social problem.

Alcoholism should be looked upon as a psychic illness rooted in a personality disorder or immaturity. As in the psychoneuroses, with which alcoholism has much in common, the patient is usually unaware of the particular personality problems from which he has sought relief through the escape and anxiety-relieving mechanisms which alcohol facilitates. Theoretically, therefore, the object of treatment should be directed toward preventing the patient from desiring alcohol rather than toward restraining him from it. While it is exceptionally uncommon for an addictive alcoholic to become a moderate social drinker, the goal of achieving total abstinence for those who come to treatment should not be regarded as the sole criterion of success. In some, total abstinence does not bring about overall improvement in social adaptation; it may result in social deterioration. A number of chronic alcoholics may learn to restrict their drinking within the framework of the social mores and successfully reinstate themselves in their family and social life. The personality characteristics that typify this group and the supportive forces that sustain this

balance between limited abstinence and social functioning remain to be determined. For the most part, however, total abstinence has proved more effective in rehabilitation.

The patient should be approached with the attitude that his disorder is one of personality rather than of morality. The emphasis should be not on the alcoholism but on the individual in whom it occurs. Psychiatric treatment should have a basic routine program of active physical exercise, constructive occupational work, agreeable social relaxation, and psychotherapy. The patient's mental life and experiences should be reviewed for the purpose of discovering the main factors which have caused him to become dependent on alcohol. One must, therefore, obtain a thorough understanding of the patient as a person and of his particular life situation. Orthodox psychoanalytical techniques are usually not practicable with the addictive drinker, because of his instability and low tolerance to stress. Because of these characteristics, he usually resumes drinking whenever painful unconscious material begins to come to the surface. A constructive analysis of his personality difficulties must be accompanied by a prolonged reëducational effort.

The alcoholic is usually a dependent personality and therefore needs continuous support over a long period of time, frequently for years. Frequently, too, he is a hostile, anxious, guilt-ridden person. Primitive or restraining measures that increase the patient's sense of being wronged and stir aggressive and resentful feelings should be avoided. The therapist should not condone his patient's alcoholic habits, yet he should not be critical. His attitude should be objective and impersonal. It should be remembered that the patient's rationalized reasons for his alcoholism are not the real reasons. It is often necessary to carry out the treatment in an institution, although in one where the patient can lead as normal a life as possible.

In those instances in which there is

a demonstrated dependent relationship upon a protecting person, often the mother, wife, or lover, who provides the alcohol and gives in to the insatiable demands of the alcoholic, this individual must also receive treatment in order to break the pathological bond that perpetuates the habit. Better results are secured in special institutions for alcoholics where planned psychotherapy is used. Psychotherapy is of course possible only in the habitué whose intellectual equipment is still sound. If dementia has occurred, he must usually be committed to an institution where he can no longer secure intoxicants and where both the patient and society may be protected from the results of his intellectual and moral defects.

Group psychotherapy of alcoholics is employed with greater frequency. The experience of being with other similarly afflicted people seems to make the alcoholic accept more readily treatment in the group environment. The interpretations offered by other members make the attainment of insight easier and less frightening.

ALCOHOLICS ANONYMOUS.   Alcoholics Anonymous, established in 1935 in Akron, Ohio, and conducted by former alcoholics, has produced many temporary and even prolonged cures of alcoholic addiction. Although it was organized without psychiatric guidance and its movement is largely limited to a social-religious program it has been of great value in reorienting many addicts in a socially efficient way of life. Despite the fact that this program is very heavily weighted with an unrealistic optimism, it has constructively utilized many principles of group psychotherapy.

As a rule, members of Alcoholics Anonymous are above the average in intelligence, education, and social status, and their attitude toward the addict is tolerant and constructive. The organization offers the confirmed addict an opportunity to escape from his former psychosocial isolation, from the feeling that no one really understands or cares about him and that he can trust no one. In his group, the addict has a sense of belonging, of being understood and accepted, and of sharing common convictions. By means of his allegiance to the group, the member develops a religious fervor, and when he answers a call to aid another alcoholic at the cost of inconvenience and self-denial, his religious devotion is constructively internalized. An inspirational and mass-suggestion approach is an important feature.

By arousing a deep desire to help others and by creating a sense of responsibility for doing so, the organization contributes to the addict's cure. The opportunity to talk about himself in the group meetings affords the addict an opportunity for narcissistic satisfaction, for self-expression, and for therapeutic catharsis. The program of Alcoholics Anonymous ignores the cause of the alcoholic's addiction and focuses directly on the drinking itself.

Unfortunately, certain individuals addicted to alcohol are unwilling to join this organization. The reasons for their lack of motivation for this group affiliation remain unclear. Some do so as a denial of the addiction, while others appear to have competing loyalties, are perpetuating a defense of self-sufficiency against dependent strivings which would arouse shame, or are prone to develop intolerable anxiety in group situations.

DISULFIRAM OR ANTABUSE THERAPY.   In 1948 two Danish investigators, Jens Hald and Erik Jacobsen, in search of a vermifuge, tried disulfiram (tetraethylthiuram disulfide). They observed that persons who had ingested this substance previous to the consumption of alcohol showed symptoms which differed quantitatively and qualitatively from those present in the common picture of alcoholic intoxication. The discomfort after alcohol consumption in persons taking this drug was so great that these investigators decided to use it as a remedy for alcoholism. It is believed that the discomfort is caused by interference with the excretion of acetaldehyde, an intermediary product in the oxidation of alcohol.

When a patient who has taken 0.5 to 1 gm. of disulfiram within the preceding

12 hours partakes of alcohol, he experiences within 5 to 15 minutes a feeling of heat in the face soon followed by an intense vasolidation of the face and neck, the skin of which may assume a purple-red color. At the same time, the conjunctiva is injected, and the patient suffers from tachycardia. These symptoms are soon followed by headache, dsypnea, dizziness, chest pain, nausea, palpitation, and vomiting. There is an initial rise of blood pressure followed by a fall, perhaps to 80 mm. Hg. The discomfort following the imbibition of alcohol so long as disulfiram is in the blood is so great that the patient does not care to drink. The dose of disulfiram should be individualized, but usually 0.5 gm. once a day, preferably in the morning, is sufficient. Rarely 1.0 gm. is required. Initial treatment with a drug possessing such serious toxic potentialities should be under constant medical supervision. Cardiovascular complications, including myocardial infarction, may occur. Although it was originally believed that persons suffering from marked disease of the liver, coronary disease, arteriosclerosis with hypertension, or diabetes should not receive disulfiram, experience with a large series of patients suggests that the only important contraindication is cardiac decompensation. There have been several reports of psychoses occuring during the use of the drug.

Formerly the administration of disulfiram was not begun until after an abstinence from alcohol for one week, but in recent years disulfiram has been given even when the patient is intoxicated. In such instances, the initial dose is one-half or less of the usual one (7.5 mg. per kilogram of body weight) and is given with an antihistamine drug, such as 25 mg. of Promethazine, and 5 gm. of sodium chloride in one-half glass of water.

Disulfiram therapy must be considered as a variation of the conditioned reflex aversion method. In contrast to other forms of conditioned reflex methods, the unpleasant effects not only are present each time the patient takes a small but adequate dose of disulfiram and drinks alcohol, but they actually increase with continued ingestion of the drug. If continued, it probably helps to overcome the craving for alcohol. For the treatment to be successful, however, it is necessary for the patient to have a real desire to be helped, to be willing to take the drug with consistency, and to coöperate in psychotherapy. Daily uninterrupted administration of disulfiram makes it physiologically impossible to continue to use alcohol as a defense mechanism. To remove this protection, however, without at the same time eliminating its need by psychotherapy can scarcely lead to a cure of the patient. As long as the basic difficulties which led to the alcoholism are not resolved, the desire for alcohol persists and, along with it, an unwillingness to take the medication.

Calcium carbamide (Temposil) has actions similar to disulfiram but appears to be excreted more rapidly so that its effectiveness is short lived following its ingestion. Calcium carbamide is considered a safer medication than disulfiram, because when taken with alcohol it produces fewer hypotensive and electrocardiographic changes. Furthermore it appears more acceptable to patients, because the associated side effects are less.

BIBLIOGRAPHY

Arky, R. A., Abramson, E. A., and Freinkel, N.: Alcohol hypoglycemia. Metabolism, *17*:977–987, 1968.

Carpenter, J. A., Moore, P. K., Snyder, C. R., and Lisansky, E. S.: Alcohol and higher order problem solving. Quart. J. Stud. Alcohol, *22*:183–222, 1961.

Curlee, J.: Alcoholism and the "empty nest." Bull. Menninger Clinic, *33*:165–171, 1969.

Davidson, E. A., and Solomon, P.: The differentiation of delirium tremens from impending hepatic coma. J. Ment. Sci., *104*:326–333, 1958.

Dott, A. B.: Blood alcohol levels and intoxication. J.A.M.A., *214*:2196, 1970.

Graw, R. G., Jr., Buckner, C. D., and Eisel, R.: Plasma exchange transfusion for hepatic coma. Transfusion, *10*:26–32, 1970.

Gross, M. M., Halpert, E., Sabot, L., and Polizoes, P.: Hearing disturbances and auditory hallucinations in the acute alcoholic psychoses. J. Nerv. Ment. Dis., *137*:455–465, 1963.

Himwich, H. E.: The physiology of alcohol. J.A.
M.A., *163*:545–549, 1957.

Isbell, H., Fraser, H. F., Wikler, A., Belleville, R.
E., and Eisenman, A. W.: An experimental study
of the etiology of "rum fits" and delirium tremens. Quart. J. Stud. Alcohol, *16*:1–33, 1955.

Johnson, L. C., Burdick, A., and Smith, J.: Sleep
during alcohol intake and withdrawal in the
chronic alcoholic. Arch. Gen. Psychiat., *22*:406–
418, 1970.

Kaim, S. C., Klett, C. J., and Rothfeld, B.: Treatment of acute alcohol withdrawal state: Comparison of four drugs. Amer. J. Psychiat., *125*:
1640–1646, 1969.

Koller, K. M., and Castanis, J. N.: Family background and life situations in alcoholics. Arch.
Gen. Psychiat., *21*:602–610, 1969.

Levy, M. S., Livingstone, B. L., and Collins, D. M.:
A clinical comparison of disulfiram and calcium
carbamide. Amer. J. Psychiat., *123*:1018–1022,
1967.

Panmill, F. C., and Smith, J. A.: The chronic alcoholic. J.A.M.A., *171*:2299–2303, 1959.

Pattison, E. M.: Critique of abstinence criteria in
treatment of alcoholism. Int. J. Social Psychiat.,
14:268–276, 1968.

Spitzer, R. L., Cohen, G. M., Miller, J. D., and
Endicott, J.: The psychiatric status of 100 men
on skid row. Int. J. Social Psychiat., *15*:230–234,
1969.

Victor, M.: Alcohol withdrawal syndrome: Theory
and practice. Postgrad. Med., *47*:68–72, 1970.

Victor, M., Herman, K., and White, E. E.: A psychological study of the Wernicke-Korsakoff syndrome. Quart. J. Stud. Alcohol, *20*:467–479,
1959.

Winokor, G., Reich, T., Rimmer, J., and Pitts,
F. N., Jr.: Alcoholism. III. Diagnosis and famil-
ial psychiatric illness in 259 alcoholics. Arch.
Gen. Psychiat., *23*:104–111, 1970.

Chapter 13

Brain Syndromes Associated with Infection

GENERAL PARALYSIS

The brain syndrome associated with syphilitic meningoencephalitis, known as general paresis, general paralysis of the insane, or dementia paralytica, is a disorder produced by progressive syphilitic meningoencephalitis leading to a degeneration of brain parenchyma with an infiltration of interstitial elements. Clinically, general paresis is characterized by a comprehensive but variable syndrome of neurological and mental disturbances associated with fairly constant serological changes.

History

Although Haslam of Bethlehem Hospital, in a monograph entitled "Observations on Insanity," described in 1798 the associated mental and physical symptoms that occur in general paresis, the credit for its recognition as a clinical and pathological entity belongs to the French psychiatrist, A. L. J. Bayle, who published his thesis in 1822 at the age of 23. An opinion that paresis was caused by syphilis was first expressed in 1857 by Esmarch and Jessen. At first this theory received little credence. The development of the Wassermann reaction indicated the existence of syphilis in practically all cases of paresis. Any remaining doubt that syphilis is the sole determining cause was dispelled in 1913, when Joseph W. Moore at the Central Islip (New York) State Hospital and Hideyo Noguchi of the Rockefeller Institute demonstrated the *Treponema pallidum* in the brains of paretics. It is now possible to demonstrate treponemata in fresh paretic brains taken at necropsy and studied by darkfield illumination. They may also be discovered in brain tissue obtained by puncture in living paretics.

In 1917 Wagner-Jauregg of Vienna found that artificial fever induced by inoculation with malaria resulted in an arrest of the paretic process and an improvement of the patient. In 1943 penicillin was found to be an active spirocheticidal agent and has since then proved to be the effective means of treating both general syphilis and neurosyphilis.

Frequency and Pathogenesis

Prior to 1920, 8 to 10 per cent of the patients committed to public hospitals in the United States were suffering from general paresis, whereas at the present time less than 1 per cent of the patients admitted for the first time are suffering from this disease. This decline in admissions is probably a result of both a decrease in syphilis and earlier and more adequate treatment.

The *Treponema pallidum* is one of the few microörganisms which can penetrate the blood-brain barrier with ease. It is now believed that during the period of generalized spirochetemia this invasion of the neuroaxis occurs in most, if not all, patients infected with syphilis. In the majority of cases, this original invasion never produces symptoms, physical signs, or changes in the cerebrospinal fluid; the organisms which have penetrated the nervous system are spontaneously eliminated by obscure immune processes not yet understood. The reason for the development of paresis in some luetic individuals while others remain free from the disease is not known, but perhaps the incidence is determined by the virulence of the infection and by immune factors in the host. There probably is not a special neurotropic strain of treponema.

Paresis occurs four times more frequently in men than in women. The cause for this strikingly higher incidence in men is uncertain, since the probable ratio of primary syphilis infection among men as compared with women is not greater than 2 to 1. Parenchymatous neurosyphilis is also much less frequent among Negroes than among white subjects in spite of the greater incidence of syphilis among the former.

Pathology

The basic pathology of paresis is a chronic syphilitic meningoencephalitis in which two pathological components—inflammation and degeneration—are at work. The process, with its progressive degeneration of nerve cells, begins largely in the frontal region, but as the disease progresses, any part of the cortex, cerebellum, or bulb may become involved.

Microscopically the perivascular lymph spaces of the vessels are crowded with proliferated endothelial cells, occasional mast cells, and, most important of all, lymphocytes and plasma cells. The pia mater is similarly infiltrated with lymphocytes and plasma cells. A sprouting of the capillaries produces increased vascularity, while the "cuffing" of these capillaries by the perivascular infiltration mentioned gives rise to one of the important histopathological features of paresis, although it is not confined to general paralysis but occurs also

in epidemic encephalitis and in trypanosomiasis. The ganglion cells are cloudy and suffer degeneration, and many disappear, particularly in the middle layer of the frontal cortex. It has not yet been determined whether the degenerative changes are caused by the action of the spirochetes themselves or by their toxic products. The usual cortical architecture, with lamination and column formation of the neuron cells, is disorganized. The glia is proliferated. Scattered about through the cortex are numerous cylindrical-appearing cells known as rod cells or "stäbchenzellen," first described by Franz Nissl.

Another constant finding in the brain of the paretic subject is the presence of iron pigment in the walls of the blood vessels and in the cortical microglia. Many pathologists consider that the presence in the rod cells of a substance giving a Prussian blue reaction is to be considered as characteristic and pathognomonic of general paresis. Spirochetes are found in about 80 per cent of the untreated cases.

Incubation Period

General paresis develops from five to 30 or more years after the primary infection with syphilis. In one-half of the cases, the incubation period is from 10 to 20 years; in one-fourth the period is under 10 years, and in one-fourth it is over 20 years. The peak in the curve of incidence occurs between the ages of 35 and 45.

Invasion of the nervous system by *Treponema pallidum* is first manifested by a rising cell count in the *cerebrospinal fluid*. Three to six months later the protein becomes elevated, and this is then followed by the development of positive Wassermann and colloidal reactions. If the nervous system has not been invaded by the end of the second year of the disease, it is unlikely that it will ever be involved.

It is established that there is a preclinical period during which the only evidence of the condition consists of spinal fluid findings characteristic of the disease. During this period the patient may be said to be suffering from *asymptomatic paresis,* the forerunner of clinical paresis.

Trauma as Etiologic Factor

The question whether trauma may play a precipitating role in the production of general paralysis in a person already suffering from syphilis is one that occasionally confronts industrial accident and other boards exercising similar judicial functions. Medical evidence and judicial precedent indicate that there is a connection between head trauma and the development or acceleration of the paretic process. The limits usually set for this causal relationship are six weeks to three months as a minimum and two or three years as a maximum. There is, however, divergence of opinion as to the severity of injury necessary for a relationship between the injury and the development of the disease.

To justify the opinion that trauma precipitated or aggravated the general paralysis, it must be shown that the trauma involved the head and was of sufficient intensity to injure the brain by concussion, or more likely by contusion. It is probable, in such a case, that the injury did not initiate the paretic process but that the trauma activated an asymptomatic paresis and caused clinical symptoms to appear. It cannot be stated whether or not, in the absence of trauma, a person in such a preclinical stage would have developed general paresis.

Symptoms and Signs

The description of syphilitic meningoencephalitis may conveniently be considered under the following headings: personality disturbance, physical and neurological signs, and serological changes.

PERSONALITY DISTURBANCE. Changes in personality and disturbed mentation commonly are the first noted signs of the illness. The clinical findings often fail to reflect the extent of the pathological process. Frequently the mental symptoms develop so insidiously that the patient's family has not recognized that a deteriorating change in personality has been taking place. The early symptoms consist largely of an extension and exaggeration of previous personality traits. Other early symptoms may be irritability, fatigue, difficulty in concentration, depression, periods of confusion, disturbed sleep, and headache. The early paretic individual is often opinionated and perhaps quarrelsome. Frequently he becomes neglectful of his dress, unkempt in appearance, inconsiderate of others, and forgetful of social amenities and proprieties and manifests an insidious breakdown of higher ethical and cultural sentiments and standards. The moderate user of alcohol may become dissipated; sexual activities may become excessive. The man whose previous life has been quite exemplary may not only suddenly show some surprising defect of character but feel no concern for his dereliction.

Early in the disease there is often an impairment in professional skill or in craftsmanship. Unaccustomed slips and failures in the discharge of ordinary duties occur. The consequences of errors are not foreseen. The patient may conceive ambitious schemes of an extremely impracticable and extravagant nature. The businessman may no longer show his former capacity for successful management and, because of failing judgment, may dissipate the resources upon which the livelihood of his family depends. There is often a contented indifference—an apathy and unconcern that at first may be mistaken for laziness. Frequently there is a tendency to drowsiness. The patient becomes incapable of submitting his impressions and conclusions to a critical examination, nor does he recognize the insidious deterioration that is going on in the intellectual, feeling, and social aspects of his personality. The man previously regarded as possessing an acute and well-trained mind and sound judgment surprises his acquaintances by his failure to grasp the finer shades of meaning or by some puerile, inept remark. Associations are characterized by their slowness, superficiality, and poverty.

A change of mood is common in the early stages, the frequent mood being apathy or depression. Sometimes the early stages are characterized by anxiety. In some cases, euphoria and expansiveness exist from the beginning, but more often these mood trends appear somewhat later. Momentary periods of confusion or an inability to grasp a situation and to act promptly and correctly lead to automobile accidents in early paretic patients whose mental disorder has not yet been detected.

Delusions occur at some period of the disease in a majority of the patients. It has usually been emphasized that the delusions are grandiose, yet not more than 50 per cent of the subjects express delusions of this nature. Expansive delusions may reach the height of absurdity. The patient may declare, for example, that he owns a trucking company, each car of which is loaded with million-dollar treasury notes. Ideas of boundless benevolence may be expressed, including fantastic schemes for the welfare of all mankind. However, delusions often are depressive, self-accusatory, nihilistic, or persecutory. Hallucinations occasionally occur but are not of diagnostic significance.

In the very early stage of the paretic process, individuals who, before the development of the psychosis, showed a definite tendency to schizoid or cyclothymic manifestations, frequently exhibit, at the onset of the mental disturbance, features suggestive of schizophrenia or manic-depressive psychosis.

The dementia of general paresis, even at a comparatively early stage, tends to be of a diffuse type, involving memory, judgment, emotional life, and conative expressions. Intelligence tests show a mental deterioration with defective reasoning and an impairment of social ability, memory, and learning. Unlike the dementia of senility, it is not at first limited largely to memory. As the disease advances, the dementia becomes progressive. Affectivity and emotional response suffer impoverishment, inadequacies of perception prevent contact with the environment, memory fails, associations become slow and limited, apperception is destroyed, spontaneous activities cease, and finally, the mental processes, devoid of conscious participation, are reduced to those at the reflex and vegetative level.

PHYSICAL AND NEUROLOGICAL SIGNS. As numerous and varied as are the mental symptoms that may exist in paresis, the physical and neurological symptoms are equally so. During the stage of onset, the patient may become easily fatigued and may lose weight. Numerous somatic complaints referred to the various bodily systems are frequent. The diagnosis in many paretic patients has been neurasthenia. Many patients complain of headache. Because of the loss of tone in the facial muscles, the lines of expression become smoothed out. This relaxation of the facial muscles, together with the blunting of emotional response, gives the facies a vacant, fatuous appearance.

Disturbances in the eye, or in its innervation or reflexes, almost always occur at some period; these disturbances vary greatly in degree. Papilledema, syphilitic retinitis, or primary optic atrophy may occur. Complete optic atrophy occurs in 2 per cent of the cases and incipient and intermediate stages of atrophy occur in 62.5 per cent. More frequent than optic atrophy are the disturbances of the pupils, which may be unequal in size, irregular in outline, much contracted, or widely dilated. Reaction to light is often sluggish or lost, as may also be the convergence reaction. The type of pupil first described by Argyll Robertson in 1869 will be found in over half of the paretic patients. This is a miotic pupil which contracts when the eyes converge and accommodates for near vision but does not contract when strong light is suddenly thrown on the eye. It is to be distinguished from Adie's myotonic pupillary response, which also is seen to be associated with absence of deep reflexes. The myotonic pupil is never miotic but is dilated, sometimes oval, and after a period in the dark it slowly contracts with exposure to light. Occasionally there may be some degree of ptosis of one lid or weakness of one of the external muscles of the eye, especially the external rectus.

A progressive weakness and incoördination of all voluntary mucles occur. There is tremor of the facial muscles, first observed in the lips when the patient attempts to speak or show his teeth. As enunciation becomes more difficult, there is an overactivity of all the facial muscles when speech is attempted. The tremor of the tongue is coarse and is best demonstrated when the tongue is protruded. This muscle weakness and incoördination lead to the disturbance of speech, which, when associated with the blandly inane facial expression already noted, constitutes a syndrome so characteristic that the experienced psychiatrist can often make a diagnosis as the patient speaks. At first this speech defect is often manifested in the form of a hesitation, drawl, or slurring. Later there is omission, reduplication, or transposition of syllables. The speech disturbances are often best demonstrated by asking the patient to repeat polysyllabic words or phrases containing labial or dental types of consonants (as "electrical artillery brigade"). As the disease progresses, the speech may become quite unintelligible. Transient, incomplete aphasic attacks may occur, at times rather early in the disease.

Deterioration in handwriting is often an early clinical symptom. Because of loss in delicate muscular coördination, it is often tremulous. There may also be reduplication or elision of letters in syllables. Later the patient may become unable to write at all from dictation, and if he attempts to form characters, he produces only an unintelligible scrawl.

Muscular incoördination gives rise also to many other symptoms. Among early ones is a tremulous incoördination of finer movements of the hand. Later the patient is unable to button his clothing or even to dress himself. Station and gait then become uncertain, all movements are clumsy, and finally, because of his weakness and ataxia, the patient is confined to his bed. The muscles of deglutition do not escape involvement, with the result that difficulty in swallowing may occur.

Disturbances of the deep tendon reflexes are the rule. More frequently these are exaggerated, in which case ankle clonus and spasticity are usually present, but if, as not infrequently happens, a tabetic process coexists, the knee jerks are absent. Disturbances of the rectal and vesical sphincters are common in the terminal stages. The bladder may become greatly distended, resulting in a dribbling of urine caused by an overflow of retention. Rupture of such a bladder may occur upon receipt of slight trauma. Trophic changes may occur in the bones, causing them to be easily fractured.

It is not uncommon for the paretic subject suddenly to develop a marked rise in temperature without evidence of infection or of additional somatic disease. These fevers are probably a result of disturbances of the heat-regulating centers.

About three-fourths of patients suffer from convulsions at some time during the course of the disease. Occasionally a convulsion, particularly of an abortive type, may be the first symptom to attract attention to the illness.

Another form of episodic attack is apoplectiform in type. These attacks are sudden in onset, are accompanied by disturbances of consciousness, and are followed by hemiplegia or more localized paralyses. These paralyses are usually temporary in nature, often clearing up without residuals in a few days. Less frequently a hemorrhage occurs, leaving a permanent paralysis.

SEROLOGY. Serological changes supply important diagnostic evidence as to the existence of general paresis. The spinal fluid changes provide the best guide to the activity of a syphilitic infection of the central nervous system and to the effect of treatment. In nearly all cases of untreated paresis, the blood serological tests for syphilis are positive. In general paresis the cerebrospinal fluid pressure may be increased, and in approximately 8 per cent of the cases it will exceed 200 mm. H_2O.

Spinal Fluid Wassermann Reaction. In untreated syphilitic meningoencephalitis, the Wassermann reaction in the cerebrospinal fluid is positive in 90 per cent of the cases with 0.2 ml. of the fluid and is always positive with 1 ml. A positive Wassermann reaction does not signify that the neurosyphilis is of the paretic type, nor does it necessarily indicate that the process is active. An increase of protein to 50 to 150 mg. per 100 ml. (normal, 25 mg.) with a disproportionate increase of globulin is the rule in paresis. The total protein and the amount of globulin are greater in general paresis than in any other type of neurosyphilis except acute meningitis. The more active the paretic process, the larger the amount of these substances. In paresis, the number of cells in the spinal fluid may remain normal or may reach 100 per cubic millimeter, the average being 25 to 50. An excess of this number indicates that a syphilitic meningitis also exists. The cell count affords the most valuable information as to the activity of the infection. It is also the first abnormality to return to normal as a result of treatment.

Colloidal Gold Test. Given a positive Wassermann reaction of the spinal fluid and other evidence of neurosyphilis, one of the most valuable tests in determining its type is the colloidal gold test described by Lange in 1912. This test depends on the precipitation and varying degrees of decolorization of a solution of gold chloride by a series of dilutions of the cerebrospinal fluid. The precipitation is considered to be caused by globulin, the curve of precipitation depending on the relative amounts of globulin and albumin present in the arachnoid fluid. Since, of the various forms of neurosyphilis, paresis shows the largest amount of globulin in the cerebrospinal fluid, the greatest precipitation of gold chloride occurs in the form which gives a first-zone curve. De-grees of precipitation show as changes from the normal salmon-red color of the solution and range through a slight change to deeper red, to lavender, violet, and red-blue, the colorless solution representing complete precipitation of the gold. An intense paretic reaction might be as follows: 5555554432; a less marked reaction might be 55432111000.

In multiple sclerosis, Schilder's disease, and other types of neurosyphilis, the decolorization curve with colloidal gold may follow that of general paresis. The colloidal gold reaction is an indication of an abnormality of the protein content of the fluid. It does not reflect the activity of the disease. This, as previously stated, is best indicated by the cell count.

Clinical Types

Because of the conspicuousness of certain presenting symptoms, different clinical types of syphilitic meningoencephalitis are usually described. Such a division into forms possesses the merit of descriptive convenience only. Some cases, too, do not fit into such a classification, and in others the symptoms may shift during the course of the disease.

SIMPLE DEMENTING TYPE. In this form, the chief symptom is an insidious, progressive dementia with few, if any, delusions and no psychomotor disturbance except the declining activity indicative of the failing interest and capacity. Following closely upon the gradual loss of ambition and of mental alertness, there appears the flabby, vacuous facies, presenting a syndrome that can scarcely be mistaken. Remissions are rather uncommon in the simple dementing form.

The following brief abstract indicates the general clinical picture often occurring in the simple dementing form.

A woman of 26 was brought to the hospital because she had become lost when she attempted to return home from a neighboring grocery store. About seven months before the patient's admission, her husband noticed that she was becoming careless of her personal appearance and neglectful of her household duties. She often forgot to prepare the family meals, or, in an apparent preoccupation, would burn the food. She seemed to have little appreciation of time and would not realize when to get up or go to bed. The patient would sit idly about the house, staring uncomprehendingly into space.

At the hospital the patient entered the admission office with an unsteady gait. There, by way of greeting, the physician inquired, "How are you today?" to which she replied in a monotonous, tremulous tone, "N-yes-s, I was-s op-er-a-ted on for 'pen-pendici-ci-tis." She never made any spontaneous remarks and when, a few days after her admission, she was asked if she were sad or happy, she stared vacantly at the physician and, with a fatuous smile, answered, "Yeah." The patient sat about the ward for hours, taking no interest in its activities. Sometimes she would hold a book in her lap, aimlessly turning the pages, never reading but often pointing out pictures like a small child and showing satisfaction when she found a new one to demonstrate. Neurological examination showed dilated pupils that reacted but slightly to light and on convergence. There was a tremor of lips and facial muscles on attempting to speak. The protruded tongue showed a coarse tremor. All deep tendon reflexes were hyperactive. The Wassermann reaction was strongly positive in both blood serum and cerebrospinal fluid. There were 24 cells per milliliter of spinal fluid. The colloidal gold curve was 5555543210.

EXPANSIVE TYPE. The expansive form, while no longer emphasized as distinctly characteristic, is regarded as one of the most important of the clinical types. In the early stages, the patient is self-satisfied and has a superficial good humor, but becomes easily irritated. If handled with good-natured and tactful suggestion, he is quite amenable, but if interfered with, his resentment may lead to violence. Although his grandiose ideas may be most absurd, the paretic patient sees nothing incredible in them.

The following report illustrates the defective judgment and grandiose ideas of the expansive type:

M., aged 41, a roofing salesman, was transferred to a state hospital from the jail to which he had been sentenced for violation of the motor vehicle laws. The prodromal symptoms of the patient's oncoming disease were apparently slight. The informant, his sister, who had seen him but infrequently, stated that she had not noticed any change in him except that for a year he had seemed somewhat "worried." While driving his car, he disregarded the collector at a toll bridge and drove across the structure at high speed. When overtaken by a police officer, the patient was found to have no license to drive an automobile, the permit having been revoked several years previously. Three days later, while awaiting trial for this offense, he was again arrested for driving an automobile without a license. He was given a short sentence in jail, where a physician soon recognized the patient's disorder and had him committed to the hospital.

On arrival at the admission office of the hospital, he told the office attendant that he was going to give her a million dollars because she was "a nice lady." As he was being questioned for the usual admission data, he began to boast of his wealth, claiming that he had three automobiles, thousands of dollars in the bank, a "diamond watch," and much other valuable jewelry. His son, he said, was lieutenant governor of the state, was soon to be governor, and later would be president of the United States. After having expressed various absurdly grandiose plans, he added, "I have another plan, too. I'm going to the wardens of the prisons in this state and all the other states and I'm going to buy the prisoners. I'll have an agreement with the warden to take their prisoners and put them to work on farms, and I'll charge each prisoner $300 for doing it and for getting him out of jail. I made $105,000 with prisoners just last week, and when I get going, I'm going to make plenty of money." The neurological signs were all consistent with syphilitic meningoencephalitis, and the serology was in all respects typical of the disease.

As a subgroup of the expansive type may be mentioned an excited or galloping form. Included in this subgroup are those who show great motor excitement, often with confusion. Some of these patients run a rapid course, quickly exhaust themselves, and die within a few weeks after the appearance of the excitement.

DEPRESSED TYPE. The depressed forms are those characterized by melancholia and frequently by hypochondriasis or by nihilistic delusions. Some of these patients have ideas of persecution and many have ideas of unworthiness and attempt suicide. In spite of the depression, there is often a certain element of apathy, and observation usually detects some dementia.

CIRCULAR TYPE. Interesting, but not particularly common, are the circular forms of paresis presenting alternations of mood that in their course and clinical manifestations resemble manic-depressive psychosis. It has been suggested that the organic disease is superimposed on a cyclothymic personality.

TABOPARESIS.   Patients with neuro-syphilis show not only evidence of the parenchymatous involvement of the brain seen in general paresis, but also symptoms and signs of involvement of the posterior columns met with in tabes dorsalis. The coexistence of both of these diseases is known as taboparesis. The symptoms of tabes usually precede those of paresis.

The taboparetic patient manifests not only the mental symptoms of general paresis, but also the ataxia and other physical evidence of tabes. Frequently there is a history of difficulty in walking in the dark, of "shooting" pains in the legs. The knee jerks are absent. Romberg's sign is present, and there is a loss of sense of position in the lower extremities. Primary optic atrophy may occur. The colloidal gold curve may be of the second zone type.

JUVENILE PARESIS.   This form, which occurs in the child or adolescent suffering from congenital syphilis, was first described by Clouston in 1877. Infection is transmitted from the mother to the off-spring by the transplacental route after the fifth month of pregnancy. It is estimated that rather less than 1 per cent of the cases of congenital syphilis develop general paresis. The age of the juvenile paretic subject at the time of the onset of symptoms corresponds approximately to the length of the incubation period in adult paresis. The child will generally, therefore, be from 5 to 20 years of age at the time of onset of symptoms. In about one-third of the cases, there is retardation of physical development. Many, perhaps 40 per cent, are found always to have been feebleminded. In those who have been markedly feebleminded, the onset is usually so vague that it is impossible to set a time of onset. In the moderately feeble-minded, and in those who have a period of normal development before the onset, there is an insidious but definite failure of previously learned accomplishments, followed by a progressive dementia.

The child's history may reveal that he had attended school and had acquired knowledge with fair success until 8 to 14 years of age, when insidious dementia began to develop. Many patients show confusion and restless, purposeless behavior. Because of the impairment of intelligence and the appearance of convulsions, not a few of the cases are diagnosed as epilepsy or idiocy with epilepsy. Delusions and euphoria are much less frequent in the juvenile than in the adult form of paresis. Trophic and other neurological disturbances are often conspicuous. Optic atrophy is not uncommon. Remissions of the type seen in paresis resulting from acquired syphilis are uncommon. The average duration of the disease is four to five years. In the final stages, the child is mute, untidy, and emaciated, and lives at merely a vegetative level. Treatment is less effective than in adult forms.

The following is a fairly illustrative case of juvenile paresis.

J. C. was admitted to a hospital when 17 years of age. The first pregnancy following his parents' marriage terminated at seven months, the child dying almost immediately. The patient was the next child in order of birth. His early development was said to have been normal. He attended school from 6 to 13 years of age and is said to have been promoted each year. The first symptoms appeared in October, when, as his father explained, the boy "became draggy and droopy" and "didn't want to serve his paper route as before." In December, the teacher reported that he was failing in school. In the spring, the patient "began to talk funny and was thick-tongued." At practically the same time, the parents noticed a weakness of the left leg and arm. His difficulty in walking increased, his speech became almost unintelligible, and he occasionally soiled himself.

On admission to the hospital, the patient was found to be of rather small stature but fairly well nourished. He walked somewhat in the manner of a mechanical doll, with his elbows pressed close to his ribs, his forearms extended straight before him, and his fingers separated. His steps were short and shuffling, with his feet widely separated as if to maintain his balance. His pupils were widely dilated (the right more than the left), were irregular, and did not react to light, but showed a little contraction on convergence. Both nerve heads were found to be somewhat atrophic. His tendon reflexes were exaggerated, there was a bilateral Babinski reaction, and he showed tremor of the fingers. Coördination in fine movements was defective. Attempts to secure the finger-to-nose tests were unsuccessful, as the patient could not be made to comprehend the instructions. The Wasser-mann reaction was positive on both blood and spinal fluid. The latter contained 19 cells and an excess of globulin and show a colloidal gold curve of 5555422210.

Mentally the patient's manner suggested that of a high-grade idiot. His facial expression was smoothed-out, and he frequently exhibited a silly grin. He coöperated in the eager, ineffective manner of a mentally defective and responded to all questions with "Huh?" He could not utter a single intelligible word but obeyed simple requests, such as "Shut your eyes," "Close your mouth." The Wassermann reaction on the father's blood was found to be positive.

Because of the active effort now made to ascertain if pregnant women are infected with syphilis and the efficacy of treatment with penicillin, cases of congenital syphilis are relatively rare. Juvenile paresis is therefore now an uncommon disease.

Course and Prognosis

If not treated, syphilitic meningoencephalitis leads inevitably to dementia and death. If not arrested within a reasonable period, it produces a permanent but varying degree of dementia and economic dependence. In the absence of treatment, death usually occurs from two to five years after the first appearance of symptoms. The course may be interrupted, however, by spontaneous remissions in slightly over 10 per cent of the untreated cases. The clinical improvement that may occur in these remissions may seem almost miraculous. Remissions are more frequent in those cases in which the onset has been comparatively sudden and stormy. The duration of the remissions is quite variable, extending from one or two months to five or six years. The average life expectancy in the untreated patient is four years.

The prognosis in the treated patient depends upon the promptness and thoroughness of treatment. Active treatment with adequate doses of penicillin during the asymptomatic stage should prevent the development of clinical symptoms in at least 85 per cent of the cases. If treatment is begun in the early clinical stages, 60 per cent or more of the patients will improve sufficiently to return to work. It is generally believed that a spinal fluid that is negative after three years from the date of infection will not become positive. In hospitals where patients are admitted in all stages of the disease, the number recovering rarely exceeds 30 per cent, the death rate is 20 to 30 per cent, and further progress is arrested in 30 to 50 per cent of the patients.

Diagnosis

Paresis has been confused with Alzheimer's disease, Pick's disease, multiple sclerosis, senile dementia, cerebral tumor, or other diseases producing cerebral damage, particularly to the frontal lobes. The spinal fluid findings constitute the most important differential criterion.

Treatment

Penicillin is the treatment of choice for syphilitic meningoencephalitis. A course of penicillin, repeated if necessary, is effective in a large proportion of both symptomatic and asymptomatic forms of the disease. The patient should receive a course of penicillin intramuscularly totaling 12,000,000 to 15,000,000 units. Different types of penicillin are used by different clinics. Many physicians use 600,000 units daily of procaine penicillin G, given intramuscularly for 20 days.

The results of the spinal fluid tests serve as a guide for both the activity of the paretic process and the effect of treatment. The spinal fluid should be examined four to six months after the completion of treatment. The first change in the cerebrospinal fluid following penicillin therapy is a reduction in the number of cells, which usually reach normal limits within six months. This is followed by a drop in total protein level. If the increased cell count has reverted to normal or near normal, the amount of protein has decreased, and the patient seems improved, no further treatment is needed. The complement-fixation reaction and results of the colloidal test may not revert to normal for several months or years and cannot be used to gauge adequate treatment. If the cell count and protein value remain high, a second course of treatment is mandatory. The second course should be the same as, or more intensive than, the first one. When the response is favorable, the spinal fluid should be examined at intervals of four to six months for the first year after treatment, then yearly until the spinal fluid is no longer abnormal. Less reliance is placed upon clinical features than upon spinal fluid changes as a guide to further treatment.

In greatly overactive patients, as well as in those with prominent affective components, it is often well to precede the administration of penicillin by a course of electroshock treatments.

SYPHILITIC MENINGITIS

The differentiation of the meningovascular forms of syphilis from meningoencephalitis is clinically important, as the symptoms, course and prognosis are quite different in the several conditions.

It is customary to divide syphilitic meningitis into three types, depending on the site of selective involvement.

BASILAR MENINGITIS. In this form, the inflammatory process is concentrated around the base of the brain. Basilar meningitis, which is one of the commonest forms of neurosyphilis, usually develops from one to three years after the primary infection. Thickening and infiltration of the pia mater occur in the cerebellopontine angle and in the interpeduncular space. With the infiltration of the former region, the sixth, seventh, and eighth nerves are affected, and as exudative processes occur in the latter space, the second and third nerves are involved.

Headache and perhaps dizziness appear; the patient shows mental hebetude, impairment of memory for recent events, sleepiness, difficulty of comprehension, clouding of consciousness, confusion and delirium, and occasionally stupor. The degree of disturbance of consciousness and of impairment of the more strictly intellectual functions varies roughly with the extent to which intracranial pressure is increased, as well as the degree to which the cortex is involved. The mental symptoms, if present, are usually so clearly of an organic type, are so obviously associated with neurological signs, and yield so quickly to treatment that comparatively few patients reach the mental hospital. Signs resulting from involvement of the optic nerve and of the nerves controlling the extrinsic muscles of the eye appear early and are perhaps fluctuating and inconstant at first. Ptosis, diplopia, strabismus, pupillary disturbance, papilledema, and choked disc are therefore present. Loss of corneal reflex, facial anesthesia, peripheral facial palsy, deafness, or signs of involvement of other cranial nerves may occur. Even in the absence of treatment, the mental symptoms may disappear, only to reappear shortly.

VERTICAL MENINGITIS. This type of cerebral syphilis usually occurs later than the more focal forms of syphilitic meningitis and involves the meninges of the convexity rather than of the base of the brain. Severe paroxysmal headache, often worse at night, is common. Dizziness is frequent. Sometimes the mental symptoms are so indefinite and are combined with such an ineffectiveness of personality that the patient is thought to be neurasthenic. More frequently there occur irritability, loss of ability for sustained effort, progressive hebetude, slow thinking, inertia, amnesia, and other signs of intellectual impairment. There is often much irregularity in the impairment of intellectual functions, some being retained much better than others. The nucleus of the personality is less impaired than in syphilitic meningoencephalitis. Retarded speech, brief attacks of aphasia, and other speech difficulties occur. Generalized or jacksonian convulsions may appear, and hemiplegia is not uncommon. Confusion, delirium, and stupor may be present in relatively acute cases. Paranoid reactions may exist, but here, as in the other types of nonparenchymatous forms of brain syphilis, there are less disturbance of behavior, judgment, and social reactions, and fewer delusional trends, than in paresis.

ACUTE SYPHILITIC HYDROCEPHALUS. This is a relatively rare form of neurosyphilis and is not characterized by selective involvement. Signs and symptoms include headache, nausea, vomiting, choked disc, stiffness of the neck, and Kernig sign. The symptomatology is caused by an excessive formation of cerebrospinal fluid and an impairment of the absorption of the fluid resulting from the inflammatory reaction.

Diagnosis

Syphilitic meningitis is accompanied by a positive Wassermann reaction in both blood serum and cerebrospinal fluid. Cells are markedly increased, there is an excess of albumin, and globulin is present. Typically, the precipitation of colloidal gold is greatest in the second zone, giving what is called the "luetic curve" (0123443210).

Treatment

The treatment of meningeal and vascular forms of neurosyphilis is the same as that of the meningoencephalitic form, i.e., with penicillin. Treatment with this antibiotic is usually followed by excellent results unless vascular or meningeal inflammation has already caused permanent damage to the nervous tissue. Routine laboratory examinations of both blood and cerebrospinal fluid should be made every six months.

THE ENCEPHALITIDES

Behavioral disturbances occur both during and after the acute phases of cer-

tain viral encephalitides. Glaser and Pincus have suggested that there may exist a predilection of certain forms to affect mainly the temporal lobe and particularly its medial portion associated with the limbic system. Thus, both acute and subacute inclusion body encephalitides, presumably due to herpes simplex, measles, and rabies, have such a predilection. It is thought that the unique histometabolic features of the limbic system render it susceptible to such infectious processes. The particular biochemical and metabolic features of the limbic system are reviewed in Glaser and Pincus' article.

The symptoms are affective, with anxiety and apprehensiveness associated with outbursts of rage or terror and their behavioral concomitants. So, too, one may note any of the exaggerated ego defenses, described earlier, to protect against such affective arousal.

While not occurring widely today, the best studied of the encephalitides is Type A, von Economo's epidemic encephalitis.

EPIDEMIC ENCEPHALITIS

An infectious disease of the brain which appeared in Rumania in 1915 but was first described and identified in 1917 by Constantin von Economo of Vienna spread to America in 1919 and subsequently attracted much attention both because of its devastating epidemiological features and because of its remarkable symptomatological polymorphism. Von Economo termed the disease lethargic encephalitis, but as it was not always characterized by lethargy, it has become generally known as epidemic or Type A encephalitis. No cases of the acute form have been reported since 1925, but the disease continues to have clinical interest, since chronic forms are still seen.

ETIOLOGY AND PATHOLOGY. It seems to be clearly established that the etiological agent was a filterable virus, although its mode of transmission is not known. The most common pathological lesion existing in this form was characterized by a cuffing or infiltration of the perivascular spaces in the brain with lymphocytes. While this may have existed in the cortex, hypothalamus, or even peripheral nerves, by far the most frequent site was the basal ganglia. Ganglion cells degenerated and many disappeared. In the chronic cases, which are the only ones now being seen by pathologists, the chief findings are loss and degeneration of neurons, especially in the substantia nigra, which may be grossly pigmented, as well as gliosis. The virus probably remains active in the nervous tissue for years, much in the manner of the *Treponema pallidum* in neurosyphilis.

SYMPTOMS. Since the acute form of this type of encephalitis is not now seen, little description of it will be given. Not even excepting syphilis is there a disease involving the central and peripheral nervous system capable of such polymorphic manifestations. Following the general symptoms of any infectious disease, there appeared the evidences of an invasion of the nervous system in which any one of its functions might be disturbed. The acute forms tended to fall into two ambitendent types: the hypersomnic-ophthalmoplegic and the irritative hyperkinetic. In the first or negative type, the most conspicuous symptoms were drowsiness with gradations to lethargy, stupor and coma, slowness of intellectual function, paralytic phenomena of cortical origin, aphasia, agraphia, astereognosis and loss of limb sense caused by paralytic lesions in the parietal cortex, ptosis, strabismus, and other disturbances of the ocular apparatus as well as other paralytic phenomena indicative of localization in the brain stem. The lethargy and other sleep disturbances were often the most striking symptoms of the acute form. The patient might remain in a deep sleep for days or weeks. If aroused, he promptly fell asleep again. In the irritative, hyperkinetic or positive type there were restlessness, irritability, excitability, insomnia, jacksonian or generalized convulsive seizures, and other irritative phenomena. Hyperkinetic phenomena resulting from involvement of the basal nuclei occurred in the acute form of the

disease and were of a great variety. Among them were tremors, myoclonias, and athetoid and choreiform movements.

Chronic Phase. Following the great epidemic mentioned, many patients who had survived the acute phase continued to show symptoms that at first were ascribed to residual lesions. Gradually, however, it became apparent that these symptoms were not stationary and that a continued, chronic activity persisted. Other patients who had supposedly recovered began, after intervals of months or years free from symptoms, to develop parkinsonism or other evidence of a continuing process. Also during the years since the epidemic, many persons with a history of some previous infection, perhaps diagnosed as influenza but with no associated acute encephalitic symptoms, developed chronic encephalitis. Others with no history of previous infection insidiously developed an encephalitis that was chronically progressive from the onset.

The symptoms of a chronic encephalitis of the von Economo type are varied and depend upon the areas in which the progressive inflammatory-degenerative changes take place, although the extrapyramidal basal motor nuclei are the most frequent sites. The most common syndrome is parkinsonism (cf. Chapter 19). Tremors, tics, myotonias, and athetoid and choreiform movements are frequently observed. In addition to these dyskinesias and hyperkinesias, there may be paroxysmal symptoms such as disturbances in rate or rhythm of respiration and gasping or yawning. One of the most frequent paroxysmal phenomena is oculogyric crises in which the eyes are spasmodically turned upward owing to the periodic activity of certain neural mechanisms. Narcolepsy and epileptic attacks may occur. Excessive flow of saliva, seborrhea, and obesity are not uncommon.

The psychic manifestations of the acute phase of epidemic encephalitis presented the general characteristics of an acute organic type of mental reaction of toxic infectious origin, viz., clouding of the sensorium and impairment of the capacity for apprehension, for elaborating impressions, and for activating memories. Most patients showed delirium, although in a considerable number the delirium was easily overlooked because of the more obvious stupor, some degree of which occurred in the acute stage of nearly all cases. In a rather large proportion of cases, emotional alterations continued after the acute phases and often constituted the only evidence of a lack of recovery. Among such mood alterations were irritability, explosive reactions, stubbornness, and apathy.

Intellectual defects did not usually follow the disease except when the infection occurred at a very early age—usually four years or younger.

Behavior Disorders. In children the chronic stage of epidemic encephalitis was often associated with serious alterations in character and behavior, the severity of which bore no relation to that of the acute stage. In some cases, in fact, it was difficult to obtain any clear history of an acute attack. The restless overactivity, emotional irritability, and impulsiveness of the early period were followed in a certain number of cases by lying, stealing, running away, cruelty, gross sexual offenses, and other behavior comparable in many outward manifestations to that exhibited by the psychopathic child. The troublesome behavior disorders shown by the encephalitic child were of every variety and usually in a setting of constant hyperactivity. The behavior or the adequacy of the social adjustment showed no correlation with the neurological signs. The child's personality, too, might be completely changed, yet his intellectual functions might not be affected.

There seems to be reason for believing that psychogenic factors may have played a certain role in the production of these behavior disorders. Not infrequently, for example, the laity looked upon "sleeping sickness" as something mysterious and was therefore prone to suspect that its victim might somehow be peculiar. Such children soon became aware of this attitude. If, too, the victim suffered from strabis-mus, tremor, narcoleptic attacks, or from parkinsonism with its absence of expressive movements of the face, its rigidity of posture and gait, and its slowness of speech, other children often called him "crazy" or "dumb," or with taunting nicknames made him the laughing-stock of his associates. Under these circumstances the child's feelings of inferiority and insecurity led to all sorts of undesirable defense reactions to his handicaps. During convalescence, in some instances, the child was overprotected, his training was neglected and faulty, and regressive tendencies were permitted or encouraged.

DIAGNOSIS. As already stated, acute cases of Type A encephalitis are no longer seen in the United States. A considerable number of patients, however, who exhibit the sequelae of the disease are still seen. The most common manifestations are tremor, rigidity, and slowness of voluntary movements, which combine to form a neurological picture resembling in some ways the hepatolenticular degeneration of Wilson and, in others, paralysis agitans. Chronic epidemic encephalitis does not, of course, show the corneal pigmentation (Kayser-Fleischer rings), a mixed static and intention tremor, and the evidence of liver disease seen in Wilson's disease.

In degenerative parkinsonism, one does not see the bizarre postures and gaits, the muscular spasms such as oculogyric crises, the coarse tremors, or the behavioral peculiarities frequently seen among the sequelae of epidemic encephalitis.

PROGNOSIS. From 10 to 50 per cent of the patients died during the acute phase of epidemic encephalitis, usually from respiratory paralysis. Of the survivors, roughly 75 per cent, within a period varying from a few weeks to six years, developed signs of a continuing infection, manifested by neurological, endocrine or metabolic disturbances, or by behavior, mood, or other personality disorder.

TREATMENT. Atropine, stramonium, and scopolamine have long been used for postencephalitic parkinsonism. Artane (trihexyphenidyl), which is similar to atropine in chemical composition, and other antiparkinsonian agents may also be used. The initial dose of Artane should be 1 mg. the first day, the amount being gradually increased, according to response, to 6 to 10 mg. daily. Rabellon is also helpful. These drugs are more effective in relieving rigidity and associated asthenia than in controlling tremor. Today, L-dopa is prescribed for patients with severe post-encephalitic parkinsonism. Its use is detailed in Chapter 19. Benzedrine sulfate, administered orally two or three times a day, in doses of 25 mg. is useful in reducing oculogyric crises and for asthenia.

OTHER ENCEPHALITIDES

While acute forms of von Economo's disease are no longer seen, one should remember that there are other forms of neurotropic virus infections that may cause such mental and neurological symptoms as drowsiness, confusion, stupor or coma, and other focal symptoms such as convulsions, hemiplegia, aphasia, ataxia, cranial nerve palsies, tremor, chorea, athetosis, and rigidity. Among such forms of encephalitis are St. Louis encephalitis, equine encephalitis, and the occasional cases of encephalitis associated with measles, infectious mononucleosis, various enteroviruses (Coxsackie, echo, polio, mumps, and herpes), and vaccination against cowpox. Residual psychiatric effects of infection with both eastern and western types of equine encephalomyelitis have been reported in the United States and Canada; also, residuals have occurred following Japanese B encephalitis contracted by United States military personnel in Japan and Korea since 1950.

In both eastern and western forms of equine encephalitis, infants and children have been more prone than adults to infection. In the former, sequelae have been virtually universal and most severe in infants under one year of age, who suffered persisting mental retardation, spasticities, and hemiplegias. Similar residuals have been observed with the western type

in infants as well. In one series approximately 25 per cent of adults affected who were followed over time showed impairment of higher intellectual functions with difficulty in abstract thinking and planning.

ACUTE BRAIN SYNDROME ASSOCIATED WITH SYSTEMIC INFECTION

In the case of the mental disturbances resulting from, or associated with, the infectious diseases that have thus far been mentioned, the infecting organism is located in the brain or its coverings. In many instances, however, mental disturbance may be associated with infections in which the infecting agent does not invade the central nervous system. Such temporary disturbances may result from many severe infections, such as typhoid fever or pneumonia, and appear especially during the febrile period and most frequently in the form of delirium.

MENINGOCOCCAL (EPIDEMIC) MENINGITIS

Probably the most important form of meningitis encountered by the psychiatrist is epidemic cerebrospinal meningitis. Actually the meningitis is but part of a septicemia caused by infection by meningococci. Delirium with confusion, muttering, rambling talk, disorientation, and restlessness usually occurs early in the course of the infection, but the acuteness of the mental symptoms depends on whether the disease is fulminating, acute, subacute, or chronic in type. At first the delirium may be nocturnal or exist only when the patient is undisturbed. In the acute cases, the patient is usually restless or even noisy and violent. In unfavorable cases, a terminal coma develops, appearing very early in the fulminating forms. In the subacute case, drowsiness, confusion, and mild delirium occur. Recovery may be complete or there may be special sense deprivations accompanied, perhaps, by various types of motor paralysis and a varying degree of mental defect. The resulting mental change may consist merely in moroseness, inability to concentrate, impairment of memory, and irritability, or, especially when the disease occurs in infants, there may be a serious arrest of intelligence.

The diagnosis is established by the existence of the above signs of diffuse cerebral dysfunction with the presence of signs of meningeal irritation, including a stiff neck, Kernig and Brudzinski signs, and often of a purpuric rash, hyperesthesia, and hyperalgesia. Spinal puncture shows a purulent fluid under increased pressure with a predominance of leukocytes. On Gram staining, the meningococcus may be cultured or tentatively identified as a diplococcus. The sugar and alkaloids of the cerebrospinal fluid are decreased.

Parenteral administration of 3.0 to 4.0 gm. of diethanolamine sulfisoxazole (Gantrisin) intravenously as a 0.5 per cent solution in physiologic saline should be the initial treatment. The same total amount should then be given daily in three divided doses four hours apart intravenously if the patient cannot retain oral medication. If he is able to do so, the patient may receive 1 gm. every four hours following the initial dosage given either intravenously as indicated above or as a 4.0 gm. dose by mouth. The drug should be continued for two to five days following symptomatic and clinical improvement. It is desirable to maintain a blood sulfonamide level of 10 to 12 mg. per 100 ml. This level should be checked regularly to prevent overdosage. Sulfadiazine is also highly effective as a therapeutic agent but requires alkalinization of the urine with its administration so as to prevent precipitation of the drug in the renal tubules.

Penicillin has been used, but the results are less satisfactory than with the sulfonamides unless large doses in the neighborhood of 1,000,000 units are given every two hours intramuscularly.

TUBERCULOUS MENINGITIS

In both children and adults, the onset of tuberculous meningitis is usually insidious. The previously active child begins to tire easily, appears weary, is irritable, peevish, and disinclined to talk or play. Sleep is often restless and disturbed by mild delirium. As the intracranial pressure increases, difficulty of grasp, clouding of consciousness, and confusion begin to appear, and headache increases. For a time, the patient, if roused, may for a short period be fairly well in touch with his environment, although he usually resents any disturbance. Some adults exhibit an agitated confusion. As the lethargy increases, the patient is no longer capable of recognizing friends and sinks into coma.

A diagnosis of tuberculous meningitis is made in the presence of signs of diffuse cerebral dysfunction as described above, with clinical evidence of meningitis indicated by a stiff neck, Kernig or Brudzinski responses, or both, hyperreflexia, patellar and ankle clonus, and Babinski reflexes. Later such signs may disappear with deepening coma. Cerebrospinal fluid is usually clear, with slight increase in pressure. A thin coagulum will develop if the fluid is allowed to stand. Tubercle bacilli may be found in the coagulum. The cells in the fluid are increased to 25 or more per cubic millimeter. Protein is elevated while glucose content is diminished.

Current treatment with streptomycin and isoniazid has been most gratifying. Intrathecal medication is unnecessary. With adults, streptomycin in the dosage of 1.0 gm. may be given intramuscularly in two divided doses in conjunction with 8 to 10 mg. per kilogram of body weight of isoniazid by mouth. This regimen should be continued for periods of six months or more after obvious clearing of the infection. The isoniazid may be decreased by 5 mg. per kilogram as improvement ensues. The clearing of the infection is indicated by the rise in the glucose content of the cerebrospinal fluid. Para-aminosalicylic acid may be given as well. In children, 1 gm. of streptomycin is given intramuscularly with isoniazid 10 mg. per kilogram daily in divided doses. When the cerebrospinal glucose has increased, the same dose of streptomycin is given twice weekly for one or two months, followed by sulfone (Promizole) by mouth for several years (0.25 to 8 gm.). Corticosteroid in the form of prednisone, 80 mg. per day in four divided doses, should be given but after a few days or a week a stepwise reduction in dosage is indicated depending upon the clinical course and changes in the spinal fluid. The use of intrathecal corticosteroids is advisable in those cases in which the diagnosis is made late in order to prevent the development of fibrinous inflammatory exudates which would hasten the blockage of flow of the cerebrospinal fluid.

Close observation is required in order to detect signs of intoxication with isoniazid and streptomycin. The symptomatology of toxicity with isoniazid is described in Chapter 18. Deafness and other disturbances have been observed with streptomycin. It has been shown that the prognosis for survival is related to the time of initiation of therapy and the severity of the illness. The state of consciousness, the degree of abnormality detected in the electroencephalogram, and the increase in cerebrospinal fluid protein with decrease in glucose provide indicators of the latter.

ACUTE (SYDENHAM'S) CHOREA

Sydenham's chorea is now regarded as an infectious encephalitis involving both the cortex and basal ganglia. It is thought that it results from the factors which produce rheumatic fever or from similar factors. It is probably a rheumatic encephalitis and represents an exudative stage of cerebral involvement similar to the exudative changes which may be observed in the joints and heart. It seems certain that a streptococcus is involved in the process. The involuntary, jerky movements, the muscular incoördination, and the grimaces are important symptoms of the disease, but only its mental aspects will be considered here.

SYMPTOMS.   In addition to an easy mental fatigability, many psychic symptoms may be associated with chorea. One of the most constant of these is an emotional instability. The choreic child becomes preoccupied, sensitive, irritable, restless, quarrelsome, and resentful of correction. Insomnia, night terrors, and sleepwalking may occur. Heedlessness and impairment of attention and of concentration are frequent; there is also an apparent inability to remember. The majority of these children are tearful, cry at the slightest provocation, are peevish and fretful. Many show a lack of concern for ordinary duties and obligations. Occasionally there may be considerable depression. The facies is sometimes described as wistful in expression. Selfishness and disobedience are common, and many feel that the somewhat frequent association of behavior disorders and delinquency with the disease is more than a coincidence. Sometimes the behavior disturbances are not unlike those following encephalitis or trauma of the head. Delirious episodes may occur. Unfortunately the family may fail to appreciate the seriousness and significance of the disease and therefore may scold and punish the child for the emotional and other rather trying behavior characteristics. Such ill-advised treatment tends to aggravate the emotional behavior and reactions. At best, the disease often leads to undesirable defense reactions. Chorea sometimes occurs for the first time, or recurs, in young women, associated with their first pregnancy.

DIAGNOSIS.   A history of rheumatism or of repeated attacks of tonsillitis and the presence of heart disease or of high fever may be helpful in establishing the diagnosis. It must be differentiated from hysteria, tics, athetoid movements, and from a restless, general hyperactivity. Sydenham's chorea usually continues for two or three months and occasionally for longer periods. Relapses are not uncommon. The disease occurs much more frequently in girls than in boys. There is much to suggest that a postinfectious encephalopathy may exist following chorea and that it is accompanied by permanent personality changes in the form of hyperkinetic or neurotic symptoms and peculiarities of character or temperament.

TREATMENT. One of the most essential requirements of treatment is physical and mental rest. The earlier the child is put to bed, the shorter, usually, will be the course of the disease. The disturbing presence of other persons should not be permitted. Treatment in a hospital away from disturbing home influences is often wise. Sodium salicylate and aspirin have long been used. In children over 13, fever therapy induced by means of the air-conditioned, thermostatically controlled hypertherm has been recommended by some as a means of shortening the course of the illness. The patient may be given daily treatments for two hours with temperatures from 104° to 105° F. Usually eight to ten treatments are given. Some pediatricians advise against fever therapy if cardiac damage exists. Such sedatives as bromides, chloral, or sodium amytal may be required if restlessness is marked. Since the chorea is merely a symptom of the rheumatic infection, the treatment of the latter must be continued until all criteria indicating its arrest are satisfied.

DELIRIA

Depending on their temporal relation to the febrile stage of the infection, the deliria with infectious diseases are known as prefebrile (initial) delirium, febrile delirium and postfebrile delirium.

PREFEBRILE DELIRIUM. Initial or prefebrile delirium is a delirium that rather infrequently develops during the incubation or prodromal period of infectious diseases before there has been any rise in temperature. The cause of the delirium can naturally not be ascertained until symptoms diagnostic of the infection appear. Such deliria may be marked and often imply a serious prognosis.

FEBRILE DELIRIUM. The delirium oc-

curring during the febrile period of an infection is often spoken of as febrile delirium. The intensity of the symptoms is dependent less upon the height of the fever than upon the integration of the personality and the importance of psychogenic factors. The forms of this, as of other delirioid reactions, are determined largely by individual personality factors. In milder degrees, there may be merely restlessness, sensitiveness to light or noise, and disturbing dreams. In the more severe cases, there will be hallucinations, confusion which may become extreme, indistinct muttering, stupor, twitching, carphologia, coma, and death.

POSTFEBRILE DELIRIUM. Postfebrile delirium may be merely the continuation of a previous delirium into the postfebrile period of an infectious disease, or it may be a delirium making its first appearance after the temperature has returned to normal. Consciousness is clouded to a variable degree, sometimes even to the point of stupor. In cases showing great prostration after the fall of the fever of infection, the symptoms may be of an extreme severity, constituting what H. Weber in 1866 described as collapse delirium. In this there is clouding of consciousness or a stuporous state, sometimes marked confusion and great motor excitement that appear to be motivated by fear and may increase even to violence and destructiveness. The stream of talk may be an incoherent flight of ideas. Emaciation and exhaustion progress rapidly, and a typhoid state, followed by stupor and coma, may develop. Death occurs in a few days in most of these malignant types of delirium, although a few patients recover after a prolonged sleep.

Treatment of Delirium

The treatment of delirium is primarily the treatment of the infection, toxic state, or other disturbing factor that led to the reaction. This does not mean, however, that the delirium itself should not be actively treated. Occasionally a beginning delirium may be aborted by reducing environmental stimulation, applying an icecap to the head, the reassurance of the nurse, or the administration of chlorpromazine or a hypnotic, such as paraldehyde. Precautions should be taken to prevent accidental injury or suicide. Unless carefully supervised, the delirious patient, usually disoriented and in some cases in intense fear, may unknowingly wander into danger or may attempt to escape imaginary enemies by suicide. Measures which tend to support his contact with his environment will lessen his fearfulness and anxiety. Such measures are the presence of close family members or familiar articles from his home in the room and a quiet environment with continuous light in the room day and night. Changes of environment or of physicians or nurses are apt to be disturbing. Greatly preferable to mechanical restraint are continuous baths or cold wet packs.

The patient should receive an abundance of nourishment which should include a liberal amount of proteins and of carbohydrates. Chlorpromazine given by mouth or by intramuscular injection in doses of 25 to 50 mg. is often effective. Other phenothiazines may be used as well. Multivitamin preparations are usually advisable. Sodium chloride, or other salts, and glucose, administered orally or intravenously, should be given liberally, if needed, to restore normal acid-base equilibrium. Caffeine may be advisable as a cardiac stimulant. The administration of sedatives should, if possible, be limited to the night. From 10 to 15 cc. of paraldehyde may be given in ice water, tea, or wine. Bromides and the barbiturates should be avoided. Chloral hydrate (7½ to 15 grains) may be used.

After the patient's recovery, the physician may be able to give considerable retrospective interpretation of delusional and hallucinatory experiences.

POSTINFECTIOUS MENTAL DISORDERS

These disorders differ somewhat from the postfebrile deliria just described. Delirium is not usually a conspicuous symptom, consisting, when it occurs, of a mild confusion and fleeting hallucinations. Rather more typical of the postinfectious mental disorders are states of easy exhaustion, reduced attention, restless irritability, difficulty in thinking, suspiciousness, anxious depression, and hypochondriacal ideas. The patient is frequently easily frightened, over-sensitive to light and noise, morose, complaining, and preoccupied with his physical sense of weakness and debility. A state of physical exhaustion and prostration exists and is doubtless an important factor in the development of the disorder. If there has been a prolonged subvitaminosis, there may be a retrospective falsification of memory suggesting Korsakoff's syndrome, which may be complete even to the existence of polyneuritis. On rare occasions, some degree of mental enfeeblement follows. Although the outstanding symptoms in the post-infectious disorders may be mental, their cessation depends upon the recovery of the patient's physical health.

ACUTE VIRAL HEPATITIS. With the increased recognition of acute viral hepatitis in recent years, the occasional association of mental disturbances with this infection has been observed. In some instances, this is a coincidence, as has been noted in public mental hospitals in which mild epidemics of infectious hepatitis have occurred. Occasionally, however, the infection releases a psychotic disturbance in poorly integrated personalities.

TRICHINIASIS. Trichiniasis is scarcely comparable to the infections which have just been discussed, yet mention may be made of the fact that occasionally mental disturbances occur in this disease if the young nematodes invade the cerebrum. The symptoms are those of the toxic-organic syndrome—confusion, cloudiness, disorientation, delirium, hebetude, and, at times, confabulation. Occasionally signs of focal neurological disturbances are noted.

BIBLIOGRAPHY

Glaser, G. H., and Pincus, J. H.: Limbic encephalitis. J. Nerv. Ment. Dis., *149*:59–67, 1969.

Hahn, R. D., et al.: Penicillin treatment of general paresis. A.M.A. Arch Neurol. & Psychiat., *81*:557–590, 1959.

Herzon, H., Shelton, J. T., and Bruyn, H. B.: Sequelae of western equine and other anthropoid-borne encephalitides. Neurology, *7*:535–548, 1957.

Infections of the Nervous System. Proceedings of the Association for Research in Nervous & Mental Diseases. Vol. 44. Baltimore, Williams & Wilkins Co., 1964.

Merritt, H. H., Adams, R. D., and Solomon, H. C.: Neurosyphilis. New York, Oxford University Press, 1946.

Mulder, D. W., Parrott, M., and Thaler, M.: Sequelae of western equine encephalitis. Neurology, *1*:318–327, 1951.

Von Economo, C.: Encephalitis Lethargica. Its Sequelae and Treatment: Translated by K. O. Newman. New York, Oxford University Press, 1931.

Chapter 14

"As for this disease called divine, surely it too has its nature and causes whence it originates, just like other diseases, and is curable by means comparable to their cure."

Hippocrates

Brain Syndromes Associated with Convulsive Disorders (Epilepsy)

The term *epilepsy,* derived from the Greek word meaning to seize or fall upon, has long been applied to a group of explosive reactions formerly believed to constitute a disease *sui generis.* The name has persisted, although it is now generally agreed that epilepsy is not a disease entity but a symptom complex characterized by periodic, transient episodes of alteration in the state of consciousness which may be associated with convulsive movements or disturbances in feeling or behavior, or both.

ETIOLOGY, TYPES, AND SYMPTOMS

Physiologically, epilepsy may be regarded as a disturbance in the electro-physiochemical activity of the discharging cells of the brain, a disturbance that may be produced by a variety of irritative stimuli impinging upon them from within or from without. This physiological disturbance may be expressed in the form of (1) a change in electrical potential as recorded in the electroencephalograms, (2) varied disorders of consciousness, (3) disordered functioning of the autonomic nervous system, and (4) convulsive movements or psychic disturbances. The nature of the disturbance of the internal milieu which, in so-called idiopathic epilepsy, alters the activity of the cortical neurons or of basal gray matter and precipitates an abnormal discharge of electrical energy in the brain is unknown. There is much to suggest that biochemical changes which increase the excitability of neurons may be the pathophysiological abnormality. Epilepsy, therefore, is probably neurogenic rather than psychogenic, although psychogenic factors may precipitate a seizure in a person who has a tendency to them.

Precipitating Factors

Although it appears that, in the majority of patients, the attacks are not precipitated by obvious external stimulation, in some they are always induced by a specific type of physical or perceptual stimulation. The arousal of anxiety either through some immediate interpersonal conflict or through fantasy of such a conflict often acts as a precipitating factor. In patients whose attacks originate in such a manner, psychiatric management may be helpful. In other cases specific sensory stimuli act as the precipitants.

Sudden sounds, occasionally listening to music, or flickering lights (as when driving through an avenue of trees in sunlight, watching sunlight on water, or watching television, rapidly moving the hands before the eyes) may induce seizures. Seizures induced by flickering lights are now designated as *photogenic epilepsy.* In some instances, only complex visual stimuli prove excitatory. Prolonged reading has initiated an attack, which commences with "clicking" or movement of the jaws. Some patients are able to terminate such an attack if they discontinue reading with the initiation of the jaw "clicking."

In female epileptic patients, the occurrence of a seizure in association with the menstrual period is common, but it is not known in what way the premenstrual hormonal interplay acts to precipitate attacks. The final metabolic derangement that results in a seizure is probably not the same in all patients or even the same at all times in any one patient. If the equilibrium of the internal milieu is in delicate balance, an attack may be precipitated by a minor physiological disturbance, such as that produced by hyperventilation.

Electroencephalography

Although the occurrence of an abnormal discharge of energy in the cerebral cortex coincident with epileptic attacks has only relatively recently been proved by electrical methods, Hughlings Jackson (1834–1911), the father of clinical neurology, conceived the idea nearly 100 years ago that such a discharge must be the basis of epilepsy. In 1929 Hans Berger of Jena discovered that by perfecting technical methods of amplification he could record through the intact skull the changes in electric potential already known to accompany cortical activity. The electroencephalogram (EEG) indicates alterations in electrical, and thus physiological, activity within the brain. Further study showed that normally about 10 electrical impulses originate in the brain every second, and that when these currents are recorded in the electroencephalogram they show a pattern of voltage and frequency (height and rate of the waves) more or less characteristic of the individual.

In epilepsy there are paroxysmal bursts of abnormal cortical activity with resulting changes in the rhythmic pattern of the EEG, indicating abnormalities in both rate and voltage of these currents. For this reason Lennox introduced the term "paroxysmal cerebral dysrhythmia" as applicable to epilepsy. Although abnormalities are to be observed in the electroencephalogram in many conditions other than epilepsy, in this disorder these abnormalities tend to assume certain patterns. Further, these patterns are distinctive for certain types of seizures. The electroencephalogram reveals the presence of these dysrhythmic discharges but fails to reveal their pathogenesis. When the focal discharging lesion is in the parietal, occipital, or frontal lobes, the symptomatology is largely neurological; if the disorder is in one or both temporal lobes, the symptomatology is largely psychiatric or that of psychomotor epilepsy.

Electroencephalographic studies of cerebral epileptic foci indicate that occipital foci are most common in infancy, rolandic between the ages of 3 and 6, and temporal between the ages of 5 and 12. The clinical course varies with each type. In children bilateral and multiple foci are frequent and the discharges synchronous. Such foci may remain stable over time, migrate, or spread. It is often difficult to relate the clinical phenomenology to the observed electroencephalographic foci. The morphology of the electrical discharges also may change over time. Thus, poorly organized "spike-and-wave" forms present at birth become more clearly evident after a few months of life. Tonic-clonic discharges become organized later, clonic between the ages of 3 and 6 months and tonic between 18 months and 2 years.

It is generally estimated that 5 to 10 per cent of normal persons exhibit abnormalities of their electroencephalograms similar to those seen in epileptics. It is believed that such persons are predisposed to epilepsy, although the disturbance in cortical electrodynamics as represented by the EEG is not so serious as to result in seizures unless the cerebrum suffers some pathological alteration. It has also been found that about 85 per cent of persons with a history of epilepsy show abnormalities of electroencephalographic rhythm during a 15-minute recording in the in-

terval between convulsions as compared to
10 per cent in the average population.
When such abnormalities of the EEG exist
in the interparoxysmal period, they tend
to be of the same general type as those
observed in the form of seizure from which
the patient usually suffers. These types
will be described later. There are, however, undoubted epileptics in whom abnormal tracings have never been obtained
even by repeated examinations.

It will thus be seen that the electroencephalogram has its limitations. Although
the finding of seizure discharges creates a
presumption that clinical seizures have occurred or will occur, a negative report (no
seizure discharges) does not rule out
epilepsy. This is because (a) seizure discharges can be present in the depths of
the brain and not appear in standard recordings from the surface of the head, and
(b) discharges may occur so infrequently
that there is almost no likelihood of one
occurring during the relatively short period of recording required in a routine
examination. In the waking state, but
more especially during sleep, seizure discharges occur, as evidenced by the electroencephalogram, that are not immediately
associated with clinical symptoms. Eighty
per cent of patients with a history of convulsive epileptic seizures have nonconvul-
sive seizure discharges while asleep. When
not asleep, only 35 per cent of this group
have subclinical seizure discharges.

Idiopathic and Symptomatic Epilepsy

In many instances clinical seizures develop in persons with preëxisting cerebral
dysrhythmia but in whom no visible or
otherwise demonstrable alteration of cerebral tissue can be discovered. For this reason seizures of unknown origin have long
been known as *idiopathic epilepsy*. About
77 per cent of all epileptics fall among
those in whom no cause of the condition
can be found. Cases in this group tend to
manifest themselves early in life. In other
instances tumors, trauma, inflammation,

chronic localized encephalitis, or other discoverable lesions precipitate seizures in a
person who may or may not have had a
preëxisting cerebral dysrhythmia. Those
seizures in which a cerebral lesion either
brought out a subclinical dysrhythmia or
produced seizures in the absence of preexisting dysrhythmia are known as *symptomatic or acquired epilepsy*. A growing
recognition of the multiplicity of etiological and contributing factors continues
to displace the traditional idiopathic versus symptomatic point of view.

Frequency of Epilepsy

It is generally estimated that the incidence of epilepsy in the United States is
1 in 200 of the population. Because of the
development of new drugs in recent years
for the treatment of the disorder, fewer
patients than formerly require institutional care. The incidence in males is
slightly greater than in females, probably
because of the greater frequency of head
trauma in the male both at birth and in
adult life.

Age of Onset

Idiopathic epilepsy may develop at any
age but a majority of the cases appear between the ages of 10 and 20. Not a few
occur before 10 years of age, but the first
appearance of a seizure after 20 requires
study by all known methods before the
conclusion is reached that it is idiopathic.
Infantile convulsions appearing without
obvious cause should be regarded with
apprehension. It is reported that infantile
convulsions associated with fever or other
physical disturbance increase the chances
of epilepsy five times.

Inheritance

The exact degree to which heredity influences the development of seizures is
controversial. The prevailing opinion to-

day is that the inheritance of epilepsy is multifactorial (polygenic) across the whole series of cases. In some instances the genetic role is significant; in others exogenous factors provide the predominant factor in predisposition and precipitation of the cortical convulsive discharge. It is now thought that the genetic factor is expressed principally in the tendency to produce spontaneous paroxysmal cerebral electrical discharges with an inclination for spreading of such discharges. Epilepsy is more common among relatives with nonfocal electroencephalographic abnormalities than those with focal distortions. Lennox, Gibbs, and Gibbs found from an electroencephalographic examination of parents of epileptics that these parents had abnormal brain waves much more frequently than did control persons. In the opinion of these authors, the "presence of abnormal brain waves in the parents of epileptics is presumably evidence that the cerebral dysrhythmias associated with epilepsy are inheritable and that parents who show such cortical dysrhythmias are 'carriers' of the disorder." These authors found that 60 per cent of the near relatives of noninstitutionalized epileptics had dysrhythmia and 2.4 per cent of them had a history of seizures. Of their controls, 10 per cent showed dysrhythmia. Of course none had seizures.

It has been found that among identical twins idiopathic epilepsy occurs eight times more frequently in both individuals than it does in both of fraternal twins. It is estimated that epilepsy occurs about five times more frequently among near relatives of idiopathic epileptics than it does in the general population. The existence of a predisposition to the disease in the child of an epileptic is often demonstrable in the form of cerebral dysrhythmia. There is also a striking likeness of brain-wave abnormalities in epileptics with the same heredity. A person afflicted with epilepsy who marries a nonepileptic may, however, expect only one child in 50 resulting from the union to suffer from convulsions.

The psychiatrist is frequently asked concerning the advisability of marriage for the epileptic or the probability that his children may inherit the disease. The following factors tend to minimize the chances of the disease in the child of an epileptic: a family history devoid of epilepsy or migraine for the spouse as well as the patient, a minimal abnormality of their electroencephalograms, some acquired condition that is at least partially responsible for seizures, late onset of the illness, and a normal mental endowment. The genetic factor in epilepsy is probably no greater than it is in many other common diseases.

Types of Seizures and Their Symptoms

Three major types of clinical seizures are usually described: grand mal, petit mal, and psychomotor seizure or psychic equivalent. Heredity is of importance in determining the pattern of seizure. The seizures of all types are irregular and unpredictable. There are many variants of epilepsy which, because they depart so far from the "usual" forms of seizures, are apt to escape recognition. Loss of consciousness with or without convulsive spasm is the criterion of epilepsy. It is probably not sufficiently appreciated that in many attacks consciousness is not lost but is merely disturbed. The patient may be aware of all that is going on around him, may hear and understand what is being said, but is for the time being unable to collect his thoughts or reply to a question. Not rarely the occurrence of a major epileptic fit suddenly renders clear the meaning of obscure minor events that may have existed for years. These may have been myoclonic, local muscle spasms, defects of attention, "absences," dreamy states, or brief periods of mental inhibition when mental processes seemed to be arrested and the mind a blank. The form that epilepsy takes depends not so much on the pathological features of the lesion as on its site and the violence of the neuronal discharges in the neighborhood of the lesion and the extent of their spread to the rest of the brain.

GRAND MAL. The grand mal seizure with its intense spontaneous neuronal activity is the most dramatic of the epileptic manifestations. Seizures of this type tend to be accompanied by an increase in speed and voltage of brain waves, which are recorded in the electroencephalogram as sharp spikes, often at the rate of 25 per second.

Aura. From a moment to several seconds before the loss of consciousness, about half of the patients with a grand mal type of attack have an *aura,* or warning, that a seizure is immediately imminent. The aura is not really a premonition but the first manifestation of the neuronal discharge. The form of the aura depends primarily upon the site of the epileptogenic focus. Lesions of the precentral region generally give rise initially to motor phenomena and of the postcentral region

to sensory phenomena. The aura may consist of numbness, tingling, or uncomfortable sensations, of a feeling of distress in the epigastrium, perhaps passing up toward the head, or of a hallucination of the special senses, such as flashes of light, certain noises, or olfactory hallucinations. The aura is usually affectively unpleasant. Sometimes the aura is motor in nature and consists of a twitching or stiffness in a certain group of muscles preceding the loss of consciousness.

Tonic Phase. The loss of consciousness is sudden and complete. The patient falls at once, and, as he rarely has any opportunity to protect himself, he may sustain serious injuries. As he falls, the entire voluntary musculature goes into a continuous contraction, remaining in this *tonic* phase from 10 to 20 seconds. The muscles of the chest often contract at the same time as do those of the larynx; air is thereby forcibly expelled and results in

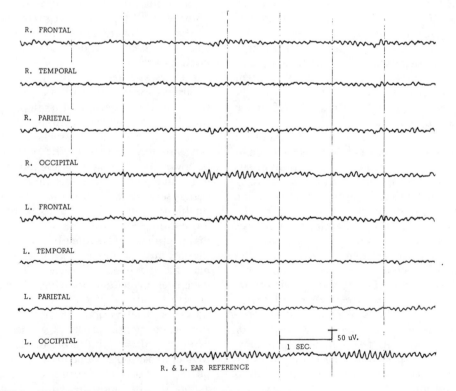

FIGURE 1. Normal adult record characterized by 11 c.p.s. alpha rhythm, which is not prominent in the occipital areas.

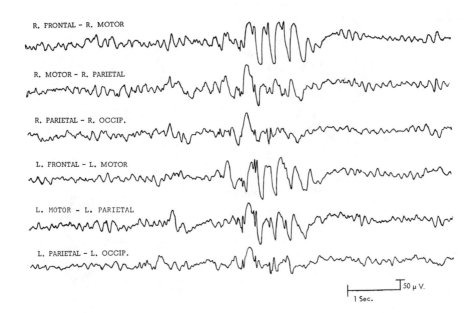

FIGURE 2. One of a number of types of tracings found between attacks in patients with grand mal epilepsy. The record shows a burst of irregular, slow waves and atypical spike and wave discharges from all areas.

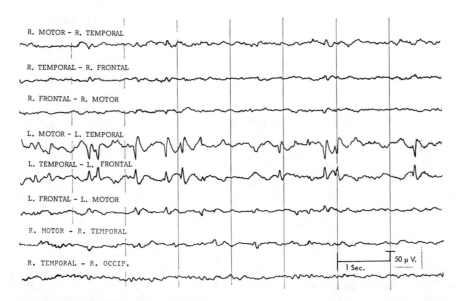

FIGURE 3. Spike discharges from the left anterior temporal lobe seen between attacks in a patient subject to psychomotor seizures of temporal lobe origin.

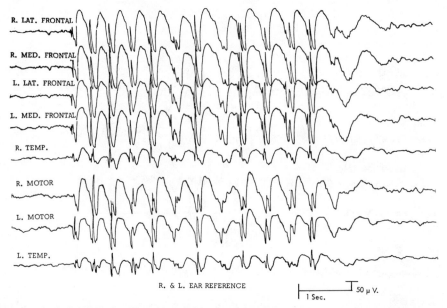

R. LAT. FRONTAL

R. MED. FRONTAL

L. LAT. FRONTAL

L. MED. FRONTAL

R. TEMP.

R. MOTOR

L. MOTOR

L. TEMP.

R. & L. EAR REFERENCE

1 Sec.

50 μ V.

FIGURE 4. A short clinical petit mal attack accompanied by continuous 2-per-second spike-and-wave discharges. Both the attack and the electrical discharges begin and end abruptly. (Records by courtesy of Dr. E. Goldensohn.)

the peculiar sound known as the epileptic cry. At first the face is pale, but as the muscles rigidly contract, the superficial veins become engorged. At the same time the chest becomes fixed and the aeration of the blood ceases, thus adding to the cyanosis of the face. During this tonic phase and for a variable period afterward, the pupils are dilated and do not react to light and the corneal reflex is absent. The Babinski reflex is present and the tendon reflexes are absent or decreased. During the general muscular contraction, the bladder is often emptied and occasionally the rectum.

Clonic Phase. The tonic stage is followed by intermittent or *clonic* muscular contractions, at first rapid but gradually growing less frequent. If at this time the tongue happens to fall between the teeth during a relaxation, it may be bitten when a clonic contraction follows. As respiration returns, the saliva, which could not be swallowed, may become intermixed with air and thus appears in a foam, perhaps tinged with blood.

Coma. In the *postconvulsive coma,* the pupils are rigid, tendon reflexes are absent, respiration is stertorous, the face is congested and covered with perspiration, and the lips are cyanosed. If an arm or leg be lifted and then released, it drops heavily as in a state of flaccid paralysis. If left undisturbed, the patient may sleep for an hour or two, complaining of headache, fatigue, and perhaps of a painful tongue on awaking. As the patient emerges from the coma, he is often bewildered and may perform semiautomatic acts, move aimlessly about, exhibit chewing movements, fumble at his clothing, or attempt to remove it. Sometimes clouded states persisting for a few days may develop after several successive convulsions. They are more frequent in men than in women.

Some patients have convulsions during sleep as well as in their waking hours, while in some patients the convulsions are always nocturnal. Many have their seizure just as they are falling asleep. It should be remembered that occasionally an epileptic who is subject to nocturnal seizures is suffocated by burying his face in a pillow during a convulsion.

Status Epilepticus. Sometimes a patient may pass from one seizure into another without intervening recovery of consciousness. This condition, known as *status epilepticus,* always involves danger to life. It is sometimes precipitated by abrupt withdrawal of medication, particularly if the patient has been receiving phenobarbital. It may follow alcoholism or excessive fatigue, but frequently no precipitating factor is evident. It is not rare after cerebral operations on epileptics. If preventive measures are not taken, the temperature may rise to dangerous heights. The patient may become profoundly exhausted, lapse into coma, and die from cardiac dilation or pulmonary edema.

PETIT MAL. Abortive seizures of various degrees and types occur, in all of which there is usually some disturbance of consciousness. The most frequent of the minor forms is that of petit mal, which is characterized by a transient interruption of the stream of consciousness. The electroencephalogram of petit mal consists of a slow, round wave followed by a quick, sharp spike. Groups of these alternately slow and fast waves occur three times a second. It is the most distinctive of any of the epileptic brainwave records. The details of these minor attacks differ widely among individual patients, but the most frequent form consists of a loss of consciousness lasting from 5 to 30 seconds. They begin and end abruptly and are without warning or sequel.

The patient does not fall. He may become pale, with his posture fixed, his eyes staring and expressionless; his attention cannot be secured; he may suspend his occupation and, through loss of muscle tone, drop whatever article may be in his hand. Usually there is a little rhythmic twitching of eyelids, eyebrow, or head. After a few seconds, consciousness abruptly returns and the patient resumes his activities. Most patients recognize that an attack has occurred, but some remain unaware of this "absence."

The onset of petit mal is usually between four and eight years of age. After 18 years of age it tends to disappear or to be replaced by other types of seizure. Petit mal attacks usually occur much more frequently than grand mal seizures. From one or two to a few hundred attacks may occur in a day. The two forms frequently coexist. Two of every three children with petit mal subsequently develop grand mal.

Many children with petit mal are often socially and emotionally maladjusted. This maladjustment often appears to be explained on the basis of an impaired parent-child relationship which affects the child's personality formation. The impaired relationship apparently grows out of a conscious or unconscious parental rejection. The lack of basic security occasioned by the impaired parent-child relationship tends to extend and pervade all relationships. Sometimes the child, believing that all adults are like his parents and that all experiences will be frustrating, develops a pattern of antagonism and rebellion.

Usually included in the petit mal form are myoclonic twitches in which single contractions of the flexor muscles of the arms occur without loss of consciousness, as well as akinetic attacks in which there is a sudden falling with muscular hypotonia. Like the classic petit mal, the latter two forms show a wave-and-spike rhythm of electrical discharge. Formerly the term pyknolepsy was given to what was believed to be a special type of seizure allied to petit mal. It is now considered to be a true petit mal. The name should therefore be dropped.

In recent years a significant increase in excretion of urinary amino acids has been found in many with petit mal.

PSYCHOMOTOR EPILEPSY. Of greatest importance to the psychiatrist is psychomotor epilepsy, since it is characterized by trance-like attacks and confusional episodes which often lead to its misdiagnosis as schizophrenia or psychoneurosis. It is much more common in adults than in children, although in minor forms of the condition the attacks are very similar to those of petit mal. They differ from petit mal, however, in various ways. The attacks last longer, from one-half to two minutes, and are frequently associated with movements of the muscles concerned with mastication, swallowing, or speech, so that the patient may smack his lips, chew, or make incoherent verbalizations. Also, the clouding of consciousness is greater than in petit mal, with amnesia persisting for one-half to several minutes after the attack. In other instances, either brief episodes of automatic thought formations of a delusional nature and auditory or visual hallucinations may take place. In the case of the former, the patient may report only an amorphous repetitive and ill-defined thought, a crystallized thought percept, an internally located voice usually in the head but sometimes in the abdomen or elsewhere or placed in the external environment. The visual hallucinations also may be apprehended either internally or externally. Finally, the electroencephalographic record is not similar to that of petit mal and its focus is the anterior pole of the temporal lobe.

Some patients describe brief affective states of fear, vague alarm, terror, rage, and occasionally well-being or pleasure. The patient's behavior is appropriate to his mood. Other episodic but sustained moods may be in the form of extreme irritability, depression, ill humor, or bad temper. Sometimes the psychomotor seizure takes the form of a clouded state characterized by confusion, bewilderment, excitement with hallucinations, outbursts of violence, or occasionally ecstatic moods with religious exaltation. Clinically the clouded state suggests a delirium with liberation of aggressive and, occasionally, self-destructive impulses. Acts of violence may be committed in these automatisms and may be of a strikingly brutal nature, the patient pursuing his crime to a most revolting extreme.

These furors are characterized by their suddenness, absence of premeditation and of precaution, and amnesia for them. The extraordinary degree of discrimination and judgment displayed in the psychomotor attack often gives the patient's acts a misleading appearance of deliberation. It may be difficult to accept the fact that the author of the crime was not responsible for his acts. Usually these psychomotor seizures continue for only a few minutes, but they may go on for hours or even days. Sometimes the seizure may assume the form of a fugue. Occasionally the patient may report feelings of loneliness, strangeness, or typical "déjà vu" phenomena as if he had undergone the same experience in the dim past. Psychomotor seizures may occur in pure form, but in many cases grand mal seizures may also be present. Their frequency increases with age.

Many children with temporal lobe epilepsy exhibit outbursts of catastrophic rage. In Gunsted's recent study of children with this behavioral expression, it appeared that such rage attacks had beginnings in three separate age periods. Those associated with hyperkinesis commenced before the fourth birthday. The majority of children without hyperkinesis but with the episodic rage attacks had onset between 7 and 11. Onset after that was not usually associated with outbursts of rage. In the first group many remitted until late adolescence or early adulthood. It seems probable that disappearance of this type of behavior with epilepsy may be related to increasing inhibition due to cortical control and related to superego development.

In most patients with temporal lobe discharge sex behavior tends generally to be marked by a lack of libidinal and genital arousal, although a few have episodic expressions of excessive drive.

The episodic behavior disturbance of many with temporal lobe convulsive discharges has been likened to the schizophrenic reaction. Yet serious affective disturbances do occur as well. From his studies of a series of cases, Flor-Henry suggests that temporal lobe epilepsy of the dominant lobe predisposes to psychotic behavior; this is most likely to be schizophrenia-like. That of the nondominant lobe is more likely to be associated with affective reactions. Yet frequent psychomotor attacks seem to suppress such abnormal behavior.

Probably to be included among the psychomotor epilepsies is the syndrome known as *epilepsia cursiva* ("running fit"). This is an episodic alteration of awareness associated with running. Consciousness may be clouded to a variable degree. Sometimes the running fit occurs immediately after a grand mal seizure. There may or may not be an aura. The duration of the running is brief. Frequently one finds a history of conflicts with members of the family that seem to have acted as precipitating factors.

The distinguishing feature of the electroencephalogram in the psychomotor seizure is the presence of spike seizure discharges at the rate of four to eight a second. It is believed that the focus of electroencephalographic activity is the anterior part of the temporal lobe. There is an increasing tendency to use the term *temporal lobe epilepsy* as a synonym for the psychomotor type, or to refer to the seizures characterized by hallucinations, memory disturbances, and automatisms as "temporal lobe" in preference to "psychomotor." Penfield and his co-workers, by stimulation of the cortex of the temporal lobe in patients with temporal lobe epilepsy, produced complex hallucinations, vivid memories, and dreams that were often identical with the content of the seizures.

A 10-year-old girl was brought to the clinic by her mother after she had suffered a number of episodes of loss of consciousness. These were described by the mother in the following way.

She awakened with a headache, seemed listless, and then was noticed by her mother to develop a twitching movement of the left side of her mouth and eyes. Her arms assumed an "odd," stiff position and became unresponsive. This condition persisted 5 minutes, to be followed by another similar episode 10 minutes later in which she urinated and defecated. These attacks were followed by five others preceded by an aura of "fear"—as the child stated, being "scared." The patient had total amnesia for the attacks.

Physically, no abnormalities were noted. An electroencephalogram showed a right occipitotemporal focus of high voltage, 31 per second activity aggravated by hyperventilation. Other studies were negative. Psychiatric and psychological examinations at this time showed no pathology. She was treated with phenobarbital and Dilantin in increasing doses, with reduction in the occurrence of attacks and in their intensity.

For years she reported only daily brief episodes of "scary feelings." It was necessary to increase the dosage of the anticonvulsant medication, and Mebaral was prescribed as well. At age 14 she was admitted to the hospital with an acute delirious state due to barbiturate over-dosage. Following this hospital admission, her mother noticed a character change in that she became resentful and hostile, expressed the attitude that she was disliked, and seemed depressed. Then "slow spike waves" were observed over the left temporal region during periods of sleep.

At this time she commenced to have episodes of loss of consciousness, occurring without warning and with subsequent amnesia, in which she suddenly rushed away from her place of work, walking rapidly and aimlessly through the streets, impulsively removing her stockings and placing them in her purse or suddenly staring blankly, smacking her lips, giggling foolishly, and then mumbling incoherently. High-dosage combinations of various anticonvulsants failed to control these seizures. Due to her progressive social disability and withdrawal, in spite of medical therapy, a craniotomy with resection of the right temporal lobe was performed when she was 20 years old. Following the operation she was free of seizures and resumed her work on treatment with Dilantin alone.

Behavior Disorders with Cerebral Dysrhythmias

Some children without clinical evidence of the classic forms of epilepsy but with cerebral dysrhythmia on encephalogram suffer behavior disorders. Such children may complain of headaches, be moody, have temper tantrums or attacks of rage, scream or cry unreasonably, and appear distractable, overaggressive, fearless, or lacking in shyness. Their attention span is often limited, and in formal psychologic tests wide scatter is often seen—a finding common in the brain damaged. Children with such symptoms should be examined electroencephalographically. They respond well to treatment with *d*-amphetamine, methsuximide (Celonten), or acetazolamide (Diamox).

Narcolepsy

The term *narcolepsy* was introduced in 1880 by Gélineau to describe a "rare neurosis characterized by an invincible need for sleep, ordinarily of short duration, occurring at longer or shorter intervals of time, often several times a day, forcing the subject to fall to the ground or to lie down in order to avoid falling." It has often been described as a variant of epilepsy. Probably, however, this is not the case, and it should be considered as a special clinical type in a group of sleep disorders. In many cases a history of previous epidemic encephalitis has been obtained. In some instances narcolepsy may be a sequel or a continuing form of that disease.

Narcolepsy is characterized by a sudden, irresistible desire to sleep. Regardless of the situation in which he may be placed or of the activity in which he may be engaged, the patient falls fast asleep. The sleep is apparently natural; the patient may be awakened, but the period of sleep usually lasts from seconds to 30 minutes. After he has awakened the patient usually states that he feels refreshed. Nocturnal sleep is not modified. The condition is most frequent in young male patients. Sexual impotence, obesity, and lymphocytosis are often associated symptoms. It is generally believed that some anatomical pathologic condition, the result of localized encephalitis, trauma, or neoplasm, exists in the gray matter surrounding the third ventricle at the level of the ocular nuclei or in the hypothalamus. Lesions of the hypophysis may be secondary.

Cases supposed to be psychogenic have been reported. Psychometric studies in certain groups of patients with the narcoleptic syndrome have shown a common background of emotional conflict. The individuals felt themselves to be caught in a life pattern which they resented but felt obligated to conform to it. Frustrated in their efforts to achieve an autonomy in another pattern of their own choosing because of their dependent emotional attachments, those affected develop the narcoleptic complex which relieves the anxiety of open conflict.

Many consider narcolepsy as a syndrome that may occur in several pathological states. It is probably not a disease *sui generis*. Electroencephalographic records do not show the cerebral dysrhythmia of epilepsy. When the individual is alert, the electroencephalogram appears normal. On the other hand, a large proportion of patients with the syndrome demonstrate the electrical patterns of REM (rapid eye movement) sleep in connection with narcoleptic attacks and at the beginning of nocturnal sleep, suggesting that the attack represents an aberrant diurnal expression of paradoxical sleep. Similar EEG findings occur with nonsleeping attacks of cataplexy as well. Since REM sleep is specifically inhibited by d-amphetamine, it is not surprising that this drug is the treatment of choice. Because of the EEG findings, some regard narcolepsy as a reversible dysfunction of the pontine system and not as a paroxysmal convulsive disorder.

Yoss et al. have reported that the pupillographic studies of those with narcolepsy show characteristic spontaneous changes. In darkness the untreated narcoleptic has smaller pupils which frequently change in size as waves of pupillary constriction and dilatation occur. In contrast the non-narcoleptic presents large pupils which seldom change in size. It is thought that these pupillary changes reflect decreased wakefulness. They are reversed when patients are treated with the amphetamines. Pupillography may be used to assess the appropriate therapeutic dosage of such agents.

Narcolepsy does not respond to bromides, phenobarbital, or other sedatives, but, as mentioned, it is controlled by d-amphetamine sulfate (10 to 50 mg. twice daily) or racemic amphetamine sulfate (10 to 50 mg. twice daily). Methylphenidate hydrochloride (Ritalin) given in 5-mg. doses also has been useful. If taken after midday, such drugs may produce insomnia.

DIFFERENTIATION FROM HYPERSOMNIA. Since this disorder may have psychogenic determinants or may be confused with hypersomnia as a symptom of an emotional disturbance, careful psychiatric evaluation is indicated in all suspected cases. Psychogenic hypersomnia differs in that the patterns of drowsiness or sleepiness last for several hours rather than for 15 to 30 minutes and are often associated with a history of disturbed nocturnal sleep, obesity, and the personality characteristics of passivity, with anxiety aroused by any situation threatening expression of criticism or anger to others. Such situations, particularly when the emotional outburst might be directed toward the person to whom they hold a strong dependent relationship, are the usual precipitant of the hypersomniac period. In hypersomnia, in contrast to narcolepsy, the amphetamines are unlikely to be useful, but their use may enhance the possibility of working out psychotherapeutically the psychodynamic conflict. Psychotherapy is reported to be helpful in certain instances.

Cataplexy

Apparently related to narcolepsy are the paroxysmal attacks known as cataplexy in which, under the influence of emotional excitement, there are paralysis of voluntary movements and postural collapse of the whole body. The patient suddenly loses power and tone of all skeletal muscles, his knees give way, and he sinks helplessly to the ground. Many patients are unable to speak during the episode, although consciousness is fully preserved. Laughing, in particular, appears to provoke an attack, although anger, anxiety or annoyance may act similarly. Narcolepsy and cataplexy are probably allied reactions, since cases of a transitional nature, including narcoleptic attacks provoked by emotion, are observed. The attacks of narcolepsy and cataplexy constitute what is often spoken of as the narcoleptic-cataplectic syndrome. As mentioned previously, the cataplectic attack is accompanied by the electroencephalographic pattern of REM sleep. With REM sleep there occurs a sudden and profound fall in muscular tonus demonstrable in the electromyogram. The treatment of cataplexy is the same as for narcolepsy.

Epileptic Personality

Reference is often made to a so-called epileptic personality. The idea, however, of an epileptic personality as a precursor and an essential background of epilepsy has been discarded. Undoubtedly, some epileptic children are overly aggressive, irritable, restless, overactive, moody, stubborn, oversensitive, and shy, and may manifest such conduct disorders as lying, stealing, fighting, sex misbehavior, cruelty, and destructiveness. By no means do all epileptic children show these characteristics. If they exist they are probably a result of bad home environment and of the frustrations, social rejection, state of insecurity, constant anxieties, and other emotional difficulties arising from the child's handicap.

Psychiatrists whose contacts with adult epileptics are limited to institutionalized patients usually assert that the epileptic patient has a rigid, unpleasant, irritable, self-centered personality given to rage on frustration. On the other hand, physicians who see no epileptics except those met in the office and clinics report that their patients do not exhibit more undesirable traits than do persons free from the disease. Undoubtedly, however, the patient who feels that he is handicapped through his disorder, who is constantly struggling for a place in his community, who fears exposure and is convinced that he is destined to be an abnormal member of the family has periods of irritability and depression. The sense of resentment that he often feels may produce unhappiness, add to his problem of adjustment, and perhaps create antisocial tendencies. Discouragement and hopelessness may lead to contraction of interests and mental slowness. The religiosity shown by some epileptics may have its origin in a search for security, solace, and self-esteem.

Epileptic Deterioration

Although the mean intellectual functioning of those with idiopathic epilepsy tends, as a group, to be less than that of their unaffected relatives, their intellectual functioning still falls within or close to the average. In fact, a third of the group exceed the performance of their unaffected relatives on appropriate tests. Nevertheless, continued and uncontrolled seizures are considered to impair intellectual functioning.

In a certain number of epileptics, the range of interests narrows as the convulsive reaction continues. A psychic slowness develops; attention, intellectual processes, and emotional responses become increasingly dull; and comprehension and memory become impaired. The patient suffers from a poverty of ideas, shows a tendency to stress the trivial as much as the important, to become circumstantial in his ideational expression, to disregard the interests of others; and to become selfish, affectively self-satisfied, boastful, lazy, and careless in appearance; his facies is characterized by expressionless vacuity. His speech comes to be slow and monotonous, with but little variation as to accent or tone, and his vocabulary becomes limited.

The degree to which dementia progresses, if it occurs, varies greatly. In extreme cases this dementia is great, the patient existing at a purely vegetative level, having no interest in, and no intelligible communications with, his social environment. Dementia is a much more frequent outcome in those who develop epilepsy in early childhood than in those in whom it appears in later years. Deterioration occurs less frequently if the patient was mentally normal at birth and if his seizures are of the petit mal or of infrequent grand mal types. It is more frequent in institutionalized patients than in the noninstitutionalized ones. Of the latter, about one-third show some degree of mental impairment, although in only about 10 per cent is it so gross as to be immediately evident.

It is possible that deterioration may, in fact, be the result of the repeated anoxia and increased intracranial pressure that accompany repeated convulsions. In part it may be the result of the prolonged toxic effect of drugs; in considerable part it may be a response to the problems and situations which the very nature of the disease creates. The social and intellectual ostracism from which the epileptic often suffers, the deprivation of normal educational advantages, his feelings of inferiority, and his discouragement and hopelessness lead to a contraction of interests and to an impoverishment of personality.

The following case is fairly illustrative of the type of epileptic that enters institutions for mental disorders:

T. C. was admitted to a state hospital at the age of 31. He was described by his family as having a rather bad temper, being somewhat stubborn and inclined to boast. At 17 he began to suffer from mild seizures with loss of consciousness but without generalized convulsive movements. Not until age 27 did seizures occur more than two or three times a year. At that time they began to occur once or twice a month. At 29 the seizures became more severe, with marked convulsive movements and longer periods of unconsciousness. Because of a seizure at his place of employment, he lost his position in an ice factory. Unable to find other employment, the patient became somewhat depressed, worried, irritable, and "hard to get along with." His seizures became more frequent and severe.

One day following a period of moody preoccupation, during which he seemed unaware of his wife's presence, he said to her, "Catherine, I've done good today. I've made my fortune." He then added, "Call the doctor and the priest, I'm afraid I am going to die." That night he walked about all night, talking constantly about becoming rich, quoted passages from the salesmanship instructions issued by a concern for which he had recently attempted to canvass, and paid little heed to his environment.

The following night he became so uncontrollable that, at his family's request, he was taken to the police station, and on the following day, he was committed to the state hospital. When he was brought to the institution, he shouted in a loud tone, "I drank a lot. I don't need that fellow. I thought an awful lot of that fellow. I think an awful lot of my mother. I told them plenty. I said, 'No! No!'" At intervals he struggled violently to escape from the two officers who were holding him. When asked any questions he would shout, "None of your business."

On examination at the hospital, he was noted to be a tall, ungainly individual, his large ears standing out prominently nearly at right angles to his skull. The conformation of his facies suggested that he was a biological variant. He remained clouded for about six weeks, at times apparently hallucinated, sometimes preoccupied, mute, and having to be tube-fed, again talking in a loud, angry tone. He was usually to be found in his room, frequently with his prayer beads hanging from his mouth, often nude, and when approached would spontaneously make such remarks as: "I'm—I'm trying to solve the problem. I'm trying to find the solution. Irish! Irish! Captain I, an eye for an eye, and a tooth for a tooth. I've tried to save my soul."

After this prolonged clouded state, the patient remained clear for two months, occasionally suffering from a convulsion. Four months after admission he again became cloudy. At times he was stuporous, at times excited, and on several occasions attempted suicide. Nine months after admission he was paroled to his family, and for seven months he remained well except for occasional light convulsions. At the end of that period, while attending church, he suddenly arose during the services and began to pray loudly. He held a crucifix high above his head, and when led from the building, seemed much confused. The patient was then returned to the hospital, where the clinical course was much like that of the first residence.

DIAGNOSIS

If the attack is witnessed by the physician or by a trained observer, the diagnosis of the typical grand mal, with its unconsciousness and sequence of tonic cramp, cyanosis, clonic convulsive movements separated by intervals of gradually increasing length, stertorous breathing, perhaps automatic activity, stupor, and hebetude, is comparatively easy. In the case of petit mal or of an atypical and incompletely developed seizure, the diagnosis may be difficult. One should inquire for a history of migraine and of fainting attacks, and ascertain if any disturbances of consciousness have been accompanied by biting of the tongue, relaxation of the sphincters, or injury to self. If observed by the physician, the discovery of fixed, dilated pupils, of loss of the corneal reflex, and the presence of a Babinski reflex may confirm suspicion as to the epileptic nature of the paroxysm. The diagnosis of epilepsy is, however, not always easy. Attacks of loss of consciousness, of muscle-twitching, of feelings of faintness, or of unreality will usually suggest epilepsy, but often a diagnosis must be based on retrospective facts found by careful questioning of the patient and observers.

The electroencephalogram is of assistance in establishing a diagnosis, but the evidence supplied by it must be supplemented by clinical observation. It must be remembered that about 5 per cent of the persons who never suffer from seizures of any kind show minor dysrhythmia in the EEG, and occasionally the EEG in such normal persons may be characteristic of the records made in epileptics between attacks. This is particularly true in the relatives of epileptics. In rare instances an epileptic with definite clinical seizures may in intervals between convulsions show an entirely normal EEG. It is estimated that the chances are nine in ten that any disturbances of consciousness occurring in a person with a positive EEG are epileptic. Activation of the abnormal electrical potentials may be induced occasionally by hyperventilation, or by small doses of metrazol intravenously. It is of interest that mescaline and diethyl lysergic acid diethylamide (d-LSD-25) are incapable of activating the attacks or the typical electroencephalographic abnormality in those who have temporal-lobe seizures.

Hysterical patients with attacks resembling epilepsy usually have normal electroencephalograms. The seizures of the hysteric occur in the presence of others, and there is often some fairly obvious gain or domination to be secured by the paroxysm. The hysterical person rarely injures himself in a seizure. It is important to remember the makeup of this type of individual with his tendency to histrionic poses and simulation of symptoms. Although there may be a history of an emotional disturbance just prior to an epileptic convulsion, any dramatic staging of a seizure points strongly toward hysteria. The hysterical seizure is usually grotesque in its manifestations, lacks the characteristic "march" of phases seen in epilepsy, and is not accompanied by ocular signs indicated in the previous paragraph, by sphincter incontinence, Babinski sign, or so deep a loss of consciousness. In hysteria there is never any biting of the tongue as in epilepsy.

There may be difficulty in the differential diagnosis of temporal-lobe epilepsy and hysterical amnesic periods with automatism. The presence of psychogenic factors and the absence of the psychomotor type of electroencephalogram will point to the latter. It is often said that no epileptic attack is "motivated" and that no motivated act is epileptic.

Also to be differentiated from the temporal lobe or psychomotor seizure are acute anxiety attacks manifested in the *hyperventilation syndrome,* particularly common in those with anxiety phobic neurosis. The hyperventilation syndrome and its diagnosis are described fully in Chapter 25 on the psychoneuroses.

Syncopal attacks associated with progressive slowing of the electroencephalogram may be induced in a high proportion of healthy adults by the Weber or Valsalva maneuver. In this maneuver the subject inhales deeply and then strains against a closed glottis as forcefully and long as he is able. This syncopal attack appears similar to others induced in situations of acute hypoxia which have been observed experimentally in low-pressure chambers; such attacks might occur in airplane travel with sudden decompression. They differ from grand mal in that the subject suddenly loses consciousness and muscular tonus, sliding to the floor. Then there occur several bilaterally synchronous coarse clonic movements, generally in the upper limbs. With more severe attacks there may be extensor thrusts of the legs, but there is no *tonic phase.*

The diagnosis of syncope versus epilepsy is often complex. The loss of consciousness in epilepsy is primarily caused by paroxysmal discharges within the brain, while in syncope it results primarily from a fall in blood pressure. In syncope a cause —postural, emotional, or physical—seems apparent. In syncope there is a fairly long warning. The patient often comments "I feel faint," and adopts some protective action, such as sitting. Pallor and hot or cold sweating are apparent. Consciousness usually returns without any confusion or sequel except sweating. The epileptic's loss of consciousness is usually followed by drowsiness and frequently associated with headache. In a Stokes-Adams attack, syncope and a convulsion may be closely linked. Here a rapid fall of blood pressure caused by cardiac arrest produces convulsions through cerebral anemia.

COURSE AND PROGNOSIS

Today the average epileptic enjoys an incomparably brighter prognosis than he did 25 years ago. Credit belongs mainly to the widespread availability of the electroencephalograph for diagnosis, to an ever-expanding group of nonsedative drugs that in many cases suppress epileptic phenomena, and to an increasing education of the public concerning the disorder with a resulting lessening of the rejection and social stigma from which the epileptic suffers.

With temporal lobe epilepsy, the outlook for improved clinical, social, and psychological adaptation in those resistant to drug treatment and a localized spike-discharging focus in the EEG is best following temporal lobectomy. In such cases, as Taylor and Falconer report, the best outcomes were associated with pathological evidence of mesial temporal sclerosis in which there had occurred early onset of epilepsy associated with febrile convulsions. Overall, improvement relates most closely to relief from seizures.

Most epileptics are intelligent and normal persons apart from their attacks and are quite able to earn a living. In a large percentage of the patients seen by the private physician, deterioration does not occur at all; if it does, it is but slight. The prognosis is least favorable if the onset is in childhood. The prognosis as to recovery is worse in petit mal than in grand mal, but, contrary to general opinion, the mental life does not suffer so much in petit mal.

To a considerable extent, the prognosis is dependent upon the promptness of diagnosis and treatment. Both rate and extent of deterioration vary greatly but tend to be influenced by the age of onset, the frequency of seizures, and the effort made to maintain wholesome, constructive, satisfying, unselfish interests and constant employment. The emotional handicap produced through faulty attitudes such as shame or overprotectiveness on the part of the patient's family may operate against recovery. In its more malignant forms, the deterioration may proceed until the patient lives at an essentially vegetative level. A few epileptics become psychotic and require care in a hospital for mental diseases. However, with the anticonvulsant drugs now available, complete control or total abolition of grand mal seizures can be secured in 80 per cent of the patients.

TREATMENT

General Management

One of the fundamentals of treatment is the maintenance of optimum physical health. Physical and mental activities should be encouraged, especially those that afford a combination of muscular exercise, intellectual interest, and pleasure. It should be remembered that conscious or unconscious parental rejection may seriously warp the developing personality of the child. He should not be the object of oversolicitous fear and overprotection. Petit mal attacks, even if frequent, should not prevent attendance at school, nor should infrequent major attacks. The epileptic patient should be employed, but at a job where his own safety or that of others would not be jeopardized should he suffer a seizure. If possible, safety should not be purchased at the cost of active participation in life.

Although it is usually necessary to raise the seizure threshold through medication, psychiatric treatment should not be omitted, particularly when there is evidence that emotional arousal precipitates repeated seizures. Recently, behavioral therapy in the form of an "extinction technique" has been successful in the treatment of a case of "musicogenic" epilepsy. Emphasis should be placed upon the relief of emotional or other psychic stress and upon the promotion of a normal life within the limits of the patient's psychobiological equipment. He should be given an opportunity to preserve his self-respect, develop his abilities, and maintain social usefulness. Many epileptics tend to daydream and to indulge in idle dissipations that increase the frequency of their seizures and hasten deterioration. The epileptic should be encouraged to plan his own work, studies, and activities. Sustained work is often a difficult habit for him to establish but one of great importance.

There has often been an unnecessary restriction of the epileptic's diet. Ordinarily he should eat the same food as other members of the family, but attacks may be precipitated by hypoglycemia. The patient should therefore not go too long without food. The ingestion of an abnormal amount of fluid at one time may precipitate an attack. Food should be moderate in amount, and alcohol should be avoided.

It is agreed that an epileptic whose disorder is not well controlled should not be permitted to operate a motor vehicle. In many states a known epileptic is forbidden by law to operate one. In recent years there has been a tendency to be more permissive in the case of persons with well-controlled epilepsy. In 1949 the Wisconsin legislature, with the support of the state medical society, enacted legislation to allow the person with controlled epilepsy to drive a motor vehicle subject to the following provisions: When the epileptic can present medical certification that he has been completely free of attacks for two years, he can obtain a driver's license. This license is automatically renewable every six months upon application and medical certification that the patient's condition has remained under complete control during the previous six months.

It is reported that, during the period 1949 to 1957, 553 licenses to operate a motor vehicle were granted, 96 licenses were denied after review by the medical review board, and but one accident occurred during the period because of the occurrence of an epileptic seizure in a driver.

Drug Therapy

The aim in treatment is to give medicine which will counteract the explosive tendency of the brain cells. For over 60 years bromides, first suggested in 1857 by Sir Charles Locock, constituted the principal form of medication. They have now been largely displaced by newer drugs.

Phenobarbital, or phenylethylbarbituric acid, first recommended by Hauptmann in 1912, is one of the drugs most widely used for raising the convulsive threshold of the epileptic. In persons 12 or more years of age, one may begin with a dose of 0.1 gm. once a day. In adults this may, if necessary, be increased to 0.3 to 0.4 gm., administered in divided doses. In children under five, 0.05 gm. may be used. If the seizures are nocturnal, it may be given at bedtime. If they are diurnal, it may be taken in the morning. Should seizures be frequent and severe, the patient may receive the drug three times a day. Even ordinary doses may produce drowsiness at the beginning of its use, but this effect usually disappears in a few weeks. Toxic doses may produce apathy, slow mental reactions, ataxia, slow speech, and muscular weakness. A sudden discontinuation of its use usually leads to an increase in the number of seizures and even to status epilepticus. Phenobarbital, nevertheless, is usually the most effective drug in alleviating grand mal seizures and least frequently produces toxic symptoms. It is of little value in petit mal, which should usually be treated by Tridione. Methylethylphenylbarbituric acid (Mephobarbital or Mebaral) acts similarly to phenobarbital but is more effective with certain individuals. For adults the dosage is 0.3 to 0.6 gm. daily.

In 1937 Merritt and Putnam introduced sodium diphenylhydantoin sodium, generally known as Dilantin, an anticonvulsant that has proved of great value. Not being a hypnotic, it does not cause drowsiness, as is so often the case with phenobarbital. The usual dose is a 0.1-gm. capsule three times a day. The maximum amount that adults tolerate is approximately 0.6 gm. daily. If necessary for the control of seizures, this may be increased somewhat. In psychomotor seizures, it is the most efficacious of the antiepileptic drugs and in grand mal may be effective in some cases in which phenobarbital has failed. There is apparently a synergy between phenobarbital and Dilantin sodium that makes the combination more effective than when either drug is used alone. In toxic amounts, Dilantin causes gastric distress, a symptom that usually ceases after one or two weeks of treatment. Less frequently it causes dizziness, ataxia, tremors, nystagmus, diplopia, drowsiness, and hyperplasia of the gums. Its sudden, complete discontinuance may induce status epilepticus.

Initially all patients with this form of convulsive disorder should undergo trials on phenobarbital and Dilantin and the combinations of the two. In instances where seizures remain uncontrolled or where several forms of seizures occur, other drugs and their combinations may be tried.

Another anticonvulsant which is now rather extensively used is Mesantoin. The usual doses are 0.1 gm. three times a day for children and 0.2 gm. for adults. Since it may be toxic, blood counts should be made once a month. Combined with Dilantin or phenobarbital, it may be effective in cases resistant to other drugs. Its combination with Tridione is to be avoided.

Trimethadione, introduced in 1945 under the trade name Tridione, has been found to produce gratifying results in the treatment of *petit mal* but may aggravate other types. The starting dose of trimethadione is 0.3 gm. three times a day for adolescents and adults. Gradual increases in dosage are carried out until a therapeutic effect is obtained, the optimal dosage being usually between 1.5 and 2.7

gm. daily. In children under two years of age, 0.15 gm. two or three times is the initial dosage, with increments of 0.15 gm. Toxic symptoms in the form of skin eruptions, "glare phenomenon," a photophobia in which objects appear to shimmer and vision is blurred, drowsiness, dizziness, and headache may occur. Toxic action on the blood-forming elements of the bone marrow followed by death has been reported. For some persons, paramethadione dimethylethyloxazolidine dione (Paradione) is more effective than Tridione. N-Methyl-α-phenylsuccinimide (Milontin) may also be used for petit mal, though it is less effective than the diones. For adults, the dose is 0.9 to 3.0 gm. daily, and for children, 0.6 to 1.8 gm. daily.

Another drug which has been increasingly employed in therapeutically resistant convulsive disorders since 1949 is Phenurone (phenacetylcarbamide). This may be used in both *grand mal* and *psychomotor seizures,* but seems to be more effective in the latter type. It may be given in 500 mg. doses three times a day. After the first week of treatment, an additional 500 mg. may be taken on rising. One-half the adult dose is recommended for children from 5 to 10 years of age. It seems to be especially useful in combating drowsiness and lethargy in patients who are affected in this manner by phenobarbital and other drugs. Patients receiving Phenurone should be watched carefully for the possible development of serious damage to the hematopoietic system and to the liver.

Primidone (Mysoline) is safer than Phenurone and is reported to be of much value in the treatment both of psychomotor epilepsy and grand mal. Dosage range is from two to eight 250-mg. tablets a day.

Acetazolamide (Diamox) has been reported useful for all convulsive forms. The initial dosage is 0.25 gm. three times daily by mouth. This dosage then is gradually increased by a similar increment up to 1.0 gm. daily. Since hematuria and agranulocytosis have been observed during its administration, urinalyses and blood counts should be made recurrently.

It should be kept in mind that the phenothiazines and the aminodibenzal antidepressants (imipramine and its analogs) may activate epileptic foci and probably are contraindicated in the treatment of those with convulsive disorders even when there are severe behavioral accompaniments.

Patients with all types of seizures show some improvement under anticonvulsant therapy, and those with focal and grand seizures respond best. Phenobarbital and Dilantin usually give the best results in seizures of those types.

Because of the danger of status epilepticus, anticonvulsive drugs should not be withheld abruptly. The occurrence of *status epilepticus* constitutes a medical emergency and is best handled in a hospital. Prolonged status epilepticus may lead to irreversible cerebral changes and even death.

The patient must be placed under heavy sedation and kept in that condition for 24 hours. Diazepam (Valium) has been recommended recently as a highly effective drug for this condition. It may be administered in one or more intravenous or intramuscular injections of 10 mg. in 100 ml. In some instances 100 mg. has been given in a slow intravenous drip daily.

Others prefer to use a solution of amobarbital sodium, 1.0 gm. in 20 ml. for injection, given slowly intravenously at the rate of 1 or 2 ml. per minute until the seizure stops and deep sleep results. Sleep is maintained with a continuous intravenous drip of 0.5 gm. amobarbital sodium (Amytal) in 500 ml. of isotonic saline solution. The patient should be turned every half hour to prevent hypostatic and aspiration pneumonia. Mild Trendelenburg position is maintained, and mechanical aspiration of secretions is often necessary. Oxygen is given through a nasal catheter when indicated. Additional sedation may be obtained without depressing respiration with the use of paraldehyde suppositories, each containing 4.5 ml. of paraldehyde, repeated every four hours. A parenteral preparation of

Dilantin is now commercially available and may be injected either intramuscularly or intravenously. This has been found valuable in status epilepticus in a dosage not to exceed 500 mg.

Surgical Therapy

In those patients with severe temporal lobe epilepsy, difficult to control by pharmacological agents, consideration should be given to surgical excision of the convulsive focus. These operations have little likelihood of success when electroencephalographic studies show approximately equivalent seizure discharges in both temporal lobes. The best outcome from temporal lobe excisions occurs when epileptiform activity is delimited by the EEG to one temporal lobe or appears in the opposite side only as synchronous, lower-voltage transmitted waves. Following operation patients customarily are continued on medication for at least one year. If control is maintained, an attempt is made then to reduce dosage gradually. Postoperative mortality in patients with uncomplicated epilepsy has been less than 1 per cent. Large excisions accompanied by vascular complications occasionally are followed by quadrant defects in the visual fields, or occasionally by hemiplegia or aphasia. Approximately two-thirds of patients treated in a large series had satisfactory results, the majority being free of seizures and the remainder suffering only isolated attacks.

BIBLIOGRAPHY

Bandler, B., et al.: Role of sexuality in epilepsy. Psychosom. Med., 20:227–234, 1958.

Barrow, R. L., and Fabing, H. D.: Epilepsy and the Law. New York, Paul B. Hoeber, Inc., 1956.

Blumer, D.: Hypersexual episodes in temporal lobe epilepsy. Amer. J. Psychiat., 126:1099–1106, 1970.

Duvoisin, R. C.: Convulsive syncope induced by the Weber maneuver. Arch. Neurol., 7:219–226, 1962.

Ferguson, S. M., Rayport, M., Gardner, R., Kass, W., Weiner, H., and Reiser, M. F.: Similarities in mental content of psychotic states, spontaneous seizures, dreams, and responses to electrical stimulation in patients with temporal lobe epilepsy. Psychosom. Med., 31:479–498, 1970.

Flor-Henry, P.: Schizophrenic-like reactions and affective psychoses associated with temporal lobe epilepsy: Etiological factors. Amer. J. Psychiat., 126:400–404, 1969.

Forster, F., et al.: Modification of musicogenic epilepsy by the extinction technique. Trans. Amer. Neurol. Assoc., 90:179, 1965.

Gastaut, H., Nagud, R., Poiré, R., and Tassinari, C. A.: Treatment of status epilepticus with diazepam (Valium). Epilepsia, 6:167–182, 1965.

Goldstein, N. P., and Giffin, M. E.: Psychogenic hypersomnia. Amer. J. Psychiat., 115:922–928, 1957.

Hill, D., et al.: Personality changes following temporal lobectomy for epilepsy. J. Ment. Sc., 103:18–26, 1957.

Koch, G.: Die Erblichkeit der Epilepsien. Psychiat. Neurol. Neurchis., 66:153–183, 1963.

Millechap, I. G., Jones, J. D., and Etheridge, J. E., Jr.: The abnormal aminoaciduria in petit mal epilepsy. Neurology, 16:569–572, 1966.

Needham, W. E., Bray, P. F., Wiser, W. C., and Beck, E. C.: Intelligence and EEG studies in families with epilepsy. J.A.M.A., 207:1497–1501, 1969.

Ounsted, C.: Aggression and epilepsy. Rage in children with temporal lobe epilepsy. J. Psychosom. Res., 13:237–242, 1969.

Passonant, P., and Cadilhac, J.: EEG and clinical study of epilepsy during maturation in man. Epilepsia, 3:14–43, 1962.

Rechtschaffen, A., and Dement, W.: Studies on the relation of narcolepsy, cataplexy and sleep with low voltage fast EEG activity. In Kety, S. (ed.): Disturbances of Consciousness. Proceedings of the Association for Research in Nervous and Mental Diseases. Baltimore, Williams & Wilkins Company, 1965.

Robertson, E. G.: Photogenic epilepsy: self-precipitated attacks. Brain, 77:232–251, 1954.

Schwarz, B. E., Bickford, R. G., Mulder, D. W., and Rome, H. P.: Mescaline and LSD-25 in activation of temporal lobe epilepsy. Neurology, 6:275–280, 1956.

Stevens, J. R.: Psychiatric implications of psychomotor epilepsy. Arch. Gen. Psychiat., 14:461–471, 1966.

Taylor, D. C., and Falconer, M. A.: Clinical, socioeconomic and psychological changes after temporal lobectomy for epilepsy. Brit. J. Psychiat., 114:1247–1261, 1968.

Yoss, R. E., Moyer, N. J., and Ogle, K. H.: The pupillogram and narcolepsy. Neurology, 19:921–928, 1969.

Chapter 15

Brain Syndrome Associated with Intracranial Neoplasm

Brain tumors with accompanying mental disorder are more frequent than indicated by the diagnostic statistics provided from hospitals. Summaries of the total incidence of intracranial tumors found at autopsy in patients in mental hospitals in the United States give a figure of 3.7 per cent against that of 2.35 per cent for patients without diagnosed psychiatric disorder in general hospitals. Meningiomas are found much more frequently in autopsies performed on patients in mental hospitals than in the general hospitals. The number of brain tumors discovered at necropsy is much larger than the number diagnosed correctly ante mortem. Probably in only a minority of early cases of brain tumor are the mental symptoms so pronounced as to form a conspicuous part of the clinical picture of the neoplasm, although there are few cases that remain entirely free of manifestations of mental disorder. There is need to recognize that the initial symptoms of tumor may be masked by preëxisting or concomitant mental and emotional disturbances. There is a great statistical disparity as to both the frequency and the nature of mental symptoms in brain tumor. Clouding of consciousness and disturbance of memory occur most frequently. There is, however, no symptomatic picture which may be considered characteristic of a brain tumor.

Symptoms

The genesis, pathological structure, neurological signs, and electroencephalographic records of brain tumor will not be discussed. Generally speaking, the symptoms and signs of brain tumor fall into three groups: (1) signs of increased intracranial pressure; progressive impairment of consciousness and energy with headache, vomiting, and papilledema; (2) focal neurological symptoms and signs determined by the location of the tumor; (3) psychiatric symptoms, which tend to fall into two types.

Of the latter, symptoms of the first type, which often appear early, perhaps before those caused by increased intracranial pressure or focal neurological symptoms determined by the site of the tumor, are psychogenically determined by the characteristics of the patient's premorbid personality structure and his particular stresses, conflicts, and defenses. In some cases the first and, perhaps for a time, the only symptoms may be psychiatric and consist of accentuations of personality tendencies. Some patients show a loss of inhibitions with blunting of social or moral sense, egotistic tendencies, shamelessness, and even gross sexual or other misbehavior.

Psychiatric symptoms of the second group stem from cerebral damage incident to the tumor and to increased intracranial pressure.

Among early symptoms may be absentmindedness, later becoming an obvious memory defect, especially for recent events, easy fatigability, a raising of the threshold of consciousness, disturbances of sensorium, difficulty of grasp, impairment of calculation and of reasoning abilities, defective attention, hebetude, drowsiness, confusion, and disorientation. Psychomotor retardation is not uncommon. Fluctuations of consciousness may occur. Sometimes the patient may confabulate as in Korsakoff's psychosis. Loss of libido is common.

Temporal lobe tumors are frequently mistaken for schizophrenic disorders. Often they present paroxysmal motor, affective, and perceptual disturbances. These may be crude and disagreeable olfactory or gustatory hallucinatory experiences. The disturbances are characteristically repetitive, and although the patient is absorbed in, and may suffer anxiety with, the experience, he is usually capable of perceiving the existence of both the present environment and the hallucination. Either then or later he is able to distinguish the experience as ego alien— outside his usual personification of self-functioning. "Déjà vu" phenomena occur with such tumors, but more frequently patients describe emotional reactions and transitory experiences of strangeness, loneliness, or dreamy states. Also noticed are episodic and short-lived affective states consisting of feelings of dread, terror, or overwhelming fear. Some patients have reported either unexpected angry affect or feelings of well-being.

Motor automatisms may take place in which the patient may carry out sudden aggressive or assaultive actions or other complex performances for which he has no memory.

Frontal lobe tumors are particularly likely to produce symptoms affecting the functioning of personality over time. Slow-growing meningiomas compressing the frontal lobe are among the most frequently undiagnosed tumors of the brain that produce symptoms of a psychiatric nature. Tumors in this area produce insidious and subtle changes in personality functioning.

A flattening of affect coupled with a growing apathy concerning personal and business affairs is frequent. Other emotional disturbances are instability, irritability, depression, and anxiety. Euphoria and facetiousness ("witzelsucht" of Oppenheim) are probably a little more frequent in tumors of the frontal lobe but are not specific for any one location in the brain. It well may be that this lightness of spirit and tendency to be witty is merely a defense reaction against the threat to the integrity of the organism by the destructive growth.

Occipital lobe tumors are associated more frequently with unformed simple visual hallucinating experiences which consist of flashes of light or of colored lights. Moving objects may be hallucinated. Complex visual and auditory hallucinations are more frequent in tumors of the temporal lobe. Olfactory hallucinations in the form of disagreeable odors may occur in the case of tumors on the undersurface of the hemispheres.

It is generally agreed that tumors of the *corpus callosum* are accompanied by intellectual impairment, difficulty in concentration and in thinking, and failure to respond to stimuli, particularly to auditory stimuli.

The conspicuousness of the symptoms and, to some extent, their nature are determined by the rate of growth of the tumor. In the case of slowly growing meningiomas, there may be simply a slowly developing mental deterioration. In rapidly developing gliomas (spongioblastomas), there may be an active delirium suggesting a toxic state, with confusion, disorientation, and perhaps stupor. In those that develop unusually rapidly, both the mental and neurological signs may suggest an inflammatory lesion.

Diagnosis

If increased intracranial pressure appears suddenly and develops rapidly, mental symptoms are usually produced and may be severe. If pressure increases slowly, there may be no mental symptoms. Many tumors, because of their site and the particular structures they injure, produce neurological signs of great localizing value. Mental symptoms by themselves have, however, little or no value in localizing a tumor of the brain. It is stated that mental symptoms are nearly twice as frequent in the case of supratentorial tumors as in infratentorial growths. If the brain tumor causes convulsions, difficulty may arise in evaluating the mental symptoms, with the result that they may be attributed to idiopathic epilepsy. Convulsions occur in about 8 per cent of the cases and may be either of grand mal or petit mal type. Seizures are rare in cerebellar tumors and most frequent in those of the parietal and temporal lobes.

Difficulty in diagnosis may also arise if the patient suffered from cerebral arteriosclerosis prior to the appearance of the mental symptoms. If the patient suffers from sensory or motor aphasia or from apraxia by reason of the location of the tumors, the resulting inability of the patient to communicate his ideas adequately may make it difficult to determine the presence or extent of mental symptoms. In the terminal phase the patient may be stuporous and lose control of both rectal and vesical sphincters.

The electroencephalogram is an invaluable aid in detecting those tumors present in "silent areas" or not productive of increased intracranial pressure early in their course. The use of the electroencephalogram has been recommended as a routine procedure for patients admitted to mental hospitals. However, its serial application is necessary in many instances to insure detection of tumors. Metrazol for activation of the electroencephalogram is valuable, particularly for the diagnosis of temporal lobe tumors.

More recently cerebral arteriography and the use of radioactive scanning devices have expanded the diagnostic potential of the neurosurgeon, particularly in determining the localization and extent of the tumor mass. The latter technique, particularly, promises to extend current knowledge of neoplastic growth and its diagnosis.

BIBLIOGRAPHY

Bailey, P.: Intracranial Tumors, 2nd ed. Springfield, Ill., Charles C Thomas, 1948.

Mulder, D. W., Bickford, R. G., and Dodge, H. W., Jr.: Hallucinatory epilepsy: complex hallucinations as focal seizures. Amer. J. Psychiat., *113:* 1100–1102, 1957.

Patton, R. B., and Sheppard, J. A.: Intracranial tumors found at autopsy in mental patients. Amer. J. Psychiat., *113:*319–324, 1956.

Soniat, T. L. L.: Psychiatric symptoms associated with intracranial neoplasms. Amer. J. Psychiat., *108:*19–22, 1951.

Waggoner, R. W., and Bagchi, B. K.: Initial masking of organic brain changes by psychic symptoms. Amer. J. Psychiat., *110:*904–910, 1954.

Chapter 16

Mental Disorders Caused by or
Associated with Head Trauma

With the mounting occurrence of accidents incident to industry and traffic and with the enactment of industrial compensation laws, there has been a marked increase in traumatic mental disorders and their medicolegal importance. For these reasons, the relationship of head trauma to the development of mental disorders often presents an important and difficult problem. Frequently the difficulty of this problem is accentuated by the fact that the clinical picture may be complicated through the personality response activated by loss or impairment of mental functioning following brain injury, with appearance of psychogenic symptoms or by exaggeration or overdetermination of symptoms expressive of impaired brain function.

In order to arrive at an accurate diagnosis, it is necessary to make detailed mental and neurological examinations and to obtain a precise history of the patient's mental status prior to his injury. The opinion popularly entertained that injuries to the head are a frequent cause of mental disorders is an error. Undoubtedly severe trauma to any part of the body may occasionally serve as a contributing or precipitating agent in schizophrenia and manic-depressive psychosis in persons predisposed to these respective reactions. At times, too, trauma of the head, without recognizable injury to the brain, may activate an asymptomatic paretic process and lead to clinically active syphilitic meningoencephalitis. Such psychoses, however, are not included among the traumatic mental disorders.

The mental disturbances associated with head trauma are divided into those caused by acute brain disorder and those caused by chronic brain disorder. This classification will be explained as these disorders are considered.

ACUTE DISORDERS CAUSED BY, OR ASSOCIATED WITH, HEAD TRAUMA

The acute (at times subacute) disorders following trauma of the head tend to fall into the following syndromes:
  (a) Concussion
  (b) Traumatic coma
  (c) Traumatic delirium
  (d) Korsakoff, or amnesic-confabulatory, syndrome

Concussion Syndrome

In concussion, there is a momentary physiological interruption of cerebral processes because of head injury, but there are no histological changes or clinical signs. Recovery is rapid and complete. There is not only amnesia for the moment of injury but also for a period, usually seconds or moments, before the injury. Concussion follows the impact of a severe, functionally paralyzing force upon the head, especially of a force that causes abrupt acceleration or deceleration. In recent years it has been suggested that concussion may be the result of the cavitation phenomenon in the cellular fluids. Experi-

264

ments show that an impulse applied to the skull by a severe mechanical blow or by an underwater explosion produces first a momentary positive pressure wave followed by a negative one. Although this negative wave is sustained for only an infinitesimal period of time, it apparently causes minute bubbles to form momentarily in the cellular fluids. This phenomenon of cavitation, with its molecular-disrupting action, produces a momentary generalized cortical electric discharge that renders the patient unconscious. This discharge is followed by a depression of function.

Brains of animals subjected to concussion and examined by fine techniques several days after the trauma have disclosed histological changes in nerve cells. These suggest that some of the remote symptoms following concussion may develop on the basis of nerve cell changes taking place some time after the concussion. The period of unconsciousness may be momentary or may continue for hours. Many patients vomit as they regain consciousness. There is apparently no relationship between the severity of the concussion as measured by the duration of unconsciousness and the severity of the psychiatric sequelae. In regaining consciousness, the patient may wake up suddenly or may pass through a state of clouded consciousness and confusion. He will subsequently have a loss of memory (post-traumatic amnesia) for this period, even though he seems alert and able to carry on a conversation. Usually recovery is complete in a short time, but occasionally a chronic personality disorder may follow.

Contusing and lacerating injuries do not in themselves produce concussion, although they may be associated with it. On the other hand, a severe injury may be sustained without concussion. The diagnosis of uncomplicated concussion can be made only in retrospect. Only after the regaining of consciousness can one be sure that no organic sequelae will follow. Although cerebral concussion is an acute syndrome, there is frequently an after-math of variable, even prolonged, duration. These postconcussion symptoms will be discussed on page 270.

Traumatic Coma

Severe concussion without injury, or, more frequently, concussion accompanied by contusion (a mechanical disruption of tissue usually accompanied by minute capillary hemorrhages) or by laceration (a gross tearing of tissue) may produce prolonged coma. Coma is, of course, characterized by absence of response on stimulation. It may last for hours or for several days, the duration depending upon the degree and extent of the injury. In the absence of localizing signs of laceration or of pressure (as by subdural hemorrhage), coma for more than 24 hours usually means a major contusion. Following coma there is a period of stupor, restlessness, and clouding of consciousness, from which the patient may emerge into clear consciousness or at times pass into traumatic delirium. Coma is often interrupted by intervals of semistupor. Prolonged coma is frequently followed by a period of delirium succeeded by a longer period of amnesia or by the amnesic-confabulatory syndrome known as the Korsakoff syndrome.

Traumatic Delirium

If delirium follows the suffering of head trauma, it usually begins during the gradual emergence of the patient from traumatic stupor or coma. The underlying cause may be concussion, contusion, laceration, hemorrhage, or increased intracranial pressure. In a majority of cases, delirium is mild and consists of haziness, irritability, dreamy fabrications, restlessness, and mild disorders of the sensorium. The patient does not grasp the finer points of situations and events of his surroundings. Although most of the time he may realize that he is in a hospital, he does not remember how he came to be there, may not recognize persons about him, and may not understand why he is detained. Other patients may be definitely bewildered. Not a few are apprehensive and fearful. In some cases the delirium is concerned with the patient's occupation. Many patients are resistive, noisy, irritable, uncoöperative, and verbally abusive. Some patients are belligerent, demanding, and aggressive. If hallucinations occur, they are usually visual. In the more severe cases, there may be such confusional excitement and a tendency to wander about that restraint becomes necessary. Violent, impulsive outbursts making the patient dangerous to himself or others may occur. As their noisy delirium subsides, some patients remain talkative and show a perseveration of words. At times, after the stage of irritability, the emotional state may be characterized by a childish elation and happiness. As in delirium resulting from other causes, the course may be characterized by fluctuations between relative clearness and confusion. In some instances, the syndrome may be that of a twilight or dream state instead of delirium. With or without preceding delirium, various degrees of post-traumatic defect may follow major contusions with their diffuse degeneration of ganglion cells.

Delirium continuing for more than a week suggests considerable damage. An estimate of the final residual defect should not be given for at least six months. Delirium or coma of more than a month's duration usually means serious tissue destruction. An estimate of the final deterioration and other results of tissue destruction should not be made until 12 to 18 months after the injury. The final mental defect will usually not be as serious as early symptoms suggest.

Korsakoff, or Amnesic-Confabulatory, Syndrome

A relatively frequent syndrome following head trauma is that first described by Korsakoff as associated with chronic alcoholism. The most striking feature of this syndrome is confabulation, although this is accompanied by disorientation and impairment of perception and recent memory. The fabrication of memory may be a mixture of truth and fiction or purely new fabrications. Suggestive questions may often elicit contradictory statements. The patient may superficially appear alert but on closer examination it will be found that perception is greatly deranged. Many patients with the Korsakoff syndrome show serenity and mild euphoria or even facetiousness but readily become irritable on questioning. The polyneuritis resulting from thiamine deficiency and seen in some instances of Korsakoff syndrome does not occur in the post-traumatic symptom complex. Since polyneuropathy is not present in the syndrome originally described by Korsakoff, the term "amnesic-confabulatory syndrome" is more appropriate. The symptoms are of shorter duration following trauma than in the alcoholic Korsakoff syndrome.

In practice it will be found that the acute and subacute symptoms of traumatic mental disorder do not usually occur in such distinct classificatory types as have been described. In severe cases one often observes mixed and transitional reaction types. Delirioid and Korsakoff symptoms are particularly apt to be associated.

Treatment of Acute Traumatic Mental Disorders

Except for the surgical procedures required in the case of definite injuries to the head, operative interference is to be avoided. The patient should be closely watched for any signs of increased intracranial pressure, and also for the occurrence of any complication.

The initial objective is to quiet the patient. Rest in bed and as limited a use of sedatives as possible are important. Narcotics are contraindicated. In the acute stages, careful note should be made as to the state of awareness and the presence or absence of signs of injury to the cerebral substance. Vital signs should be recorded at intervals of two to four hours. Fluids and a soft or liquid diet may be administered if the patient is conscious and able to swallow. With the presence of coma, either feeding by a nasal tube or the administration of parenteral fluids is indicated. Fluids and salt should be restricted but not to the point of leading to dehydration and acidosis. The fear of cerebral edema should not lead to their over-restriction. Patients with simple concussion require at least 24 hours of observation and may then return to their usual activities. The period of bed rest and convalescence of patients with more severe injuries is determined by the reaction of the patient to the treatment. It is important that the severity of the injury not be overemphasized or the period of hospitalization unduly prolonged. There should be a gradual increase of activity with continuance of convalescence at home through the medium of graduated exercises. Active work should be deferred for two to three months following discharge from the hospital. Patients should be advised that alcohol tolerance is diminished following head injury.

Of utmost importance in the treatment of the acute traumatic mental state is the continued awareness of the possibility of severe complications. Such changes in the vital signs as slowing of the pulse and respiration, fluctuating states of consciousness, or the development of signs of focal disturbances of the brain, including paresis, suggest strongly the possibility of serious pathology. In particular, the possibility of *subdural hemorrhage* must be kept in mind.

Subdural Hematoma

Following injury to the head, subdural hematoma is said to occur in 1 to 10 per cent of individuals. In a series of 3100 consecutive autopsies of psychotic patients, 8 per cent showed evidence of subdural hemorrhage. Subdural hematoma may be associated with any variety of psychotic reaction but occurs particularly in the senile, epileptic, alcoholic, and paretic individual. Such patients are especially prone to head injury.

Subdural hematoma consists of a collection of blood between the dura and arachnoid in the subdural space. The bleeding in this space is of venous origin and follows tearing of small veins reaching the subdural space. The fluid in the space may be admixed with cerebrospinal fluid if the arachnoid tears. Blood extravasated into this area fails to be absorbed and eventually is organized and encapsulated by the dura. Fibroblasts proliferate from the inner surface of the dura and invade the clot when in contact with the dura. Capillaries extend into the clot and gradually absorb the liquefied fluid. If the clot is small, it may become completely organized, but if large, fibroblasts may form an encapsulating membrane by growing both along the inner surface of the clot and on the surface adjacent to the dura.

Subdural hematomas may occur either acutely following the head injury or at later periods. In either case the symptomatology may be brought to the attention of the psychiatric consultant. Headache is invariably present. Perhaps most important is the variable state of consciousness. Following recovery from the initial coma, the patient becomes irritable or confused. His mental status frequently changes from day to day or even from hour to hour. Focal signs of cerebral damage are not present in more than one-half of the cases. The most frequent signs are hemiplegia or central facial weakness. In chronic cases the symptoms are similar, but in addition, slight to severe intellectual impairment is usually noted. The initial trauma may not be remembered.

Cerebrospinal fluid is usually bloody and under increased pressure. Roentgenologic examination of the skull may or may not show evidence of a linear fracture. The electroencephalograph is often helpful in defining an abnormality on one or the other side of the brain. The diagnosis is firmly established only by placing a bur hole on both sides of the skull with discovery of the characteristic hematoma.

Other complications that may follow head injury in the acute phase are extradural hemorrhage, intracerebral hemorrhage, subdural hygroma, and cerebral thrombosis. When a subdural hemorrhage or other traumatic vascular lesion is suspected, neurological and neurosurgical consultations are immediately indicated.

CHRONIC DISORDERS CAUSED BY OR ASSOCIATED WITH HEAD TRAUMA

A definite classification of mental disturbances caused by, or associated with, head trauma into a group of acute disorders and a group of chronic disorders is somewhat arbitrary, but in general there are two groups of syndromes both in respect to their temporal relation to the trauma and in respect to clinical features. The chronic disorders may also be divided into two subgroups. One subgroup consists of those disorders presenting symptoms which are the direct result of the trauma, and the other, those in which the syndrome is only a secondary result of the head trauma. The following classification of the chronic traumatic disorders is therefore suggested:

I. Caused primarily by head trauma:
   Post-traumatic personality disorders
   a. of adults
   b. of children
   Post-traumatic defect conditions
   a. traumatic encephalopathy of pugilists (punch drunk)
   b. traumatic convulsive disorder (traumatic epilepsy)
II. Caused secondarily by head trauma:
   Psychoneurosis with head trauma

CHRONIC MENTAL DISORDERS CAUSED PRIMARILY BY HEAD TRAUMA

Psychopathology which occurs following lesions of the brain is now regarded not only as an expression of changes that the patient's personality undergoes as the result of cerebral lesions but also as an expression of the efforts of the brain-damaged personality to adapt to these defects and to the demands that can no longer be met because of these defects. In his work on persons with brain injuries consequent to war wounds, Goldstein emphasized that various types of symptoms must be evaluated and understood in this context if a rational therapy is to be applied in the treatment of individuals with chronic disorders resulting from head injury.

Symptoms

The effort of such patients to find the new adjustment necessary because of the head injury results in three types of symptoms: The first expresses the conflict that the individual faces. The second reflects the tendency to build up substitutive performances so as to adapt to the demands of the environment in the most effective manner under the circumstances of the defect consequent to the injury. A third group of symptoms is the direct result of the impairment of the brain functioning itself. In the third group, the defect may be ameliorated by training, and it is here in particular that the impairment of the "abstract attitude" described by Goldstein is to be found.

Among the symptoms exposing the patient's defect is that now commonly known as the *catastrophic reaction*. Confronted with a problem he cannot solve, the brain-injured individual becomes suddenly anxious and agitated and may appear dazed. A change in his color may appear, he fumbles at the task, and he may present other evidences of autonomic disturbances, such as irregular pulse and changes in respiratory rate. If he was initially in good spirits, he now becomes evasive, sullen, irritable, and even aggressive. The catastrophic reaction develops simultaneously with the attempt to perform the task in which he fails, and not following the performance. Thus it does not represent the patient's response to the awareness that he has failed. As a consequence of such catastrophic reactions, a definite behavior pattern evolves in many of those with brain injury. Some, when confronted with tasks they cannot solve, lose consciousness. Others avoid exposing themselves to such situations by isolating themselves from individuals, or by avoiding tasks through apparent inability to understand directions. Some brain-injured individuals attempt to prevent upsurges of anxiety by continuous activity, which exposes the patient's inability to adopt a reflective attitude, to take himself for granted, or to place himself in the position of a detached spectator. The over-activity may be of the type commonly spoken of as "occupational delirium" and seen in patients with dementia. Certain patients appear to be unable to follow directions and carry out tasks. Essentially they avoid the task in the anxious expectation of precipitating the unpleasant catastrophic response. Others adapt themselves through an excessive orderliness. This may express itself in a meticulousness not only in relation to one's own property but also to that of others in the home.

The brain-injured person tends to suppress knowledge of his disability. Such denial, according to Goldstein, is more easily achieved in the patient with complete destruction of some function than in the individual with incomplete disturbance.

In addition to the efforts of the brain-injured person to avoid the catastrophic reaction by restricting his environment, his brain defect expresses itself through evidence of increase in the threshold of excitability, with the result that greater stimuli are required to bring forth responses. At the same time, the patient may appear unusually susceptible to exposure to various external stimuli because of his easy distractibility. Owing to his difficulty in discriminating between the object to which he is exposed and the background or setting in which the object is presented, the brain-injured patient suffers doubt and anxiety in his perceptions of common objects presented under ordinary circumstances. Thus his capacity for solving problems is impaired as a consequence of this perceptual weakness.

Goldstein has described what he terms the *abstract attitude*. He defines this as the capacity to assume a mental set voluntarily; to shift from one aspect of a situation to another; to retain simultaneously several aspects of a situation; to break up and isolate the whole into its constituent parts; and to abstract common properties, plan ahead ideationally, and think or behave symbolically. The *concrete attitude*, on the other hand, is a form of thinking fixed and unable to proceed beyond the stimulus of an immediate experience or object. To him the brain-injured person is impaired in his ability to assume the abstract attitude and has difficulty in moving easily from the abstract to the concrete.

Post-traumatic Personality Disorders

Although these personality disturbances are primarily a result of injuries to the cranial contents, psychological factors usually participate to a varying degree. A decision as to the relative importance of the brain injury, of environmental factors, and of the previous personality pattern of the patient is not always easy. Sometimes the impression is gained that the patient has always had an immature attitude or, as a result of the accident, has reverted to such an attitude, accompanied by a reluctance to face former responsibilities. Again, the mental symptoms appear mainly or entirely psychogenic and merge into a neurosis secondary to the trauma (accident neurosis).

Among the names applied to the personality syndrome caused directly by the head injury are "postconcussion syndrome," "post-traumatic general cerebral syndrome" (Foerster), "minor contusion syndrome" (Symonds), "traumatic constitution" (Meyer), "traumatic psychopathic constitution" (Ziehen), "traumatic encephalopathy," and others. In adults this primary post-traumatic personality syndrome may assume two forms: a milder and more frequent form known as post-concussion syndrome or postconcussional neurotic state, and a more serious disturbance to which the name post-traumatic personality disorder is applied in a narrower and more specific sense.

POSTCONCUSSION SYNDROME.   Whether the injury that preceded this syndrome was mild or severe, the presenting symptom is anxiety. Other symptoms are headache, vertigo, fatigability, oversensitivity to strong sensory stimuli, insomnia, impairment of memory and of ability to concentrate, a narrowing of interests, a lessening of spontaneity, aggravation of symptoms by heat, excitement, or exertion, and a reduced tolerance of alcohol. Headache and vertigo are aggravated by quick movement, by stooping, or by psychological tension. Many patients are emotionally labile, irritable, and easily moved to tears. Many complain of decreased sexual potency. Some become "head-conscious." This is perhaps to be expected, since the head is the most significant part of the body image. Head injury, therefore, is more commonly experienced as a form of psychic trauma than injury to almost any other part of the body. If the injury occurred under conditions of discontent or dissatisfaction, psychogenic symptoms are particularly likely to follow.

Diagnosis and Prognosis.   The chief problem in the diagnosis of the postconcussion syndrome is to determine when a postconcussional headache and other symptoms having an organic basis cease to be a result of organic causes and are carried on by psychological influences. The relative importance of psychogenic and physiogenic factors is often difficult to determine. If the headache is paroxysmal, throbbing, and aggravated by postural alterations or physical exertion, it may be that it persists from an encephalopathic rather than from a neurotic state. The same is true if mental functions tend to be sluggish and if the emotional status

is sanguine and not characterized by gloom, ready annoyance, and apprehension. If the symptoms are definite and constant and are not modified by suggestion, and if the patient's interest is in rehabilitation and not in indemnification, they are probably not of psychogenic origin. The postconcussive or neurotic state is discussed elsewhere in this chapter. Most, but not all, patients with the postconcussion syndrome recover if complications of psychoneurotic symptoms are not too numerous or too severe. Recovery may be delayed for one or two years.

Treatment.   In certain respects, the most important aspects of therapy are careful and adequate surgical and medical treatment at the time of injury, combined with subsequent discreet management in adjusting the patient to his symptoms and to the general situation with which he is confronted. Too early return to strenuous labor should be discouraged, yet too long a rest may lead to a secondary neurotic syndrome. Nearly every patient with concussion should have supportive and suggestive psychotherapy.

POST-TRAUMATIC PERSONALITY DISORDER OF ADULTS.   In some instances, the most conspicuous sequel of head trauma is a change from the original personality makeup of the patient. The amiable, placid individual may become irascible, irritable, and impulsive. He may become quarrelsome and subject to outbursts of rage, aggression, and motor excitement. Family and other obligations and responsibilities are disregarded. Ambition and initiative are lost. The patient becomes petulant, resentful, self-centered, willful, and selfish. Some become morose and tend to develop paranoid reactions toward persons about them. Others lose all interest in activities and withdraw from social contacts. Not uncommonly, some degree of organic mental deterioration accompanies these changes in the psychological structure of the personality.

POST-TRAUMATIC PERSONALITY DISORDERS OF CHILDREN.   In general, children withstand head injury better than adults. However, brain-damaged children may present serious behavior problems. Children without serious destruction of brain tissue may show much disorganization of behavior. The behavior disorders are similar to those seen following the epidemic encephalitis of the 1920's but they are more severe and of poorer prognosis. The previously normal child becomes disobedient, distractible, impulsive, aggressive, destructive, cruel, quarrelsome, and antisocial. Constant restlessness and overactivity are the rule. There may be some degree of intellectual deficit. The child is dominated by instinctive and emotional impulses and shows no regard for the welfare of others. Although there is little impairment of original intellectual capacity, the child does not concentrate, shows little interest in school work, and does poorly in the classroom, where he is intolerably disruptive. The usual methods of training and discipline are ineffectual, and eventually the most serious delinquents become institutionalized.

Although the emotional disorders seen in the brain-injured child probably have organic roots, they certainly have psychogenic ones. Because of his handicap, the child is in need of emotional support. Parents' feelings and their attitude toward his handicaps may greatly influence his behavior. Some parents may manifest a smothering overprotectiveness and others may be unsympathetic and rejecting. An impatient attitude and unjustified blame by the teacher increase the child's anxiety and result both in more disturbed behavior and in less ability to learn. Environmental pathology becomes, therefore, the crucial determinant of the disturbances in behavior.

Post-traumatic Defect Conditions

Mental deterioration (dementia) following severe head trauma may or may not have been preceded by traumatic delirium. It frequently happens that, as consciousness returns following delirium, an impairment of former mental capacity becomes manifest. In milder forms, this may consist only of loss of initiative, mental slowing, loss of sense of responsibility, and impairment of ability to recognize abstract relationships. In somewhat more serious disturbances, memory is impaired, attention is reduced, reaction time is slowed, and defensive confabulations may be expressed. Judgment is impaired and finer affective feelings are blunted. Social values are not appreciated. Tasks that were formerly performed easily become difficult or impossible. The patient may consider himself normal, although it is apparent to his intimates that he has never been the same since his injury. The degree of dementia varies greatly according to the site of the lesion, the nature and extent of the injury, and its secondary results (atrophy, meningoencephalic adhesions, distortion of ventricles). A permanent mental deterioration to a degree requiring institutional care is uncommon after contusion. If laceration has been extensive, the dementia may be great and associated with epileptiform seizures, paralyses, aphasia, deafness, and other neurological signs.

Difficulty sometimes arises in differentiating post-traumatic mental deterioration from psychoses of arteriosclerotic origin complicated by head injury. Careful inquiry should be made as to any symptoms of arteriosclerosis existing before the injury. The possibility that the confusion of arteriosclerosis or of a cerebral attack may have led to the injury should be kept in mind.

Severe, chronic dementia is hopeless, yet caution should guide the therapist in expressing a prognosis in acute or subacute cases, since with time many patients show a surprising improvement.

Traumatic Encephalopathy of Pugilists (Punch Drunk)

A chronic post-traumatic personality disorder first described by Martland is that to which he gave the name "punch drunk." This syndrome occurs among pugilists who have sustained repeated severe blows on the head over a period of at least a few years. The more skillful the fighter, the greater is the probability that he will either escape the causative injuries or remain relatively free from them for a considerable period of time. The disorder probably results from successive and accumulative petechial hemorrhages and foci of necrosis deep in the cerebrum. The patient shows an insidious impairment of skill, a slowing of muscular action, a little uncertainty in equilibrium, slight confusion, and deterioration in attention, concentration, and memory. Speech becomes thick and hesitating. The patient "continuously simulates a person who is just a little drunk." Most patients are voluble and euphoric. Confusion and defects of memory become more marked, and intellectual impairment continues to a disabling degree. The tremor, propulsive gait, and mask-like facies of the parkinsonian syndrome may appear. The symptoms progress for approximately a year, then become stationary. The degree of deterioration depends upon the extent and degree of brain injury.

Traumatic Epilepsy

One of the sequelae of brain injury may be epilepsy. There is so wide a variation in statistics as to the incidence of epileptic seizures following head injury—4.5 per cent (Sargant) to 34 per cent (Denny-Brown)—that they are probably of little value. Study of 279 American personnel who sustained wounds of the brain in World War II showed that 36 per cent developed seizures within two years after injury, and 41.6 per cent within three years after receipt of penetrating brain wounds. The incidence is greatest in patients who suffer a penetration of the dura. Penfield showed that the most frequent epileptogenic lesions in post-traumatic convulsive state are cerebrodural or cerebral cicatrix and focal atrophy. Epilepsy is therefore more common after penetrating than after closed injuries and is not the result of generalized damage to the brain. Seizures do not develop after a simple concussion.

A lesion causing the convulsive state does so as a result of irritation of adjacent areas of the brain. The pattern of the attack and the march of motor phenomena during the seizure may betray the epileptogenic point of origin. Electroencephalography may be of much value in localization of the lesion. In the typical focal or jacksonian seizure, consciousness is not lost. Clonic twitches develop in one part of the body and spread consecutively to other parts of the same side. In a large percentage of cases, however, consciousness is disturbed in the manner of either the petit mal or grand mal seizure. There may also be the same paroxysmal periods of depression, exaltation, or fugues. Mental deterioration may be slight or extreme.

CHRONIC MENTAL DISORDER SECONDARY TO HEAD TRAUMA: PSYCHONEUROSIS

Although a later chapter will be devoted to a description of the psychoneuroses, those associated with head trauma have features sufficiently significant to justify special mention of them in a discussion of mental disorders following head injury. It is not generally considered that traumatic neuroses are the direct result of anatomical or physiological changes produced by the trauma, yet a subjectively disturbing postconcussion syndrome or other post-traumatic symptoms may facilitate or become the nucleus for neurotic attitudes. In some individuals the traumatic incident sets off a stress reaction, with the typical symptoms described later in this book. If the trauma occurred at a time, or in a setting, in which anxiety-producing factors such as economic insecurity, occupational dissatisfactions, family tensions, or inability to secure work existed the neurotic response is more likely. The circumstances under which the trauma was sustained—compensable accidents, in contrast to accidental falls in the home or injuries in sports—may have a significant etiological relation. There is also a contributing element in the fact that the head, particularly the brain, is an organ on which the patient sets particular value. If, therefore, the injury is followed by dizziness and headache, or if other physical symptoms are associated with it, a sense of insecurity and an associated anxiety may readily develop.

Complicating situational stresses arising from, or relating to, the injury tend not only to create but also to perpetuate the neurotic symptoms. Feelings of discontent or of grievance predispose to their development. Fear, suggestion, and wishful thinking may all be important psychological factors in the production of symptoms.

Diagnosis

The onset of psychoneurosis associated with head trauma occurs not at the time of injury but at a variable period after it. Frequently there is a history that the patient recovered from the organic symptoms produced by the trauma and was about to return to his usual employment, or even resumed work for a brief period, when a return of headache, dizziness, and other symptoms rendered employment impossible. This period between the time of the injury and the appearance of neurotic disability is often described as one of "incubation and contemplation." The patient who has had a resentful, dissatisfied attitude toward his work and was protected from resuming former responsibilities by reason of the acute physical symptoms that followed the head trauma is prone to the development of a neurosis. With the loss of the protecting physical disability, other means of avoiding a return to a distasteful situation must be sought. This means is readily provided by a return of headache, vertigo, impairment of memory, fatigability, irritability, and other symptoms. Likewise, both the man who is fundamentally covetous and indolent, or who was harassed by debts or other financial obligations before his injury, and the apprehensive, suggestible man fearful of losing compensation by

return to work may develop similar psychoneurotic symptoms to assure a continuation of compensation. The sympathy and solicitude of friends, lack of occupation and interest, suggestive examinations, misdirected treatment, continued compensation, and other subconscious motivations tend to fix the symptoms. Various factors, such as fears related to the injury, head-consciousness, and accentuation and elaboration of preëxisting conflicts concerning occupational and financial problems, contribute to the development of anxiety, which is often a conspicuous symptom. Other symptoms are physical and mental fatigability, depression, apprehension, neurasthenic and hypochondriacal reactions, and a volubility and elaboration in expression of complaints. Symptoms tend to be vague, numerous, and inconstant.

Undoubtedly the organic concussion syndrome, with disturbance of consciousness, subsequent dizziness, and the feeling of insecurity connected with it, facilitates the production and suggests the nature of neurotic symptoms. As organic symptoms continue, they often tend, therefore, to acquire an overlay of psychoneurotic ones. Frequently, indeed, the post-traumatic concussion syndrome becomes the basis for psychological elaborations of a hysterical type. As a result, psychogenic symptoms coincide or may be interwoven with organic sequelae of head injuries. With this tendency of neurotic attitudes to crystallize around the nucleus of head injuries, the differentiation between organic and psychogenic symptoms is not always easy; every combination of organic and psychiatric symptoms may, in fact, exist. The relative significance of these two groups may be a matter of personal opinion.

Treatment

Since the pretraumatic personality and the setting and circumstances of the accident are often more significant than the severity of the injury in producing post-traumatic mental disability, apprehension should not be manifested either by the physician or the patient's relatives. Prolonged rest in bed after head injury suggests that the injury is serious, engenders anxiety, and predisposes to the development of the post-traumatic syndrome. The stay in a hospital should not be prolonged, and the patient should return to his work as soon as practicable. Planned activity even before return to regular employment is desirable. Reference has already been made to the fact that occupational and home worries and concern for compensation favor the persistence of symptoms. Gain from the injury in any way deters recovery. A speedy settlement of any compensation question is advisable. Since the association between head injury and psychiatric factors is close, the "preneurotic interval" between the injury and the development of the neurosis is one in which preventive psychotherapy is advisable.

Rehabilitation of the brain-injured should commence immediately after the patient has become conscious. Such patients are often highly fearful and suggestible. Explanation as to the nature of the injury and reassurance as to outcome should be given. Efforts should be made to avoid inquiry concerning symptoms that are not spontaneously presented. As soon as the patient is able, he should move about, and a carefully planned program of progressive activity should be established. Such a program should not overtax his capacities intellectually, emotionally, or physically.

Those with chronic defects require more than a regimen of occupational therapy, games, and exercises, even though such activities assist in restoring self-confidence and an awareness of capacity for performance. Treatment is most effectively managed in hospitals with well-established departments for rehabilitation, including occupational, recreational, and vocational therapies.

Many advances have been made in the methods used in the reëducation of those with chronic brain damage, particularly of those who manifest, in addition to disturbances of the abstract attitude, specific defects in the field of language, motor disabilities, and perception, as Goldstein has indicated. Such patients require a careful psychological evaluation and then retraining by skilled persons. There is a continuing need for the insight of the psychiatrist and his assistants in dealing with the emotional problems of patients. However, in addition to this type of therapy, the utilization of the psychologist trained in the pedagogy of the brain-injured, and also of the social worker if there are particular family needs, must be considered. The outcome varies according to the severity of the lesion and the pretraumatic personality of the individual. In some cases, intellectual tests may fail to reveal serious disturbances, yet when the patient has returned to work his impairment in judgment and capacity for work may be demonstrated. Here the well-established rehabilitation center, with the opportunity for testing performance in a workshop, is most useful in determining the eventual capacity of the individual for an occupation and the proper type of vocation for the future. In those rare cases of dementia with severe personality change, the prognosis is grave.

BIBLIOGRAPHY

Association for Research in Nervous and Mental Diseases, Vol. XXIV: Trauma of the Central Nervous System. Baltimore, Williams & Wilkins Company, 1945.

Critchley, M.: Medical aspects of boxing. Brit. Med. J., *1*:357–364, 1957.

Denny-Brown, D.: Disability arising from closed head injuries. J.A.M.A., *127*:429–436, 1945.

Eisenberg, L.: Psychiatric implications of brain damage in children. Psychiatric Quart., *31*:72–92, 1957.

Goldstein, K.: After-effects of Brain Injuries in War. New York, Grune & Stratton, 1942.

Ingram, T. T. S.: A characteristic form of over-activity behavior in brain-damaged children. J. Ment. Sci., *102*:550–558, 1956.

Strauss, A. A., and Lehtinen, L. E.: Psychopathology and Education of the Brain-Injured Child. New York, Grune & Stratton, 1947.

Walker, A. E., Caveness, W. F., and Critchley, M.: The Late Effects of Head Injury. Springfield, Ill., Charles C Thomas, 1960.

Walker, A. E., and Erculer, F.: Head Injured Men. Springfield, Ill., Charles C Thomas, 1968.

Chapter 17

Brain Syndromes Associated with Endocrine, Metabolic, and Nutritional Disturbances

Although their relations are complex and imperfectly understood, and although the psychological and physical interrelations consequent to endocrine, metabolic, or nutritional derangements are poorly correlated, it is apparent that mutually influencing reactions occur among the central nervous system, mental and personality functioning, and the endocrines.

It is reasonable to assume that interactions between emotional and metabolic processes may produce endocrine disturbances, and these, in turn, may affect cerebral functions and mental reactions. The psychological consequences of a given hormonal action are not uniform. A certain hormonal change may or may not have a psychological effect. If it does produce an effect, it is not necessarily the same in all cases but will depend upon the previous personality organization of the individual and upon all the other influences acting upon the personality.

It is not clear, however, whether endocrine abnormalities will in themselves produce a psychosis. Some endocrine disturbances produce changes in brain function by influencing brain metabolism, but this is no indication that such changes are related to disturbances in behavior. This is well illustrated when thyroid function is considered. Although psychotic and other types of reaction occur in association with hyperthyroidism, it has been shown by recent work that the cerebral metabolic rate is not elevated from normal in this condition. On the other hand, in myxedema there are a reduction of oxygen consumption by the brain and a retardation in expression at the psychological level.

In the evaluation and management of the personality disorders associated with metabolic and endocrine disturbance, the degree of stress consequent to the metabolic shift and the rate of change of bodily functions secondary to that shift must be weighed against the constitutional and experiential development of the specific individual. The time in development at which such changes take place is highly significant.

Preceding the onset of personality disorder, there exist chemical, metabolic, physiological, and sometimes anatomical changes. This is in contrast to what is now known of the functional psychoses and neuroses. Such changes are perceived, and must be adapted to, by the specific individual in his own environment.

When endocrine disorder produces gross changes in the body, creating psychological and social stresses which vary from one person and culture to another, the adaptation is particularly difficult because the body image is disturbed. Thus the patient may see himself as deformed, inadequate, or sexually misidentified and may, in turn, suffer ridicule or attack. He then develops feelings of shame and inadequacy. His responses may be anxiety, hostility, guilt, or social withdrawal, or all of these.

In those instances in which the metabolic change induces largely subjective perceptions, there is likely to result only a shift in the affective life and the level of the drive. It is clear that the symbolic significance of change induced by the metabolic shift depends on the ego attitude toward the body and its functions, derived during psychosocial development. Thus young women exposed to the masculinization resulting from an adrenal tumor develop anxieties as to their sexual role and functions, associated with activation of sexual fantasies and doubting, an attitude which would not be observed in the young child who has suffered since birth with the symptom complex due to adrenal hyperplasia.

ADRENAL DISORDERS

Cushing's Syndrome

In his original descriptions in 1932 of what has come to be known as Cushing's syndrome, Harvey Cushing called attention to the frequent coexistence of mental symptoms. It is now recognized that these occur in approximately a fifth of those with the syndrome. Originally thought to be associated with a basophil adenoma of the pituitary gland, Cushing's syndrome now is regarded generally as the result of adrenocortical hyperfunction with either neoplastic or hyperplastic expression in the adrenal glands.

The diversity of the associated personality disturbances is such as to indicate that they represent the defensive adaptations of the individual to the endocrine imbalance and also, to a considerable extent, to the disfiguring alteration in the patient's appearance. Thus, as the illness progresses, the patient may change from an attractive young woman to an obese and bearded lady whose activities are restricted by weakness and easy fatigability.

A reactive depression is the most frequently encountered response. In relatively few patients is it associated with psychomotor retardation. Other patients, without depression, are anxious and have crying spells, or are agitated or stubborn in their behavior. Irritability, paranoid ideation, and rarely a florid schizophrenic response are seen. Less than a fourth of those with associated personality disturbance suffer serious personality decompensation with psychosis. Obviously this syndrome presents symptoms similar to those induced by the administration of cortisone, other adrenal steroids, and corticotropin as is discussed in an earlier chapter.

DIAGNOSIS. This is made with observation of the complaints of marked weakness and easy fatigability and an often painful adiposity, which may develop rapidly, with characteristic distribution of fat in the areas of the face and neck (moon face) and trunk. The combination of supraclavicular fat pads and dorsal kyphosis due to osteoporosis sometimes gives a humped posture. There may be depressed purple streaks over the abdomen, thighs, and upper arms, with increased susceptibility to bruising. There is a diminished carbohydrate tolerance due to increased gluconeogenesis from protein, sometimes with diabetes. Hypertension and peripheral edema may occur. Women, the most frequently affected, are usually amenorrheic and show masculinization, with deepening of the voice, hirsutism, growth of the clitoris, and acne. Men are often impotent. The definitive diagnosis is established by laboratory evidence of increased excretion of 17-hydroxycorticoids in the urine. Also helpful are the findings of an eosinophil count below 50 per milliliter, lymphopenia, neutrophilia, polycythemia, and glycosuria and evidence by x-ray of osteoporosis.

TREATMENT. Abolishment of the adrenal hyperfunction by subtotal resection of the adrenal gland or removal of an adrenal tumor usually relieves both the personality and physiological disturbances. However, the return to health is not immediate and requires time. Those who develop hypoadrenalism after surgery and in whom substitution therapy proves inadequate often have persistence of the personality disorder. Others, particularly young women who have suffered severe disfigurement due to hirsutism, bony deformities, and the scars of acne also are apt to have a stubborn perpetuation of symptoms.

Adrenogenital Syndrome

The virilizing effects of excessive secretion of adrenal androgens, whether due to bilateral hyperplasia at birth or an adrenal tumor (often carcinomatous) occurring later in life, have serious consequences for personality development. The condition is frequently associated with psychosis.

When the syndrome develops in women after puberty with the physical deformity resulting from overgrowth of sexual hair, deepening of the voice, absence of breasts, enlargement of the clitoris, and amenorrhea, it leads to marked anxiety. Female patients particularly are preoccupied with their masculinized appearance, develop doubts as to their gender and sexual role, often become depressed and withdrawn socially, and are obsessed with thoughts of homosexuality or guilt relative to masturbation.

DIAGNOSIS. This is established definitively by demonstration of increased secretion of adrenal androgens and 17-ketosteroids. Other forms of precocious sexual development and hermaphroditism may be distinguished by special differential analyses of steroid secretions.

TREATMENT. Small doses of cortisone suppress the virilizing activity of the adrenals. If this treatment is given in early life, the female patient develops normally and at puberty matures and menstruates regularly. Removal of a tumor or partial adrenalectomy is the treatment of choice for those late in life.

Pheochromocytoma

Accompanying this rare medullary tumor of the adrenal or of other chromaffin tissues, there occur many symptoms suggesting the existence of anxiety neurosis. These symptoms are due to increased se-

cretion of norepinephrine and epinephrine by the gland.

Symptoms, which may exist for a few weeks or years, appear in some instances to be precipitated by emotionally charged incidents, and in others by physical exertion or changes in posture. They are variable in frequency, duration, and severity, and are spoken of as occurring in attacks by over half the sufferers. During such acute episodes the patients suffer apprehension, pounding headaches, sweating, palpitation, tremulousness, pallor or flushing of the face, pain in the chest, nausea or vomiting, and paresthesias in the extremities. High levels of hypertension with hyperglycemia and glycosuria occur during such acute paroxysms.

The differential diagnosis from primary psychiatric disturbance is made in the presence of hypertension, either transitory or persistent, the palpation or radiographic visualization of a tumor in the adrenal areas, and the patient's response to provocative and blocking pharmacologic tests. Histamine phosphate given intravenously provokes a rise in blood pressure within two minutes with some of the symptoms of the paroxysm. The adrenergic blocking agent Regitine, given to patients with sustained hypertension, will lead to a fall of blood pressure to within normal limits within three or four minutes. Such tests must be administered with care; their indications vary with the nature of the accompanying hypertension.

THYROID DISORDERS

Hyperthyroidism

In the mental disorders associated with hyperthyroidism—an association in which there is a striking interaction between emotional and metabolic processes—it has long been noted that a special type of personality seems usually to have existed before the clinical signs of Graves' disease were apparent. This disease arises largely in sensitive, impressionable persons who react keenly to life, have a marked feeling of insecurity, and an unusual sense of responsibility. The general hypermotility, emotional excitability, and alertness to every sound and impression, the tendency to walk, talk, and eat rapidly, and the mild anxiety, apprehensiveness, and irritability commonly observed in Graves' disease and characterized by the laity as "nervousness," represent in many ways but an exaggeration of a previously existing pattern of response to ordinary life problems. In other words, these persons have been anxious individuals with psychiatric problems giving rise to tension. In them it is frequently impossible to tell where anxiety stops and hyperthyroidism begins.

Psychiatric studies have shown that, usually long before the onset of the clinical symptoms of hyperthyroidism, patients who succumb to this illness have suffered emotional and psychological maladjustment. The majority of those who have examined groups of patients indicate that the basic need of such patients is for the satisfaction of an exaggerated dependency relationship. With chronic frustration, their response is aggressive and leads to the welling up of death wishes toward the person from whom they had hoped to obtain gratification. As a means of adapting to such wishes, the patient may respond by an over-depressed relationship to the significant person or turn away from this person and attempt a striving at self-sufficiency which is often premature. Women with the illness have many conflicts and fears in relation to childbirth; yet at the same time they manifest a strong desire for children. The dependency needs are satisfied while the child is small, but when the time comes for the child to seek its own independence, the mother responds often with anxiety and anger or with the reaction formation of anxious over-concern. These psychological defenses are not specific for the hyperthyroid patient and may be seen in many other conditions. Nevertheless, the strivings of individuals with this type of personality structure relate well to those observations that show that the psychiatric problem frequently precipitating the hy-perthyroid activity is the loss of a key person in the patient's life.

Although the usual mental symptoms associated with hyperthyroidism are those of tension, overactivity, and emotional instability already mentioned, in many untreated acutely thyrotoxic patients a psychotic reaction appears. In extreme cases a fairly typical manic excitement may develop as if in accordance with the increased tempo of all organic processes. In other instances there may be an acute hallucinatory delirium accompanied by great restlessness and insomnia. Other patients present depressed, anxious, agitated reactions. Paranoid states with systematized delusions may occur. In general the symptoms manifested are exaggerations and caricatures of the previous personality. It will usually be found that persons with recurrent hyperthyroidism after thyroidectomy are still struggling with serious and unresolved personality difficulties.

The treatment of hyperthyroidism is often a joint task for the psychiatrist and the internist. The internist directs his efforts to the restoration of the metabolic rate to normal limits. The function of the psychiatrist is to aid patients who are disturbed emotionally in accepting the need for therapy through bringing insight to their denial of symptoms. Continued psychotherapy is indicated for those hyperthyroid patients who present clear evidence of psychological maladjustment prior to the onset. Here psychotherapy is an important adjunct in bringing about a permanent euthyroid state with reduction in emotional and psychological symptomatology.

Myxedema

Although Ord, in 1877, first proposed the term "myxedema," Gull, four years earlier, had presented a paper entitled, "On a cretinoid state supervening in adult life in women." Accompanying mental changes were noted in the early descriptions of the disease. Among the most frequent mental symptoms are slowness and difficulty in apprehension, thought, and action. These retardations, together with indecision and listlessness, may suggest depression. Memory may be impaired, the defect being more marked in respect to recent events. Speech is frequently slow, and changes in articulation may occur. Recently these clinical findings have been interpreted as the result of impairment of the level of awareness leading to defects in attention, concentration, endurance, and conceptual use without sensory activation. In cases showing such manifestations, there is associated an electroencephalographic abnormality with diminution in mean frequency and voltage, resulting from impaired cerebral metabolism. The serial subtraction test is said to expose the defect in awareness most effectively. Associated with their hebetude, many patients show an unusual fretfulness, irritability, and a paranoid trend. The clinical picture is determined largely by individual emotional and personality factors. There may, therefore, be paranoid characteristics, delusions of persecution, and hallucinations. Mild degrees of thyroid insufficiency are not infrequently seen in middle-aged persons who complain of fatigue, pains, and headache and are pessimistic.

Treatment with thyroid extract not only relieves the symptoms but corrects the electroencephalographic disturbance in those without permanent cerebral damage. Treatment with the extract should be initiated with caution; such treatment is best carried out in a hospital under careful observation and should be commenced with low dosages of 15 mg. daily. The dosage may be increased to 0.1 to 0.2 gm. of thyroid extract daily. The sudden changes in metabolism are particularly dangerous for those with cardiovascular disorders.

PARATHYROID DISORDERS

Hypocalcemia

The most common cause of hypocalcemia is the removal of or damage to the parathyroid glands during thyroidectomy. Psychological symptoms are observed in such patients in addition to the characteristic clinical signs of paresthesia, cramps, carpopedal spasms, tetany, or laryngeal stridor. The most common symptoms are those of depression, memory loss, disturbance of deep reflexes, and emotional lability. Such symptoms may persist for years, yet are often quickly relieved by correction of the hypocalcemia with the administration of calcium salts orally and with vitamin D; the dosage is carefully controlled by regular determination of the serum calcium. Parathyroid hormone has not been effective for such control.

Hyperparathyroidism

Although uncommon, psychiatric symptoms do occur in patients with hyperparathyroidism owing to adenomatosis of these organs. Usually the presenting picture has been that of an acute brain syndrome (delirium) or evidence of a behavioral change expressed with depressive or paranoidal psychotic manifestations. Initially the patient's history of illness is one of anorexia or listlessness. Later there occur apathy, weakness, insomnia, anorexia, nausea, and vomiting. A useful clue of the primary etiology is a history of previous renal calculi or peptic ulcer. The diagnosis will be made by evidence of hypercalcemia, abnormally low phosphatemia, and the electrocardiographic changes of prolonged P–R interval. Recovery follows, after surgical removal of tumor, in those without existing personality abnormality.

PANCREATIC DISORDERS

Hypoglycemia

It is now recognized that spontaneous—in distinction from therapeutically induced—hypoglycemic states may occasionally exist. At times the clinical picture of such hypoglycemic attacks may be dominated by mental symptoms, usually transitory in nature. There is no single psychic syndrome characteristic of the condition. Among the many mental phenomena that may be prominent are the following: apathy, irritability, restlessness, anxiety, negativism, somnambulism, confusion, disorientation, fugue states, delirium, syncope, stupor, or coma. Thinking may be confused and retarded and speech may be disturbed. Grasp may be impaired and emotions unstable. Hallucinations and delusions may be present. The patient may complain of weakness, fatigability, and hunger. He perspires and may suffer from tremor, unsteadiness of gait, diplopia, and convulsions. There is no recollection of the attack. There is a tendency for the symptoms to appear after exertion or when the patient is hungry. Complete relief from the symptoms follows the administration of sugar. Hypoglycemia should always be suspected as the cause of any mental symptoms appearing in a diabetic who is receiving insulin.

DIAGNOSIS. The diagnosis of spontaneous hypoglycemia is made on evidence of depression of the blood sugar level. Since the periods of the condition are transient, it is often difficult to establish its presence by simple study of the fasting blood sugar. A definitive diagnosis is evident if the blood sugar level during an attack falls below 50 or 60 mg. per 100 ml. If the attack is convulsive in nature, the blood sugar may be elevated following the seizure. Glucose tolerance tests have limited value but may suggest the diagnosis if the blood sugar level falls to 50 mg. per 100 ml. three to five hours after the stimulating dose of glucose. When hypoglycemia is not demonstrated by these means, a 24- or 48-hour fast should be instituted and blood sugar determinations made at periods of 12, 18, and 24 hours. With the onset of symptoms and their prompt alleviation by the use of intravenous glucose, the diagnosis is established. Electroencephalographic changes occur in association with such attacks and show local or widespread dysrhythmias which again are relieved on ingestion or intravenous administration of glucose.

ETIOLOGY. Once the diagnosis of hypoglycemia is established, its etiology must be determined. Although the majority of such patients will be found to suffer from hyperinsulinism caused by islet cell tumors of the pancreas, the functional cases with an associated neurosis are of particular interest to the psychiatrist. It has not been determined whether this type of condition may occur as a somatic manifestation of a psychoneurosis or whether the majority of these cases fall into the group of *induced hypoglycemic states* symbolic of a sadomasochistic neurotic conflict. A number of such cases of induced hypoglycemia have been observed, usually in women and most frequently in nurses who have had experience with the utilization of insulin. The diagnosis was established on one occasion by tagging the insulin used by the patient with radioactive phosphorus and then detecting the excretion of the radioactive material in the urine the following day. In some instances the patient suffered from diabetes and had numerous unexplained attacks of hypoglycemia, though denying the use of insulin.

The following case history illustrates such a problem and its management:

The patient, a 44-year-old married nurse, with a history of episodic attacks of hunger, weakness, sleepiness, sweating, vertigo, and occasionally unconsciousness, was referred for study. The attacks were always aborted by eating. They were so severe that six months previously the patient had to give up a fast. Another physician had diagnosed an islet cell pancreatic tumor and advised surgery. The patient refused operation, stating that she had gained weight and was not suffering any pain. She consulted other physicians in an attempt to obtain a different diagnosis. She expressed her fear to these physicians that if operated upon she would become diabetic and require insulin.

A careful medical examination failed to reveal any evidence of tumor. The patient sustained a fast without the development of hypoglycemia. In view of previous experiences with patients who had induced hypoglycemia, the patient's room was searched while she was having a diagnostic test and several bottles of insulin and a syringe were found. At this point a psychiatric examination was requested.

In consultation the patient reported that her mother, who had died two years previously, had been a diabetic and had been nursed in her terminal illness by the daughter. The patient had lived a restricted life and had entered nursing to relieve herself of her loneliness. Some four years previously she had undergone a hysterectomy performed by a physician who had advised her that she had an islet cell tumor.

Following the initial psychiatric interview, the patient stated that she proposed to sign out of the hospital. Since it was considered that her condition was dangerous in the sense that she was exposing herself to a potentially major surgical procedure, the psychiatric consultant concluded that it was advisable to suggest the possibility of induced hypoglycemia to the patient. This was done by informing her of the conclusions reached by the medical service on the basis of finding the bottle of insulin and the previous experience of the hospital with others with similar conditions. The patient was gently told that, if this was the case, she must have some underlying emotional problems which had led her to the desperate expedient of the self-administration of insulin and that she might therefore wish to solve the major conflicts which had driven her to such action. The suggestion was met by immediate denial. When seen the following day, the patient asked assurance that any information given by her would be considered inviolate. When this was given, she broke down, cried, and gave the following information.

She stated that her drive for the self-administration of insulin began about four months previously during the period of a fast when she felt weak and unable to continue her work. Believing that she might obtain a dispensation from a religious fast from the physician who had removed her uterus some years earlier, with whom she worked and toward whom she had a strong positive attachment, she asked if he would assist her in securing a dispensation for medical reasons. He replied that he would do so if he found her to be suffering from hypoglycemia. Shortly before blood was to be drawn for the determination of its sugar content, the nurse, without the knowledge of the physician, took her first injection of insulin. Naturally, hypoglycemia was found. The physician therefore gave her the desired recommendation that dispensation be granted from the obligation of fasting before communion.

The nurse then revealed that she had developed a feeling of depression after her hysterectomy. She feared that she had not healed properly and wondered whether she would develop a cancer. Her father had died of cancer and had suffered from fears relating to mental disease. He was given insulin to relieve his depression. The patient herself had given insulin in mental hospitals and recalled her anxiety on being shown the brain of a patient who had died during insulin shock therapy. Throughout her life she had felt hungry, had been an extremely heavy eater, and had felt weak when she fasted. The patient had always devoted herself to the care of her mother and an aunt and had spent months at home each year nursing them for their various ailments. The mother had written her that she should provide nursing services not only for herself and the aunt but also for her brothers, if she really loved her family. She always seemed fearful of losing the love of her relatives. Perhaps it is not surprising that upon the death of her parents she expressed the sentiment that her brothers "beat her out" of her patrimony.

The nurse declared that she had devoted the same amount of attention to the care of her physician's patients as she had to her own family. She admitted that her response to his insistence on evidence of hypoglycemia by blood test prior to supporting her request for a medical dispensation had been one of anger and resentment. On the other hand, she felt so anxious concerning the possibility of losing his respect and good will and so guilty in relation to the church that she felt obliged to continue the self-administration of insulin when faced with another medical examination. Following these revelations, which were responded to with sympathetic interpretation of her emotional reactions and their origin, the patient returned home to her profession and made a satisfactory adaptation, with no recurrence of the hypoglycemic attacks.

Acute Pancreatitis

A very high proportion of patients who suffer recurrent bouts of acute pancreatitis in the course of a continuing relapsing disease of the pancreas develop an acute psychotic brain syndrome with these attacks. The majority of such patients are confirmed alcohol addicts. Their symptoms are most frequently hallucinatory, either auditory or visual, with memory deficits, difficulty in concentration, agitation, fearfulness, and, in some, confabulation. Often confused with delirium tremens, this toxic delirious state may be identified by the principal complaint of abdominal pain, usually associated with vomiting. The patient invariably has an elevated serum amylase level. Although associated with chronic alcoholism, the condition may occur in periods of long abstinence and is found in those with cirrhosis of the liver, diabetes, calcification of the pancreas, or malabsorption syndromes.

There is some reason to believe that impairment of pancreatic activity affects brain and associated mental functioning through metabolic mechanisms that are altered in an unknown manner. Supporting this possibility is the reported occurrence in some patients of severe depression that has antedated other symptoms of pancreatic carcinoma by months.

The hallucinatory brain syndrome associated with acute pancreatitis resolves rapidly over a 10-day period as the pancreatitis subsides.

Carcinoma of the Pancreas

Symptoms of depression, anxiety, and premonition of serious illness are among the most frequent presenting complaints of patients with carcinoma of the pancreas. From 10 to 20 per cent of patients have such symptoms. These symptoms are often noted before other signs and symptoms, which may present from one to four years later. A six-month interval is common. The insomnia associated with the depression has often proved unresponsive to prescription of ordinary hypnotics. The majority of patients with carcinoma of the pancreas, studied by Fras et al., tended to repress their rage responses and also suffered more significant loss of object relations in the immediately preceding months than did patients with other abdominal tumors. The relationship remains unclear between the physiological effects of this tumor growth as contrasted with others, the personality of the patient, and the potential precipitating factor of object loss.

PITUITARY DISORDERS

Acromegaloid Personality

Manfred Bleuler has called attention to the fact that, while acromegaly does not in itself lead to a psychosis, it is quite regularly accompanied by an alteration of personality. This change consists mainly of a lack of initiative and spontaneity and a change in mood. Some patients show brief periods of moodiness without apparent cause, sometimes manifesting cheerfulness, self-satisfaction, and elation, with passivity and indifference. Again, the mood may at times be anxious, resentful, tense, and unpleasant. In advanced acromegaly, even without increased intracranial pressure,

there are slow reactions and a slowness in the stream of thought. There is no intellectual impairment except that referable to apathy and slowness of thought and action. The patient's social attitude is usually characterized by egocentricity, lack of consideration for and interest in other people, impatience, irritability, and oversensitivity during social contacts. Bleuler does not mean that this type of personality is specific to acromegaly, but he speculatively raises the question whether the endocrine disturbance of acromegaly and the emotional and other psychological disturbances may not, as in other fields of psychosomatic medicine, be merely different aspects of a single life process. To support this hypothesis, Bleuler calls attention to the fact that it is now conceded that psychogenetic factors are of importance in many forms of hyperthyroid disorders, in Cushing's disease, and in other endocrine derangements.

METABOLIC DISTURBANCES

Porphyria

This condition, first described in 1911 by Günther, is a constitutional metabolic disorder resulting in the production of abnormal types of porphyria which appear in the urine. Porphyria is classified as the erythropoietic (congenital) type and the hepatic type. Of the latter there have been described acute intermittent, cutaneous, hereditary and mixed, latent hereditary, idiosyncratic cutaneous, and acquired forms. The congenital type is seen only in childhood, and the mixed has mostly dermatological symptoms. The acute intermittent type is the one with which mental symptoms are most frequently associated. In this form acute attacks are precipitated often by such agents as the barbiturates, sulfonal, trional, chloroquine, and even alcohol. Hexachlorobenzene, a fungicide, has been implicated as a causal agent in one acquired form.

The acute intermittent type is commonly familial and thought to be inherited through a mendelian dominant trait. Congenital porphyria, on the other hand, appears to be transmitted as a mendelian recessive.

Biochemically, it has been suggested that inhibited synthesis of purines with overproduction of porphyrins and their precursors takes place as a consequence of poisoning of the succinate glycine cycle. In this cycle, α-amino levulinic acid is the common precursor of both porphyrins and purines. Inhibition of the oxidative deamination of this acid may block purine synthesis and lead to overproduction of the porphyrins. The biochemical explanation remains to be confirmed. Dean recently has stated that in the acute intermittent type the urinary porphobilinogen and α-amino levulinic acid levels continue at high levels for years, in contrast to the mixed or variegate form. On the other hand, coproporphyrin and protoporphyrin excretions in the stool are raised only during the acute attack, in contrast to the condition in the mixed form.

Pathologically the changes in the nervous system consist of patchy areas of demyelination with or without the destruction of axis cylinders, particularly in the spinal nerves. Retrograde degeneration of the motor cells occurs in the central nervous system and the sympathetic ganglia. These findings are inconstant and nonspecific. In rapidly fatal cases no changes may be evident in the central nervous system. The liver may show fatty degeneration, cirrhosis, or cell injury. In the hematopoietic type the bone marrow is hyperplastic and normoblastic. Splenomegaly and hemolytic anemia exist. The teeth may be reddish brown, as are the bones, as a result of uroporphyrin deposit.

Symptoms and Signs

Porphyria occurs much more frequently in women than in men. The disease may be suspected in a patient who presents a combination of abdominal, neurological, psychiatric and, at times, dermatological symptoms. The acute attack often starts with colicky abdominal pain, sometimes associated with nausea, vomiting, and constipation. The gastrointestinal symptoms often suggest appendicitis, with the result that laparotomy is performed. The patient continues to complain bitterly of abdominal pain and becomes anxious, irritable, argumentative, and perhaps obviously psychotic. As the disease progresses, the patient loses much weight and may become quite cachectic.

Psychiatric manifestations are varied and may be the most prominent presenting symptoms. They are probably due to a direct, possibly reversible, metabolic effect of the disease. They usually precede the neurologic symptoms. Agitation, depression, and disturbances of memory and of the sensorium, with delirious and psychotic-like hallucinatory and delusional experiences, are among the most common symptoms.

The neurological manifestations are greatly varied. Perhaps the most frequent are motor weaknesses, which may be irregularly distributed but are most frequent in the extremities and less so in the muscles of the trunk and abdomen and in the muscles innervated by the cranial nerves. Of the latter, the facial and oculomotor muscles are most often involved. The motor weaknesses may be accompanied by severe pain and paresthesias, but there is usually little or no objective sensory disturbance. The paralysis is flaccid, and tendon reflexes are usually absent or depressed. Convulsions may occur. Cases of both receptive and expressive aphasia have been reported. Bulbar involvement with dysphonia, dysphagia, tachycardia, and respiratory and vasomotor dysfunction may occur.

Tachycardia develops in some cases within a few days of onset of the initiating psychiatric and abdominal symptoms and precedes usually by several weeks the onset of neuropathy. When the latter occurs the tachycardia increases as the neurological signs expand, disappearing as they subside. It has been suggested that the tachycardia may be due to autonomic cardioneuropathy.

The following case report illustrates the acute intermittent form.

A woman registered for examination at a medical clinic at the age of 40 with a history of five attacks of pain in the right upper quadrant of the abdomen during the previous eight months. The attacks of pain were described as continuing from a half hour to two hours. Results of the general physical examination were essentially normal. A cholecystogram made at this time was reported as disclosing nothing abnormal. A brief note by the medical consultant suggested the existence of an emotional disturbance associated with an unsatisfactory marital relationship. The diagnosis of porphyria was not made at this time.

A history was obtained of brief attacks of pain in the right upper quadrant of the abdomen recurring periodically over a period of 11 years. The present attack began 10 days before the patient's visit to the clinic. This attack was more severe than usual, was accompanied by fever, and persisted much longer. The severity of the pain was such that for the first time the patient allowed her physician to administer narcotic agents by hypodermic injection. These consisted of one tablet of scopolamine and morphine administered nine days before admission and 100 mg. of meperidine hydrochloride (Demerol) on the following days, when she was placed in a hospital elsewhere. No further sedatives were administered. Penicillin was given and plans were made to remove her gallbladder after the fever had subsided. The patient and her family, because of their religious beliefs, were opposed to this or any surgical procedure. Four days before her clinic visit her family noticed that she wrote unusual letters and displayed peculiar, incessant to-and-fro movements of her hands and arms to the extent that she had no rest. She withdrew from contact with others. The day before her admission to the clinic she refused to accept food or fluids.

At the time of her registration, the patient held herself in a rigid position, with her right arm stiffly raised in a cataleptic pose. Her hands were clenched tightly, and her eyes were closed, and she muttered incoherently. When she was spoken to, she closed her eyes more tightly and repeated in a rhythmic way, "Are they laughing at her?" She resisted attempts to change her position by strong muscular contractions wherever she was touched. When she was left alone, she opened her eyes; occasional jerky, sucking movements of her mouth were observed. Results of the neurological examination were essentially negative. With great difficulty she was examined by a surgeon, who found no evidence of an acute abdominal lesion.

The patient's history was obtained from the husband. She was the eighth of 11 children. The father was alcoholic until 15 years before his death at 85 (four years prior to the time of this report). The parents' attitude toward surgical treatment had always been, "What God put there was meant

to stay." The patient had repeatedly refused cholecystectomy. She had been in good health except for the repeated attacks of pain in the right upper abdominal quadrant previously mentioned. Information about the patient's relatives indicated that in general they had lived to advanced age and had been free of abdominal complaints and mental symptoms.

During her first seven days in the hospital, repeated physical examinations failed to disclose abnormalities except for the behavior disturbance. The patient's temperature remained persistently elevated between 99.6° and 102.8° F. Oliguria was present. The specific gravity of the urine was 1.030. Grade 4 albuminuria was noted. The value for urea nitrogen was 68 mg. per 100 ml. of blood. After the subcutaneous administration of fluids, the output of urine increased and there occurred a decrease in the content of albumin in the urine and a rapid decrease in the level of the blood urea nitrogen. On the third hospital day, qualitative study of the urinary porphyrins showed no uroporphyrins, but the presence of coproporphyrin. On the fourth and fifth hospital days, the patient was mute. On the sixth day she was either crying out incoherently or whispering and muttering unintelligibly. On this day the diagnosis of porphyria was established by the detection of porphobilinogen in the urine. (Quantitative porphyrin test, 24 units; uroporphyrin, none; porphobilinogen, 2.6 Ehrlich units; coproporphyrin, 333 μg.)

The patient's rectal temperature reached 105° F on the seventh hospital day. She remained withdrawn, mute, and uncommunicative until the twelfth hospital day, when she began to talk irrelevantly. Visual and auditory hallucinations occurred on the fourteenth hospital day. She sang and talked incoherently and screamed for long periods. She soiled and smeared herself with feces. She spoke of being crucified, of sinning so terribly that she would never be forgiven, and of committing sexual misdemeanors. On the nineteenth hospital day, results of qualitative tests for urinary porphyrins were reported negative. The behavior disturbance remained unchanged.

Electroshock treatment was initiated on the twentieth hospital day. Immediately after this treatment, the patient inquired as to where she was and what she was doing. She declared she wished "to get better." Following the second electroshock treatment she began to eat without assistance. She declared that she had burning sensations (paresthesias) and complained of pains in the distal portions of her extremities. Her verbal production still indicated suspicion and misinterpretation of her environment.

Six electroshock treatments were administered between the twentieth and thirtieth hospital days. After the fourth treatment the patient's temperature again became normal. She was oriented and was able to recall recent and past events except for the period of acute illness, although she did not recall her fright and some of the hallucinations which occurred in this period. At this time there was slight increase in the sensitivity of her feet to touch and pinprick. She was returned to her home 33 days after admission.

DIAGNOSIS. The diagnosis depends upon the finding in the urine of uroporphyrin or porphobilinogen, or both, in excess. Porphobilinogen is found only in patients showing combined abdominal and nervous manifestations. With the excretion of large amounts of uroporphyrin, the urine attracts attention because of its characteristic red, port-wine color. Spectroscopic examination readily permits identification of the uroporphyrin. It is important to stress the fact that the presence of reddish urine is by no means a general rule. Frequently a fresh urine specimen is nearly normal in color, while in other instances it is light yellow or dark amber. When porphyria is suspected, it is unwise to discard a sample of urine merely because it fails to show the characteristic port-wine color. Such specimens should be kept in the light; they will then darken, and appropriate laboratory tests for uroporphyrin may be performed. Porphobilinogen may be detected in fresh urine by means of the Ehrlich aldehyde test. Excessive coproporphyrin may be found in such urines. Recently α-amino levulinic acid has been found also.

The triad of variable abdomen pain, gradually increasing paralysis of the arms and legs, and toxic-organic mental symptoms should suggest the possibility of this rather uncommon and frequently misdiagnosed disease.

PROGNOSIS. The outlook for life is relatively good in the erythropoietic and in the dermatological or photosensitive types; in the intermittent acute variety the mortality is relatively high, particularly in those with symptoms referable to the bulbar nervous system.

TREATMENT. Chlorpromazine is the most helpful remedy thus far available in the treatment of acute porphyria. It does not affect established paralyses, may not prevent fatalities from bulbar or respiratory paralyses, and does not appear to influence porphyrin metabolism directly.

At the outset it may be necessary to give as much as 100 mg. four to six times in 24 hours intramuscularly; however, it is usually possible to reduce this dose quite rapidly and often to discontinue it entirely. There are some cases in which a small maintenance dose is necessary. Electric shock therapy has been tried in several patients with psychotic symptomatology, and the response has been variable. Conflicting reports have been expressed concerning the effectiveness of cortisone and of corticotropin (ACTH). Alcohol, barbiturates, and other toxic agents should be avoided. It is important also that emotional stresses be alleviated, as these are often decisive in precipitating attacks.

Hepatolenticular Degeneration

This rare condition, described by S. A. K. Wilson in 1912, is associated almost invariably in its later course with evidence of personality disorder. In some instances, emotional lability or even gross behavioral deviations are the most prominent early symptoms. It has been, and is, most likely to be confused with schizophrenia, with paranoid, hypomanic, and depression reactions, and with hysteria.

Hepatolenticular degeneration is the result of chronic copper intoxication. It is caused by an inherited metabolic defect causing abnormal storage of copper in the liver, brain, and kidneys. The inheritance occurs as an autosomal recessive with gene frequencies computed at 1/200 and 1/500. It is associated with a deficiency of the copper-containing globulin ceruloplasmin in the blood. Ceruloplasmin does not appear to be a transport protein for the metal.

Characterized by degenerative changes in both brain and liver, it is associated in over half of those affected with a characteristic greenish yellow ring seen on the undersurface of the cornea near its margin (the Kayser-Fleischer ring). Hepatolenticular degeneration appears to be inherited as a recessive character and represents a primary metabolic defect.

SYMPTOMS.   The illness may occur in a rapidly progressive form, which commences most commonly in childhood and early adolescence, terminating in death after a few months or several years. Emotional lability of the pseudobulbar type (forced crying and laughing), thought of as childishness, and behavioral disorders occur with the development of dysarthria and dysphagia, slowing of voluntary movements, rigidity, and dystonic movements. The acute type is often associated with fever.

Those cases developing in later adolescence or early adulthood more frequently run a prolonged course, without fever, and are characterized by tremulousness, titubation, later contractures, and sometimes convulsive seizures, with eventual evidence of general cerebral insufficiency. These are the patients whose personality disturbances resemble the schizophrenic, hypomanic, and hysterical reactions. Untoward expressions of hostility, temper tantrums, antisocial behavior, and delusional and hallucinatory experiences may occur. The tremor is characteristic, most often involving the distal portion of the extremities. It becomes progressively more violent. When the arms are extended, it appears as though the patient were waving his hands (wing beating).

There is usually little evidence of hepatitis, although occasionally jaundice may precede the illness. The liver is seldom enlarged.

DIAGNOSIS.   In addition to the various clinical symptoms and the presence of the Kayser-Fleischer corneal ring, there exist an increased urinary excretion of copper and amino acids and a diminution in serum ceruloplasmin. While a concentration of less than 20 mg. per 100 ml. is almost always diagnostic of the disorder, occasional patients with severe liver disease have normal ceruloplasmin concentrations. So, too, a biochemical diagnosis of Wilson's disease may be made in asymptomatic members of families carrying the pathogenic gene. This diagnosis allows the institution of early preventive therapy, as Sternlieb and Scheinberg have reported.

Determination by whole body reactivity for three or four weeks after intravenous injections of 60 Cu of prolonged retention of the metal, in the absence of cirrhosis, has been demonstrated as determinative of carrier status. Combined external probe radioactivity studies of uptake of copper in liver and muscle have been suggested as a means of determining whether the individual is a homozygote or heterozygote carrier. Minor symptoms of nausea and anorexia may precede or accompany the neuropsychiatric disturbance. More recently it has been found in x-ray studies that many patients with Wilson's disease have osteomalacia with pseudofractures and marginal bone fragmentation resembling the changes in the Fanconi syndrome.

PATHOLOGY.   There is gross degeneration of the lenticular nuclei, particularly in the putamen and caudate nuclei. Histologically, neuronal degeneration with loss or pathological changes is found not only in the cells of the basal ganglia but also in those of the cerebral cortex and cerebellum. There are generally nodular cirrhosis of the liver and splenomegaly. Excessive deposition of copper is found in the brain, liver, Descemet's membrane of the cornea, and other organs. It appears that an excessive absorption of copper takes place from the intestinal tract. It has been suggested that the excessive copper is toxic due to a blocking effect on coenzyme A or a related enzyme which leads to disturbed pyruvate metabolism.

TREATMENT.   The preferred treatment today is by penicillamine (cuprimine), a chelating agent which promotes excretion of copper. It should be prescribed as D-penicillamine in divided oral doses totaling between 1 and 4 gm. daily. It is necessary to maintain an effective negative copper balance in order to bring about continuing therapeutic improvement. This requires repetitive copper balance studies at six- to twelve-month intervals to determine necessary changes in dosage of penicillamine and intake of copper. On carefully regulated regimens with continued penicillamine therapy and reduction of copper intake, a recession of psychiatric, neurologic, and hepatic symptoms takes place, along with a rise in capacity to perform in psychological tests. Since this agent sometimes causes fever, cutaneous eruptions, and, less commonly, hematological and renal reactions, close medical supervision is needed. With continued penicillamine therapy there are a regular recession of neurological symptoms and a variable response in the psychiatric and hepatic disturbances. The Kayser-Fleischer rings recede and the cupriuria diminishes.

In patients sensitive to penicillamine one may prescribe weekly intramuscular injections of 2,3-dimercaptopropanol (BAL or British anti-lewisite) in doses of 1.0 to 1.5 ml. of 10 per cent solution in peanut oil, to be given indefinitely. In order to reduce the absorption of copper in the diet, 20 mg. of enteric-coated capsules of potassium sulfide should be given with each meal, in association with a diet low in copper-containing foods.

VITAMIN DEFICIENCY SYNDROMES

In recent years it has been recognized that there is a common factor operative in various mental and neurological phenomena which had been previously regarded as unrelated entities. This common factor is a vitamin deficiency, particularly a deficiency of vitamin B. The localization of the pathological process produced in different parts of the nervous system by the deficiency determines the neurological signs and releases the mental symptoms. The nature of the symptom or syndrome depends upon the particular member of the B complex in which the deficiency is relatively greatest and upon the part of the nervous system predominantly affected by the deficiency. If the deficiency of nicotinic acid is greatest, the clinical picture produced is that of pellagra. If, as is not rare, a peripheral "neuritis" is also observed, a deficiency of thiamine exists associated or if a Korsakoff syndrome is also. If, because of chronic alcoholism, the

patient suffers from thiamine deficiency, he may suffer from a painful thiamine neuropathy, or "alcoholic neuritis." If at the same time there is a nerve cell degeneration in the cerebral cortex resulting from deficiency of another member (or members) of the B complex (probably niacin), the patient will present an alcoholic Korsakoff syndrome.

Wernicke's Syndrome

In 1881 Wernicke described a syndrome consisting of ophthalmoplegia, memory loss, confabulation, apathy, progressive dementia, ataxia, clouding of consciousness, and even coma. It is now known that it is invariably associated with thiamine deficiency and that usually there is a deficiency of niacin also. Because of the thiamine avitaminosis, there is an impaired oxidation of pyruvic acid, which is formed during the breakdown of glucose. As a result, pyruvic acid accumulates in the blood.

Wernicke's "encephalitis" mainly affects chronic alcoholics but has also been described in pernicious anemia, hyperemesis gravidarum, and gastric cancer, and in prisoners of war. Delirium usually precedes its development. The Wernicke syndrome, formerly observed occasionally in pernicious vomiting of pregnancy or after abdominal or pelvic operations when solutions of glucose were administered in considerable amounts, is now seen much less frequently, apparently because thiamine is given with the glucose as a usual procedure. This syndrome has almost disappeared since 1942. This disappearance is ascribed to the fact that enrichment of bread and flour began in that year.

The pathological changes are mainly in the brain stem and involve the mammillary bodies and the regions adjacent to the aqueduct and to the third and fourth ventricles. The lesions are characterized by various degrees of necrosis of both nerve cells and nerve fibers, together with reactive changes of microglia and astrocytes, alteration of small blood vessels, and, in some instances, petechial hemorrhages.

The ocular disturbances take the form of horizontal and vertical nystagmus and various degrees of paralysis of conjugate gaze and of the external recti.

H. B., aged 62, a chronic alcoholic who had been arrested many times for drunkenness, was taken to a general hospital because of confusion and difficulty in walking. There was a history that following a long alcoholic debauch he had been taken into custody by the Salvation Army. For several days the supervision of this organization made it impossible for him to secure alcohol. He then remained at its hotel for several days more, performing light duties until his physical disabilities made employment impossible. Soon after entering the general hospital he became confused, restless, demanding, and was noisy at night. He was then transferred to a psychiatric hospital where the confusion soon subsided. On neurological examination, he showed marked bilateral ptosis, his pupils reacted very slightly to light, and he was totally unable to follow a light in any direction. His speech was thick and slurred; there was a great defect in coördination of his extremities; all tendon reflexes, except the biceps, were absent. The calves of both legs were tender, and he was unable to walk unaided. A diagnosis of Wernicke's syndrome plus peripheral neuritis was made. He was at once placed on large doses of thiamine. He soon began to improve, but the evidence of ophthalmoplegia did not completely disappear for seven months.

If the thiamine deficiency produces peripheral neuropathy, cardiac hypertrophy, myocardial weakness, and edema, the clinical manifestation is that of beriberi, a form of deficiency without mental accompaniment. Beriberi may, however, be associated with Wernicke's encephalopathy. An uncomplicated thiamine deficiency without any associated neurological phenomena may produce a neurasthenic syndrome characterized by feelings of weakness, easy fatigue, emotional instability, irritability, moodiness, quarrelsomeness, forgetfulness, apathy, mild depression, and vague fears. These symptoms soon disappear after the intake of thiamine is increased.

In nutritional encephalopathy, there is almost never a single vitamin deficiency. In the same individual one may see delirium tremens (the cause of delirium tremens is uncertain, but it is probably a result of a disturbance of cerebral metabolism incident to vitamin deficiency), Korsakoff's psychosis, nicotinic acid encephalopathy (pellagra), and the Wernicke syndrome. There may also be a neuropathy in the form of an "alcoholic neuritis."

Pellagra

Pellagra was first described in 1735 by a Spanish physician, Gasper Casal, under the name *mal de la rosa*. He attributed the disease to a poor diet, but not until 1915 was its dietary origin conclusively demonstrated by Goldberger. In 1937 it was discovered that nicotinic acid (niacin) is the pellagra-preventive vitamin. The principal deficiency, therefore, is in nicotinic acid, although it appears that the disease may also result from a deficiency in the amino acid, tryptophan. Usually there are also other associated deficiencies, particularly of thiamine and riboflavin. Often, too, there is a deficiency of ascorbic acid. Many of the neurological symptoms in pellagra are presumably a result of the associated thiamine deficiency.

Pellagra occurs most frequently in communities where the prevailing low economic status leads to extensive nutritional deficiencies. Isolated cases occur among chronic alcoholics whose food has consisted largely of alcohol and has therefore been deficient in vitamin B complex. It is not rare in aged, destitute people who, living alone and in deprivation, suffer from vitamin deficiency. Sporadic cases may also occur in persons suffering from intestinal lesions that interfere with the absorption of food.

It should not be forgotten that pellagra may develop in persons who are already psychotic. This was formerly common in institutions for mental diseases. With more abundant and better-balanced diets, such institutional cases are no longer common.

MORBID ANATOMY. There is but little experimental evidence indicating that uncomplicated niacin deficiency results in injury to the nervous system. In well-developed cases, neuronal and capillary changes are found distributed throughout the neuraxis, usually most marked in the cerebrum. In the frontal lobes and in the hippocampus, the ganglion cells lose their Nissl substance and may eventually disappear. There may be proliferation of glia cells and of capillary endothelium. The similarity of these changes to those of Meyer's "central neuritis" and to those of Wernicke's syndrome has long been noted. There now seems reason to believe that the same factor is common to all these conditions, that the histopathological changes in all of them are caused by thiamine deficiency or by a polyavitaminosis of the vitamin B complex, since it is known that single vitamin deficiencies rarely if ever occur. Until the pathological changes become somewhat advanced, they are reversible.

SYMPTOMS. The early mental symptoms of pellagra are often regarded as psychoneurotic and consist of vague headache, irritability, difficulty in concentration, forgetfulness, restlessness, apprehension, and a feeling of inability for mental or physical effort. These early symptoms are followed by those of an organic syndrome and consist of memory defects, confusion, disorientation, intermittent delirium, Korsakoff's syndrome, and dementia. Some patients show a manic excitement, while others may be depressed, anxious, apprehensive, or paranoid. Although organically released, the particular type of such reactions will be determined by the patient's previous personality pattern. Later in the disease there may be evidence of irreversible neurological impairment resulting from advanced encephalopathy. This may be in the form of stupor, convulsions, incontinence, muscular rigidity, irregular involuntary movements, hypertonia, defective sensation, and muscle paralysis.

Mild mental symptoms are usually the first evidence of pellagra, but after some months these are followed by stomatitis and by glossitis; the tongue is red and painful and the papillae are atrophic. Digestive disturbances with achlorhydria and diarrhea are common. An early erythema of the skin is followed by coarse scaling and a deep red-brown pigmentation. The dermatitis occurs characteristically on the extensor surfaces of the extremities and on the vulva and inner surfaces of the thighs.

PROGNOSIS. If treatment is begun early before irreversible neuronal changes have taken place, the prognosis is good, but in neglected cases, permanent impairment of memory and persistent dementia result.

TREATMENT. Mild, ambulatory cases of pellagra are relieved by 100-mg. doses of niacin or niacinamide given three to six times a day. In extremely severe cases the patient should receive 1200 to 1500 mg. a day for several days. Sodium nicotinate may be given intravenously or intramuscularly in 100-mg. doses. Parenteral liver extract given intramuscularly in doses of 20 cc. three to five times daily is indicated in severe cases. Since a thiamine deficiency usually coexists, this vitamin should also be given. The patient should receive from 40 to 200 gm. of powdered brewers' yeast daily, best tolerated in iced milk. The diet should be liberal and include a quart of milk daily, wheat germ, lean meat, liver, and such vegetables as lettuce, spinach, asparagus, fresh peas, cabbage, and tomatoes. Diets high in carbohydrate and fat are contraindicated. The patient should receive and retain a well-balanced diet of approximately 4000 calories daily.

Pernicious Anemia

Although Addison in his original descriptions of pernicious anemia in 1849 and 1855 spoke of the occasional "wandering of the mind," the mental disorders associated with the disease have received less attention than have the associated neurological disturbances incident to the accompanying degeneration in the spinal cord, first recognized by Lichtheim in 1886. Mental symptoms of depression, anxiety, loss of libido, irritability, poor concentration, and impaired memory occur from moderate to severe and have been noted in as high as a third of untreated patients.

In Shulman's recent study of those depressed with pernicious anemia, there occurred a high incidence of personal or familial history of depression. These symptoms are probably secondary to disturbances in cerebral metabolism. With the effective and early treatment now available, these symptoms are encountered less frequently. Mental symptoms may be present alone or in association with cord disturbances.

MORBID ANATOMY. Degenerative foci in the white matter of the brain similar to the degenerative plaques in the cord were first demonstrated by Barrett, although they are not always present. Areas of degeneration occur also in the gray matter, the pyramidal cells undergoing disintegration, with the presence of rod cells and other changes, particularly an increase in glia, increase in lipoid products in cells, swelling and proliferation of intimal cells in cerebral blood vessels, and miliary hemorrhages. The pathological changes, both in their location and in their nature, are suggestive of those found in Wernicke's encephalopathy.

SYMPTOMS. The time of onset of mental symptoms in relation to the course of pernicious anemia is variable. Although any associated psychosis was formerly thought to be a terminal condition, it is now recognized that mental symptoms may also occur early, even before the typical blood picture of pernicious anemia is established. Except sometimes in the case of confusion, there is no relationship between the degree of anemia and the intensity of the mental symptoms. Although there is no mental syndrome characteristic of pernicious anemia, the mental picture tends to fall into one of the following groups: acute delirioid state, paranoid condition, affective reaction, and organic deterioration. Probably the organic changes release a psychosis, the type of which is predetermined by previous psychogenic factors and psychological mechanisms.

Organic Deterioration. In patients with the organic deterioration syndrome, there is a gradual disintegration of intellectual functions, with impairment of memory and judgment and, at times, periods of confusion.

TREATMENT. Symptoms of delirium and memory impairment improve with liberal doses of liver extract or with vitamin B_{12}. Both should be administered parenterally. During the first week of treatment, 30 μg. of vitamin B_{12} or its equivalent as liver injection USP should be given intramuscularly each day. Thereafter the same dose is given twice weekly. After two months, if the response is satisfactory, a single injection every other week is sufficient.

The depressive states with pernicious anemia are unrelated directly to vitamin B_{12} deficiency. But recovery from the physical effects of the illness leads to relief of the affective reaction.

Acute Vitamin Deficiency Syndrome

Chronic mental syndromes frequently accompany cases of chronic avitaminosis, particularly in thiamine deficiency, but acute mental syndromes are quite uncommon. Jolliffe, however, called attention to what he named "acute nicotinic acid deficiency encephalopathy." This syndrome is characterized by delirium, sucking and grasping reflexes, cogwheel rigidities, and irregular jerking movements of the extremities. This readily disappears after treatment with niacin.

EXHAUSTION DELIRIUM

At times acute, confusional, delirioid reactions accompany marked states of exhaustion. Since such reactions are not associated with infection, they may best be considered in a discussion of acute syndromes resulting from disturbances of metabolism. Exhaustion delirium is not common but it may occur occasionally, associated with hemorrhage, unusual and extremely prostrating physical exertion, starvation, prolonged insomnia under conditions of stress or emotional tension, and debilitating effects of emotional tension and effects of a chronic wasting disease such as carcinoma. This acute hallucinatory confusion (*"confusion mentale"*) was described by Chaslin under the term "primary mental confusion" and by Meynert under the designation "amentia," a term still applied to this syndrome by English and German but not by American psychiatrists, who occasionally employ the word as synonymous with feeblemindedness.

The onset is usually with insomnia, some clouding of consciousness, mild confusion, difficulty in collecting one's thoughts, perplexity, perhaps of a distressed type, vague fears, restlessness, illusions, fleeting hallucinations, and changing delusions. The patient's mood varies with his thought content. The environment appears obscure and distorted. As the condition increases in severity, the patient becomes more bewildered; his perceptions are more impaired; he misidentifies persons and objects and becomes disoriented. Sometimes speech is of a question-and-answer form. Frequently the patient may seem to be groping in a mental fog, as if attempting to differentiate his confused, dreamlike world from that of reality and gain a point of contact with his previous normal life. Sometimes he may be comparatively clear for a period, only to return to his previous confusion.

This confusional toxic-exhaustive state may continue for several weeks, but recovery finally takes place. After his recovery, the patient may be able to give considerable retrospective interpretation of his delusions and hallucinatory experiences.

BIBLIOGRAPHY

Bleuler, M.: Endokrinologische Psychiatrie. Stuttgart, Georg Thieme Verlag, 1954.

ENDOCRINE DISORDERS
Adrenal

Moorhead, E. L., Caldwell, J. R., Kelly, H. R., and Morales, A. R.: The diagnosis of pheochromocytoma. J.A.M.A., *196:*1107–1133, 1966.

Trethowan, W. H., and Cobb, S.: Neuropsychiatric aspects of Cushing's syndrome. Arch. Neurol. & Psychiat., *67:*283–309, 1952.

Pancreas

Fras, I., Litin, E. M., and Pearson, J. S.: Comparison of psychiatric symptoms in carcinoma of the pancreas and those in some other intra-abdominal neoplasm. Amer. J. Psychiat., *123:*1553–1562, 1967.

Rynearson, E. H.: Hyperinsulinism among malingerers. Med. Clin. N. Amer., *31:*477–480, 1947.

Schuster, M. M., and Iber, F. L.: Psychosis with pancreatitis. Arch. Int. Med., *116:*228–233, 1965.

Parathyroid

Denko, J. D., and Kaebling, R.: The psychiatric aspects of hypoparathyroidism. Acta Psychiat. Scand., *38,* Suppl. 164, 1964.

Reilly, E. L., and Wilson, W. P.: Mental symptoms in hyperparathyroidism. Dis. Nerv. Syst., *26:*361–363, 1965.

Thyroid

Flagg, G. W., Clemens, T. L., Michael, E. A., Alexander, F., and Wark, J.: A psychophysiological investigation of hyperthyroidism. Psychosom. Med., *27:*497–507, 1965.

METABOLIC DISORDERS

Porphyria

Ridley, A., Hierons, R., and Cavannaugh, J. B.: Tachycardia and neuropathy of porphyria. Lancet, *2:*708–709, 1968.

Hepatolenticular Degeneration

Goldstein, N. P., Ewert, J. C., Randall, R. V., and Gross, J. B.: Psychiatric aspects of Wilson's disease (hepatolenticular degeneration): Results of psychometric tests during long term therapy. Amer. J. Psychiat., *124:*1555–1561, 1968.

Goldstein, N. P., Tauxe, W. N., McCall, J. T., Gross, J. B., and Randall, R. V.: Treatment of

Wilson's disease (hepatolenticular degeneration) with penicillamine and low copper diet. Trans. Amer. Neur. Assoc., *94*:34–37, 1969.

O'Reilly, S., Weber, P. M., Pollycove, M., and Shipley, L.: Detection of the carrier of Wilson's disease. Neurology, *20*:1133–1138, 1970.

Sternlieb, I., and Scheinberg, I. H.: Prevention of Wilson's disease in asymptomatic patients. New England J. Med., *278*:352–359, 1968.

Walshe, J. M.: Wilson's disease. Biochem. J., *111:* 8P-9P, 1969.

NUTRITIONAL DEFICIENCIES

Shulman, R.: Psychiatric aspects of pernicious anemia: A prospective study. Brit. Med. J., *3:* 266–269, 1967.

Chapter 18

Brain Syndromes Resulting from Drug or Poison Intoxication

As described in Chapter 9, toxic substances may interrupt the multiple processes of general cerebral metabolism in a variety of ways. The associated clinical syndrome is that of cerebral insufficiency with various symptomatic expressions, depending upon the degree and suddenness of interruption of ego functions, the extent of permanent cellular damage, and the varieties of adaption to loss of function peculiar to the individual personality.

Such brain syndromes are frequently complications of modern medical therapy or represent the secondary effects of suicidal attempts, self-medication, or industrial poisoning. Again, in this day of heavy pollution of the environment through open disposal of industrial wastes, the syndrome may result from intake of toxic quantities of substances through inhalation, ingestion, or absorption.

Removed from this chapter is the description of the acute and chronic brain syndromes consequent to experimentation with, dependence upon, or habituation or addiction to the now widely abused sedatives (the barbiturates and other "minor tranquilizers"), stimulants such as the amphetamines, and the hallucinogens. The description of these clinical syndromes and their outcome and the treatment of intoxication by these substances will be found in Chapter 27.

Cortisone and ACTH

These agents may produce a wide variety of mental disturbances, resulting, ap-
parently, from their direct effect upon the central nervous system, although the precise pathogenetic mechanisms are not yet determined. The total energy exchange of the brain as measured by cerebral metabolic rate does not seem to be altered by ACTH or by cortisone, yet these hormones disturb enzymatic reactions by altering the electrolyte and water patterns of the body. In general, the mental reactions do not exhibit the type of confusion, disorientation, and sensorial disturbance characteristic of toxic psychoses. Nearly all patients receiving the drugs show an increased joviality and optimism. Among the common disturbances are affective ones varying from depression to hypomania, also from apathy to panic, and even inappropriateness of affect. Feelings of depersonalization, or a sense of detachment or strangeness in awareness of one's body image, may occur. Disturbances of speech are frequent and may vary from mutism to flight of ideas. Illusions and hallucinations may occur, as also do delusions of depressive, grandiose, or persecutory types. A wide variety of motor disturbances may appear, including immobility, pressure of activity, and regressiveness. In general the type of mental disturbance produced by the drug seems to be determined by the basic pattern or structure of the patient's personality. Complete spontaneous recovery occurs upon discontinuance of the drug. In prolonged cases, lucid intervals of gradually increasing frequency and duration may occur until a normal state is fully established.

Experience has shown that the occurrence of a psychiatric disturbance with use of the corticosteroids does not indicate that a similar disturbance will take place if the steroid is withheld and then administered again at a later date. Nor is there clear evidence that these reactions are related to dosage.

Isoniazid

With the increasing use of this drug for the treatment of tuberculosis, a number of cases of mental disturbance have been observed associated with its administration. The clinical picture is that of an acute, toxic, confusional disorientation for time, place, person, and situation, restlessness, and auditory or visual hallucinations. It is usually preceded by muscular twitching, hyperreflexia, difficulty in micturition, constipation, and sometimes convulsions. Occasionally this toxic state is followed by signs of an organic cerebral impairment of the Korsakoff type. It has been stated that the toxic mental symptoms are related to the plasma level of the drug and that the majority of psychotic reactions occur in patients receiving more than 8 mg. of isoniazid per kilogram of body weight daily. Pyridoxine in large doses may prevent the appearance of isoniazid neuritis. This agent is not effective in reversing symptoms once they are established.

Sulfonamides ("Sulfa" Drugs)

The administration of sulfa drugs may at times cause headache, dizziness, confusion, bewilderment, inability to concentrate, and hallucinosis.

Thiocyanates

The continuing use of thiocyanates in the treatment of hypertensive disease with the occurrence of toxic mental symptoms must be kept in mind. Levels of blood thiocyanate that exceed 15 mg. per 100 ml. are likely to produce toxic reactions. It has been shown that thiocyanates are converted to cyanide in the body, and this cellular poison probably leads to depression of utilization of oxygen by inhibition of cytochrome oxidase. The consequent oxygen lack in the cerebral cortex leads to the production of the delirious reactions as well as to other symptoms, such as convulsions, ataxia, aphasia, and paraplegia. The usual toxic mental symptoms are incoherent muttering, slurring of speech, confusion, disorientation, auditory and visual hallucinations, restlessness, agitation, resistance, ideas of persecution, and convulsions. Several deaths have been reported. In addition to withholding the thiocyanate, a trial with methylene blue or sodium thiosulfate is probably worthwhile. It has been suggested that hydroxycobalamine (vitamin B_{12}) may serve as a potent antidote.

CLINICAL REPORT. The following case illustrates thiocyanate intoxication:

A 59-year-old housewife, admitted as an emergency case, complained of "pain all over." She claimed she was paralyzed, yet tossed restlessly about on the ambulance cot. She was confused and unable to give a coherent story. Her daughter said the illness started with a severe dizzy spell that had occurred two months earlier. Her home physician had found that her blood pressure was "over 300," and had prescribed some red tablets. She had continued to take the medicine until she came to the hospital, although at no time had a blood test been made. Three weeks prior to admission, general weakness, tremor of the hands, somnolence, tinnitus, and blurring of vision had developed. These symptoms had become progressively more severe in the meantime.

On physical examination, the patient complained volubly of unbearable tenderness in all her muscles. Her systolic blood pressure was 150 mm. and the diastolic 80 mm. Hg. There were narrowing and sclerosis of the retinal arterioles. No neurological deficit was detected, although the weakness she described was confirmed.

The concentration of thiocyanate in the blood was 17.6 mg. per 100 ml., and a diagnosis of thiocyanate psychosis was made. On mental examination, she was depressed, withdrawn, negativistic, and distractible. Delusional, self-derogatory thinking was disclosed by her statements that other patients regarded her as a germ carrier and her physicians thought she was a nuisance and wanted to "fumigate" her. Hallucinations were not evident. She spoke haltingly and cried easily. She was disoriented as to time but not as to place or person. She was unable to repeat more than five digits forward and none backward. Simple multiplication was impossible, and she was unable to subtract serial sevens. Her memory was severely impaired for both recent and past events.

With a high intake of fluid, the signs of toxic delirium subsided rapidly. The concentration of blood thiocyanate decreased to 8.7 mg. per 100 ml. by the eleventh day in the hospital, and there was only mild residual tenderness in the calves of her legs. When she was dismissed on the twentieth day, her blood pressure was 150/90, and she was free of symptoms.

Lead

ETIOLOGY. Of the various metallic poisons, lead is the one with which mental symptoms are most frequently associated. Both the source of intoxication with lead and the clinical picture differ considerably in adults and children. With adults the inhalation of toxic lead compounds is the major means of intoxication. Recently, the necessity of considering lead encephalopathy as a complication of chronic alcoholism has been suggested by discovery of this condition in individuals consuming large quantities of illicitly produced alcohol in communities of the southern United States. For the most part, patients with the lead encephalopathy–alcohol withdrawal complex have come from the lower socio-economic black groups in these communities. In infants poisoning occurs through the eating or chewing of lead-containing paint, often picked up in flakes peeling from woodwork or painted surfaces. The habit of *pica* in children is frequently associated with mental deficiency, but it occurs also in children of good intellectual endowment who show some emotional disturbance. In adults the history of exposure in industry or building to paint spraying, burning of lead in salvage operations, the oxygas cutting of red lead, of painted steel, and of older structures during dismantling, as well as vocational employment in bronze, solder, or type metal or in the modern industrial practices of enameling and glass manufacture should suggest the possibility of exposure to poisonous, lead-containing vapors.

SYMPTOMS. Mental symptoms associated with lead poisoning tend to be of two types: (1) acute delirious episodes; (2) progressive mental deterioration. The delirious type may occur in either acute or chronic poisoning. It is of sudden onset and is characterized by confusion, insomnia, restlessness, tremors, fear, outbursts of violence, visual hallucinations, and delusions which are frequently persecutory in content. Convulsions may occur and may be accompanied by a delirium in which the patient experiences terrifying visual hallucinations. In the chronic form, apathy or depression, speech defect, forgetfulness, and at times confabulations suggesting the Korsakoff syndrome are frequently observed. The progressive mental deterioration may suggest general paresis. Occasionally the clinical picture is one of neurasthenia; the patient is irritable and depressed and complains of weakness, fatigability, and dizziness. In association with the mental disturbances there is usually a history of colic, constipation, and vomiting. The former is frequently more severe in adults than in children. In adults, black deposits may be seen around the gum margins of pyorrheic teeth. This is seldom visible in children. There is usually an associated hypochromic anemia with basophilic stippling. In children there may be a mild renal glycosuria. Coproporphyrinuria commonly accompanies intoxication with lead. Roentgenograms will demonstrate dense radiopaque bands going into the shafts of long bones in children. The spinal fluid protein content is increased to levels between 15 and 200 mg. per 100 ml.

The chronic encephalopathy of children is characterized largely by failure of cerebral maturation and demonstrates itself in defects in attention, judgment, self-control, and visual learning. For those children who survive, a high proportion suffer irreversible brain damage that limits maturation. The major threat to the life and mentality of the children is increased intracranial pressure. Such children may be verbally facile but find it difficult to learn the techniques of reading, writing, and arithmetic. In both adults and children, a characteristic peripheral neuritis is frequently seen. The most used muscle groups are affected rather than those supplied by individual nerves. Thus weakness of the extensors of the wrist occurs in adults and of the dorsiflexors of the feet in children. All tendon reflexes are lost, but sensation remains intact.

TREATMENT. Treatment commences with removal of the patient from exposure to and absorption of lead. Since there is no antidote to lead, therapy must be directed to relief of the symptoms and elimination of lead from the body. Increasing the output of water is the simplest method of increasing the output of lead. Treatment with calcium disodium versenate (ethylene-diaminetetraacetic acid, EDTA), a chelating agent which has the capacity of forming stable, water-soluble complexes with metals, is now recommended to promote the loss of lead from the body. It may be given intravenously and by mouth, 1 gm. to 15 kilograms of body weight per day. One-half the 24-hour dose can be administered at intervals of 12 hours in 250 to 300 ml. of 5 to 10 per cent glucose solution. A test dose of 10 per cent of this amount is recommended. Treatment should be continued for three to four days, followed by an interval of three days, and a total of three or four courses should be given. The level of lead in the blood should then be determined. If the concentration of lead is excessive (0.08 mg. or above per 100 gm.), the course of treatment should be repeated. These interrupted courses of therapy should be repeated until the blood level of lead has fallen below 0.06 mg. per 100 gm. Since lead is stored in the skeleton and may be released later at dangerously high levels, it is recommended that levels of lead in the blood be determined subsequently at intervals of four to six weeks and that further courses be given when dangerous rises are observed. Neurosurgical decompression of the skull may be required in patients with evidence of medullary compression.

In addition to the specific therapy described above, patients with lead encephalopathy will require the general measures used in the care of the delirious states. Those with neuropathy should receive orthopedic protection of the weakened muscles and ligaments. In chronic lead poisoning, alcohol is to be avoided; a high-calcium diet supplemented by vitamin B_1 is indicated.

Mercury

Among the mental symptoms manifested by patients suffering from chronic mercury poisoning are irritability, timidity, discouragement, loss of self-confidence, fear, and occasionally outbursts of extreme anger. Less frequent are apathy, drowsiness, and impairment of memory. Chronic mercury poisoning results from the inhalation of volatile mercury for long periods of time. The hazardous trades are those concerned with the production of mercury and its derivatives, the manufacture of scientific apparatus, preparation of hatters' fur, felt hat making, the extraction of gold from silver by amalgamation, and the application of antifouling plastic paint to the hulls of ships. There is usually a moderately fine but later coarse jerking tremor of the orbits, lips, tongue, fingers, and limbs. Sometimes contractions of the limbs occur. The tremor is often intentional and subsides during rest. Weakness of both flexor and extensor muscles of the hand and forearm has been reported. No specific therapy is available for chronic mercury poisoning, although dimercaprol (BAL) has been used in those with acute poisoning. Recovery results following withdrawal from exposure.

Manganese

Workers in manganese may suffer from permanently disabling mental and neurological symptoms. Among the principal neurological symptoms are those of extrapyramidal involvement, including the basal ganglia. Gait and speech disturbances usually exist. Also present are tremors of the tongue and of the extremities and muscular weakness. About 20 per cent of the cases show mental symptoms, including restlessness, elation, and uncontrollable laughter or crying. There is no specific therapy available for manganese poisoning.

Carbon Monoxide

The gas which most frequently produces mental disturbances is carbon monoxide. The deleterious effects of this substance, which is inhaled either intentionally or by accident from the exhaust fumes of automobiles or, more infrequently, in illuminating gas or gas produced through the defective combustion of coal in stoves or furnaces, are caused by anoxemia of the brain. Carbon monoxide combines with hemoglobin to form carboxyhemoglobin, a stable compound which prevents the blood from absorbing oxygen. In those patients who die after several days, the central nervous system shows ischemic changes of the nerve cells as well as areas of softening, particularly in the cerebral cortex and the basal ganglia. Serious mental sequelae of carbon monoxide poisoning are infrequent in relation to the number of acute intoxications.

Mental symptoms following acute poisoning occur only in cases in which the intoxication has been extreme and unconsciousness complete. Of persons developing mental symptoms, about two-thirds pass directly from the comatose condition into states of confusion and delirium. In the remainder there exists a clear period of a week or more between emergence from the coma and the appearance of mental symptoms, among which are apathy, lack of initiative, and indifference to duties and responsibilities. Some patients continue to show confusion, bewilderment, and impairment of memory, with Korsakoff-like confabulations. Amnesia lasting from six to nine months may occur. In extreme cases, the patient sinks to the level of vegetative existence, with incontinence, unresponsiveness, and inability to carry on any voluntary activity. Occasionally a patient suffers from auditory aphasia. At times neurological complications may occur, owing usually to degenerative changes in the putamen or globus pallidus. Frequently, therefore, there is a modified parkinsonism, with stiffness of extremities caused by muscular hypertonia. Most patients with mental sequelae of carbon monoxide poisoning begin to improve within a few weeks after exposure and completely recover within two years. Those who have not recovered within that period of time remain in a state of mild or severe mental enfeeblement.

Attention has been called to the immediate and the delayed forms of mental sequelae arising from acute carbon monoxide anoxemia. Persons repeatedly subjected to moderate or minimal toxic amounts of the gas for periods ranging from several months to many years may develop mental and nervous symptoms. Among these manifestations are emotional instability, depression, agitation, anxiety, impairment of grasp and of memory, and at times confusion. Other symptoms are headache, vertigo, neuromuscular pains, digestive disturbances, dyspnea, and palpitation.

Carbon Disulfide

The extensive use of carbon disulfide in the manufacture of rayon has resulted in the production of toxic psychoses through its destructive effect upon the lipid content of neural tissue. Among the most commonly observed early symptoms are insomnia, bad dreams, fatigue, impotence, listlessness, and loss of memory. Neurologically there may be symptoms referable to almost any part of the central and peripheral nervous system. Among them are tenderness of nerve trunks and areas of hyperesthesia followed by loss of touch and pain sensation. Signs of irritated motor nerves include fibrillary twitching and spasmodic contraction of nerves. Among motor signs are early fatigue, weakness, and flaccid paralysis. Basal ganglia symptoms may include parkinsonism, thalamic syndrome, and choreoathetosis. Diminution and loss of corneal and pupillary reflexes are common.

Other Drugs

Several other drugs may occasionally produce delirium, particularly belladonna, chloral hydrate, and paraldehyde. Of these, belladonna probably leads most frequently to toxic symptoms. Occasionally patients, especially children, may develop delirium following the introduction of atropine into the eye. In addition to the usual physiological symptoms, the patient manifests a delirium marked by fear, excitement, and visual and auditory hallucinations. Prolonged use of chloral hydrate may lead to a delirium lasting two or more weeks.

Recently there have been noted both acute and chronic symptoms of cerebral insufficiency in individuals exposed to organic phosphorus insecticides which may irreversibly inhibit cholinesterase.

BIBLIOGRAPHY

Cheatham, J. S., and Chobot, E. F., Jr.: The clinical diagnosis and treatment of lead encephalopathy. South. Med. J., *61*:529–531, 1969.

Cummings, J. N.: Heavy Metals and the Brain. Springfield, Ill., Charles C Thomas, 1959.

Gilbert, G. J., and Glaser, G. H.: Neurologic manifestations of chronic carbon monoxide poisoning. New England J. Med., *261*:1217–1220, 1959.

Jenkins, C. D., and Mellins, R. B.: Lead poisoning in children. Arch. Neurol. & Psychiat., *77*:70–78, 1957.

Karpinski, F. E., Rieders, F., and Gersh, L. S.: Calcium disodium versenate in the therapy of lead encephalopathy. J. Pediat., *42*:687–699, 1953.

Pleasure, H.: Psychiatric and neurologic side effects of isoniazid and iproniazid. Arch. Neurol. & Psychiat., *72*:313–320, 1954.

Ritchie, E. A.: Toxic psychosis under cortisone and corticotrophin. J. Ment. Sci., *102*:830–837, 1956.

Chapter 19

Chronic Brain Syndromes Associated with Diseases of Unknown or Uncertain Cause

DEMYELINATING DISEASES

Although demyelinization within the nervous system occurs as the consequence of vascular lesions, infectious illnesses, and nutritional and toxic disturbances, this type of pathological lesion is not the primary phenomenon in these disorders. Multiple sclerosis and the various forms of diffuse sclerosis (encephalitis periaxialis diffusa of Schilder, encephalitis periaxialis concentrica of Balo, and the several forms of progressive cerebral sclerosis) form the group of primary demyelinizing disorders. The etiology of these structural disturbances of the nervous system is unknown. Their importance to the clinical psychiatrist springs from the concomitant personality disturbance noticed in the course of the illness, or the behavioral abnormalities often confused with other disturbances of personality. Their differentiation is important for therapeutic and prognostic reasons.

MULTIPLE SCLEROSIS

Despite the fact that multiple sclerosis is definitely a structural disease of the nervous system, in a considerable percentage of patients personality problems are present at the onset or during the course of the disease. Both in multiple sclerosis and in Parkinson's syndrome enough concomitant psychiatric symptoms

may be present to mask the organic picture, with the result that a psychiatric instead of a neurological diagnosis is made. Psychotic symptoms that require commitment are, however, rare.

There is no characteristic syndrome determined by the organic pathology of the disease. The general nature of the symptoms tends to be dependent upon the personality makeup of the individual patient. Not rarely, therefore, we see paranoid, depressive, hypomanic, or expansive reactions. Previous personality patterns of these types may, through the damage sustained by the personality at the organic level, become exaggerated. As a compensating psychological reaction to the disorganizing, destructive effect of the disease, one often observes a pathological complacency, cheerfulness, and even euphoria. These symptoms occur so frequently that they have often been erroneously regarded as a particular feature of the disease process itself.

Sometimes the patient's reaction to his disability is marked by an irritability or emotional instability that seriously disturbs interpersonal relationships. Impaired control over the expression of laughter and of crying resulting from bilateral upper motor neuron defects is often a significant feature. The emotional instability is associated with the clinical impression of intellectual impairment. If the explosive and forced laughing or crying occurs, the patient does not feel any affect such as the emotional signs suggest. A few patients manifest serious behavior disorders. These are occasionally observed in patients who are impotent but nevertheless have an increase in sex urge. Emotional lability and intellectual impairment are often found in patients with marked neurological disability.

Examination of cerebrospinal fluid will reveal some abnormality in cell count, total protein, or colloidal reaction in a majority of the cases. The electroencephalogram is abnormal in half of the patients, although there is no pattern specifically diagnostic.

Therapy today is directed to symptomatic relief and restoration or maintenance of social and motor skills.

DIFFUSE SCLEROSIS

The most common type is that known as Schilder's disease, which occurs as a rapidly progressive disorder productive of various mental symptoms, convulsions, loss of vision, and motor or sensory defects. Fatal cases show extensive demyelinization of the cerebral hemispheres. The signs and symptoms are inconstant from patient to patient and depend upon those areas of the cortical hemispheres involved. Headache, vomiting, and vertigo are common. Memory defects, apathy or irritability, personality changes, or confusion with disorientation and dementia may occur. The neurological signs are extensive. Cortical blindness is common. Hemianopsia, optic atrophy, and choked discs have been observed. All varieties of motor and sensory disturbances, with the associated defects in neurological examinations, may occur. Occasionally these conditions are confused with brain tumors caused by the increase in intracranial pressure. Early in the course of these illnesses they have been confused with hysterical or schizophrenic reactions. The spinal fluid shows no consistent changes. In the majority of instances, these illnesses are clinically progressive and terminate fatally following the development of dementia and quadriplegia with decerebrate rigidity. Remissions occasionally occur. Treatment consists presently in providing symptomatic care and nursing.

PARALYSIS AGITANS

In his "Essays on Shaking Palsy," published in 1817, James Parkinson, himself a victim, described the disease of late middle life now known as paralysis agitans. With its degenerative lesions of the extrapyramidal system, particularly of the corpus striatum and substantia nigra, the neurological symptoms are the conspicuous features of the clinical picture. A similar symptom complex may be induced by viral infections (encephalitis), trauma, or such toxins as manganese, carbon monoxide, and the phenothiazines. In almost all instances, toxin-induced parkinsonism is reversible.

The chronic progressive muscular rigidity, the immobile facies, the posture of flexion of neck, trunk, and extremities, the poverty of movement, and the slow, rhythmic tremor affecting the extremities to varying degrees constitute a striking syndrome. In many cases there are no mental symptoms. Most patients present a good-natured complaisance, but some, in reaction to their disability, are irritable, peevish, and dissatisfied. Depressive reactions with obsessive-compulsive features are among the most frequently observed personality responses to this disorder. The fact that the patient finds himself in a continuously contracting environment in which he becomes more and more dependent on other members of the family creates many emotional problems.

The discovery by Hornykiewicz of the diminution of neurotransmittor dopamine in the corpus striatum and substantia nigra, where norepinephrine is absent, instigated the series of therapeutic trials with dopa (the precursor of dopamine), a substance capable of passing the blood-brain barrier.

Levodopa $(3-(3+4\text{-dihydroxyphenyl})\text{-}$ L-alanine) has been discovered to be the most effective agent for the relief of the parkinsonian syndrome, modifying particularly rigidity and bradykinesia. In some it reduces tremor, postural instability, dysphagia, and sialorrhea, as well as depression, dementia-like symptoms, and impotence.

The optimal therapeutic dose of levodopa for each individual must be carefully assessed through gradual administration of increasing dosage. It is usual to commence administration with 0.5 to 1 gm. daily in divided doses, increased by 0.125 to 0.75 gm. every three days to tolerance. The average daily therapeutic level is 1 to 6 gm. given at three or more times with food.

The common side effects are nausea, vomiting, anorexia, postural hypotension and cardiac arrhythmias, and involuntary movements. Some patients develop severe agitation and hallucinations as well as restlessness and insomnia, which are relieved by withdrawing the medication.

The drug should not be given when a sympathomimetic amine is contraindicated. Concomitant treatment with monoamine oxidase inhibitors is contraindicated, but the tricyclic antidepressants have been used effectively with levodopa to treat depression with parkinsonism. Pyridoxine, in small doses, has been used to relieve the torsion dystonias and choreoathetoid movements sometimes induced by levodopa. Levodopa may be given with the solanaceous drugs and the synthetic antispasmodics.

Drugs of the solanaceous group have been used for over 80 years in the treatment of this disease. Hyoscine hydrobromide in doses of 0.3 or 0.6 mg. three times daily by mouth is the most commonly prescribed medication.

Of several synthetic antispasmodic drugs, trihexyphenidyl (Artane) is now widely employed. The initial dose is 1 mg. on the first day, increased to 1 to 2 mg. daily up to a total of 4 to 8 mg. divided into three or four doses. Elderly patients usually can take only 1 to 2 mg. daily. Toxic effects of these drugs are dryness of the mouth, excessive mydriasis, gastrointestinal upsets, and rarely a delirious reaction. In cases of severe muscle rigidity, contracture, and spasm, the powerful muscle-relaxant action of benztropine methanesulfonate (Cogentin) may prove helpful. It is longer acting than other antispasmodics and can be taken in doses of 0.5 to 1 or 2 mg. in older patients and 1 to 4 mg. in younger patients, usually once a day on retiring. Procyclidine hydrochloride (Kemadrin) is one of the newest of the synthetic antispasmodic drugs. It combines antirigidity action with a strong cerebral-stimulating action that is helpful in patients with somnolence and depression. The initial dose is usually 2.5 mg. three times daily, gradually increasing to 5 mg. three times daily. Another antiparkinsonian drug which has been increasingly employed is orphenadrine hydrochloride (Disipal). The average dose is 50 mg. three times a day. It is a harmless preparation with minimal side reactions. Its chief drawback is the tendency for the good effects to wear off in the course of months.

For those patients with an associated depressive reaction and its related symptoms, imipramine (Tofranil) or its analogs should be prescribed in doses of 25 to 50 mg. three or four times daily. This agent not only is effective in relieving the affective complications but also has proved useful in modifying rigidity and bradykinesia. It contrasts with agents of the phenothiazine group, then, which may induce parkinsonian-like states.

The surgical procedure of chemopallidectomy has proved of value in selected patients, particularly in relieving tremor or rigidity and other motor disabilities.

HUNTINGTON'S CHOREA

Huntington's chorea is a degenerative disease of the central nervous system resulting from a dominant mutation. The first distinctive description of the disease was given in 1872 by Dr. George Huntington, whose father and grandfather had practiced medicine at East Hampton, Long Island, for a period conjointly covering 78 years and had observed families among the adult members of which an incurable chorea had existed for generations. No person not descended from a progenitor so tainted has ever been known to develop the disease. It is inherited as a pure mendelian characteristic. It behaves as a dominant, with the result that there is a probability of 0.5 that the offspring of a sufferer will develop the disease. Kennedy quotes over 1000 cases in the United States as having been traced to three individuals who emigrated from an English village in 1630. Its organic basis was demonstrated by Alzheimer. The essential pathology consists of a slow degeneration of the cells of the caudate nucleus, of the putamen, and of the cerebral cortex.

Symptoms

The onset of Huntington's chorea is insidious and, generally speaking, occurs between the ages of 30 and 45 years. Frequently a change of character antedates or accompanies the appearance of the choreiform symptoms. The patient may be irritable, obstinate, and moody and lack initiative. In other cases the picture may be one of fatuous euphoria. Esthetic and ethical senses are blunted. Many patients become fault-finding, spiteful, irascible, and even destructive and assaultive. These emerging personality traits adversely affect their relations in marriage, their family, and their vocation. There is an increasing lack of spontaneity in activity, of concern as to the disease, and of solicitude as to obligations of conscience, affection, or ideals. Suspiciousness, jealousy, and paranoid trends, even to the extent of well-developed delusions of persecution, appear. Some patients experience hallucinations. With the increasing emotional deterioration, there is a coincident impairment of attention, memory, and judgment. Interest in life becomes progressively narrower. There is also a poverty of ideas and a disorderliness of thought. The dementia may become extreme.

Before the choreiform movements are clearly manifest and as muscle tone increases, with twitching, bobbing movements, and inability to remain still, accidents are frequent, owing to falls or collisions with objects. Complaints of soreness and stiffness of joints, weakness, and arthritis are common at this stage.

The choreiform movements usually appear first in the upper extremity, neck, and face. These involuntary movements are clumsy, irregular, jerky, stretching ones. In the early stages it appears as if the patient were merely inattentive or careless in his movements, which gradually increase in intensity and incoördination. The contractions of the facial muscles result in grimaces while those of the tongue, lips, and respiratory muscles lead to a hesitating, explosive, poorly articulated type of speech which, in advanced cases, is difficult to understand. The choreiform movements result in a shuffling, dancing type of gait associated with irregular movements of the trunk. The movements usually cease during sleep. As the disease progresses, there is interference with swallowing, walking becomes impossible, and the patient may become bedridden. The tendon reflexes are increased. Suicide is not uncommon.

The diagnosis usually remains undetermined from onset of symptoms for from one to over ten years.

R. A. was admitted to a mental hospital at the age of 56. The familial incidence of Huntington's chorea was striking. The maternal grandmother, a maternal uncle and his daughter, the patient's mother and four of the patient's siblings exhibited definite symptoms of Huntington's chorea. Two members of the family committed suicide after they had developed the disease. Prior to her illness the patient was apparently an attractive, well-adjusted person. She was a Girl Scout leader and took part in community affairs. Shortly before she was 35 years of age she began to show an insidious change of personality. She discontinued her church, Girl Scout, card club and other activities; she lost interest in her family and at times wandered away from home, returning at night but giving no information as to where she had been. In this same period she began to drop articles and to show twitching of her hands.

The patient became neglectful of her personal appearance, refused to comb her hair, bathe, or change her clothes. She refused to launder soiled garments and would hide them in closets or corners. The choreiform movements increased in extent, and she occasionally fell. At times she showed temporary alertness and interest in anticipation of a visit from her daughter, but after one or two days she drifted back into her former seclusiveness and deteriorated habits.

On many occasions she threatened and even attacked her husband, sometimes with a knife, and on one occasion inflicted a four-inch scalp wound. She became profane and her favorite term in addressing her husband was, "You G-d-fool." She was subject to tantrums in which she would threaten to jump from a window. She came to be known to the children in the neighborhood as "the old witch on the third floor." Finally, the choreiform movements became so extreme that it was difficult for her to go up and down stairs and she often fell.

On arrival at the hospital, her facial expression was vacant and she showed such uncoördinated and choreiform movements of her legs that she had difficulty in walking without assistance. There were gross choreiform movements of the head and all extremities. Her constant grimacing, blinking of her eyes, and twitching of her fingers were quite striking. The coördination of her hands was so poor and the movements of her head were so extreme that she had difficulty in eating. Her speech was explosive and difficult to understand. Although somewhat irritable, demanding, and distrustful, she adjusted to the hospital environment without serious difficulty.

Treatment

Treatment is directed toward relief of symptoms and emotional support. Oral fluphenazine given in increasing daily doses until the initial toxic symptoms of parkinsonism appear (usually 6 to 8 mg. daily) will reduce the choreic activity and improve the mental status in the majority of patients. Some report this drug more effective in treatment of women than men. Haloperidol has had similar therapeutic effect.

The average duration of life is 15 years.

LUPUS ERYTHEMATOSUS

The psychiatrist practicing in the general hospital now frequently encounters lupus erythematosus disseminata as a condition with various reaction formations, or with delirious and psychotic manifestations. This condition, once considered rare, is now frequently diagnosed on the medical services because of the increasing awareness of the symptomatology and a better knowledge of the tissue and cellular pathology, including the existence of the now well known "LE cells."

Lupus erythematosus disseminata is one of the group of conditions now known as diseases of the collagen tissues. In lupus the primary damage is to the subendothelial connective tissue of capillaries, small arteries, and veins, and the endocardium and synovial membranes. Approximately 85 per cent of all clinically recognized cases occur in women. The onset of the illness usually takes place in childhood but is most commonly recognized during adolescence and early adult life. The pathological changes are found in the ground substance and collagen which serves as a matrix and binding substance for the capillaries and small blood vessels in various parts of the body. Gross thickening is found in the endocardial and pericardial tissues, while the small arteries and arterioles of various organs, including the brain, show a fibroid degeneration and necrosis in the connective tissue matrix of the vessel wall. In certain of the affected areas of connective tissue, the intercellular ground substance shows deep metachromatic staining or the presence of eosinophilic masses, thought to be a result of the swelling and fibroid degeneration of collagen fibers. Certain deep purplish staining material found in some of the affected areas has been identified histochemically as desoxyribonucleic acid. This is apparently the abnormal chromatin material found in the so-called LE cells of the blood and bone marrow on dry smears.

In one series of cases, 50 per cent presented delirious or psychosis-like phenomena at some time during the course of their illness. Another small group developed neurosis-like symptoms, while a considerable number had neurological signs at one time or another.

The early symptoms of the condition are easy fatigability, malaise, and fever. The so-called butterfly rash that occurs across the bridge of the nose and on the cheeks, often considered a traditional lesion of the disease, is not present or necessary for the diagnosis of systemic lupus erythematosus. Commonly the initial signs are those of migratory reactions of joint and fibrous tissue simulating rheumatic fever or rheumatoid arthritis. Examination sometimes discloses anemia, lymphadenopathy, and edema, or signs indicating pathology involving the pleura, lungs, heart, pericardium, or gastrointestinal tract. The differentiation of the illness from rheumatic fever or rheumatoid arthritis is suggested on finding hematuria. The LE cell is found in stained blood of bone marrow smears, particularly those made from clotted blood or the buffy layer of heparinized blood. They consist of phagocytes containing masses of chromatin material which stain deep purple with Wright's or Giemsa stain. When the LE cell test, the fluorescent antibody test, and complement-fixation tests are employed, almost every case will show a positive reaction to one of the three. Usually there are leukopenia, elevation of sedimentation of the erythrocytes, and occasionally intermittently or falsely positive serological reactions for syphilis.

At the onset of the illness, anxiety is often evident, and the patient may manifest personality changes which are frequently considered to be reflective of the personality structure. Phobic, depressive, and schizophrenic pictures have been seen as well as delirioid reaction. The psychiatric disorders have been thought by many to be related to the use of steroid therapy in the course of this illness. The psychotic reactions are usually apparent some 12 days after the institution of steroid therapy, with a maximum of 30 days and a minimum of two. It must be concluded, however, that the steroid therapy per se is not related to the occurrence of the disturbance of mental functioning. In one group of patients, a large number recovered from the initial deliroid psychotic reaction only to have an active recurrence of lupus at a later time. The majority, when placed on an equivalent dose of

ACTH or cortisone, did not again present the mental aberration. Exacerbation of the lupus erythematosus itself, rather than the usage of the steroids, appeared to increase the possibility of the occurrence of psychiatric disturbances.

Although remissions may occur, and cortisone and ACTH have proved effective in inducing prompt improvement, most sufferers ultimately die from renal insufficiency and intercurrent pneumococcal or streptococcal infection. The majority who present psychotic disturbances have characteristic lesions in the cerebral hemisphere at autopsy.

The behavior disturbances associated with this illness often require protective hospitalization and careful nursing. Cortisone and ACTH should be administered. The former is usually given in dosages of 0.025 gm. every six hours intramuscularly. Cortisone may be administered orally 0.15 to 0.30 gm. in four divided doses during the day. Following seven to ten days on this dosage, the agents may be gradually reduced each succeeding two or three days until a maintenance level is reached, below which evidences of clinical activity are observed to recur. The majority of the patients require a small maintenance dosage for indefinite periods. The careful collaboration of a psychiatrist and the internist is often indicated in the treatment of disseminated lupus erythematosus.

J. M.: Five months before her admission to a general hospital, this 18-year-old girl noticed fatigability, sore throat, and fever associated with pain on movements of the ankles, fingers, and joints. These symptoms improved. About four weeks before admission she suffered nausea, loss of appetite, and intermittent vomiting. Eleven days before admission she developed double vision on lateral gaze, at first intermittent, but later constant. A few days later her vision was blurred. On admission her temperature was 98.8° F., pulse 82, respiration rate 14. She had lost 22 pounds in weight.

At this time her behavior and mental status were not unusual. She appeared thin, showed some unsteadiness in standing, and had double vision on lateral gaze, but otherwise there seemed to be no conspicuous physical disturbances. Her urine contained albumin; there was evidence of liver dysfunction with a positive cephalin flocculation test. Electroencephalogram was abnormal with disorganization and slowing in the temporal areas and periods of low voltage, 4 to 7 per second activity. At this time the sedimentation rate equaled 82 mm. per hour. Bilateral papilledema developed. A medical consultant suggested that the patient had either rheumatoid arthritis or possibly disseminated lupus erythematosus. An internal carotid arteriogram was normal. Treatment was commenced with cortisone. The spinal fluid contained 460 mg. of protein per 100 ml. The patient's symptoms increased, particularly those referred to the joint pains. When she finally received 100 mg. of cortisone daily two months after admission, her symptoms subsided quickly. She was then discharged to her home on cortisone, 75 mg. daily.

She remained well at home until three months later, when she became very elated and overactive. She spoke of her body and brain shrinking; she said that she was becoming a baby again and would shortly die. Her return to the hospital was precipitated by a series of convulsions. She then seemed quiet and rather suspicious, but occasionally she called out for help in a loud voice. She failed to recognize certain physicians who had treated her before. The cortisone dosage was reduced from 125 to 75 mg. and her symptoms remitted.

Later the patient recounted that the psychotic disturbance occurred when she had the impression that she "was getting much better on the cortisone. I was getting stronger. About 8 p.m. when I was watching television I suddenly got the feeling that I was going to change into a baby. Previously I had talked to my relatives about this, but they didn't pay any attention to it. I felt that I was going to be bald, that all my hair was inside of my head, and that they couldn't operate to let the hair out. I felt that I was cramped up and couldn't move." (At this point she assumed the fetal position.) "I felt that I was going to die like a girl that I knew while in the hospital. I was in a dream." She declared that she felt that, when blood was being drawn from her arm, the purpose was to drain every drop of blood from her. "I felt that all the people in the ward were German spies. One of them had an Irish accent, but I felt it was a German accent. They were trying to electrocute me. When my mother came to visit me, I tried to push her off the bed so that she would not be electrocuted, but she didn't understand this. I felt that all the nurses were traitors—German spies." She seemed to interpret the slightest remark or facial expression as something of significance to her; she was frightened when the doctors approached her. Her sensorium was clear.

Some five days later the psychotic picture disappeared. A blood smear showed LE cells. The encephalogram performed at the time of the behavior disturbance revealed an increase in the abnormality. The patient was discharged on 75 mg. of cortisone daily.

Because of increased weakness, joint pains, and general debility, she was readmitted to the hospital seven months later. At this time no psychotic disturbance was evident, although she was carefully followed by a psychiatrist. She was from time to time preoccupied by a fear of death and freely called for psychiatric help when most anxious. No recurrence of psychiatric symptoms took place on elevation of the daily dose of cortisone to 87 mg. Following another period at home, she returned to the hospital two months later with hemiparesthesia and expired shortly thereafter. Necropsy disclosed the typical pathology of lupus erythematosus.

BIBLIOGRAPHY

Bowman, L.: Diffuse Sclerosis: Encephalitis Periaxialis Diffusa. Bristol, John Wright & Sons, Ltd., 1934.

Greenfield, J. B., et al.: The pathology of parkinsonism. J. Nerv. & Ment. Dis., 122:200–201, 1955.

Heine, B. E.: Psychiatric aspects of systemic lupus erythematosus. Acta Psychiat. Scand., 45:307–326, 1969.

Hornykiewicz, O.: Dopamine and brain function. Pharm. Rev., 18:925–964, 1966.

Huntington, G.: On chorea. Med. and Surg. Reporter, 26:317, 1872.

James, W. E., Mefferd, R. B., and Kimball, I.: Early signs of Huntington's chorea. Dis. Nerv. System., 30:556–559, 1969.

Malamud, N., and Saver, G.: Neuropathologic findings in disseminated lupus erythematosus. Arch. Neurol. & Psychiat., 71:723–731, 1954.

McCaughey, W. T. E.: The pathologic spectrum of Huntington's chorea. J. Nerv. & Ment. Dis., 133:91–103, 1961.

O'Brien, C. P., DiGiacomo, J. N., Fahn, S., and Schwarz, G. A.: Mental effects of high dosage levodopa. Arch. Gen. Psychiat., 24:61–64, 1971.

O'Connor, J. F., and Mosher, D. M.: Central nervous system involvement in systemic lupus erythematosus. Arch. Neurol., 14:157–164, 1966.

Parkinson, J.: An Essay on the Shaking Palsy. London, Sherwood, Neely & Jones, 1817.

Ross, A. T., and Reitan, R. N.: Intellectual and affective functions in multiple sclerosis. Arch. Neurol. & Psychiat., 73:633–677, 1955.

Whittier, J. R., and Koreny, C.: Effect of oral fluphenazine on Huntington's chorea. Int. J. Neuropsychiat., 4:1–3, 1968.

Yahr, M. D., DuVoisin, R. C., Schear, M. J., Barrett, R. E., and Hocher, M. M.: Treatment of parkinsonism with levodopa. Arch. Neurol., 21:343–354, 1969.

Chapter 20

"We are not ourselves when nature, being oppress'd
commands the mind to suffer with the body."

Shakespeare

Disorders of Psychogenic Origin

In the preceding chapters there has been discussion of mental disorders associated with diffuse impairment of cerebral tissue function. It was pointed out that if the brain lesion is reversible, the associated mental reactions are temporary and recoverable, with no residual damage to the personality. On the other hand, if the damage to cerebral tissue is not fully reversible, a variable but permanent impairment of its function, with resulting disturbance of memory, judgment, orientation, comprehension, and affect, will result.

Several of the chapters to follow are devoted to a discussion of disorders that today may not be related to specific anatomical or physiological abnormality of the brain. Yet for the schizophrenic and affective psychoses there is gathering evidence of cerebral dysfunction related to the dynamics of inter- and intraneuronal biochemical events. While genetic and constitutional predispositions may exist, the symptomatic expressions of these conditions represent the result of symbolic, emotional, and interpersonal factors acting on the organism overtime. These disorders may be divided into four groups:

1. Psychotic disorders;
2. Psychophysiological autonomic and visceral disorders ("psychosomatic" disorders);
3. Psychoneurotic disorders;
4. Personality disorders.

Psychotic Disorders

These disorders are characterized by a varying degree of personality disorganization. To different degrees, too, the patient may break with reality or fail to test and evaluate it correctly. As a result, his capacity for effective work and for adapted relations with other people is temporarily, and in some instances permanently, impaired or destroyed.

Psychophysiological Autonomic and Visceral Disorders

In this group are included disorders in which organ and visceral symptomatology is produced by emotional factors acting through the autonomic nervous system. Such a visceral expression of affect may serve to prevent the individual from becoming conscious of it. Long-continued deranged physiological states of viscera produced in this way by emotional factors may eventually lead to structural changes—to peptic ulcer, for example.

Psychoneurotic Disorders

These disorders represent either a symptomatic expression of "anxiety" or the psychological mechanisms unconsciously and automatically adopted to control it. Material disorganization of the personality does not occur, and there is no gross distortion or falsification of external reality as seen in the psychoses in the form of delusions and hallucinations. General types of psychoneuroses are recognized, the form being determined by the way in which the patient attempts to deal with the threatening danger felt in the conscious area of his personality but arising from the unconscious portion.

Personality Disorders

Disorders in this group are characterized not by mental or emotional symptoms but by developmental defects or pathological trends in the personality.

In disorders included in this classification, the personality, in its efforts at adjustment to internal and external stresses, utilizes patterns of action or behavior, and not measures or symptoms expressed in the mental, somatic, or emotional spheres.

Chapter 21

"Though this be madness, yet there is method in it."

Shakespeare

Schizophrenic Psychoses

SCHIZOPHRENIC REACTIONS

Although the variety of behavioral expressions designated as the schizophrenic reactions are relatively easily described and, in their grosser expressions, recognized with ease, even by the unexperienced, neither their definition nor the etiologic factors predisposing to them or precipitative of them have been universally agreed upon.

Because of the heterogeneity of the manifestations, it may be more accurate to speak of the group of schizophrenias rather than to think of each group of disordered reaction as a single disease entity. There is, therefore, an increasing inclination to think of schizophrenia as a term for a number of somewhat similar patterns of reactions to life situations that the individual has found too difficult to meet.

Symptomatically, the schizophrenic reactions are recognizable through odd and bizarre behavior apparent in aloofness, suspiciousness, or periods of impulsive destructiveness and immature and exaggerated emotionality, often ambivalently directed and considered inappropriate by the observer. The interpersonal perceptions are distorted in the more serious states by delusional and hallucinatory material. In the most disorganized forms of schizophrenic living, withdrawal into a fantasy life takes place and is associated with serious disorder of thought and profound habit deteriorations in which the usual social customs and personal care are disregarded.

It is generally considered that the schizophrenic is incapable of effectively harmonizing his drives and inhibitions through mature adaptations and defenses. He had failed to develop a satisfying concept of his body and a clear or stable self-concept. He is often unclear in his goals, or his aspirations are so demanding or inflexible that they exceed his talents, persistence, and drive to mastery. Thus he is deficient in his capacity to assess clearly the realities of the world. Interactions with others are characterized by immature processes of communication, thought, and adaptation.

In psychoanalytic terms, the schizophrenics represent those who have failed to evolve the ego integrative processes or strengths necessary to resolve flexibly conflicts between their (id) drives and overdemanding superego attitudes and the aspirations of the ego ideal. They are thus defective in the capacity to adapt to the social demands confronting them and to their own drives and they thereby lack a harmonious self-concept and ego ideal with clear goals and motivations. Much of their adaptation is made, instead, through partially satisfying regressive or fixated infantile behavior.

Evolution of Concept

Although not so called, the clinical picture we now know as schizophrenia has long been recognized. In 1849 John Conolly (1794–1866) of Hanwell Asylum in England, the champion of "no restraint," stated in his Croonian Lectures: "Young persons not infrequently fall into a state somewhat resembling melancholia, without any discoverable cause of sorrow, and certainly without any specific grief; they become indolent or pursue their usual occupations or recreations mechanically and without interest; the intellect, the affections, the passions, all seem inactive or deadened and the patients become utterly apathetic."

The term dementia praecox (démence précoce) was first used by the Belgian psychiatrist Morel in 1860 in the case of a boy of 14 who previously had always been "first in his examinations, and that without effort and almost without study. . . . Unconsciously he lost his cheerfulness and became sober, taciturn, and showed a tendency to solitude." The boy showed a "state of melancholy depression and a hatred of his father even with the idea of killing him. . . . The young invalid progressively forgot all that he had learned, and his brilliant intellectual faculties entered into a very disturbing period of arrest. A kind of inactivity bordering on stupidity replaced his former activity and when I saw him again it looked as if a transition into an irrecoverable state of dementia praecox was taking place."

Morel interpreted this disorganization of personality as an arrest of development, to be included with mental deficiency as a "variety of intellectual, physical and moral degeneracy" resulting from heredity.

The next step in the history of dementia praecox was Hecker's description in 1871 of *hebephrenia,* although the term had previously been used by Kahlbaum. "The characteristic features of hebephrenia," wrote Hecker, "above all are: its appearance in connection with puberty, the succession or changing appearance of various forms (melancholia, mania and confusion), the very quick termination in a psychic enfeeblement and a characteristic form of final deterioration the evidences of which can be seen in the first stages of the disease." He considered hebephrenia to be a progressive disease of puberty and adolescence.

Another step in the development of the dementia praecox concept was the description of *catatonia,* or *"tension insanity,"* by Kahlbaum in 1874. He described catatonia as "that condition in which the patient sits quietly or completely mute and motionless, immovable, with a staring countenance, the eyes fixed on a distant point and apparently completely without volition, without any reaction to sensory impresssions, sometimes with a full fledged cerea flexibilitas as in catalepsy." Kahlbaum assumed that catatonia was the symptom of a structural brain disease.

In 1896 Kraepelin offered the proposition that a common denominator exists among such apparently unrelated syndromes as the hebephrenia of Hecker, the catatonia of Kahlbaum, and many paranoid psychoses. By defining dementia praecox as a distinct syndrome, he introduced order into what had been a clinical chaos so far as observation and classification had been concerned.

In 1906 Adolf Meyer developed the thesis that dementia praecox is not a disease entity but rather a type of reaction developing in certain personalities as a result of progressive difficulty in adaptation and that the accumulation of faulty habits of reaction lead to a "habit deterioration."

Another landmark in the history of dementia praecox was the introduction by Eugene Bleuler (1857–1939) in 1911 of the term *"schizophrenia."* Following Bleuler's suggestion, the designation *dementia praecox* has been supplanted by the name *schizophrenia* (splitting of the mind), since the disharmony or "split" of the psychobiological expression of the organism that we call mind, and the breaking up of a former normal synthesis of thought, feeling, and activity, are now considered more characteristic and distinctive of the reaction than are symptom-complex and outcome as stressed by Kraepelin.

Conceptions of Schizophrenia

Since present conceptions of schizophrenia are largely based upon the formulations of Kraepelin, Bleuler, Meyer, and Freud, a brief presentation of their respective formulations is added.

Kraepelin, through his keen observations, gave an excellent clinical description of the disorder and classified it into types (hebephrenic, catatonic, and paranoid). Bleuler and Meyer, on the other hand, greatly advanced the psychiatric understanding of schizophrenia by their interpretation in dynamic terms of the symptomatic manifestations observed.

KRAEPELIN'S FORMULATIONS   As previously indicated, Kraepelin brought together varied mental syndromes that he concluded were manifestations of a single disease entity. To these he gave the name *dementia praecox,* a term previously having a more limited application. He thought these clinical syndromes arose from the same disease process, since they had in common the following features: a beginning in adolescence or early adulthood and a progression toward a similar state of "dementia." Similar morbid processes were, Kraepelin assumed, the causes of the various clinical features. These causes, he believed, might be either a degenerative disease of the brain or metabolic disturbances that produced autointoxication. He believed, too, that injury to the germ plasm might be of significance in its development. Kraepelin was of the opinion that the clinical results of these processes consisted of a weakening of emotional and volitional reactions and a loss of harmonious connections among emotional, volitional, and intellectual reactions. He gave an extremely comprehensive and lucid description of the clinical features of dementia praecox but was critical of any attempt to explain the behavior of the patient on a psychological basis.

BLEULER'S FORMULATIONS.   Bleuler came to the conclusion that it was misleading to compare even the extreme deterioration of what Kraepelin called dementia praecox with the state of mind of the mentally defective or with that of organic deterioration caused by severe brain atrophy. Therefore the label "de-

mentia praecox" could no longer be considered satisfactory. He pointed out that the patient's psychological reactions to his environment are complicated and differentiated, quite different in kind from the elementary, simple reactions of feebleminded persons and those with organic brain disease. Bleuler believed, therefore, that the disease was not one of *de-*mentia, a state of diminished mind, but a disharmonious state of mind in which most contradictory tendencies, thoughts, and potentialities existed together, so that the harmony of the personality was split. According to this conception, the outcome of the disease was not necessarily one of deterioration, as Kraepelin had maintained, and the diagnosis had nothing to do with the course. Bleuler was the first to point out that it was not only interesting but extremely important to consider seriously and from a scientific point of view the content of the patient's thoughts, of his trends, of his instincts, and of everything that he did. He noticed that if the patient's hallucinations and delusions were thoroughly studied, they could be connected with his life history, with his early hopes and fears, and with early relationships with parents and siblings.

Prior to Bleuler's time, it was believed that every mental symptom was caused by an underlying physical disorder. Psychological symptoms, such as delusions, hallucinations, mannerisms, and catatonic musculature signs had been looked at in the same way as aphasia, apraxia, or reflex disturbances. Influenced by the firm and prevailing belief that all psychoses, and even neuroses, were of somatic origin, Bleuler hesitated to conclude that all the morbid manifestations in schizophrenia, or that schizophrenia itself, was of a functional nature and could be understood psychologically. He therefore distinguished between primary and secondary symptoms. He designated as *primary signs* those that he considered were the direct manifestations of a hypothetical somatic morbid process; these included a peculiar loosening of the associational links in thinking, a morbid ambitendence and ambivalence that dominated the affective life of the patient, and a tendency to replace reality by fantasy, a quality that was responsible for the various manifestations of autism. Among the *secondary symptoms,* or those that he believed were of psychic origin, were delusions explainable by the patient's frustrations and hopes, a part of the hallucinations, the mannerisms, the catatonic muscular symptoms, and a large part of the complicated attitudes that others had called deterioration or dementia. He believed that the secondary symptoms were attempts at adaptation to the primary disturbance.

After Bleuler had become convinced of the importance of psychological influences in the morbid picture of schizophrenia, it became clear to him that the disorder should be treated by psychotherapy. He stressed that a sound, strong, and personal relationship between nurse and patient and between physician and patient would exercise a beneficial therapeutic influence.

In 1897 Bleuler left Rheinau and became professor of psychiatry in Zurich and director of the Burghölzli Clinic. Here Bleuler and his first assistant, Carl Jung, became acquainted with Freud, who spent a period at Zurich. As a result, Bleuler developed a great interest in psychoanalysis at a time when few psychiatrists had accepted Freud's teachings. He concluded that, to a large extent, schizophrenic symptoms could be understood by the same symbolization that Freud had discovered in dreams and in neurotic developments. Although Meyer, probably justifiably, criticized Bleuler's conception of schizophrenia as assuming an unwarranted dualism of mind and body, Bleuler's monograph on the subject is nevertheless one of the classics of psychiatry.

MEYER'S FORMULATION. Meyer's dynamic conception of schizophrenia and his naturalistic behavioral approach in its formulation appeared earlier than Bleuler's work. He emphasized the clinical picture of schizophrenia, not as an autonomous disease entity, but as a maladaptation logically understandable in terms of the patient's experiences and life history. He emphasized the concepts of habit deterioration and of reaction types. The schizophrenic reaction, he believed, can best be understood as a habit disorganization resulting from a progressive maladaptation, in which there takes place "a substitution of inefficient and faulty attempts to avoid difficulties rather than to meet them by decisive action." The result is disorganization of the personality and final withdrawal from reality. Many of the clinical symptoms represent abortive and "twisted" attempts at balance and reconstruction. He expressed the opinion that the failure to find any structural or physiological changes in neurons excludes an organic etiology, although he believed that an inferior constitution as well as a great variety of pathologic conditions of a physical nature may add to the individual's load of handicaps.

Meyer was one of the first to emphasize that the interest should be not so much in a classificatory diagnosis as in the facts and factors at work in the individual patient and in his assets. Although admiring Kraepelin's description of the reaction, Meyer did not subscribe to his invariably unfavorable prognosis of a progressive intellectual deterioration.

At the present time, the concepts of Kraepelin, Meyer, Bleuler, and Freud are all considered inadequate. There exist a number of new working hypotheses, which will be discussed under the section on etiology.

Epidemiology

The schizophrenic psychoses are recognized in all cultures in which mental disorders have been subjected to thorough study. Cultural forces appear only to modify the clinical phenomenology of these reactions in terms of the content of delusional and hallucinatory material. Thus in Western society, religious and sexual delusions were more common a century ago than in the present. These psychoses occur in all socioeconomic strata, although several epidemiological studies have suggested a correlation between higher prevalence of illness and lower socioeconomic status.

At this time the schizophrenics are the most prevalent of the major psychoses. In a recent examination of the existing material on prevalence and incidence, Mishler and Scotch conclude that at any moment 0.3 per cent of the general population are suffering the disturbance, 0.15 per cent of the population are likely to experience its development, and 0.02 per cent are admitted to hospitals with schizophrenia for the first time. Schizophrenic reactions now constitute approximately 25 per cent of the first admissions to public mental hospitals in the United States. Owing to the chronicity of these reactions, some 60 per cent of the population of state hospitals is made up of patients with this syndrome. Calculations made from various epidemiological surveys give the morbid risk for the syndrome as 1 per cent. Morbid risk is defined as the total risk of becoming manifestly ill for all persons surviving the age period of 15 to 45 years, when the disease is customarily recognized.

More recently Deming, working with data derived from the annual statistical reports of the State of New York, applied to the 1960 data a recursion formula which hypothesized that (1) for every schizophrenic recognized in the hospitals of the state of New York there were three living in the community; (2) the proportion of males living in the state that had a first hospital admission as a schizophrenic is 1 in 68 and of females is 1 in 62; (3) that the proportion of people of all ages from birth on that have already had an admission as schizophrenic or will live long enough to have one is 1 in 46 for males and 1 in 39 for females.

Deming's calculations are based on experience in New York where diagnoses of schizophrenia by psychiatrists are recognized as exceeding those elsewhere in the United States as well as abroad, judging by various transcultural studies.

Etiology

Personality development and maldevelopment are dependent upon the genetic and constitutional endowment of each individual. Impinging upon that endowment are the early maternal and later family transactions that dynamically bring about the unfolding of various ego and superego functions and the ego ideal of each individual. As the personality growth of each individual ensues over time, social opportunities and stresses must be met which act upon the growing individual and may serve as precipitants of disorder, including schizophrenic disorder.

THE GENETIC FACTOR. Accumulating evidence from numerous twin studies carried out in the United States, Great Britain, Japan, and the Scandinavian countries demonstrates that monozygotic twins are found to be concordant for schizophrenia about four times as often as dizygotic twins.

The most impressive evidence for the influence of a genetic factor is the statistical data of Kallmann obtained from the extensive study of twins. Kallmann found that if the disorder exists in one of monozygotic twins, it occurs also in the other twin in 85.8 per cent of the cases. However, the expectancy for a dizygotic twin partner is 14 per cent, equivalent to that of siblings. Kallmann interpreted his findings to indicate that there exists a genetic predisposition to schizophrenia.

Although the concordance rates for schizophrenia were much lower in monozygotic twins in later studies which sampled total populations rather than those of identified patients in psychiatric hospitals, nevertheless the rate for monozygotes always remained greater than for the dizygotic twin pairs. Also, the risk of schizophrenia for children of those with this condition approximates 15 times that of the general population. When both parents are schizophrenic, up to a third of the children have been found schizophrenic as well.

Various criticisms have been given to

studies of twins. It has been pointed out that such studies lack information on the early biological and family experiences of the twins and have not weighed the psychodynamic forces in twin development that are believed to tend toward mutual identification between twins rather than for the growth of separate identities.

Thus a shared fetal cross-circulation may be found in monozygotic but not in dizygotic twins. Sufficient emphasis has not been placed upon studies of those factors that protect one of a monozygotic twin pair from schizophrenia in at least 15 per cent of the cases. It may be expected that important insights would come from examination of the supportive environmental factors useful in reducing the risk of the reaction in the spared twin.

In one sample of monozygotic twins almost a half had never been separated more than a single day, whereas three quarters of the dizygotic twins had this experience. So, too, monozygotic twins are often dressed alike, and even their parents mistake the individual identities. Yet in studies such as those of Inouye in Japan, where culture dictates that twins be separated and one be reared by someone else than the mother, the frequency of occurrence of schizophrenia in both monozygotic twins remains higher than in dizygotic twins reared separated from birth. Furthermore, studies of adopting parents have shown that they are less likely to have pathology than the primary parents. Occurrence of schizophrenia in cases of adoption thus supports influence of the genetic factor.

Heston suggests that in genetic research on schizophrenia one must consider the schizoid but nonpsychotic person as well, because 45 per cent of the siblings, parents, and children of schizophrenics are found to be either schizoid or schizophrenic. On his computations he estimates that about 4 per cent of the general population will be affected by the schizoid-schizophrenic personality complex. He would explain this distribution on the hypothesis of a defect in a single auto-somal dominant gene. The majority of geneticists have supported genetic transmission of predisposition to schizophrenia as polygenic, the illness being regarded as a threshold trait. At any rate the genetic contribution to the schizophrenic complex now appears well established. The manner in which that contribution is expressed in the biological make-up of the individual remains unclear, as do the environmental processes which lead to its clinical presentation.

BIOLOGICAL PREDISPOSITION. That constitutional weaknesses exist is suggested by data indicating that schizophrenic mothers have a higher incidence of deviant fetal growth in terms of perinatal mortality and malformations in the newborn than mothers from the population at large. Also, careful physical and psychological investigations of groups of children considered to have childhood schizophrenia have shown that a majority present in their motor, postural, sensori-perceptual, and conceptual performances indications of delayed or uneven functioning. These impairments are described in greater detail later in this chapter in relation to childhood schizophrenia. Whether these impairments are due to delays in maturation as a consequence of a defect in genetic endowment or to unrecognized brain damage in early life has not been ascertained. Some would exclude from the schizophrenic reactions all children showing such defects.

Consistent physical abnormalities are not associated with schizophrenia; yet in the past clinicians have suggested that there existed instability in function of the autonomic nervous system. Largely such inferences arose from observation of the pupillary dilatations and presumed vasomotor phenomena of the extremities usually seen in certain catatonics with coldness and cyanosis of limbs. So, too, it has been reported by Maricq and others that there is an abnormal subpupillary capillary plexus clearly visible in the nail folds of schizophrenics exceeding the findings of mental defectives and the healthy.

The sweat of schizophrenics has been thought to exude a peculiar odor. The substance causing the odor has been identified as trans-3-methyl-2 hexenoic acid. Most recently Feinberg has reported that stage 4 electroencephalographic sleep value as recorded in schizophrenic patients occurs in approximately 50 per cent of actively ill schizophrenics. This finding, too, is unspecific, as such sleep abnormality is discovered in severe depression. There exist today no specific biological tests which discriminate the schizophrenic from others.

The numerous experimental studies directed toward the finding of constitutional, metabolic, endocrine, and other physiological defects have yet to produce any significant data that have been subject to verification. These findings then remain irrelevant to clinical practice, as they offer, as yet, no useful theoretical diagnostic or therapeutic tools.

Areas of investigation now most actively pursued are concerned with the intermediate metabolism of cerebral glucose. Gottlieb, Frohman, and Beckett hypothesize that schizophrenics are deficient in their capacity to utilize available energy in reaction to stress owing to metabolic defects in the Embden-Meyerhof scheme. They have reported that an abnormality exists in schizophrenic plasma which leads to abnormal production of pyruvate. Attempts to isolate and characterize this plasma fraction goes on in several laboratories. Also, it is suggested that the presence of a malcontrolled protein in the blood contributes to the illness by selectively altering neuronal transmission.

Numerous groups have reported the urinary excretion of abnormal metabolites, the most recent being that of a mescaline-like derivative by A. J. Friedhoff and E. Van Winkle. Yet it is now known that this substance, dimethoxyphenylethylamine (DMPE 4) is also nonspecific—in fact the metabolites of chlorpromazine and other phenothiazines will produce "pink spots" in chromatographic procedures, and so will the urine of healthy individuals who drink tea.

Heath has proposed that there exists a structural abnormality in the septal region of the brain, the area shown in animal experiments to be concerned with alerting and repetitive activity assumed to be pleasurable. He has described a spike and slow wave electroencephalographic discharge as consistently recurrent in the septal area of some schizophrenic patients during periods of abnormal behavior—an abnormality tending to disappear as the patient seemed to improve. But similar EEG activity has been recorded from the septal area in patients with other conditions as well as from the brains of various animals.

Arguing from the disturbance of cognitive functioning with loosening and fragmentation of associations as the central clinical feature of schizophrenia, Elkes has hypothesized that there co-exists a disturbance of information processing by the brain. He has suggested that the defect exists in the integration of the subsystems subserving attention and motivation in the selective organization of sense data. The interaction between sensory information and stored affectively charged memory traces suggests to him that the limbic system as a first order monitoring group for sensory data as regards pleasurable or aversive control may be involved, as well as the highly discriminating inhibiting processes concerned with specific altering and attentions mediated by higher brain stem structures and defections. So, too, his hypothesis suggests that such defective subsystem functions must be interpreted in terms of biochemical or pharmacological abnormalities which presumably would operate on terms of brain mechanisms (synaptic transmission) in such subsystems and particularly the neuronal integrating nets.

Several hypotheses have been offered regarding dysfunction in the synaptic transmitters. Heath has suggested that brain cell antibodies attach themselves to the septal region and impair synaptic transmission there. Specifically he has suggested that an immunoglobulin designated *taraxein* obtained from serum of acutely ill schizophrenic patients, when administered to healthy volunteers, will induce EEG changes similar to those he discovered in the brains of schizophrenics. Critics point out that the latter findings are not specific for schizophrenia. Also, his work remains to be replicated.

Others are of that opinion that the abnormal defect rests in an altered metabolism of the biogenic amines necessary for synaptic transmission. Thus it has been suggested that abnormal metabolism of dopa leads to formation of 3,4-dimethoxyphenylethylamine (DMPEA) endogenously, which is capable of inducing psychotic disorganization. The dopaminergic transmitters are believed to exist in the basal ganglia including the limbic system. It is of interest that L-dopa relieves parkinsonism where dopamine deficiency is known to exist in the structures, and the phenothiazines in high doses may induce parkinsonian states and yet act effectively as therapeutic agents in schizophrenia.

FAMILY TRANSACTION. Whatever biological abnormality the future schizophrenic may bring with his birth, his personality unfolds over the years of infancy, childhood, and adolescence as the consequence of the ongoing transactions between his parents and those others who relate with him and thus influence his emotional and cognitive maturation.

The range of such impairments in the conditions designated as childhood schizophrenia is wide; a considerable number show very little evidence of early retardation in development of sensorimotor, perceptual, and conceptual deficit. However, in cases in which studies have been made of the family unit and its functioning, it appears that gross personality disturbances in parents are more likely to be associated with minimal impairment of physiologic growth of the child, and minimal pathology in the parents is found to be associated with maximal physiological retardation in the schizophrenic child.

The family transactions induced by the interplay between the child's capacities determined by his physiological equipment and the expectations of the parents then appear to play an important role in the achievement of a healthy unfolding of personality and in the arrest or inadequate development of ego attitudes and functions. Thus a child who, as the result of delayed maturation of motor development, fails to acquire skill in language, walking, and other coordinated movements may set up anxieties in certain parents with high expectancies and investment in his future that are reflected in the parental relationship, the parents pushing the child beyond his capacities while, at the same time, overprotecting him. In other children, without evidence of physiologic deficit, it has been postulated that the parental investment in the child is disturbed from the beginning, as the child represents an expected source for emotional satisfaction, or the living out of gratifications not obtained in life by one or other of the parents.

Psychoanalytic theory has held that the earliest periods of mother-infant relationship must be deficient, since the adult pathology of the schizophrenic suggests a regressive withdrawal to infantile emotional behavior in the omnipotent behavior, infantile rage reaction, and inability to perceive reality. In partial support of this hypothesis, the several direct observational studies of mothering of their infants by schizophrenic women seem to show that the mothering process was impaired by their affective depression. Such women did not play with and fondle their infants as do other mothers, although they did carry out well the usual procedures for nurture and bodily cleanliness of the child. Their infants, in turn, appeared irritable and depressed. It is probable that the restriction of affective and playful stimulation of the infant impedes the development of those early sensations that establish the body percept and the beginnings of ego attitudes of security, trust, and aggressiveness, upon which must unfold the capacities for self-control and later autonomous independence.

That deprivations of early mothering may bring about enduring defects in capacity to socialize and even to carry out sexual activities effectively now has received strong support from studies in primates and mammalian species, typified in the work of the Harlows. The animal experiments suggest that the timing and duration of the important mother-infant interaction may determine a permanent deficit in capacity to socialize—in other words, a fixation from which one may surmise only unstable substitutions or restitutive adaptations may be made. If the effects of early maternal deprivations are indeed significant to evolution of the schizophrenic process, such questions demand solution, as they hold the clues to both rational prevention and treatment.

If the early infant-mother relationship is so critical to the establishment of these ego assets, of necessity one must seek an explanation for the occurrence of schizophrenia in one or several children mothered by the same woman while others of her children develop with little evidence of psychopathology. Stabenau and Pollin discovered that in families in which some children became ill and others were spared, there was evidence of intense family crises at the time of birth or in the ensuing months which affected the mother and her relationship with the newborn and later with the ill child. Such crises were identified as the development of depression in the mother with feelings of guilt owing to her hostility toward the new child, the birth of another sibling within two years, dislike of the child's physical characteristics, or the projective identification of the child in terms of certain unpleasant characteristics of the parents.

The consequences of the lack of early constancy in the mothering process, according to Burnham, is to impair the child's capacity to maintain a stable representation with the needed person in the latter's absence. The need for the mother is intensified and yet there is fear of her loss—the need-fear dilemma. The schizophrenic thus develops a special vulnerability to separation which becomes the crucial factor in establishing and maintaining satisfactory interpersonal relations.

Childhood shyness and the later shut-in life with limitation of friendships, characteristic of the preschizophrenic, perhaps have their origins in the seeking of security in early clinging, coupled with fearfulness of loss. It remains as an undifferentiated perception of relations to others and stems from the child's failure to develop trust and certainty in his own autonomy. The later social relations with others are thus permeated by intense ambivalence, with inability to integrate this perception of need-fear with the consequent love-hate affects.

It is unlikely that disturbances in the early mothering process alone are capable of explaining the full range of schizophrenic psychopathology, such as the impaired sense of identity often associated with a confused sexual role, the use of primitive processes of thought and communication, the lack of ability to discriminate fantasy from reality, and the defects in establishing and maintaining object or interpersonal relations. These failures of development are more likely to rest on later deficiencies or distortions in the process of personality development.

From the various studies of family dynamics of the past decade, it has been found with significant frequency that schizophrenic patients have spent their childhood in seriously disturbed family groups in which both parents gave evidence of personality disturbance. In the Lidz studies, two-thirds of the families contained one parent who was found to be schizophrenic. Such family groups are unintegrated and relate through conflict in which the parents oppose each other by derogating and defying the wishes of the spouse and by efforts to win the children to their side to obtain from them the emotional support not found in the spouse. In other families, the parental relationship is disordered in that one parent has a serious personality deficit, shown in domineering, brutal, aggressive, or alcoholic behavior, while the other passively accepts his behavior or is absent when the child is exposed to an unwholesome environment. Such parents often are doubtful of their own sexual roles; some have been homosexual, and others were in conflict over control of incestuous desires.

Caught in such family groups, the children are unable to find those conflict-free periods of personal interactions and play that establish a sense of personal security, ability to share, and to repress effectively hostile, aggressive, and sexual drives. Nor do they find the sources of sound personal or sexual identification. But most important for the understanding of the schizophrenic reaction are the series of events that impair the evolution of mature communication and thought.

Bateson put forward the hypothesis that the origins of the schizophrenic defects in communication rest upon a "double bind" transaction between two persons. Thus the schizophrenic may be seen as fixed in an intense emotional relationship with a parent who, by the contradictions between her verbal remarks and behavior, makes it impossible for the former to discriminate properly or to respond for clarification, as his questioning is treated as a threat to the needed relationship by the parent. A concrete example is a schizophrenic adolescent who, tied to his mother verbally, is encouraged to use initiative in his school work, yet when he attempts to leave the home to visit the library, he is told he must not do so as the parent needs him and will become ill in his absence. Such a "double bind" restricts and confuses the development of clear communication, since the parent's position is inconsistent and also limits the son's helpful socialization with others, from which he might learn progressive social discriminations and develop the potentiality for evolving other healthy relations. Whether the "double bind" is characteristic of schizophrenic families alone or has special features for such families is not known.

Others have also been struck by the family milieu as the source of the irrationality of thought of the schizophrenic. Of particular interest in terms of the thought disturbances are the studies of Wynne, Singer, and their associates, who have offered new proposals as to their classifications and have studied family transactions through the medium of conjoint family therapy as they relate to the specific defects. Their work is reported later in the section on Psychopathology, Thought and Communication.

Johnson describes the process as taking place dynamically in that the growing child repeatedly has been the recipient of intrafamilial hostility and at the same time has identified with parents who themselves excessively use projection, denial, or conscious lying in their relations within the family. Upon this background there are often found discrete assaults upon the child, aggressive or sexual acts, that the child must deny and repress in order to preserve his dependent relationship with the parent. Later the parent reinforces the child's fear and guilt by utilizing subsequent incidents to establish the child's responsibility for the earlier trauma and to escape from his own culpability. Thus the mounting denial and repression of his own internalized rage leads eventually to breakdown, with psychotic withdrawal or impulsive sexual and murderous aggressive acts.

Failure to acquire social skills early narrows the probability of acquisition of emotional relations with extrafamily members in adolescence and adulthood; this again limits the probability of enhancing the personal skills and perceptual discriminations and sense of personal autonomy demanded for an effective social and heterosexual adaptation in adult life.

Onset

The age of onset is from late childhood to late middle age, although the most frequent age is adolescence and early adult life. Although uncommon, it is not so rare in children (3 to 13 years) as was formerly believed. The more fully the previous history is taken, the more frequently there will be found a previous manifestation not merely of schizoid traits, but even of phenomena that were nearly or quite psychotic in nature. The high incidence during adolescence is not unnatural.

There is probably, however, no specific relationship between schizophrenia and puberty, which is normally a period of turbulence, of emotional cross-currents, and of struggle to adapt emergent, maturing urges to the demands of a restraining world. At that time, the individual is precipitated into a critical emotional period without preparation or understanding. He is perplexed by new problems, particularly those pertaining to sex, religion, vocation, and social relations. He may be plagued by a desire for independence or crippled by a too prolonged dependence. Self-consciousness, sensitiveness, moodiness, vague yearnings, sudden outbursts, defensive attitudes, the tendency to indulge in strange fancies, to project inadequacies, and to be irritable are traits often particularly marked in adolescence, and frequently, especially in its early course, similar characteristics are met with in schizophrenia.

Psychopathology

Although there is a striking contrast between a normal, well-integrated individual and the person reacting with a malignant form of schizophrenic psychosis, there is frequently no abrupt transition from the schizoid type of personality to the manifest psychosis. Certain disharmonies of thought, of habits, and of interests may have long existed. In adolescence there might have been a tendency to loneliness and perhaps to slight depressions. Colorfulness of personality may seem to have been lost. There may have been a vagueness of thinking, a blandness of affect, a tendency to projection of topics touching a special personal sensitivity and perhaps a tendency to be jealous of those more happily adjusted.

Even the person in the so-called *"early"* *stage* of schizophrenia has frequently been mentally sick for a considerable period before his personality disturbance is diagnosed as such. The patient's family has not usually appreciated the nature or significance of any personality change. The *mode of onset,* except in the catatonic type, is often a gradual evolutionary process, and there may be a transitional "preschizophrenic" phase of a year or two.

A variety of subjective experiences, associated with and/or induced by mounting anxiety and terrifying fears of personal dissolution, precede the earliest observed behavioral changes and oddities that bring the schizophrenic to treatment. He becomes aware of increasing tension, confusion, and distractibility in conversations with others and of his inability to maintain a train of thought in such human transactions. Outwardly this will be noticed as blocks or breaks in conversation, sometimes related by the closely observant to the introduction of abstract materials. At such times the schizophrenic may not speak or respond appropriately to his companions; he may look fixedly away, or he may appear to stare, as he does not regularly blink his eyes in his attempts to hold his attention. At the same time his sensitivity to extraneous sights or sounds may seem magnified, and his responses thereto intrude into these transactions, producing a degree of distractability. If he is questioned then or later, he may speak of having a "temporary blackout," a "trance," a "blank spell," or a division of attention that he cannot control. These episodic periods of blocking have been dubbed by Polatin as "microcatatonic" periods.

There occurs as well difficulty in maintaining perceptual constancy as concerns both his own body and the external world. He may sense his body and its parts changing in size or shape, shrinking or swelling, or he may visually record such variability in his perception of the bodies of others or of inanimate objects. He attempts to establish constancy by building up pictures or fantasies. Auditory perceptions, too, are uncertain; too loud, too removed, too undifferentiated and thereby frightening, uninformative, or confused. His perceptions from inside his body become preoccupying: borborygmi, flatus, muscular aches and pains, and the variable constancies and changes in the genitalia preoccupy and frighten him. He often attempts to deal with them by complaining hypochondriacal requests for assistance or by attempts at denial. In the later stages of the illness the concern over his body may lead to an impulsive rejection through mutilation. He may spend much time staring into a mirror or may alternately undertake strenuous efforts to build up his body through exercise or dieting.

The schizophrenic then misperceives his body and its parts as repulsive, ugly, or threatening. His gender is felt as uncertain, and, if he dares sexual explorations, they become polyperverse as a means of attempting to identify his proper role. It is the mounting and terrifying anxiety, the defects in attentions, and the perceptual distortions that perhaps lead to the increasing uneasiness in his interpersonal contacts. The uneasiness, in turn, produces in the members of his family, his few friends, and even strangers that uncanny and eerie response which experienced clinicians often refer to as the "praecox feeling."

During the early stage there may be no single feature that is pathognomonic of the disease. In some instances, the early symptoms are more suggestive of a psychoneurosis than of a psychosis. A common early symptom is an aloofness, a withdrawal behind barriers to an area in which, if access to it could be gained, would be found loneliness, hopelessness, hatred, and fear. Frequently the patient seems preoccupied and dreamy; his friends may speak of him as appearing "far away." He does not empathize with the feelings of others and manifests little concern about the realities of his life situation. His plans for his future are often vague and unrealistic.

The schizophrenic suffers from a feeling of rejection and from an intolerable lack of self-respect. The characteristic way from which he protects himself against insult is by withdrawal from emotional involvements with other people. The resultant isolation is a protection against painful human relationships, but the loneliness contributes further to his feelings of rejection and hence to further withdrawal. The patient no longer trusts or confides in anyone. Instead of mingling with others, he remains at home, where he may sulk in his room and show an increasing indifference to members of his family, to accustomed interests, and to the demands and opportunities of his environment. It seems as if a fear of interpersonal contact had driven the patient into a state of regression and withdrawal. There may be a seemingly unexplainable deterioration in work. There are shallowness of affect, a paucity of emotional responsiveness, and an impairment in richness and variety of emotional expression.

Acquaintances may attribute to laziness the patient's listlessness and loss of spontaneity, of ambition, of interest in competition with his group, and of sustained effort in pursuit of former goals. An irritable discontent is common. The patient easily feels slighted and may begin to believe that others are talking about him. He may become ill at ease, restless, taciturn, and unapproachable. There is a lack of pleasure and satisfaction in his accomplishments, an anhedonia. He wonders what interpretation others are putting on his behavior. A superficial attitude of superiority is not uncommon. Less heed is paid to social amenities and social requirements, while former loyalties and affections become blunted. The patient becomes disregardful of, and even resistant to, conventionality. Frequently he becomes neglectful of personal care and cleanliness. Ruminations on sexual topics are usual. The patient may feel that something wrong or unusual is going on in his environment. Mysterious meanings are discovered until finally misinterpretations and suspicions may cause him to move from place to place. For a few weeks or months the new environment may be free from any suggestion of hostility; then the patient begins to feel that people are watching him or conspiring against him. Odd mannerisms or ways of acting may appear, but they cause the patient no concern.

Some patients express undue worry over their physical condition. This is especially suggestive of an approachng schizophrenia when the complaints are unusual or unlikely. The early schizophrenic is often preoccupied with abstract speculations or with metaphysical ponderings on such subjects as creation and causality, or with religious doubts, mysticism, and meaningless problems. A young truck driver who had but a seventh grade education wrote an essay entitled, "The Imperative Mind." In the very early stages, a few patients recognize that their ideas of reference and other abnormal mental experiences are unnatural; they may wish to know the meaning of their experiences and to understand their problems. Occasionally they may have some appreciation of the causes that have led to their illness. At this time they may be willing to discuss their problems. Later this desire is lost, and the patient becomes inaccessible, while in many the desire never existed. During these early stages, before the construction of an elaborate symbolic system that becomes accepted as reality, the conflicts are much less disguised, and it may often be possible to discover the problems that the patient is living out in the drama of his psychotic behavior. Occasionally the patient may show some sensorial confusion during the first few days of an acute episode.

In that group of schizophrenics now designated as "ambulatory," these indications of social withdrawal are less evident. Their dubious relationship to life is expressed in doubts as to their aims, difficulties in making decisions as to their future, the means to get on or to find a central interest. Although at times they may appear to be driving and busy, their actions are performed to prove themselves. The adolescent may date to "prove" that he can gain the attention of others as his peers do. Marriage becomes a means of "proving" that one is a man or woman or that one can "love." The relationship with children is a means of establishing the fact that one can be a mother. All activity is representative of an autistic dramatization without full affective contact with the realities of life, as though there is a continuous screen between the inner person and those with whom he relates. The existence has an "as if" quality; it is split from reality.

Sometimes the onset is sudden and precipitate. During adolescence, the loss of an only friend often precedes the gross indications of schizophrenia. Such a friend may have been the only outlet from a turbulent home life. The loss of the friend forces the future patient again to seek satisfaction in the family. This arouses increasing anxiety, and eventually panic ensues when the adolescent considers, or is unable to control, his hostility, sexuality, or his deepening despair because of being forced backwards into an isolated, lonely, unhappy life of daydreaming, hating, and fearing.

DISTURBANCES OF AFFECT. As we pass from this initial, and what might be called premonitory, stage, or stage of incubation, to the manifest psychosis, an apparent *poverty and a disharmony of feeling tone appear*. The dulling of finer feelings and an insidious narrowing of interests noted in the incipient stages become progressive. The patient is unable to feel and regulate emotions properly. There is a withdrawal of feeling or affect from external realities back into the self. As the disease progresses and the emotional impoverishment increases, the patient becomes indifferent, not merely to those sentiments and subjective values that make life worth living for the person in mental health, but, apparently existing at a vegetative level, he may be unconcerned as to fundamental comforts and needs. A few patients show, not a burned-out affectivity, but a definite, prevailing one, such as euphoria or depression. These feelings, however, usually lack depth or focus. The persistent mood, or emotional rigidity, has no relation to external circumstances or experiences.

Another disturbance of affect is one in which emotional expression is unrelated to reality. This is manifested by an emotional disharmony, often first exhibited by inappropriate smiling or laughing and silly giggling. Frequently the disharmony is between mood and conscious idea; there may, for example, be but little subjective feeling of depression even when ideas of despondency are expressed. At times experiences and ideas that should evoke a certain emotional response will produce its opposite—an emotional disconnection or dissociation. The patient, for example, may with a silly laugh speak of the death of his beloved mother. Whenever there is a display of affect by the schizophrenic, it seems unnatural and stilted, lacking in any infectious quality and often it arouses feelings of uneasiness or estrangement in the observer. At times one notes capricious, fitful, apparently causeless changes in affect and mood. This inferior affective capacity, the deterioration and impoverishment of emotional expression, and the inappropriate emotional responses to situations constitute one of the important ways in which the personality is disorganized or split, and attest the aptness of Bleuler's designation of schizophrenia.

One of the most generally accepted hypotheses advanced as an explanation of this serious disturbance in the affective life of the patient is that the affect, contrary to first impression, is not lost or destroyed but is withdrawn from the conscious, perceptive aspects of the patient's life, from matters of objective reality, and is attached to complexes and other material in the unconscious. The affect is hidden because it is fixed to highly personalized subjective constellations of ideas. According to this theory the disorganization of affect appears all the greater because it is associated with, and determined, not by one constellation of unconscious ideas, but by many complexes, among which there may be active conflict and discord. Since the affect is attached to and determined by material that is inaccessible, the emotions appear out of harmony with the contents and expressions of consciousness, although they are really in harmony with the psychic material to which the affect is attached and by which they are governed. The emotional disturbance in schizophrenia is more a displacement than a deterioration.

The emotional apathy of the schizophrenic individual may perhaps be theoretically explained in a somewhat different manner. One way by which the normal person may deal with difficult and threatening situations is by minimizing or ignoring them. It is conceivable, therefore, that the patient defends himself by building a wall of indifference around himself. Although this blunting of feeling may have arisen as a mechanism of defense against a troublesome situation in the inner world of the patient, it irradiates and becomes a general behavior pattern of the personality.

When interest and affect are withdrawn from the conscious, familiar material with which they were formerly connected and are attached to the content of the unconscious, a state known as *depersonalization* may exist. The patient has feelings of vagueness, of unreality, of detachment, or of being a spectator of life instead of taking part in it. He feels himself changed throughout in comparison with his former state. As a a result, he no longer acknowledges himself as a personality. His actions seem mechanical and automatic. The patient does not believe he is another personality (transformation of personality) but has rather a sense of loss of the limits of his own personality with its directive ego. The identification of one's own personality may become indistinct or confused. It seems to the patient that he no longer has any internal self to which he can refer forces and influences. In his attempt to rationalize this sense, the patient may come to feel that parts of his body or his mind seem strange and as though they do not belong to him. He may develop more nihilistic ideas and believe that he no longer has a body, that there is no world, or that he is dead. In addition to this change of self, the environment may seem unnatural and appear to have lost its character of reality. States of unreality are probably closely related to thought block, feelings of stupidity, fugues, dream states, and other involuntary withdrawals.

From what has been said, it will be seen that there is rarely a dominant affect in schizophrenia as is the case in manic-depressive psychoses. On the contrary, there are numerous inharmonious affects arising from conflicting desires and complexes, or the affect may be fixed to or absorbed by fantasies, by elaborate symbolic systems, and other products of the unconscious. The result is an inconsistency of affect that contributes to the peculiar disorganization of personality that charcterizes the schizophrenic patient.

Among the disturbances of affect in schizophrenia, *hypochondria* is occasionally met with. This preoccupation with the body and various subjective feelings provides a meaningful purpose as the schizophrenic loses contact with others in his social environment. The patient may then express toward his own body the same attitudes he has held toward others and use the same ego defenses. Feelings of guilt, due to sexual drives, can be centered on his genitals and lead to preoccupations with defects in genital functioning. He may express these preoccupations in such bizarre terms as "electric currents" in the genitals or as a sense of shrinking of the body. As mentioned earlier, modification of the body concept is common in the schizophrenic reaction in the early stages. In some instances, other body parts come to represent the genital areas through the process of displacement. Later, in some instances the patient's guilty anxiety becomes so great that he is led to carry out mutilative actions against his own body in those occasional fantastic acts of personal dismemberment.

ATTENTION. One result of the schizophrenic's loss of capacity for attachment of energy and interest to external objects and reality and of his autistic preoccupa-

tions is a *narrowing of attention*. Interest, and therefore attention, is centered on subjective creations, on matters within and not without the patient. This lack of attention and of concentration gives rise to the misleading impression that the patient is intellectually impaired, whereas he is intellectually inert. The replies of the schizophrenic individual are often trivial and uninformative because interests and energy are directed toward material not accessible to ordinary questioning. *Paralogia,* a condition in which the patient's reply shows that the question has been understood, but in which the answer is erroneous, is caused by the dereistic thinking to which the schizophrenic patient is particularly given.

Although active attention (concentration), as just indicated, is often disturbed, yet passive attention is much less affected, with the result that, even if the patient is living in a world of fantasy, he is still able to maintain a contact with reality sufficient for certain practical needs, yet often too inadequate for a socialized adjustment. Schizophrenics may be perplexed but rarely suffer from disturbances of the sensorium and therefore from confusion in the correct sense of the term.

THOUGHT AND COMMUNICATION. Normally, *associations of ideas* follow one another with a definite logical connection, progressing to an ultimate completeness of thought, but in schizophrenia they may be shortened, fragmented, and otherwise so disturbed as to lack logical relationship. Although the disturbances of associations in schizophrenia do not become particularly marked until serious disorganization of the personality has taken place, frequently one finds that long before any manifest psychosis developed the patient showed a loosening of the associational links in thinking. Later the patient may speak in generalities and abstractions that are difficult to grasp—a dereistic type of verbigeration rather than communicative talk. The use of eccentric, metaphorical expressions is not uncommon. Doubtless the communications of the schizophrenic patient are nearly always self-meaningful, although often their significance is not grasped by others.

In the more disorganized schizophrenic reactions, there is a tendency for associative connections to become more involved, incongruous, and at times so broken or incomplete that the patient's utterances become fragmentary, disconnected, illogical, or even unintelligible. The train of thought may not be pursued to its logical goal, with the result that thinking becomes diffuse and disorganized. Cause and effect may be interchanged. If aware of his disordered thinking, the patient may say that his thoughts are suddenly taken out of his head. Irrelevance in replies to questions, a feature that, when consciousness is clear, is particularly suggestive of schizophrenia, may be quite striking. Probably, however, irrelevance is not irrelevant to the patient and would be relevant to the listener if the latter had clues to the semantic significance of the patient's autistic productions. Set phrases may come to be used repeatedly as stereotypes. The thought productions of the schizophrenic person often become characterized by vague and unusual symbolism. It is believed that the disordered thought productions tend to express, by condensation, the various problems that concern the patient. Speech may show a curiously distorted use of language varying from a stilted and formal phraseology without apparent substance to a "word salad" of nouns and verbs having practically no articulated structure or even without apparently meaningful connection. Doubtless there was earlier a significance that became lost. Affectations in manner of speech are often observed. The patient may show a "flight into intellectualism." The following is taken from a schizophrenic production entitled "Equalitized Metabolic Demention Metabolism."

"Improper wave length—wave length changes, later visible death. That is a moving trollysis similar to circulation of life action. Born high focussating action may die through wave length charge and still live until visible death takes place.

"Education comes from radiation of action. Anyone can study all science in a compositive way. It takes a compositive mind to be able to understand. Can tell compositive minds by stromonized conception. The mind at birth takes on a birthification, becomes environmental by the radiation to it. Metabolism to dimension differ in every person is of actions of metabolism and dimension balancing. . . ."

How the thinking of a formerly well-trained mind may become disorganized in schizophrenia is illustrated in the following intellectualized rumination taken from a letter written by a man who had had a scholastically brilliant college career and after graduation had spent two years at Oxford as a Rhodes scholar.

"I'm too utterly weary from battling with my financial-religious and general-religious problems to be able to survive any shock of learning that unhintably hard-won progress supposed to have been earned in the fraternal-religious problem is illusory. For that would wreck me—in my critically exhausted condition—with horror lest humanity—contrarily from being faith-imbued joy-multipliers of Revelations All Embracing God or Unfathomably Progressive Universe—are duped victims of God's opposite faith deluding us—with illusions of immortality, a Heavenly Father and of progress—into accommodation as evil-absorbers of His unconvertible and endless agonies and struggle."

Many schizophrenics appear to show a poverty of associations and of ideas, presumably because of preoccupation with material having its source largely in the unconscious and also because of the accompanying narrowing of attention. To be ascribed to these two conditions, as well, are the casual and trivial remarks and replies of the schizophrenic so peculiar to the disorder as to have important diagnostic significance.

Elements in repressed constellations of ideas may produce various ellipses, short-circuitings of ideas, and even neologisms. These words of his own making are condensations and symbolizations of complexes with affect. Within their concealed meaning are compressed the condensations of words that refer to persons or things intimately related to the individual's particular conflict or psychic experience. The use of neologism by the mental patient always suggests a schizophrenic psychosis.

In connection with disturbances of associations, mention should be made of the fact that in early schizophrenia a fairly typical flight of ideas may occur, which later tends to develop into incoherence.

Blocking may occur as associations approach painful conflict material. It results, perhaps, from a threat that repressed material is approaching awareness. It tends to arise largely in connection with special topics, whereas neutral topics may be handled as usual.

The thinking of the schizophrenic seems directed from the unconscious, and associations and symbols are molded and directed by affective constellations and instinctive undercurrents. They then rise into consciousness as a type of thought much like that of dreams, in which one finds active the processes of symbolism, displacement, and condensation. Dereistic thinking is of the pleasurable "primary process" type of early life that tends to falsify reality, to disregard realistic, logical, and scientific thought. It is not corrected by the logic of experiences or by the demands of the external world.

The explanation for the disorders in the thinking of the schizophrenic is found in the great extent to which associations are directed by internal perceptions and associations unrelated to occurrences in the immediate environment—that is, reality. Because of their origin in the unconscious, associations are broken, are led into bypaths, are fragmented, are incongruous, do not progress, or are joined through common affects rather than through conscious, logical connection, with the result that various forms of incoherence follow. When the connections appear particularly loose, we speak of the schizophrenic's thought as being "scattered." This means that the unconscious connection of ideas is unusually marked.

From their analysis of communication in the transactions of families with a schizophrenic member, Wynne, Singer, and their colleagues have proposed a classification of forms of thinking, descriptions of the types of parental communications as they appear to relate to these forms,

and also descriptions of their methods of rating styles of communication. They, too, conceive of the family culture and its transactions as the means by which role structure, means of communication, perceiving, and thinking are experienced and psychically internalized by the growing child. Proceeding from the developmental principles of Heinz Werner that maturation proceeds from lack of differentiation through progressive states of increasing differentiation, articulation, and integration, Wynne and Singer have postulated a global, predominantly undifferentiated form of schizophrenic functioning, designated as *amorphous;* a more organized but incompletely differentiated form of thought, designated as *fragmented;* and a continuum between these two in terms of thought process, described as *mixed.* Those schizophrenics classified as *amorphously organized* communicate in sequences, broken by gaps, brevity, vagueness, and indefiniteness. Their affect is dull and apathetic and the developmental histories are associated with evidence of defects and continued failure rather than indications of repressed loss. Those considered to have *mixed thinking* qualities show areas of perceptual and cognitive clarity and have functioned fairly well periodically in certain areas of life. Their premorbid background is found to have been poor. Patients with *fragmented forms* of thought, who would generally be classified within the borderline or pseudoneurotic groups, present preponderantly difficulties in integration and articulation of experience, which under nonstressful circumstances they appear to have differentiated. They are, however, vulnerable to emotional stress and in conflict over control of powerful impulses and thoughts. Their style of thinking approximates the normal, yet there is a lack of coherent and meaningful patterns in it and in their lives; opposing impulses are held together by constricting defenses of paranoid, obsessional, and other neurotic types.

In their transactions, the families of the "amorphous" schizophrenics seriously failed to communicate attention, role structure, and forms of interpersonal relatedness and affects. The parents were vague in their expectations of each other and of others, their verbal exchanges were seldom meaningful or relevant emotionally, and they appeared out of contact with each other as well as lacking in efforts to control their own or their offsprings' behavior. In some instances one or the other parent showed these features or vacillated. On the other hand, parental transactions of "fragmented" schizophrenic patients were found to be vigorous and manipulative, with intensive interactions in which blame placing was frequent. There were common spurious agreements and fights with many shifts in position. While the parental role seemed well differentiated in some aspects, performance over time suggested poor integration, shown through shifting standards, idiosyncratic word usage, and even directfulness. Their expectations of others were shifting, so that they transmitted confusion and perplexity. Since these various studies suggest that the genesis of schizophrenic disorders derives from pathological family acculturation, their significance in terms of prevention and therapy is enormous. Still too limited and too global, lacking controls based on sufficient observation of parental transactions of those with other personality maldevelopments and of the healthy, yet these studies pioneer a promising new area of exploration in the understanding of the genesis of schizophrenia.

DELUSIONS. The dominant *ideational content* of the schizophrenic is often delusional in nature. Because the satisfactions sought by his beliefs are so highly disguised by their symbolism and because the needs in response to which the *delusions* have been created are often not apparent, the delusions of the schizophrenic often appear grotesque and meaningless. His delusions are never meaningless, however, but are specific and adapted to his peculiar psychological needs and situation and are in keeping with his particular life experiences, although they are conspicuously disregardful of reality. In referring to symbols, attention may be called to the fact that if he has artistic ability, he may show symbolic condensations in his drawings or paintings.

The tendency of the schizophrenic's delusions to be grotesque, to be loosely organized, to center around themes of persecution, of grandiosity, and of sex, to arise from autistic sources and yet to be expressed in a relatively clear setting is shown in the following letter addressed by a patient to one of the male physicians connected with the hospital in which she was under treatment:

"Dear Dr.———

"My Plan." or as mother used to call you, "The Little Plant," or else one little Plant for I was the other Plant, called "Tant." Will you please see that I am taken out of this hospital and returned to the equity court so I can prove to the court who I am and thereby help establish my identity to the world. Possibly you do not remember or care to remember that you married me May 21, 1882, while you were in England and that I made you by that marriage the Prince of Wales, as I was born Albert Edward, Prince of Wales, I am feminine absolutely, not a double person or a hermaphrodite, so please know I am England's feminine king—the king who is a king.

Your first duty is to me, and if you do not intend to do the right thing, helping me to get out of here, stop the thefts of clothing, money, jewelry, papers, letters, etc., etc.; you will please let me know so I can make some absolute change and further demand of the nations my release.

1874 Building was to have been a palace for my mother, father, myself and you, that is, if you are the one I married—so why not get busy and furnish it up as such when I go abroad. Make my trips (our trips?) short and return to America on important matters and have the right place to hold court. You and Dr. Black can take me to the equity court when I prove up my individuality and this must be done.

Sincerely,
"Tant"

Queen of Scotland, Empress of the World, Empress of China, Empress of Russia, Queen of Denmark, Empress of India, Maharajahess of Durban, "Papal authority" as a Protestant.

In the early stages of schizophrenia, the delusions may not be fixed, and the patient may at times be in doubt as to his ideas of reference or as to the hostility of his environment; later he becomes convinced that his delusions are real facts. At

the onset of his psychosis, the schizophrenic may have obsessive ideas that
prove to be the early stages of a process
that later becomes frankly one of exter-
nalization and projection.

Delusions in the schizophrenic often
serve rather effectually in subjectively
reorganizing his life situations and in
dealing with such problems as thwarted
trends and drives, frustrated hopes, biological inadequacies, feelings of insecurity,
disowned qualities, gnawing feelings of
guilt, and the affective constellations and
other contents of the unconscious. In no
other type of mental disorder are the
patient's problems, wishes, and conflicts
so thoroughly dramatized and symbolized
in fantastic form. This fact and the schizophrenic's impairment of his ability to
appreciate and test the reality of his fantasies tend to the creation of extravagant
and bizarre delusions. The role of fantasy
was well expressed by Macfie Campbell:
"Fantasy is called on to supply what real
life has denied, but the fantasies are not
woven into a structure which is compatible with a normal social adaptation."
There is a tendency to a reversion to belief
in magical cause and effect. Some patients
in their schizoid withdrawal show no evidence of delusional ideation.

PERCEPTUAL DISORDER. Clinicians have
remarked upon the hypersensitivity of the
childhood or early schizophrenic to auditory and visual stimuli as well as upon
the apparent behavioral indifference of
the chronically ill to all environmental
stimulation. The paradox in these clinical
observations is paralleled in the extensive
research on the perceptual function in
schizophrenics as compared to others.
Wider deviations have been recorded on
dimensions of sensory and perceptual behavior among the schizophrenic population than among others, but also there
has been recorded high interindividual
variability and difficulty in replication of
findings between various observers. Silverman has emphasized the necessity of
evaluating the various laboratory findings
of differentiating the various subtypes of
the schizophrenic reaction as well as its

duration. He has suggested that the
numerous findings may be interpreted,
provided that one accepts the concept,
described in earlier chapters in this book,
of a stimulus intensity control system
within the central nervous system variously operative to reduce the input of
excessive stimulations under different cognitive conditions. Attention, which defines the area of perceptual scanning, will
also be modified. Thus the nonparanoid
schizophrenics are both acutely aware of
sensory stimulation and hyperreactive to
aspects of the sensory fields generally regarded by others as marginal or irrelevant.
Silverman postulates that the hypersensitive long-term nonparanoid schizophrenics
have developed stimulus intensity reduction defenses. Also, this group, in contrast
to paranoid schizophrenics, demonstrate
little scanning behavior. To him the
chronic nonparanoid and/or premorbid
schizophrenics are characterized by greater
attention to the sensory aspects of per-
ceptual-ideational inputs and less to the
connotative attributes—particularly so if
the input stimulation is psychologically
threatening or affectively unpleasant. At
such times they exclude these aspects of
the stimulus situation fear awareness. Thus
situations to which others respond with
psychological and physiological awareness lead in these schizophrenic subgroups
to hyporesponsivity, highly variable responses, inattention, and disturbances of
set and association.

Through failure of the schizophrenic
to build up constant and realistic perceptions of himself, his parents, and others,
he reveals during his illness his shifting
perceptions of those to whom he relates.
Searles has written poignantly of the
schizophrenic's experience of his world—
of his frequent and changing misperception
or misidentification of even his closest
associates as he attributes to the others a
series of personal attributes derived from
some part characteristic—physical or psychological—of his parents.

HALLUCINATIONS. In no other form of
mental disorder do *hallucinations,* or the
projection of impulses and inner experi-

ences into the external world in terms of perceptual images, occur in the presence of clear consciousness so frequently as in schizophrenia. Their mechanism is not unlike that of hallucinations in other abnormal states, but they tend to be more highly disguised in nature and to constitute a primitive form of adjustment and therefore are of much more serious significance than is their presence in delirium or in dissociative states. It is not difficult to conceive of highly significant material in the schizophrenic's inner life as assuming hallucinatory vividness. It is but a step from the figurative "voice of conscience" to its audible perception. Unconscious material and unadjusted tendencies break through and create sense perceptions, perhaps highly symbolized, in response to psychological needs and problems. Disowned desires and feelings of guilt are projected as auditory hallucinations that, as the voice of conscience, accuse and criticize. The patient, incapable, because of his disorganized ego, of recognizing the origin or significance of his hallucinations, believes in the reality of these projected images, accepts them at face value, and reacts in accordance with what he has accepted as reality. He can no longer distinguish between subjective and objective experiences, with the result that he tends to alter reality with hallucinations and delusions. But not all the hallucinated material of the schizophrenic is accusatory. Oftentimes, as recent studies have found, the auditory perceptions are comforting, provide companionship, advice, judgments, and even sexual gratification. These hallucinated perceptions may be identified frequently by patients as representing the voices of significant persons in their lives (parents, lovers, friends) and appear to serve as a substitute for those persons. The accusatory and affectional components thus appear to represent both the actual and the desired elements in the lost personal relationship. Frequently the onset of hallucinatory experience takes place when the individual actually has lost a significant relationship or, through the isolation of the illness or hospital, is deprived of that relationship.

The schizophrenic may find his hallucinations so serviceable that he is unwilling to relinquish them, with the result that they come to constitute one of his cherished means of adjustment, and he becomes occupied not with a real but with a hallucinatory world, protected from the disturbances of reality. His hallucinations may be said to collaborate with delusions in the development of the same theme, the one by means of image symbols, the other by ideas.

But little need be said in the way of description of hallucinations in schizophrenia. They are more frequently auditory than of any other sense. Olfactory and kinesthetic hallucinatory experiences often are overlooked. Visual hallucinations are not particularly frequent and tend to be limited to acute phases of the psychosis. During their early occurrence, hallucinations are often accompanied by considerable emotional tension and may have a disturbing and disquieting influence on the patient. As time passes, they may cause but little concern and exert less influence upon behavior.

IMPULSE AND ACTION. Many of these odd, unexplained, and impulsive activities of the schizophrenic grow out of a lack of harmonious association and integration of strivings, affects, and wishes—the existence of incompatible and frequently, also, of changing objectives.

The capricious, impulsive behavior of the schizophrenic is to be looked upon as a result of an ambivalence of impulse, a contradiction of conative tendencies. The concept of ambivalence, or contradictory manifestations of impulse, of idea, or of affect, was greatly stressed by Bleuler, and considered by him to be a fundamental symptom of schizophrenia. It rests upon the principle that the true meaning of an idea, impulse, or affect is to be found in the exact opposite of that manifestly expressed. The conscious rejection and denial of expression of a desire, notwithstanding its indirect and unrecognized expression through projection in the form of hallucination or delusion, is a manifestation of the principle of ambivalence. At any rate, in schizophrenia there is a peculiar association of contradictions in mental or personality expressions. Ordinarily our behavior represents a compromise, a working harmony among diverse desires, a resultant of the contrasting considerations, forces, and motives prompting us. In schizophrenia, on the contrary, the two conflicting impulses, one of conscious origin, the other of unconscious origin, control behavior in erratic sequence, or even struggle simultaneously to direct it.

Ambivalence may be manifested by an unstable blending of love and hate, with sudden unaccountable shifts in affection and hostility, leading sometimes to impulsive episodes. Occasionally unpredictable suicidal impulses result in the unexpected death of a patient. Impulsive self-mutilation is not rare, especially in case of an adolescent masturbatory struggle.

At times a schizophrenic may consciously resist a certain impulse, but he may nevertheless carry it through into action. Unconscious and dissociated tendencies acting in this way give the patient a feeling of being forced or controlled. This feeling of being forced permits the entertainment of thoughts or the indulgence in behavior that the socially determined standards of the individual would not permit but for which the patient no longer recognizes responsibility.

ANERGIA.   A common disturbance of activity in the schizophrenic is an avoidance of concrete or spontaneous activity, a loss of initiative and purpose, and the development of a state of inaction sometimes designated as anergia. This deterioration in habits of activity may perhaps best be considered as a loss of interest and a retreat, one of the means adopted by the schizophrenic in renouncing the world with which he cannot cope. His behavior tends to become autistic and regressive. Although the normal person secures his satisfaction by expending his energy in relation to the outer world, such a way gives no satisfaction to the schizophrenic.

NEGATIVISM AND SUGGESTIBILITY.   Another disturbance is negativism, which may manifest itself in a perversity of behavior in the form of antagonism to the environment, in opposition to the wishes of those about him, and, in more marked cases, in mutism, rejection of food, refusal to swallow, or even to void urine. Presumably the patient may feel that negativism is a "safe" way of expressing hostility.

Although it is quite the opposite of negativism in certain of its objective manifestations, one occasionally meets with a *pathological suggestibility* that seems to have for its object the same purpose as negativism—a lessening of disturbing contacts with reality. It is less disturbing for the reality-evading patient blindly and passively to accept and follow whatever the environment suggests than it is actively either to oppose or to initiate contacts with reality. He may, therefore, show an automatic obedience to verbal directions without reference to their appropriateness or significance. Instead of answering a question, he may repeat it in a parrot-like manner—*echolalia*. Again, he may at once imitate the movement of a person in his immediate environment—*echopraxia*. Obedient following of the suggestion of the environment involves neither initiative nor responsible contact with others and often seems to express a mocking hostility toward them. The *waxy flexibility* of the catatonic represents this passive acquiescence to suggestions to a degree that may lead the patient to ignore physical discomfort or pain, accompanied usually by a marked disregard of his environment.

Among the disturbances of activity, *mannerisms* and *stereotypies* occupy a large place in the clinical picture. Schizophrenic mannerisms are of a wide variety. They may consist of affectations of manner, speech, gait, et cetera. Others consist of grimaces, sniffing, blowing out the cheeks, wrinkling of the forehead, tic-like movements, or elaborate methods of performing certain activities constituting a sort of ritual. Some patients assume certain postures for years. Sometimes the lips are puckered and held protruded in what is known as "snout cramp." In general, the schizophrenic's attitudes, gestures, and actions, like many of his verbal communications, appear unintelligible. The bizarre behavior of the schizophrenic has, however, a meaning for him, although its purpose and value are often obscure to others because of condensation and symbolization.

CONSCIOUSNESS AND INTEGRATION. In schizophrenia there is relatively little impairment of consciousness, orientation, or memory, although, because of lack of interest, it is sometimes difficult to test these functions. The *time sense* of schizophrenics appears impaired. Many are unable to estimate units of time with accuracy, and others state their age as that when their illness or hospitalization first occurred. One often secures incorrect replies in answer to questions as to orientation but these are because of negativism, the habit of giving casual replies in order to avoid troublesome reality, or occasionally they are due to a lack of attention associated with a certain falsification by hallucinations and delusions. Forgetting, inattention, distraction, and imaginative thoughts are used by normal persons as expedients to overcome a disappointment; these are used by the schizophrenic patient, not as substitutive reactions, but as if he were in a rut of least resistance.

Because of the disturbance in the integrative functions of the personality, leading, as it were, to a disturbance in fusion of cognitive, affective, and conative mental elements, the schizophrenic is often described as demented. This, however, is not correct, as there is no irreparable impairment of cognitive and intellectual functions. This does not mean that judgment, the capacity for making conceptual inferences, is not impaired. Rather there has occurred a disorganization of personality or a failure of even development of the ego functions of personality. The patient not only has no appreciation of the disorganization that his personality has suffered, but his concepts as to personal welfare and social relationships and pur-

pose are rendered faulty and unreliable by his introverted tendencies and his distortion of both physical and social reality through delusions and hallucinations.

RESPONSE TO PSYCHOLOGICAL TESTS. Test devices provide the means of examining a variety of responses under conditions which may be held constant and varied so as to allow the examiner to study the variables influencing response. Tests also provide an index of how the patient functions in situations of varying degrees of structure or ambiguity. In the projective techniques, for example, only limited cues are provided for what is an appropriate response. It is well to remember that social situations, like test situations, vary as to the degree to which they provide cues for appropriate social response. Some patients can function in an apparently adequate way until they are placed in a situation in which cues for appropriate action are not clearly specified. It is then that their weaknesses become highlighted.

Variability in functioning, distortions in thinking revealed in poor reality contact, overgeneralizations, unconventional and idiosyncratic thoughts, and peculiarities of language, as well as the affective disorders and disturbances of ego boundaries, are revealed in performance on the generally applied battery of psychological tests: WAIS, Bender Gestalt, Rorschach, and Thematic Apperception Tests. The performance on Stanford-Binet and similar intelligence tests by disorganized schizophrenics differs both qualitatively and quantitatively from that of subnormal persons of the same mental age level. In normal persons and in the mentally deficient, the age levels at which failures and successes are intermixed are grouped fairly closely around the determined mental age level, but in disorganized schizophrenics, as in persons suffering from many other psychoses which have led to deterioration, there is usually a spread of failures and successes at a number of age levels above and below the determined one. This phenomenon is known as "scatter."

The detection of distinctive schizophrenic features in the responses to a Rorschach test is a complex procedure because of the many variations in the schizophrenic syndrome itself. There is no set or definite pattern, and a diagnosis of schizophrenic characteristics is largely made from inference. Variation in form of responses, contamination of ideas, bizarreness, withdrawal, environmental rejection, and poor affective control are revealed with the Rorschach test. Thus, poor form of responses (F + %) indicates weakness in reality testing, the overutilization of small details reveals the trends to make unwarranted generalizations about the whole, the limited popular (P) responses the unconventional or idiosyncratic. Complete rejection of the color cards suggests apathy or emotional blunting, while impulsiveness is equated with response determined solely by color. The disturbance in ego boundaries may be reflected in the ability of the patient to apperceive movement in the inkblots, while his empathetic defect is shown by the few percepts of human movement, as are his wariness and withdrawal from human transactions.

PHYSICAL CHANGES. The more disorganized and disturbed schizophrenics sometimes show certain *physical concomitants*. One of the most frequent of these is general disequilibrium of the autonomic nervous system. This is shown by cold, bluish hands and feet, blotchy skin, and widely dilated pupils, which, when tested by a strong light, may contract momentarily but quickly dilate again. Sometimes patients in a catatonic stupor who persist in standing about in an immobile manner develop a striking edema of the lower extremities. Attacks of vertigo and of hysteriform and epileptiform seizures may occur, more frequently in the early stages. Many patients lose weight during the acute phases of the disease. Those who enjoy a favorable outcome of a schizophrenic episode often show a marked increase in weight during convalescence; however, an increase in weight without a coincident mental improvement usually denotes an unfavorable prognosis.

Malnutrition and tuberculosis have been accompaniments of chronic hospitalization of schizophrenics. With improved hospital management, active screening and segregation of the tubercular, and the use of appropriate chemotherapy, these complications may be prevented.

Types of Schizophrenia

In formulating his concept of dementia praecox, Kraepelin classified his cases into different varieties, depending on the predominant symptomatology. Although classification according to reaction type continues to be made, it must be recognized that numerous patients show at one time or another psychopathology considered characteristic of the individual groups. More is to be gained by studying each patient, evaluating his central pathology, the deficits in his life experience, and the dynamic forces inducing his particular psychopathology, and by erecting a pertinent and individualized therapy, than by attempting to categorize his illness in a vague classificatory division. Since these types or divisions are widely used, they are delineated in this section.

SIMPLE TYPE. In this type the most marked disturbances are of emotion, interest, and activity. If hallucinations occur, they are rare and fleeting, and delusions never play an important role. The disorder is usually gradual in its onset and assumes the form of an insidious change and impoverishment of personality, the significance of which is not understood by the patient's friends. In adolescence a youth who has perhaps shown much promise begins to lose interest in school or occupation, becomes moody, irritable, and indolent. His goals are no longer realistic. Shallowness of emotions, indifference or callousness, absence of will or drive, and a progressive meagerness of inner resources betray the withering of personality that constitutes the most prominent feature of this type. Neither criticism by others nor chagrin of parents appears to cause concern. Appreciation of esthetic and moral values is lost. The required period of training or apprenticeship in preparation for a profession or a skilled occupation is not completed. Many become irresponsible idlers, vagrants, tramps, prostitutes, or delinquents. In the milder cases, the social maladaptation is less serious, but the patients are considered to be neighborhood eccentrics and, although intellectually unimpaired, are capable of performing only some simple routine task under supervision. The patient remains uninterested in his environment and unimpressed by responsibilities.

A. R. was committed to the hospital when 21 years of age following his arrest for window-peeping. In describing his childhood characteristics, the patient's family stated that he "was always a little hard to understand," but was a quiet boy who never entered into rough games. His school record was excellent and he always stood high in his class. At age 17, when in the fourth year of high school, he was obliged, because of a long illness of his father, to leave school and secure gainful employment. He secured work with a large manufacturing company where he soon came to be considered the second best operative on a certain type of machine. For two years he worked steadily, seemed ambitious, and appeared to have a normal and wholesome, but not marked, interest in girls. At age 19 he gave up his position, showed no interest in securing another, and when asked if he worked replied, "What do I want to work for? I have a father and sister working and they are enough." He appeared quite self-satisfied and felt that he should have a position of importance.

At about this time he was first arrested for peeping into women's bedrooms. Through the influence of his father, the charge was dropped. He became careless of his personal appearance and remained unoccupied except for occasional periods, when he set up pins in a bowling alley. A year later he was again arrested but again was released on the intercession of his father. He came to say little unless addressed and grew antagonistic toward his father and sister. He would remain out until midnight and then come home, eat a large meal, read until 2 a.m., and sleep until noon. Finally, after his third arrest for peeping, he was committed to a hospital for mental disorders.

On arrival at the institution, the patient was found to be of asthenic physique and slightly effeminate in appearance. His emotional responses were shallow and inadequate. He showed no concern over his situation, laughed about it in a silly manner, and referred to his offense as "just a foolish idea." His hospital residence was characterized by apathy, preoccupation, and inactivity. During the summer he would at times take part in the patients' baseball games, but in winter he refused ground privileges. He never expressed any delusions and denied hallucinations. At times he would be seen, apparently much preoccupied, walking alone about the hospital reservation, laughing to himself.

Such a case illustrates how an individual is unable to complete the transition from adolescence to maturity with its adult heterosexual and social adjustments. There seemed to be a certain innate limitation to the personality. Interest became largely withdrawn from the actual world, energy was absorbed by the subjective life, and there was a diminished response to social demands.

HEBEPHRENIC TYPE. The onset of this type is insidious and usually begins in early adolescence. Occasionally the onset is subacute and is characterized by a depression that suggests an affective reaction. Usually, however, affective reactions are shallow and inappropriate. Silliness, giggling, and incongruous or inappropriate smiling and laughter are usual. Hallucinations, which are frequent, often represent the projection of repressed instinctive urges. The ideational content tends to take the form of fantasy or of fragmentary bizarre delusions rather than of elaborate or systematized beliefs. Associative processes are loose, speech is incoherent, neologisms are common, and posturing and mannerisms are frequent. Regressive features are prominent, wetting and soiling are common, and the patient eats in a ravenous, unmannerly fashion. The patient comes to lead a highly autistic life; he becomes bafflingly inaccessible and greatly introverted and withdrawn. The final disintegration of personality and habits is perhaps the greatest of any of the types of schizophrenia.

One of five children, Theresa was her mother's favorite. Greatly petted and babied by her mother, she always remained dependent upon her. She was described as having been a pretty child with a rosy complexion. She early became aware of this fact and enjoyed dressing up and strutting about to display her good looks. In spite of these signs of vanity, she was timid and shy and would blush in a self-conscious way when she realized that people were noticing her. In childhood she did not play freely with other children: "she thought herself above other children," and is described by her sisters as having in later years "a rather good opinion of herself and her abilities," and by her neighbors as "high hat."

Soon after leaving school at age 16, she began to work in a bleachery, where she remained until shortly before her commitment. She never had any girl chums and did not participate in the activities of other girls at her place of employment. Her attitude was one of "proud distance." While she was still in school there were several boys who were quite friendly toward her, but her sister said she could not remember any instance when the patient had any male callers or associates after she grew up, although she gave much attention to her clothes and personal appearance, obviously, in the sister's opinion, in an effort to attract the attention of young men. Her family described her as devoid of humor, sensitive, jealous, stubborn, willful, and easily angered. She became more seclusive, had "melancholy spells," became preoccupied, and paid less attention to her environment, and when addressed she would ask in an indifferent way, "What did you say?" She also became irritable and critical, particularly of the wife of her brother, with whose family she lived.

About six months before commitment to the hospital at age 32 she "began to grow thin and nervous" and became careless about her work, which deteriorated in quality and quantity. She believed that other girls at her place of employment were circulating slanderous stories concerning her. She complained so indignantly that X., an attractive young man employed in the same industrial plant, had put his arm around her and insulted her that her family demanded that the charge be investigated. This showed not only that the charge was without foundation but that the young man in question had not spoken to her for months. The family, however, had not suspected mental disease until six days before her commitment, when she returned from her work. As she entered the house that evening, she laughed loudly, watched her sister-in-law suspiciously, refused to answer questions, and at sight of her brother began to cry. She refused to go to the bathroom, saying that X. was looking in the windows at her. She ate no food and the next day declared that her sisters were "bad women," that everyone was talking about her, and that X. had been having sexual relations with her, that although she could not see him he was "always around." In her hallucinatory experiences she heard X. say, "Aren't you going to fire her? I've had her. She don't know it." The patient became resistive, was afraid of being killed, and at times said, "I'm dead." She stated that she was being poisoned, saw her dead mother, and heard her speak.

As the patient became noisy, did not sleep, and ate but little and then only when spoon-fed, she was committed to a private institution. Here she was uncoöperative, silly, grimaced, and whiningly repeated, "Oh, mama! mama! I want to see my father before I die." She heard voices outside her window and at night would come to the door of her room several times saying, "What is it all about? Oh, mama!" Her associations became loose; she took no interest in the care of her person or in other patients but would stand for hours with her back against the wall, her head thrust forward, fingering her hair, and unobservant of her environment.

After a residence of four months in the private institution, the patient was transferred to a public hospital. As she entered the admitting office, she laughed loudly and repeatedly screamed in a loud tone, "She cannot stay here; she's got to go home!" She grimaced and performed various stereotyped movements of her hands. When seen on the ward an hour later, she paid no attention to questions, although she talked to herself in a childish tone. She moved about constantly, walking on her toes in a dancing manner, pointed aimlessly about, and put out her tongue and sucked her lips in the manner of an infant. At times she moaned and cried like a child but shed no tears. As the months passed, she remained silly, childish, preoccupied, inaccessible, grimacing, gesturing, pointing at objects in a stereotyped way, usually chattering to herself in a peculiar high-pitched voice, little of what she said being understood. At an interview 18 months after her hospitalization, she presented an unkempt appearance, was without shoes, sat stooped far over, smiled in a silly manner, and presented a picture of extreme introversion and regression. During the attempted interview, she rarely spoke, although she occasionally replied, "I don't know" in an entirely indifferent manner and apparently with no heed to the question. The nurse reported the patient as seclusive, resistive, idle, and with no interest either in the activities of the institution or in her relatives who visited her.

CATATONIC TYPE. The catatonic type is characterized by phases of stupor or of excitement, in both of which negativism and automatism are prominent features. There may be alternation between little or no movement on the one hand to an explosive overactivity on the other. Frequently, however, a given catatonic episode may present but one phase, either stupor or disorganized overactivity, throughout its course. Again, there may be an admixture of symptoms usually thought of as belonging characteristically to one or the other phase. The most frequent age of appearance is between 15 and 25. Of the various types of schizophrenia, catatonia most frequently has a somewhat acute onset and is most frequently precipitated or preceded by an emotionally disturbing experience. The prognosis for a recovery with reintegration of personality after a catatonic episode is more favorable than in other types of schizophrenia, although after a period, perhaps after several episodes there is a tendency for the catatonic type to pass over into states approaching the hebephrenic or paranoid, with permanent disorganization of the personality.

Catatonic Stupor. Catatonic stupor, or the stupor phase, is often preceded by depression, discontent, or emotional fermentation. The patient is inclined to be uncommunicative, and his reactions become increasingly characterized by failing interest, inattention, preoccupation, emotional poverty, and dreaminess. Mute, stuporous, and with mask-like facies, the catatonic may occasionally keep his eyes closed but more frequently he stares fixedly and blankly downward. He may stand almost immobile, seldom shifting his position during the whole day. The skin of his feet may become turgid and engorged, with swelling of unsupported parts. Another catatonic may spend the day sitting on the edge of a chair or crouching on the floor. With his implicit loss of reality sense, he denies the world and actively resists the environment. He opposes any effort to move him from attitudes and positions, often constrained and peculiar, that he has assumed and may maintain for months. The patient refuses to dress or to eat, although occasionally, if he thinks he is unobserved, he will eat greedily. Saliva, urine, and bowel contents are often retained. He may not only soil clothing but even exhibit an apparent purposefulness in his annoying disregard of all cleanliness in his habits of excretion.

Gestures, grimacing, and grinning are common. The hands may be held tightly clenched and other muscle tensions may be maintained. Occasionally the physical manifestations of catatonia show some points of similarity to parkinsonian akinesia and rigidity. Catalepsy, either flexible or rigid, may be present. In this state, the patient initiates no spontaneous movements but maintains the postures into which he is passively impressed. Through automatic obedience, the patient may carry out any verbal instructions, regardless of their absurd or even dangerous nature. He shows no avoiding reaction to feinting motions before the eyes, to pinpricks, or to other painful stimuli. Although giving no indication whatsoever that he is at all aware of what is going on about him, the patient really registers the events of his environment, and when he begins to speak again, he may give a surprisingly full account of incidents occurring while he was in his stupor.

In spite of the apparent ideational poverty, there seems to be every reason to believe that ideas and representations are by no means absent, but rather are centered about a dominant ideo-affective constellation. Perhaps an analog to catatonic stupor may exist in the unapprehending, impassive response with which profound, overwhelming bereavement or catastrophe may at times be met. Both this reaction and the catatonic stupor of the schizophrenic may serve as methods of meeting situations too difficult to be met by active, resolute measures. The stupor may be thought of as a protective withdrawal from contact with surroundings that seem threatening. Again, the stupor may be compared to a retreat into an intense, trance-like preoccupation or reverie.

After a period of extremely variable duration, the patient may slowly, or at times suddenly, emerge from this profound generalized inhibition. Occasionally catatonic rigidity and negativism may terminate in response to affective stimuli. The opposite occurrence, the sudden sinking into a stuporous akinesia following an apparently trivial physical or mental event, is more frequent. Interest, affect, and behavior may return more or less closely to normal, or the patient may pass into a state of catatonic excitement.

Catatonic Excitement. Catatonic excitement is characterized by an unorganized and aggressive motor activity. It is not accompanied by emotional expression and is not influenced by external stimuli; it is apparently purposeless and stereotyped and is usually confined to a limited space. Of all schizophrenics, the excited catatonic most frequently shows impulsive and unpredictable behavior. Without warning or apparent cause, he may suddenly attack an inoffensive bystander or break a window. He destroys his clothing, remains nude, and disregards all excretory cleanliness. Negativism is usually marked. The flow of speech may vary from mutism to a pressure suggesting a flight of ideas. Attitudinizing, mannerisms, stereotypies, and grimaces are frequent. The patient may react to terrifying or ecstatic hallucinations of sight or hearing. Mystical experiences are not uncommon. Hostility and feelings of resentment are common. The patient may be sleepless, appear delirioid, refuse food, and become dehydrated and exhausted. There is often a rapid loss of weight. On rare occasions the acutely and extremely excited catatonic may collapse and die. Usually no pathologic condition sufficient to explain the cause of death is found at necropsy. In such cases, therefore, the death is ordinarily said to be a result of "exhaustion syndrome."

Probably acute catatonic excitement is often the same as the reaction that Kempf termed *acute homosexual panic*. The great activity is often accompanied by fearfulness and auditory hallucinations that accuse the patient of homosexual practices or inclinations. As previously noted, he is often assaultive.

Many psychiatrists look upon catatonic stupor as a profound regression, a dramatization of death. Attention is called to the similarity between catatonia and the instinctive immobility reaction exhibited by certain animals when confronted with a life-threatening situation. Arieti has suggested that the immobility of the catatonic has its origin in family transactions wherein criticism is directed toward action tendencies of the growing

child and is accepted by the compliant child. Catalepsy then is an expression of compliance to the demands of others. As mentioned earlier, it may symbolize an ambivalent negativism and be used to discharge hostility in a passive way.

The case of A. C., aged 32, will illustrate many of the features observed in both the excited and the stuporous phases of catatonia.

The patient's father was stubborn and self-willed, his mother was excitable and temperamental. At seven years of age he went to live with his grandparents. The grandfather, whose "word was law," suffered from epileptic seizures and subsequently died in a hospital for mental diseases; he had no understanding of the child's point of view. His seizures greatly frightened the boy. The patient was a seclusive, day-dreaming, timid, shy, and sensitive, but stubborn and self-willed, child. He still remembers with resentment how his father whipped him before another boy whom he would not thank for an apple. He was uninterested in the play of other children and spent his time either in the town library or in his own room, where he made various toys that he guarded jealously from other children, allowing only his sister, his sole confidante, to share them. At age 17 he was graduated from high school, where he had learned easily but had taken no part in extracurricular activities.

His occupational history was without significance except that his early promise of success as a draftsman and designer of airplanes and motors had not been sustained and that for eight years prior to his commitment he had earned practically nothing. At age 20 he married.

Two months before commitment the patient began to talk about how he had failed, had "spoiled" his whole life, that it was now "too late." He spoke of hearing someone say, "You must submit." One night his wife was awakened by his talking. He hold her of having several visions but refused to describe them. He stated that someone was after him and trying to blame him for the death of a certain man. He had been poisoned, he said. Whenever he saw a truck or a fire engine, the patient stated that someone in it was looking for him in order to claim his assistance to help save the world. He had periods of laughing and shouting and became so noisy and unmanageable that it was necessary to commit him.

On arrival at the hospital, the patient was noted to be an asthenic, poorly nourished man with dilated pupils, hyperactive tendon reflexes, and a pulse rate of 120 per minute. In the admission office he showed many mannerisms, lay down on the floor, pulled at his foot, made undirected, violent striking movements, again struck attendants, grimaced, assumed rigid, attitudinized postures, refused to speak, and appeared to be having auditory hallucinations. Later in the day, he was found to be in a stuporous state. His face was without expression, he was mute and rigid, and paid no attention to those about him or to their questions. His eyes were closed and the lids could be separated only with effort. There was no response to pinpricks or other painful stimuli.

On the following morning an attempt was made to bring him before the medical staff for the routine admission interview. As he was brought into the room supported by two attendants, he struggle, grimaced, shouted incoherently, and was resistive. For five days he remained mute, negativistic, and inaccessible, at times staring vacantly into space, at times with his eyes tightly closed. He ate poorly and gave no response to questions but once was heard to mutter to himself in a greatly preoccupied manner, "I'm going to die—I know it—you know it." On the evening of the sixth day he looked about and asked where he was and how he came there. When asked to tell of his life, he related many known events and how he had once worked in an airplane factory, but added that he had invented an appliance pertaining to airplanes, that this had been stolen and patented through fraud and that as a result he had lost his position. He ate ravenously, then fell asleep, and on awaking was in a catatonic stupor, remaining in this state for several days.

He gradually became accessible, and when asked concerning himself, he replied that he had had a "nervous breakdown following the physical breakdown." He referred to his stuporous period as sleep and maintained that he had no recollection of any events occurring during it. He said, "Everything seemed to be dark as far as my mind is concerned. Then I began to see a little light, like the shape of a star. Then my head got through the star gradually. I saw more and more light until I saw everything in a perfect form a few days ago." Two days later he admitted that he could remember having seen the examiner while in the stupor. He rationalized his former mutism by a statement that he had been afraid he would "say the wrong thing," also that he "didn't know exactly what to talk about." From his obviously inadequate emotional response and his statement that he was "a scientist and an inventor of the most extraordinary genius of the twentieth century," it was plain that he was still far from well.

PARANOID TYPES. The features that tend to be most evident in this type or phase are delusions, which are often numerous, illogical, and disregardful of reality, hallucinations, and the usual schizophrenic disturbance of associations and of affect, together with negativism.

Frequently the prepsychotic personality of the paranoid schizophrenic is characterized by poor interpersonal rapport. Often he is cold, withdrawn, distrustful, and resentful of other persons. Many are truculent, have a chip-on-the-shoulder attitude, and are argumentative, scornful, sarcastic, defiant, resentful of suggestions or of authority, and given to caustic remarks. Sometimes flippant, facetious responses cover an underlying hostility.

The paranoid type tends to have its frank appearance at a somewhat later age than the other forms. It is not common until after adolescence and occurs most frequently after 30 years of age. The patient's previous negative attitudes become more marked, and misinterpretations are common. Ideas of reference are often among the first symptoms. Disorders of association appear. Many patients show an unpleasant emotional aggressiveness. Through displacement, the patient may begin to act out his hostile impulses. His grip on reality begins to loosen. At first his delusions are limited, but later they become numerous and changeable. In the early stages, too, their character usually indicates more clearly the particular psychological needs or experiences that they are created to meet. Occasional remarks may supply fragmentary disclosures of the patient's preoccupations. Rejected tendencies are ideationally projected instead of undergoing repression. Delusions of persecution are the most prominent occurrences in paranoid schizophrenia, but expansive and obviously wish-fulfilling ideas and hypochondriacal and depressive delusions are not uncommon. With increasing personality disorganization, delusional beliefs become less logical. Verbal expressions may be inappropriate and neologistic. The patient is subjected to vague magical forces, and his explanations become extremely vague and irrational. Imaginative fantasy may become extreme but take on the value of reality. Repressed aggressive tendencies may be released in a major outburst; some inarticulate paranoids may manifest an unpredictable assaultiveness. Many paranoid schizophrenics are irritable, discontented, resentful, and angrily suspicious and show a surly aversion to being interviewed. Some manifest an unapproachable, aggressively hostile attitude and may live in a bitter aloofness. Auditory hallucinations usually occur, and the voices are most frequently threatening or accusatory in nature. The patient may show varying degrees of tension and may be subject to upsurges of rage that he seems unable to control. As personality disorganization proceeds, affective responses become increasingly flattened. Mannerisms, apathy, and incoherence are common. In general, paranoid schizophrenia may be regarded as a projective, regressive, defensive type of reaction. In contrast to parental transactions thought to induce catatonic behavior by criticizing action, Arieti postulates that the future paranoid is exposed to accusations of malignant intentions, deceit, and lying. Action tendencies are fostered.

The following is in many respects a rather typical case of paranoid schizophrenia.

A. B., a physician, 38 years of age, was admitted to a hospital following his arrest for disturbing the peace. Specifically, he had frightened his neighbors by hurling objects at imaginary people who, he said, were tormenting him, by beating the air with ropes, and by breaking glass in the apartment that he and his wife occupied.

The patient was born in the Ukraine. Little is known of parental characteristics. His mother is described as being "sweet and good-natured as long as things went her way, but she would have violent outbursts of temper, during which she would throw dishes and break glasses when aroused." The patient, the youngest son, is said to have been "the favorite of the whole family. He was spoiled, given his own way, and invariably the other children would be whipped for the misdemeanors of which he was guilty."

When 16 years of age, the patient came to the United States, where he continued his studies. After graduation from college, he entered medical school. His medical course continued satisfactorily until the third year, when he failed to pass a pathology course, which until that time had been one of his best subjects. For some reason, not stated in his history, he was dismissed from the first medical school he entered, but later was admitted to a second one, where he repeated the third year and was graduated.

Upon his commitment to the hospital, his wife described his personality traits as follows: "He has always been a deep thinker. Lately, however, he cannot concentrate. He is rather aggressive and is the type who insists upon imposing his own ideas on everyone else. He thinks that people have to agree with him. He is stubborn and argumentative. This trait was even referred to in his college yearbook. He is an independent thinker and is very bright. He had big plans for the future. He was formerly quite extrovertive until the last few years, when he refused to go out and mingle with people."

Soon after beginning his internship, trouble developed between the young physician and the chief resident. The former was compelled to resign but secured appointment in another hospital and completed an internship. Following this, he went to Vienna to pursue graduate work in ophthalmology, otolaryngology, and bronchoscopy. After his return to the United States, he entered private practice and was apparently successful for the first four years, although, because of various difficulties, he changed locations on several occasions. For some reason not stated in the history, the patient gave up his practice and became a medical officer in a government service. He soon began to complain that the commanding officer was "against" him. He made frequent applications of cocaine to his nasal mucous membrane, not, he said, because he was a cocaine addict but in order to neutralize the effects of chloral hydrate, which was being sprayed upon him. After a few months he was released from his appointment. He then began practice in another city, but as he believed that the spraying of chloral hydrate continued there, he remained but two months and then returned to his original place of practice. He met with but little success, as the same ideas of persecution persisted. According to his history, too, "He became forgetful and neglected his cases. He had lapses of memory and seemed to be preoccupied with his own thoughts."

The patient's wife described him as having usually preferred the company of men, "but he has quite a history as far as the opposite sex is concerned." While studying in Vienna, he became involved with a widow and married her. Two weeks after their marriage he discovered, he alleged, that his wife was unfaithful to him and was "a member of a gang of dope peddlers who tried to involve young medical students in their racket." He then returned to the United States. The following year he married again, but the couple lived together for only three months. Three years later the date was set for his third wedding, but he did not appear at a party scheduled to precede the wedding. A quarrel with the expectant bride followed, but finally the wedding took place. Soon he began to object to his wife's talking with other men and accused her of infidelity. On two occasions when she had not even been absent from home, he insisted he had seen her on the street with other men.

Four months before his commitment the patient awoke his wife and told her she must leave the house permanently the following day. He insisted that she was not his wife any longer and the next day asked if she had made her plans to leave. In view of the failure of three marriages, his accusations of infidelity in at least two of them, and his preference for the company of men, the probability at once suggests itself that at least some of the patient's personality difficulties arose from unrecognized homosexual tendencies. Further support to this assumption is added by the fact that, during the psychiatric examination after his hospital admission, he remarked that certain physical complaints from which he was suffering suggested sexual perversion. Doubtless, too, the fact that for several years he had consumed a half pint or more of alcohol daily may be of corroborative significance.

As the patient's mental disorder progressed, he developed a great wealth of delusions. He stated that he was "the link between the living and the dead," that he was a "universal medium," that a certain physician called on him by mental telepathy for added strength and skill in surgical operations. He believed that someone was hiding in a trunk in his house and so he fired several bullets into the trunk. He accused his brother of spraying him with chloral hydrate from the third floor of his house. He therefore sat behind a closed door waiting for his brother, and upon hearing a noise, shot through the door. He grew a beard because his face, he said, was being changed in subtle ways by outside influences, adding that if he wore a beard, his true identity would be known. Following his admission to the hospital, he often spent long hours in his room where he could be heard pacing the floor, moaning, or making a noise like a dog, striking his head with his fist, or pounding the wall. When asked the reason for his behavior, he explained that he was suffering tortures because people abused their powers of mental telepathy and were directing those powers toward him. He spent nearly all the day in his room where, during the fourth and fifth years of his hospital residence, he would frequently be heard shouting, screaming, and uttering noises that the attendants described as resembling the howling of a wolf. In explanation of these noises, the patient stated that there was a woman spiritualist who, in some way through persons in the hospital, was exerting a peculiar spell on him, and that by making these noises, he could drive the spirits away. His thought processes became progressively disorganized.

Thirteen years after his admission to the hospital, he wrote his ward physician a 10-page letter which he concluded as follows: "In view of the facts and their significance, and in view of the connection of tendencies and the contingent and pertinent effects, and in view of my physical condition brought about by the connected and sustained tendencies and actuating reasons behind them, I shall not consider it a mere negligence, or merely a form of criminal negligence, or merely an ethical vice, but I shall consider your interference with the anatomical and physiological requirements of my health as an outright, deliberate, well-accounted for and reasoned out criminal and dastardly endeavor at homicide."

As the years passed, he was rarely to be seen on his ward but remained in his room, where most of his days were spent in writing and reading. When approached, he was hostile and resentful in attitude. He was, however, less aggressive and less abusive in speech. As frequently happens in the paranoid schizophrenic, his prolonged institutional residence had produced a lessening of tension but little or no modification of thought content.

SCHIZOAFFECTIVE TYPE. Less frequently seen are cases of mental disorder characterized by recurring episodes that continue to show admixtures of schizophrenic and affective symptoms. The mental content, for example, may be so reality-disregarding that it seems schizophrenic, whereas the mood is one of pronounced elation or depression. Again, the affective features may stand to the fore, but the patient's behavior may be so bizarre that it must be regarded as schizophrenic. In some instances, the prepsychotic personality may have been strongly schizoid or, on the other hand, outgoing and well-socialized, yet the clinical features of the psychosis may be quite at variance or inconsistent with the early personality pattern. It is not uncommon to see depressions in schizoid individuals who, in addition to the depression, show a great deal of anxiety and many neurotic patterns. Such patients are usually refractory to treatment.

BORDERLINE OR PSEUDONEUROTIC TYPES. Both Bleuler and Adolph Meyer recognized that the onset of the schizophrenic reaction was often concealed by symptom formations considered as neurotic. The obsessive-compulsive and hysterical façades are the most commonly recognized. Hoch and Polatin have described what they term "pseudoneurotic schizophrenia," a condition frequently seen in private practice and only occasionally in the mental hospital. As the name implies, the dynamics are psychotic in character, although the symptom picture, at least in the early stages, appears neurotic. The pseudoneurotic schizophrenic usually shows a mixture of anxiety and of phobic, obsessive, depressive, and hypochondriacal symptoms. The underlying schizophrenic disorder is hidden by a façade of neurotic manifestations. Hoch and Polatin speak of the symptomatology as a pan-neurosis. A diffuse anxiety pervades all the patient's life experiences, and although he tries to force pleasurable experiences, he does not derive pleasure from anything. The neurotic manifestations constantly shift but are never completely absent. The true neurotic is usually anxious to describe his symptoms in minute detail and presses his physician with his explanations. The pseudoneurotic schizophrenic's explanations are vague, indistinct, and often contradictory, and are repeated in a stereotyped manner without details. The organization of the patient's sexuality is often chaotic. Some of these patients have brief psychotic episodes. About one-third of the patients with this misleading neurotic overlay gradually go on to a frank psychosis, although with less regression than that observed in the usual schizophrenic.

More recently, Grinker and his colleagues have attempted an analysis of the borderline syndromes and have concluded that there exist some four separate subgroups differing in behavior from those previously so classified.

The first, considered to have the least well developed ego functions and most closely related to the psychotic, express their abnormality in inappropriate and negative affect toward others, whether in individual or group relations. Usually careless in their grooming, they are immature in their sleeping and feeding behaviors. Their spontaneity was limited, and toward others their affective expression, both in verbal and nonverbal communication, was negative and expressed in occasional impulsive angry eruptions.

Their second subgroup, considered the "core" borderline category, also displayed a pervasive negative affect. However, this was "acted out" in many ways. These patients seemed to have established a reasonable personal identity but did not always act consistently with that individu-ation. They were depressed except when "acting out," participating in, or rebelling against their environment. This group may well be the same described by Hoch and Polatin as "pseudopsychopathic."

The third subgroup were individuals with blandly adaptive behavior. What was missing was the presence of positive affect—love or affection for others. Also, their self identity was uncertain. They resemble the "as-if" characters described earlier in this book.

The smallest subgroup showed some behavior exhibiting positive affection toward others. But here the feeling was directed to females and resembled that of a child-like clinging depression. Also anxiety and depression were predominant in their affective life, associated with lack of self-esteem and confidence.

In general the borderline syndrome has been found to be expressed in anger as the major affect, with infantile, dependent or complementary, but rarely reciprocal adult transactions with others. All "borderlines" have an unclear self identity, in which most characteristically they report themselves viewing or watching themselves "playing a role." Finally, depression reflected as a sense of loneliness and inability to relate to others—rather than caused by guilt or shame—seems a common element, although in the last group depression seems unassociated with anger.

Schizophrenia in Childhood

There has been much controversy as to whether childhood schizophrenia is the same as adult schizophrenia or whether it is a reactive pattern, reactive in particular to a cold emotional climate in the home during the first two years of life.

ETIOLOGY. It must be said that the causes are obscure. Theories of etiology range all the way from a psychogenic cause based on early disturbance in the mother-child relationship to a deterministic concept rooted in genetics. Bender believes that it results from "a developmental lag of the biological processes from which subsequent behavior evolves by maturation at an embryological level, leading to anxiety and secondarily to neurotic defense mechanisms." In her opinion, the fundamental pathological process is a diffuse encephalopathy for which no confirming anatomical evidence is described. Although the etiology is still debatable, there is an increasing belief that schizophrenia is the result of an interaction of constitutional and psychological factors. Perhaps childhood schizophrenia is not a separate and distinct clinical entity but rather a group of related and overlapping clinical syndromes.

Thus W. Goldfarb and others have found that the range of children diagnosed as schizophrenic includes several general clusters. On the one hand, there are those with predominant evidence of neurological or neurophysiologic disturbance who were brought up in families found by psychosocial studies to provide adequate sources for identifications and skill in communications and social awareness. On the other hand, there is a cluster of such children who show little evidence of neurological defect who were reared in disturbed families that provided inadequate roots for the growth of personal identification, communication, and perceptual and conceptual clarity.

Diagnostically these children show impairment in ego functioning. The development of a clear body image, sexual identity, and ability to conceive clearly time and space is impaired. They tend to use preferably the sensory information available from the contact receptors—touch, taste, smell—rather than the distance receptors—hearing and vision; thus they limit their capacities for anticipation and generalization and their ability to find a personal identity. It is probable, then, that a goodly proportion of the small children classified as schizophrenic might more properly be considered to be suffering from the personality disorders associated with organic brain damage. Some so classified undoubtedly fall into the group of mental deficiencies.

DIAGNOSIS. The diagnostic criteria specific for childhood schizophrenia are not definitely established. There is undoubtedly a wide variety of clinical pictures. Bender points out that some schizophrenic children are regressive, retarded, blocked, inhibited, mute, autistic, withdrawn, physically asthenic, unsocial, and unable to relate. Others develop overfast, have an exaggerated intellectual brilliance, and are overactive, precocious in language development, and excessively abstract in their thinking. In her experience, any severe psychoneurotic disorder in a child before puberty, whether it is obsessive-compulsive, so-called hysterical, or severe anxiety, is a reactive response to a deep, inherent, threatening disorder, most often schizophrenic in nature.

The older the child, the more does the clinical picture resemble that seen in adults. In such a child, therefore, we may see not only withdrawal and loss of contact and affect, but also hallucinations and delusions. The last two symptoms do not occur before eight years of age. In the older patient, the onset may be insidious or acute, the insidious type being more frequent. It may be difficult to date the beginning, although retrospectively it is often remembered that peculiarities may have been noted. It is characterized by a general reduction of interests in play and other activities. There is a gradual loss of affective contact with people, accompanied by regressive phenomena. Some patients show a tendency to brooding or to obsessive rumination on some topic ordinarily not of interest to a child. Some patients become aggressive and destructive. Self-mutilation is a common behavior seen in these children. In some instances this is expressed indirectly as accident-proneness or masochistic provocativeness. In children with these behaviors there will be found a significant history of physical abuse by the parents in the first two years of life. Many appear to be feeble-minded and are committed to an institution for mental deficiency. Any great improvement is unusual. Children having an acute onset have usually not been previously regarded as abnormal. Shortly before the appearance of acute features, there may have been an impairment of ability to concentrate, with an accompanying drop in quality of school work. The child may then begin to mumble to himself, sleep poorly, maintain odd postures, show diminished or rigid affect, become inaccessible and extremely restless, and perhaps scream and kick. Usually improvement takes place after several weeks but with a reduction of emotional and ideational expression. Subsequent acute episodes are usual, each one followed by increased personality disorganization.

The psychological problems that the child is attempting to meet with his schizophrenic reaction are those naturally accompanying, or appropriate to, childhood and are therefore different from those of adolescence or adulthood. They are also appropriate to the particular developmental period within childhood at which the onset of the disorder occurs. The symptom formation will therefore be related to the problem that has created the anxiety. In other words, much of the symptom formation is determined by the way in which the child deals with his anxiety. Bender is of the opinion that the principal problems, particularly in the small child, are those of self-identity and therefore of relating to the rest of the world and to body function and of relating to objects, for example, to play material, food, or clothes. In somewhat older children, there may be the problem of relationship to a parent, particularly the mother or siblings, or early childhood sex problems. Mental mechanisms that are normal for early childhood become points of fixation, become exaggerated by repetition, become mingled with other mechanisms, and are carried into later periods of personality development, where they constitute the psychotic symptoms of the schizophrenic child.

EARLY INFANTILE AUTISM. In 1943 Kanner described a syndrome beginning as early as ages 2 or 3 years and characterized by an extreme withdrawal and obsessiveness. To this syndrome he gave the name "early infantile autism." Because of its similarities to, and its differences from, childhood schizophrenia, its categorical place presents a challenging problem.

The prevalence of infantile autism in a general population of Great Britain is reported by Wing and his colleagues as 2.1 per 10,000 of the age group 8 to 10 years when determined on the basis of Kanner's essential features (autism and insistence on sameness). Another 24 per 10,000 have a similar syndrome but present only one of the two essential features. The male-female ratio was 2.75:1. More recently, in the United States, Treffert has found the combined prevalence rate for childhood schizophrenia and infantile autism as 31 per 10,000. Of these, 25 per cent were classic infantile autism, 57 per cent psychoses of childhood with later onset, and 18 per cent psychoses with demonstrated brain disease. To him the differences in the groups seemed less compelling than the similarities; he doubts that infantile autism should be considered as separate from childhood schizophrenia.

The striking disability in interpersonal relations and the severe obsessive-compulsive mechanisms are the pathognomonic features of autism, but the peculiarities of language and thought, although somewhat different, share the general features of schizophrenia. The amplitude of the electroencephalographic auditory averaged evoked response measured during REM sleep has been reported by Ornitz and his colleagues as significantly greater than in healthy children.

The psychotic nature of the illness becomes apparent before the end of the first, and certainly not later than during the second, year of life.

Affective contacts with mother and other persons and the ability of the child to relate himself in the ordinary way to people and situations should normally be well established by 2 or 3 years of age. In early autism there seems to be an inability to form affective ties, with a resulting lack of responsiveness. The mothers of such children complain that "the child looks right through me—he does not see me."

Almost invariably it is found that the parents of these children are intelligent and successful, often professional persons in good economic circumstances, but obsessively preoccupied with abstractions of a scientific, literary, or artistic nature. The family life is of a cold, formal type, and the child has received extremely little fondling, cuddling, or warm, genuine parental affection. The behavior of the mother toward the child is mechanical and does not convey love.

When a child with early autism is brought to a psychiatrist, his parents have usually assumed that he is severely feeble-minded. The autistic child 3 or 4 years of age usually does not talk, does not respond to people, and often has temper tantrums if interfered with. He has little ability to empathize with the feelings of others. His autistic and impenetrable aloneness shuts out anything that comes to the child from outside. If he attempts to form sentences, they are usually for a long time mostly parrot-like repetitions of word combinations that he has overheard, often long previously. He frequently refers to himself as "you" and to the person spoken to as "I." Although the child has no interest in people, he has a good relation to objects and may play happily with them for hours. He has an obsessive urge for a maintenance of sameness. Furniture must continue to be arranged in the same manner and the routine of life must be unchanged.

Although the extreme withdrawal and limited responsiveness of the autistic child suggest that he is mentally retarded, it will usually be found that he has average or even superior intellectual potentiality. The facial expression is often serious and perhaps tense but is usually strikingly intelligent. Frequently those who speak have an extensive vocabulary and a surprising rote memory.

Many of these children continue to function in an emotional vacuum and, for all practical purposes, function in a socially retarded manner all their lives. Some of them, through permissiveness and emotional stimulation, attain a normal intelligence quotient, become able to pay attention to persons, and to accept and return affection. They may even participate in environmental activities, although they often remain "peculiar."

Perhaps the primary psychopathological mechanism in infantile autism may be described as a disturbance in social perception, analogous to, but more complex than, perceptual difficulties at the sensory-motor level. The question has been raised if there may not be, parallel to intellectual inadequacy, a syndrome of affective inadequacy.

Follow-up studies of autistic children show that by 15 years of age one-third have achieved a moderate social adjustment. About half of those who possess a meaningful language by the age of 5 show further improvement, whereas only rarely does the child without ability to communicate verbally by that age show significant subsequent improvement.

Psychodynamics of Schizophrenia

Those infinitely variegated expressions of disordered personality which constitute the schizophrenic reaction are the expressions of maldevelopment of ego and superego functions. Thus there are abnormalities in perception, thought, and action, including communication, affect, and the capacity to evaluate, make judgment, solve problems, and thereby adapt to reality. Such ego attitudes as a desirable capacity for trust, autonomy, initiative, and persistence are deficient and overshadowed more often by suspicious mistrusts, personal doubting, apathetic or indifferent efforts, and their consequences in uncertainty as to sexuality and adult role. There is evidence, too, of oppressive inhibitions and restrictions as regards expressions of aggression and of sexual and dependency drives, and there are indications of overbearing superego. Aspirational demands exceed talent, opportunity, and the time needed for learning and experience in order to approach the ideal ego.

While much of the psychopathology

may be understood as the result of deficiencies, failures, or distortions in family transactions which impair the establishment within the incipient schizophrenic of dependable and meaningful models of personality functioning, this explanation alone of the weakness of development is insufficient. Inordinate aspirations, with attending feelings of deep shame at lack of achievement, and excessive burdens of guilt attached to high expectations for repression of affective displays of anger, love, or tenderness attest to learning experiences which exaggerate social demands and are internalized as hypertrophied superego functions. In many schizophrenics the arousal of rage, the physiological pressures of the sexual drive and its expressions, and the needs for dependent support, all subjected to intensive repression, are tenuously checked but from time to time are discharged impulsively and widely and in so doing widely disrupt other functions. The means by which the demanding superego and ego-ideal are structured within the schizophrenic family have not been the object of study; yet they are as crucial as the transactions which fail to inculcate capacities for stable social perceptions, communications, and thinking capacities. Here, too, one may postulate later deficiencies in extrafamilial object relations needed to modify the influence of the parental transactions in structuring the distorted superego. Consequently psychological conflict, excessive demands on the ego repressive function, and limited defenses and adaptive capacities lead to ego disruption, with regression and disruption of substitutive functions developed to cover the early defects in ego growth. The effective psychotherapeutic milieu probably owes its success as much to restructuring of the abnormal ego demands as to the development of ego functions.

Course and Prognosis of Schizophrenia

Although the onset of gross schizophrenic disorganization often occurs suddenly, careful examination of the patient's developmental history shows that there have been many indications of personality disturbances in earlier years. More often the diagnosis is made at a time when family members no longer are capable of adapting to the progressive disturbance in behavior that has proceeded insidiously over a number of years. Earlier, the indicators of childhood schizophrenia have been described. In the O'Neal and Robins follow-up of children seen in one clinic, those who became schizophrenic had more infectious diseases during the first two years of life, more hearing problems, difficulties in locomotion, and physical disfigurements than normal children have. The boys were often spoken of as having a feminine appearance. Also, the presence of antisocial behavior antedated the schizophrenic reaction in half of those who were later so diagnosed. They were physically aggressive, incorrigible, and given to vandalism and pathological lying; they also had more phobias, feelings of depression, unhappiness, and paranoid trends than other children.

Granted that schizophrenia can perhaps best be regarded as a special type of maladjustment that usually shows a tendency to be progressive and is therefore to be looked upon with apprehension, a permanent disorganization of the personality does not invariably follow. Indeed, it is now the opinion of many of the closest students of schizophrenia that acute, rather clearly psychogenic schizophrenia may at times disappear, without leaving any injury to the personality. Formerly its incurable nature and progressive course were implied in the definition of the disease, and a favorable outcome was considered presumptive evidence of an error in diagnosis. Of course, the occurrence of an obviously schizophrenic reaction should make the physician exceedingly careful in predicting that a permanently inferior type of adjustment will not be sustained. In recent years, too, there has been an increasing recognition that the episodic nature of a psychosis and the occurrence of symptom-free intermissions may not exclude its schizophrenic nature.

Occasionally one observes a schizophrenic episode of a mild, fleeting nature, with no subsequent recurrence. In many instances, however, the favorable outcome should be characterized as "social recovery" rather than as "cured" or as full recovery. By this it is meant that the patient is able to return to his previous social environment and to previous or equivalent occupation, but with minor symptoms and signs, such as irritability, shyness, or shallowness of affective responses.

From what has been said, it is evident that in any given case the effect upon the personality and future adjustment of the appearance of a schizophrenic reaction may be quite uncertain. As mentioned before, in the infantile case, the expectation of social adaptation is minimal if mutism continues until the age of five. In some cases the course is continuously progressive; in others it is intermittent. More frequently it is a question of remissions and relapses in which, although from the first interests and habits tend to be undermined insidiously, there occur periods of adjustment at a lower level for a considerable period of time.

Of committed patients who improve sufficiently to be released, about 80 per cent leave the mental hospital within the first year of residence. The expectancy of recovery falls with each year of continued hospitalization. Roughly, about one-third of those patients who are hospitalized during the first year of their illness make a fairly complete recovery; one-third improve and become able to return to outside life but remain damaged personalities and may have to return to the hospital from time to time. The remaining third will require indefinite hospital care. The introduction of the modern pharmaceutical therapies has not brought about a reduction in the number of schizophrenic patients requiring hospital care whose illness pursues a chronic course.

This differentiation of the schizophrenias by course of illness has led to a tendency to separate schizophrenia into "process" and "reactive groups." In the former are those usually who pursue a persistently chronic and disorganized course and seldom, if ever, make a social adjustment. Langfeldt separates the two groups under the designations of schizophrenia and schizophreniform psychoses. From his studies, he considers that those showing at the beginning emotional blunting, with lack of initiative and peculiar behavior, as well as those paranoid persons with depersonalization and derealization experienced as an influence from outside the self, will fall almost invariably into the group of patients with poor prognosis.

The age of onset is not of prognostic significance except that relatively late age offers a less favorable prognosis. Sex has no prognostic significance. Since onset in adolescence sometimes has seemed to occur after loss of a friendship, a study done to examine such relations suggests that one indicator of prognosis for the adolescent schizophrenic is the range and quality of his friendships. It has been found that those who pursue a course of chronic deterioration and hospitalizations have either none or very few adolescent friends. Such friendships are seldom lengthy and, if severed, are infrequently replaced. Usually the friend is either much older or younger, and the interaction between the patient and the friend is infrequent and is limited to a single form of activity. A lack of participation in group activities also expresses the same deficit in establishing interpersonal contacts beyond the family.

It will usually be found that, if the psychosis represents an insidious development and unfolding of a previous schizoid personality, the prognosis is unfavorable. Many such psychoses represent the culmination of a long period of unsatisfactory adaptation. The better adjusted the patient's prepsychotic personality, the more directly and confidently the patient has been accustomed to meet the problems and difficulties of life, the richer his interests, the more definite an external precipitating situation, and the more rapid the onset, the better the prognosis. The existence of anxiety and of an easily ascertained emotional problem makes the prognosis more favorable. With the presence of features such as those just mentioned, "spontaneous" recoveries, i.e., without therapeutic efforts by a physician, are not uncommon. Such factors as psychotic or schizoid pathology in the mother, no separations from the pathogenic family, and little "acting out" of pathology in the community recently have been correlated with chronicity. A slow, insidious withdrawal is apt to lead to an irreversible disorganization of the personality. If the ego was not strong enough to withstand routine difficulties, the prognosis is not good. If it broke only after overwhelming stress, the prognosis is better.

The prognosis is not influenced by the intelligence or previous education of the patient. Those with high personal aspirations often do poorly. An apparently "mild" case need not be an early one or of favorable prognosis. The presence of a well-marked affective element is of hopeful significance, although hypochondriasis, particularly if it is predominantly self-accusatory, is usually associated with a long-term ineffective social adaptation. Self-condemnatory hallucinations have a more favorable connotation and seem related to the patient's willingness to accept some responsibility for his behavior. The presence of cyclothymic factors in the personality background renders the prognosis more favorable. The persistence of hallucinations after an initial emotional tension has subsided is not a favorable indication. If the psychosis has existed for a year without clear-cut signs of improvement, a favorable outcome is scarcely to be expected, although it is by no means unknown.

Previous remissions should lead one to expect that a given episode will be followed by improvement. The longer the interval between attacks, the better the prognosis. In many cases of schizophrenia, regression is an important mechanism, so attempts are often made to base a prognosis on the depth of regression manifested by the patient. Infantile posture and behavior, although often of unfavorable significance, should not outweigh

other considerations in forming an opinion as to prognosis. It may be parenthetically commented that the physician whose psychiatric experience has been confined to institutions tends to develop an unwarranted pessimistic attitude in prognosis. Until recently, the mortality rate among institutionalized schizophrenic patients was estimated to be twice as high as in the normal community population.

A word should be said as to the prognosis in the different types. In catatonia, the prognosis is relatively good if the onset has been stormy and the episode is still acute. Many of these patients are restored to their prepsychotic level of adjustment for varying periods, at times for several years. The prognosis in the simple form, with its insidious marasmus of the personality developing in the absence of unusual environmental and experiential stresses, is poor. A certain number, sheltered by some normal member of the family, maintain a colorless, uneventful existence, while others become paupers, hoboes, or petty criminals. The course of the hebephrenic form tends to be one of dereistic regression and of progressive disorganization, although occasionally remissions occur before the final disorganization of personality.

The question as to whether the paranoid type of schizophrenic ever recovers is sometimes raised. The reply to this depends somewhat on a definition of terms. Undoubtedly remissions occur, and these may be looked upon as social recoveries, but they are rarely to be judged as psychological recoveries, even though the patient's adjustment during the interval is well socialized and there are no distortions of reality in response to subjective needs. In general, surly and bitter attitudes indicate the presence of a malignant process.

As for the pseudoneurotic forms of schizophrenia, Cattell reports that 60 per cent of a group followed from 5 to 20 years never required hospital treatment. The remaining 40 per cent were periodically admitted to the hospital. Only one in five developed overt psychotic symptoms, and one half of these remitted. Thus only 10 per cent evolved the well-known classical forms of schizophrenia.

Finally, both for the sake of stating the opinion of one of the greatest students of schizophrenia as to the prognosis and for emphasizing the responsibility of the physician who undertakes the care of the early case of schizophrenia, the conclusion of Bleuler must be quoted: "Although a certain number of patients become deteriorated with every treatment, and others improve even in apparently severe cases, the treatment will decide in more than one third of schizophrenic cases whether they can become social men again or not." The more individualized and personalized the care and treatment, the greater the recovery rate.

In childhood schizophrenia the importance of language facility may not be overestimated as regards future social adaptability. This condition may be confused with the aphasias of childhood owing to early brain damage.

Diagnosis

To establish the diagnosis of the schizophrenic reaction, the examiner must attend particularly to the quality of the interpersonal contact and to the perceptual and cognitive organization of the personality. Important in the contact will be the patient's ease in the interview, his ability to establish an affectively toned rapport vis-à-vis the examiner, and his capacity for sustaining attention and concentration. The examiner will note as evidence of schizophrenic organization the intrusive injection of irrelevant remarks or phrases, or blocks in the interchange. Important will be indications that the patient has difficulty in discriminating one person from another and in maintaining an affective constancy; that he tends toward overt expressions of hatred or love, mistrust or dependency; that he transfers and condenses into currently related persons the features of significant individuals from his past. He may disclose problems in discrimination of auditory and visual percepts and in evaluating his social and sexual role and his bodily perceptions. Thought processes may be revealed as too concrete, with weak conceptual ability. While often difficult to discern, disorganization of percepts and thought in the form of bizarre hallucinatory or delusional experiences with an intact sensorium will strongly suggest the diagnosis. The general sense of the examination may arouse a subjectively eerie reaction sometimes referred to as the "praecox feeling."

At times perplexing similarities are observed between schizophrenia and the psychoneuroses, between schizophrenia and other biogenetic major psychoses, particularly the manic-depressive ones, but rarely between schizophrenia and organic mental disorders. It is doubtful, too, if there is any definite demarcation between psychoneurotic and schizophrenic reactions. Again, the distinction between schizophrenic disturbances of the personality and those of the psychopath or character neurotic may be very difficult. Extreme caution should be exercised in declaring that an isolated symptom is conclusive evidence of schizophrenia, and, in evaluating a symptom, the clinical setting in which it occurs should be carefully examined. Neither should the eventual outcome be the most important determinant in diagnosis.

Many of the differential points among schizophrenia, hysteria, and dissociative reactions are discussed in Chapter 24. In addition to what is mentioned there, attention should be called to the fact that the onset in hysteria is usually more sudden and that a psychological motive is more apparent. In schizophrenic stupor, one does not discover the expression of an emotional state. In dissociative stupor, on the other hand, one may note an expression of perplexity, fear, elation, or some other affective state. The history of an insidious change in interests points toward schizophrenia. Not only are the symptoms of hysteria and of dissociation more sudden in onset, but they are more paroxysmal. The symptoms of hysteria are influenced more obviously by certain persons in the environment. Whereas the hysteric desires attention, the schizophrenic is more apt to have periods when he is preoccupied, detached, and apathetic. The hysteric uses conventional, intelligible symbols, while the schizophrenic uses individual or archaic ones. One can feel himself into the psychic life of the hysteric and of some persons with dissociative states, but with difficulty, if at all, into that of the schizophrenic.

In the early stage of schizophrenia, the differentiation from obsessive neurosis may be difficult. Sometimes schizophrenic reactions result from the release of primitive impulses that had previously been kept under control by the aid of obsessional symptoms. In schizophrenia there is usually more rumination and less tension than in the obsessive neurosis, as the patient who suffers from the latter has a strong conscious resistance to his obsessions and compulsions, a resistance that is lacking in the schizophrenic, who is not particularly disturbed by them. Often the schizophrenic, in the early phases of the disorder, expresses hypochondriacal complaints. His hypochondria lacks, however, the dramatization seen in the psychoneuroses.

Frequently one of the most difficult differentiations in mental disorders is between schizophrenia and manic-depressive psychosis. Doubtless this is a result, in part at least, of the fact that many people are not pure schizoid or pure syntonic types but rather are personality alloys and are characterized by admixtures in their personality. In addition to what is said in Chapter 22 on affective reactions, attention may be called to the fact that the onset of schizophrenia tends to be more insidious and the excitement in schizophrenia is more frequently paroxysmal, while that of the manic is more sustained; the mood of the schizophrenic rarely possesses the infectious quality seen in the manic-depressive. The delusions of the depressed schizophrenic are more grotesque than those of the depressed manic, and he is less distressed by them. Illogical remarks and incongruous statements suggest schizophrenia.

The difficulty in differentiating between these two disorders arises largely in the earlier stages of schizophrenia. With recurring episodes, the schizophrenic nature of symptoms previously doubtful becomes more apparent, with the result that confusion with manic-depressive symptomatology no longer exists. It rarely happens that a psychosis that is apparently schizophrenic in its early phases proves subsequently to be of a manic-depressive reaction type. The reverse, however, is common. There are, nevertheless, many cases of mental disorder, the recurring episodes of which continue to show a mixture of schizophrenic symptoms and of affective ones, especially depression and anxiety.

In the acute schizophrenic disorganizations the differential diagnosis as regards the acute brain syndrome (delirious reactions) is important. The schizophrenic usually presents a clear sensorium. On examination of his mental status he is oriented in all spheres; his fund of information, capacity to calculate, memory functions, and retaining ability remain intact when one examines him with patience and forbearance. However, today, with the increasing frequency of drug abuse—particularly of the hallucinogens, barbiturates and other hypnotics, amphetamines, and alcohol—many young schizophrenics are brought to treatment with the symptoms of an acute brain syndrome. Only after the symptoms and signs of that condition have subsided under treatment may one be certain of the existence of the major underlying psychopathology—schizophrenia. In these instances, the immediate therapeutic task is treatment of the toxic delirium; the next, the recognition and therapy for the schizophrenic process.

There is usually no difficulty in distinguishing schizophrenia from epilepsy, except in the instance of psychomotor attacks associated with temporal lobe convulsive foci. Occasionally, nevertheless, the schizophrenic suffers from epileptiform or syncopal attacks that to the inexperienced observer strongly suggest the seizures of epilepsy. In that case, careful inquiry should be made as to whether the seizures or the mental symptoms appeared first, and the nature of the seizure should be observed; in schizophrenia it lacks the definiteness in type and the genuine disturbance of consciousness occurring in epilepsy. Careful history and the use of the electroencephalogram should make the proper differential diagnosis.

In discussing the diagnosis of schizophrenia, mention should be made of what is often spoken of as chronic alcoholic hallucinosis. The permanent persistence in the chronic alcoholic of auditory hallucinations in a setting of clear consciousness, frequently with systematized delusions, was formerly considered as a symptom of an alcoholic psychosis. Many psychiatrists now believe that such cases are really schizophrenic reactions.

Adolescent psychoses do not belong in any special classification of their own, yet their capacity for variation in duration, intensity, and form frequently causes them to present difficulties in diagnosis. At that period one may alternatively see phases of anxiety, behavior disorder, affective disturbance, or schizophrenia. In retrospect, truancy and other forms of delinquent behavior have preceded the onset of a disorder that is subsequently diagnosed as schizophrenia. The adolescent schizophrenic frequently shows a more lively emotional response than is usual in the adult and also less incongruity of affect.

The symptomatic emphasis in adolescent schizophrenia is usually on social withdrawal, on disorders of activity, interest, and speech, and on peculiarities of manner. It must be acknowledged, however, that it is not always easy to differentiate the emotional disorders of adolescence from incipient schizophrenia. That period is normally one of emotional turmoil and instability. Much that would be regarded as pathological in later life may then be but a temporary exaggeration of normal tendencies. The adolescent, with his self-questioning and perturbing heart-searching, may verbalize his disruption of emotion and impulse without being schizophrenic. Adolescent maladjustments among shy, withdrawn personalities with feelings of inadequacy or inferiority, with evident internal conflict and family tensions, particularly with one or the other parent, are not uncommon. Poor socialization, lack of motivation, and a brooding sense of inferiority may be merely a retarded ability to integrate the new emotional drives and experiences of adolescence. Such symptoms may, however, be those of an incipient schizophrenia.

Childhood schizophrenia must be differentiated from the forms of mental deficiency, other chronic brain disorders in early years, severe childhood neuroses, behavior disorders, and familial dysautonomia. Here, the history, the physical status of the patient, biochemical and electroencephalographic data, and responses to psychological testing usually will discriminate the various conditions. Katrina de Hirsch points out that although both schizophrenic and aphasic children have limitations of visual and auditory events, the latter have specific difficulties in interpretation of spoken and printed language. In both, auditory thresholds for speech are higher. In the schizophrenic this is due to their inability to integrate meaningful material; in the aphasics it is due to problems of decoding.

Auditory memory span is very short in the aphasic as contrasted to the schizophrenic children. The latter may be able to reproduce long and complicated television commercials—a task impossible for the former. Auditory feedback is distorted in both groups.

When it comes to language as communication, the schizophrenic child is lacking in communicative intent, as evidenced clinically in his impoverished and inappropriate gestural abilities and limited verbal output. Also, the echolalia of the schizophrenic is characteristic in its high-pitched "birdlike" quality, which differs from the occasional echolalic productions of the brain damaged which more often occur as simple repetitions of words or phrases for clarification enunciated in generally normal pitch and inflection. The speech of schizophrenic children is understood and given in idiosyncratic concrete terms with intent of immediate magical power and condenses much emotionally; that of aphasic children does not demonstrate looseness of associations.

Treatment

The treatment of schizophrenia, particularly in its early stages, is undertaken with far less pessimism than formerly. Its success depends to no small degree upon the therapeutic initiative, energy, and effort of the physician, although the results will be small if the psychotic methods of thinking and feeling have become habits and established forms of adjustment. In early cases, the remission rate after treatment is about twice as high as is that of remissions occurring spontaneously.

PREVENTION. Since it has been said that schizophrenia becomes manifest for the most part only after a prolonged period of incubation, the question naturally arises as to whether a disease so disorganizing to the personality can be prevented. If it is correct that the family provides a pathogenic milieu for the incubation of and development of those ego weaknesses which evolve in an individual predisposed through genetic and/or constitutional processes, clearly early separation from the pathogenic milieu would be desirable. As of this writing, in no part of the world has this potential preventive step gained credence or been tried. Only in Japan, where culture dictates that a mother may not rear both of her twins, has one of a high risk pair had the privilege of separation and rearing in another family. Here, as Inouye has found, even if the disorder evolves, one of the twins is less severely impaired as regards pathology than is the other. In Western countries, certain high risk children born out of wedlock are adopted. The extent of protection provided by other than parental rearing remains unclear. This must be made on a prospective basis in the future, on the basis of our current knowledge of the evolution of schizophrenia.

As described before, the schizophrenic reaction is regarded now as an ego disorder. Discriminative functions are impaired. The ill person has difficulty in perceiving himself from others, and separating internally from externally aroused sensations. His adaptive functions are undeveloped, so that he is at a disadvantage in melding constructively his affects and thoughts in relation to the reality of outer social events. His integrative functions deny him an instant percept of others, a steady value system to which he may commit himself and dedicate his energy. There are impairments in his ego assets, balance of trust, autonomy, self-confidence, curiosity, personal responsibility—the social sets of empathy to humans.

All the socializing experiences which strengthen these ego functions may be regarded as preventive or therapeutic. Such experiences may occur through broadening social contacts outside the family, outside the immediate community as culture, in individual or group associations, or in therapy. They may be taken successfully when the potential or actual patient either has sufficient ego autonomy to risk separating from his family circle or is supported in his struggles by the relationship of a therapist who perceives that need.

Separation alone, prolonged social isolation in an institution, whether hospital or prison or another home, wherein the schizoid person is not afforded a stimulating contact with others, may lead to further ego disorganization and regression. Gruenberg has termed this effect, produced by prolonged and nonstimulating hospital care, the "social breakdown syndrome." Effective hospital care takes place when the staff affords healthy models for identification and offers opportunities for clear verbal communication, learning of new skills, and development of positive ego attitudes through the support of pleasurable and rewarding relationships.

EARLY STAGES. Ideally, treatment of the schizophrenic should have begun before obvious symptoms of a mental disorder are manifest. Unfortunately, this rarely occurs. The patient only occasionally seeks treatment himself, and his family, unable or unwilling to recognize that he is mentally ill, does not refer him to a psychiatrist.

Following the initial examination, decision usually must be made as to whether the patient should be treated in an outpatient department or office or admitted to a hospital. If behavior has been disturbed and promises to threaten later social acceptance, prompt admission for hospital treatment is indicated. Again, some form of hospital care is advisable when the patient is living in a home in which the family attitude is argumentative, critical, domineering, or rejecting. Social isolation at home or in a lodging and lack of vocational and social skills may suggest the advisability of day or night hospital care.

PHARMACOLOGICAL THERAPY. Whether the decision is to commence treatment on an outpatient or a hospital basis, the first therapeutic move is to provide relief of anxiety and its attendant reflections in the psychotic symptom-complex.

Phenothiazines. Administration of one of the phenothiazine derivatives is today the immediate method of choice. *Chlorpromazine,* the first of these agents to be introduced, probably is the preferred drug for the majority of patients. There are no standard rules for the administration of chlorpromazine or its analogs. For the mildly disturbed schizophrenic, initial oral dosages of 25 to 50 mg. three to four times daily may be tried for several days to ascertain the patient's tolerance and idiosyncratic responses. The drug may then be administered in doses of 100 or 200 mg. three or four times daily if the patient's condition seems to indicate this amount. Many patients may be maintained on a dosage of 400 mg. daily for indefinite periods. Some have received total daily doses of 1000 mg. or more without ill effect. If the patient is acutely disturbed when first seen, a 50-mg. dose of chlorpromazine may be tried by intramuscular injection; the drug is again given at this level, or in 100-mg. doses, every three or four hours.

The phenothiazines are indicated for all types of schizophrenia. They are of particular value in the treatment of those patients who show tension, psychomotor overactivity, agitation, impulsiveness, aggressive outbursts, destructiveness, and antagonistic, paranoid reactions. Administration to the acutely ill schizophrenic patient frequently results in the disappearance of hallucinations and delusional ideas within the first two weeks of treatment.

High dosage chlorpromazine therapy (2000 mg.) per day has been found more effective than low dosage regimens in the treatment of younger patients with chronic illnesses who have not been hospitalized for lengthy periods. But such high dosage regimens also produce a greater number of serious side effects.

The longer the schizophrenic has been ill, the less chance there is that the use of the phenothiazines will be followed by recovery. The best results are secured with patients who have not been ill for more than two years. Among these, the results will depend largely on the clinical manifestations, the degree of improvement being much greater in the overactive, disturbed patient, who improves to a degree that he becomes amenable to occupational and other activity therapies and, hopefully, to some degree of psychotherapy. Although most overactive schizophrenics who have been hospitalized for long periods of time show some improvement, not more than 5 to 10 per cent of those who have been hospitalized for more than five continuous years become well enough to leave the hospital, and an appreciable number of these will have to return at a later time. The problem of the care of the chronically ill overactive patient who does not improve sufficiently to leave the hospital has been greatly eased by chlorpromazine, however. Delusions and hallucinations may persist, but usually they are no longer disturbing to the patient. The sullen, sarcastic, and antagonistic patient is less irritable and frequently becomes quiet, coöperative, and accessible.

Of the various types of schizophrenia, the acute paranoid forms appear to respond most favorably, followed by the acute catatonic. The behavior of the chronic catatonic patients and the hebephrenics is less modifiable, although lessening of aggressive and impulsive actions usually follows the use of this drug.

Certain other phenothiazines are reported to be more effective in modifying some forms of disturbed behavior than chlorpromazine. Thus trifluoperazine (Stelazine) is said to be particularly beneficial for the withdrawn, apathetic, and depressed schizophrenic. It is administered by giving initially oral doses of 5 mg. three or four times daily; this dosage may be increased to total daily levels of 60 to 80 mg. Thioridazine (Mellaril) serves as effectively as the other phenothiazines but is less likely to produce the general run of toxic side-effects. Perphenazine (Trilafon) is indicated for those patients likely to be exposed to the sun, since its usage has not been associated with the skin photosensitivity noted with chlorpromazine and other derivatives. For some patients haloperidol and its analogs are the most effective pharmaceutical agents. More complete descriptions are given of the pharmacological actions, dosage ranges, and side and toxic effects of these agents and others, including reserpine, in Chapter 32, Pharmacological Therapy.

PSYCHOTHERAPY. In addition to the relief of anxiety and its attendant symptoms, the psychiatric therapist will be concerned with the establishment of a treatment regimen that provides over time opportunity for development of a more stable and adaptive personality. He will be particularly mindful of those weaknesses of ego identity and function that characterize the schizophrenic and will attempt to ascertain in his growing knowledge of the patient's development whether these de-

fects are due to lack or deprivation of socializing experiences or the consequence of isolation and withdrawal as the result of psychological conflict and associated emotional turmoil.

It is necessary, then, to consider, in the long term planning for treatment for the schizophrenic, the day-to-day social milieu in which he lives as well as his needs for specialized psychotherapy. Measures must be taken to strengthen his ego through restructuring the environment so that he comes in contact with other healthy persons whose interpersonal contact provides a ground in which he may develop trust, assurance, and, hopefully, some personal autonomy. The possible identifications with others than family members will clarify his confusion about his own social and sexual identity. The therapeutic milieu must be stimulating physically so as to provide an increasing awareness and perception of his own body and its functions, upon which may be established a satisfying and realistic concept of his body and its actions. Furthermore, this environment must provide a structured and stimulating social world so that there may be ingrained the sense of time and satisfactions in completeness of action and so that he may avoid the inevitable consequences of isolation. It must be emphasized that isolation leads to reduced awareness of perceptual stimulation from within and without and results in reexperiencing and becoming preoccupied with thought processes divorced from ego control, followed by regressive infantile thinking processes and hallucinatory satisfactions.

Therefore, if the patient is to be treated as an outpatient, arrangements should be made for the psychiatrist to see him on a regular schedule of appointments, with a clearly understood recognition that improvement with insight will not be quickly gained. The frequency of appointments for treatment designed to modify and improve ego function should not be less than twice weekly and often must be more. The psychiatrist should help his patient to decide if he is to continue to work or attend school, or to limit his strivings in other directions. The patient should be cautioned as to the toxic side-effects of the pharmaceuticals prescribed.

Many psychotherapists believe that the primary problem of the schizophrenic is not his anxiety about others and a consequent narcissistic withdrawal, often dating back to childhood, but fear of his own hostile, destructive tendencies. Although preoccupied, suspicious, and anxiety-ridden because of the negative impulses he feels in himself, the schizophrenic can often, at least in the early stages of his illness, be helped to relate himself to people. Frieda Fromm-Reichmann stressed that, although the schizophrenic longs for interpersonal contact, he equally fears such a closeness. Thus in office psycho-therapy, careful consideration must be given to the extent and readiness of each patient to engage in social relations with others. In many instances, aid must be provided to the withdrawn patient through planning with social service agencies and workers.

The therapist must be ever mindful of the transference distortions of the schizo-phrenic patient. The capacity of these patients to misperceive the therapist in transient roles as recapitulations of the past identification he has made with parents has been described earlier. Searles' descriptions of the multiple mispercep-tions the patients project upon the same treating person explain much of the diffi-culty of establishing a constant relation-ship with the patient. So, too, the early lack of object constancy which Burnham has emphasized affords the explanation for those defensive maneuvers used so effectively as resistances to establishing the therapeutic relationship in fear of the potential betrayal by the therapist. These defenses may vary from anxiety-producing clinging, which some therapists have diffi-culty accepting, to the avoidance maneu-vers through withdrawal, noncommunica-tion, violent counterattacks, or the use of substitute persons through acting out as a means of escaping the anxiety of the need-fear dilemma.

For the more seriously disturbed, hos-pital care is advisable. The good hospital not only protects the patient from a threatening family, social, or vocational environment but provides healthy sub-stitutes for erecting new identifications and sources for resolving conflicts as well as learning social and vocational skills previously weak or defective.

As Artiss has described in discussing *milieu therapy*, the expectancies and atti-tudes of the treatment staff are central to bringing about social rehabilitation. For each patient there must be a known goal for the various treatment efforts, and the patient must be educated in the rudi-ments of successful social behavior wher-ever he exposes weaknesses, particularly through active participation in some group. Finally, the individual patient must be placed in a situation where he has a regularly recurrent opportunity to interact with a healthy group and a responsibility to do so.

Thus, the hospital psychiatrist and many other special therapists and patients of both sexes offer opportunities to the patient for testing and establishing less anxiety-ridden relations with others. In turn, these opportunities allow the poten-tiality for reducing the confusion of per-sonal and sexual identity so characteristic of these patients. The well-regulated and structured activity of a therapeutic insti-tution provides arrangements for the reëstablishment of the patient's ego, allowing him to make clear-cut discrimi-nations between himself and the environ-ment and to refix his concepts of time and space. In the active and well-staffed hos-pital, opportunities for ego development through social interactions are made available through patient government and through group and family therapies. The use of recreational aids and physiothera-pies is dynamically important in stimulat-ing bodily activity that underlies the development of sound and satisfying body ego.

One attempts to stimulate the patient's interest and redirect it to things outside himself, detach his emotions from subjective material, inculcate healthful, socialized habits, and abstract him from his spiritual isolation. Among important aids to these ends and to the gaining of satisfaction from adaptive behavior are forms of occupational therapy chosen to meet his emotional needs. Recreation, games, music, and congenial companionships all have a common objective of promoting interpersonal relationships. Occupational therapy not only helps to reëstablish contacts with reality, but through personal contact with the therapist frequently brings a therapeutic emotional relationship. Probably, in fact, the most important tool that the occupational or other auxiliary therapist brings to the treatment situation is a genuine warmth, understanding, flexibility, and objectivity.

With a therapeutic staff trained to understand the dynamics of behavior, each aspect of the patient's pathology may be examined and each member of the staff brought to support his assets and also to confront his distortions of reality so as to assist in more effective and alternative methods of solving his social difficulties. The hospital offers a milieu in which the patient may expose his deficits and test new methods of adaptation in a setting of trust and collaboration and without criticisms, thus fostering ego growth. In such a therapeutic milieu patients may be seen to pass through several stages of change, comprised initially of adjustment to the new environment, then exposure of the adaptive responses to the emotional stresses of interhospital transactions, and finally evolution of new and more effective techniques for coping with reality.

Although many patients become permanently isolated in their own autistic lives in spite of every effort at treatment, the degree of improvement is, broadly speaking, directly proportional to the attention and treatment that they receive. There is usually a tendency to a progressive introversion and habit-deterioration.

In no instance should the patient be lost in the obscurity of chronically ill persons in a ward. It has been said that the picture seen in chronic and hopeless institutional cases is one-third a result of disease, while two-thirds is a reaction to an unfavorable and unsuitable environment. The ideal hospital would provide what the home cannot, in addition to the advantages that the patient would have received had he remained in the home.

Stanton and Schwartz have made interesting contributions to the concept of schizophrenic deterioration as a psychosocial adaptive pattern. They found it was possible to discern meaningful patterns in the occurrences in a mental hospital. They studied, for example, the symptoms of soiling and wetting, so common in chronic deteriorated schizophrenics. They pointed out that the term "incontinence" is a misnomer if by that term is meant loss of sphincter control. The so-called incontinent schizophrenic patient, Stanton and Schwartz discovered, discharges his excreta in a highly controlled manner. There are some situations in which wetting and soiling rarely, if ever, occur. On the other hand, they may take place in a specific constellation of circumstances under the pressure of an emotional need. One patient, for example, who was extremely fearful of human contact found that people left her alone when she had soiled. Another patient who craved the attentions of a mother figure soiled herself to compel attentions from a nurse.

Special Forms of Treatment

INTENSIVE PSYCHOTHERAPY. Although psychoanalytical techniques such as are usually employed in the neuroses have never been satisfactory in the treatment of schizophrenia, yet modifications have now been evolved that may successfully maintain many patients at a functioning level of social adjustment.

The establishment of a working relationship with the patient is essential to successful therapy in the schizophrenic. The relationship of the patient to the therapist is of a different quality from that seen in neuroses. It is exceedingly fragile and is subject to withdrawal on the basis of any suspicion or indication that there is a limitation of interest on the part of the physician. Breaking through to obtain the trust of the suspicious, withdrawn, highly sensitive, and perhaps disturbed patient requires infinite patience and tolerance. Rarely can the physician confine his contacts with the patient to set office hours. He must be available whenever periods of great anxiety occur. In the early stages of treatment, the patient's verbal communications may be incomprehensible to the physician, and some form of communication between the two must be established. At this stage, the therapist does not attempt to have the patient, as would be done with the neurotic, form an association with the verbalizations he is producing. Rather the therapist listens and tries to relate the patient's verbalizations to the feeling-tone of the particular interpersonal events that are reported to have preceded the distorted communications or are observed to occur in close temporal relationship. Then, when particular communications are heard, the therapist may interpret the patient's feeling directly and make it possible for him to appreciate that he is understood and will not be hurt. The patient must find in the therapist a sustaining source of security on the emergence of anxiety and hostility.

The therapist must be constantly alert to his own behavior and its possible meanings to the patient. For this reason, the therapy is conducted with the patient facing the therapist. The patient has a continuing need to check his reaction through visualizing the gestures and moves of the therapist. The latter must see himself as an active participant with his patient and must be free to disclose his own feelings and the meanings of his actions in order to clarify the patient's frequent distortions of the situation.

Contrary to the usual custom in the analytical therapy of the neuroses, the analysis of dreams is not advised. Preoccupation with dream analysis perpetuates the schizophrenic's propensity for withdrawal into fantasy living. What he needs is to face continually the emotionally toned events of everyday living and to learn socially adaptive methods of accepting them. Usually, too, the primitive impulses of the schizophrenic are so evident in their overt pathology that dream analysis will provide but little additional information. In contrast with earlier attempts to resolve delusional and hallucinatory experiences through analysis of their content, this is now recognized as unsatisfactory procedure in the therapeutic process. Rather, efforts are made to derive an understanding of the interpersonal situations that precipitate the patient's expressions of delusional and hallucinatory material and the significance of the psychopathology in terms of the affect produced in such situations. Frieda Fromm-Reichmann described this technique in some detail.

It should be remembered that there are limitations in the psychotherapy of the schizophrenic patient. Complete resolution of the schizophrenic process, fixed through indelible deprivations or traumas of early life, is rarely obtained, even by therapists of the greatest experience and patience. If, in an effort to reach the ideal, the enthusiastic psychiatrist presses his patient beyond his capacity, he may do him incalculable harm. The therapist must, of course, continue indefinitely a supportive, though distant, therapeutic relationship when the patient indicates the need.

In not a few schizophrenics, a "spontaneous" remission or recovery occurs. In such cases, the therapeutic agent usually remains unknown. In many instances it would appear that improvement followed because, for some years, the patient was able to make contact with some individual—perhaps a nurse, aide, or even some other patient—in his environment, and this interpersonal relationship became a bridge toward reality.

Group Psychotherapy. Group psychotherapy has proved useful for many schizophrenic patients. It has been administered in conjunction with individual therapy or as the sole psychotherapeutic measure. It is most likely to have value for the schizophrenic with major deficit in group living and for those inhibited in individual psychotherapy.

INSULIN COMA THERAPY. The history of the therapy of schizophrenia has been characterized by the use of various methods that temporarily had enthusiastic proponents but failed to stand the test of time. Insulin shock therapy has been largely superseded by the phenothiazine drugs in recent years. The details of its application are discussed in Chapter 33.

The percentage of remissions following insulin therapy depends largely on the previous duration of the psychosis. The recovery rate is by far the greatest in patients who have not been ill for more than six months and are thus those most likely to improve without the aid of specific therapies. Patients who have been sick less than one year will, under insulin treatment, do twice as well as those who have been sick more than one year. Full remission in patients who have been ill for more than two years is rare. Combined insulin and electroconvulsive therapy may succeed in cases in which the two treatments given separately have failed. Insulin therapy in paranoid forms produces better results than in hebephrenic or simple types. Treatment is not followed by any change in the prepsychotic personality.

ELECTRIC CONVULSIVE THERAPY. Because of the simplicity of its application, its fewer hazards, and the need for a smaller group of specially trained personnel, there has been a tendency to substitute electric convulsive treatment if some form of shock therapy is desired. Of the subtypes of schizophrenia, catatonic excitement and acute paranoid forms respond best to electroshock treatment. The results are best when affective features are present and the assets of the prepsychotic personality are good. Patients who relapse after each of two successive courses of treatment have been kept on a maintenance treatment regimen of one or two treatments a week. The use of electroshock as a maintenance treatment has been largely discontinued since the introduction of tranquilizing drugs.

PREFRONTAL LOBOTOMY. This form of treatment is not employed unless all others have failed. If it is to be employed, it should be used before emotional deterioration is advanced. If, after two or three years of active treatment that has included psychotherapy, tranquilizing drugs, and coma therapies, the patient has shown no improvement, frontal lobotomy may be recommended. Best results are secured if the patient's original personality was relatively well organized. Patients who show persistent tension, excessive motor activity, resistiveness, destructiveness, or combativeness are the most suitable subjects for this treatment. In such cases, one may at least reasonably expect that improvement will be obtained in adaptive behavior in simple situations as well as in social and ward behavior and in work activity. Mood level will be more desirable, and aggressive tendencies will be reduced. However, if the schizophrenic process has progressed to a chronic and general personality disorganization, marked by persisting emotional dulling, loss of contact with people, widespread delusions, and emotional disintegration, the results of the operation are disappointing. In fact, very few patients are helped if the disease has existed for 10 years or more. Hebephrenics rarely respond favorably. Catatonic excitement usually responds well to lobotomy, as do paranoid schizophrenic states.

BIBLIOGRAPHY

Arieti, S.: Interpretation of Schizophrenia. New York, Robert Brunner, 1955.

Artiss, K. L.: Milieu Therapy in Schizophrenia. New York, Grune & Stratton, Inc. 1962.

Bateson, G., Jackson, D. D., Haley, J., and Weakland, J.: Toward a theory of schizophrenia. Behav. Sci., 1:251–264, 1956.

Beck, S. J.: The Six Schizophrenias. Research Monographs, No. 6, New York, American Orthopsychiatric Association, 1954.

Bender, L.: Childhood schizophrenia. Psychiat. Quart., 27:663–681, 1953.

Bennett, H. S., and Klein, H. R.: Childhood schizophrenia: 30 years later. Amer. J. Psychiat., 122: 1121–1124, 1966.

Bleuler, E.: Dementia Praecox or the Group of Schizophrenias. Translated by Zinkin, J. New York, International Universities Press, Inc., 1950.

Bruch, H.: Falsification of bodily needs and body concept in schizophrenia. Arch. Gen. Psych., *6:* 18–24, 1962.

Burnham, D. L., Gladstone, A. I., and Gibson, R. W.: Schizophrenia and the Need Fear Dilemma. New York, International University Press, 1969.

Chapman, J.: The early symptoms of schizophrenia. Brit. J. Psychiat., *112:*225–251, 1966.

de Hirsch, K.: Differential diagnosis between aphasic and schizophrenic language in children. J. Speech & Hearing Disorders, *32:*3–10, 1967.

Demming, W. E.: A recursion formula for the proportion of persons having a first admission as schizophrenic. Behav. Sci., *13:*467–476, 1968.

Dunham, H. W.: Sociocultural studies of schizophrenia. Arch. Gen. Psychiat., *21:*206–214, 1971.

Edelson, M.: Sociotherapy and psychotherapy in a psychiatric hospital. *In* Redlich, E. (ed.): Social Psychiatry. Res. Publ. Ass. Res. Nerv. & Ment. Dis., *47:*196–212, 1967.

Ehrentheil, O. F., and Jenney, P. B.: Does time stand still for some psychotics? Arch. Gen. Psych., *3:*1–3, 1960.

Eisenberg, L.: The autistic child in adolescence. Amer. J. Psychiat., *112:*607–612, 1956.

Eisenberg, L., and Kanner, L.: Early infantile autism. Amer. J. Orthopsychiat., *26:*556–566, 1956.

Elkes, J.: Schizophrenic disorder in relation to levels of neural organization: the need for some conceptual points of reference. *In* Folch, P. J. (ed.): The Chemical Pathology of the Nervous System. London, Pergamon Press, 1961, pp. 648–665.

Feinberg, I., Braun, M., Koresko, R. L., and Gottlieb, F.: Stage 4 sleep in schizophrenia. Arch. Gen. Psychiat., *21:*262–266, 1969.

Freeman, T., Cameron, J. L., and McGhee, A.: Chronic Schizophrenia. New York, International Universities Press, Inc., 1958.

Friedhoff, A. J., and Van Winkle, E.: Conversion of dopamine to 3, 4-dimethoxyphenyl acetic acid in schizophrenic patients. Nature, *199:*1271–1272, 1963.

Fromm-Reichmann, F.: Psychotherapy of schizophrenia. Amer. J. Psychiat., *111:*410–419, 1954.

Goldfarb, W.: Childhood Schizophrenia. Cambridge, Harvard University Press, 1961.

Goldfarb, W.: An investigation of childhood schizophrenia. Arch. Gen. Psych., *11:*620–634, 1964.

Gottlieb, G. S., Frohman, C. E., and Beckett, P. G. S.: A theory of neuronal malfunction in schizophrenia. Amer. J. Psychiat., *126:*149–156, 1969.

Green, A. H.: Self-destructive behavior in physically abused schizophrenic children. Arch. Gen. Psychiat., *19:*171–179, 1968.

Grinker, R. R., Werble, B., and Drye, R. C.: The Borderline Syndrome. A Behavioural Study of Ego Functions. New York, Basic Books, Inc., 1968.

Harlow, H. F., and Harlow, M. K.: Learning to love. Amer. Scientist, *54:*244–272, 1966.

Heath, R. G., and Krupp, I. M.: Schizophrenia as a specific biologic disease. Amer. J. Psychiat., *124:*1019–1024, 1968.

Heston, L. L.: The genetics of schizophrenia and schizoid disease. Science, *167:*249–259, 1970.

Hoffer, A., and Pollin, W.: Schizophrenia in the NAS–NRC Panel of 15,909 veteran twin pairs. Arch. Gen. Psychiat., *23:*469–476, 1970.

Hogarty, G. E., and Gross, M.: Preadmission symptom differences between first admitted schizophrenics in predrug and postdrug era. Compr. Psychiat., *7:*134–140, 1966.

Horwitt, M. K.: Fact and artifact in the biology of schizophrenia. Science, *124:*429–430, 1956.

Inouye, E.: Similarity and dissimilarity of schizophrenia in twins. Proc. Third World Congress Psychiat., University Toronto Press, *1:*524–547, 1963.

Johnson, A. M., Griffin, M. E., Watson, E. J., and Beckett, P. G. S.: Observations on ego functions in schizophrenia. Psychiatry, *19:*143–148, 1956.

Kallmann, F. J.: Heredity in Health and Mental Disorder. New York, W. W. Norton & Co., Inc., 1953.

Kety, S. S.: Biochemical theories of schizophrenia. Science, *129:*1528–1532, 1959.

Kolb, L. C.: Psychotherapeutic evolution and its implications. Psychiatric Quart., *30:*579–597, 1956.

Kolb, L. C., Kallmann, F. J., and Polatin, P. (eds.): Schizophrenia. Int. Psychiat. Clinics, *4,* 1964.

Kraepelin, E.: Dementia Praecox. Translated by Barclay, R. M. Edinburgh, E. & S. Livingstone, 1919.

Langfeldt, G.: Diagnosis and prognosis of schizophrenia. Proc. Royal Soc. Med., *53:*1047–1052, 1960.

Lidz, T., Fleck, S., and Cornelison, A. R.: Schizophrenia and the Family. New York, International Universities Press, 1965.

Maricq, H. R.: Nailfold capillary bed in schizophrenics and the influence of institutional life. Acta Psychiat., Scand., *45:*355–366, 1969.

May, P. R. A.: Treatment of Schizophrenia. New York, Science House, 1968.

Mishler, E. G., and Scotch, N. A.: Sociocultural factors in the epidemiology of schizophrenia. Psychiatry, *26:*315–351, 1963.

Morris, G. O., and Wynne, L. C.: Schizophrenic offspring and parental styles of communication. Psychiatry, *28:*19–44, 1965.

O'Neal, P., and Robins, L. N.: Childhood patterns predictive of adult schizophrenia: a 30-year follow-up study. Amer. J. Psychiat., *115:*385–391, 1958.

Ornitz, E. M. et al.: The auditory evoked response in normal and autistic children during sleep. Electroenceph. Clin. Neurophysiol., *25:*221–230, 1968.

Pitt, R., and Hage, J.: Patterns of peer interaction during adolescence as prognostic indicators in schizophrenia. Amer. J. Psychiat., *120:*1089–1096, 1964.

Prien, R. F., and Cole, J. O.: High dosage chlorpromazine therapy in chronic schizophrenia. Arch. Gen. Psychiat., *18:*482–495, 1968.

Searles, H. F.: The schizophrenic individual's experience of his world. Psychiatry, *30:*119–131, 1967.

Shakow, D.: Psychological deficit in schizophrenia. Behavioral Sci., *4:*275–315, 1963.

Silverman, J.: Variations in cognitive control and psychophysiological defense in the schizophrenias. Psychosom. Med., *29:*225–251, 1967.

Smith, K., Thompson, G. F., and Kostner, A. D.: Sweat in schizophrenic patients: Identification of odorous substances. Science, *168:*398–399, 1969.

Sobel, D. E.: Children of schizophrenic patients: preliminary observations on early development. Amer. J. Psychiat., *118:*512–517, 1961.

Sobel, D. E.: Infant mortality and malformations in children of schizophrenic women. Psychiat. Quart., *35:*60–65, 1961.

Stabenau, J. R., and Pollin, W.: Comparative life history differences of families of schizophrenias, delinquents and "normals." Amer. J. Psychiat., *124:*1526–1534, 1968.

Stanton, A. H., and Schwartz, M. S.: The Mental Hospital. A Study of Institutional Participation in Psychiatric Illness and Treatment. New York, Basic Books, Inc., 1954.

Treffert, D. A.: Epidemiology of infantile autism. Arch. Gen. Psychiat., *22:*434–438, 1970.

Whitehorn, J. C., and Betz, B. J.: A Study of psychotherapeutic relationships between physicians and schizophrenic patients. Amer. J. Psychiat., *111:*321–331, 1954.

Wing, J. K., O'Connor, N., and Lolter, V.: Autistic conditions in early childhood. Brit. Med. J., *3:* 389–392, 1967.

Winters, E., (ed.): The Collected Papers of Adolph Meyer. Vol. II. Baltimore, Johns Hopkins Press, 1951.

Wynne, L. C., and Singer, M. T.: Thought disorder and family relations of schizophrenics. Arch. Gen. Psychiat., *9:*191–198, 199–206, 1963.

Yarden, P. E., and Suranyi, I.: The early development of institutionalized children of schizophrenic mothers. Dis. Nerv. Syst., *29:*380–384, 1968.

Zubin, J., et al.: A Biometric Approach to Prognosis in Schizophrenia. *In* Hoch, P. H., and Zubin, J. (eds.): Comparative Epidemiology of the Mental Disorders. New York, Grune & Stratton, 1961, pp. 143–203.

Chapter 22

"Moody madness, laughing wild."

Thomas Gray

"Melancholy is the nurse of frenzy."

Shakespeare

Affective Psychoses

AFFECTIVE REACTIONS

The group of affective psychoses constitutes those behavior disturbances characterized principally by increased or decreased activity and thought expressive of a predominating mood of depression or elation. Although at the ranges of disturbance the behavioral change is conspicuous, it is seldom bizarre. The abnormalities of activity, affect, and thought seem often to the casual observer to have a plausible relationship to the immediate social environment.

Psychodynamically it might be expected that the major defenses against depressive affect would be projection or denial. While one group of individuals suffer from the direct behavioral expressions of depressive affect, modified according to the weighting of guilt, shame, anxiety, or helplessness that is induced as response in the specific personality make up, in others the affective expression is obscured through the use of the aforementioned dynamisms. In some, the underlying depression is covered by a paranoidal picture in which the guilty affect is assigned by projection onto others. In another group the depression is masked or may alternate with phases of elation. These several major variants are found in the involutional and the manic-depressive psychoses respectively. In still others depression is masked by various neurotic symptoms, or by psychophysiologic responses, particularly those expressed in excessively driven oral behavior such as overeating and obesity, alcoholism, or drug dependency.

In this chapter consideration is given to the affective psychoses, the variants of the involutional, manic-depressive, and depressive psychotic reactions.

Prevalence

When one considers all affective states (psychotic, neurotic, and the masked syndromes with oral or psychosomatic symptomatology), it may well be that this category of psychiatric disability is the most prevalent. The total of depressive disorders discovered in general hospital practice is as great as or greater than all other diagnostic categories. In a recent analysis of inception of mental illness in an English city, Adelstein et al. found that the rate of 97 per 100,000 for depressive psychosis was the highest of any diagnostic category. The rate increased with age for both sexes, but women had an earlier and higher peak in the 30 to 39 year period, which was in excess of the rates between 40 and 59 in the same sex. Widowhood was associated with the high rates in the 30's. This lack of association of high rates in women during the menopausal period is surprising. In this study the diagnostic analysis did not provide discriminations of the varieties of affective psychosis. One may only conclude that in this city the rates for the involutional psychoses were lower than for the depressive psychoses.

INVOLUTIONAL PSYCHOTIC REACTIONS

The involutional psychoses tend to fall into two types. One is characterized largely by depression, the other by paranoid ideas. A depression occurring in the involutional period should usually not be included in the involutional psychotic reactions if there is a history of a previous manic-depressive reaction. In spite of the feature of depression common to both manic-depressive and involutional reactions, there are such special physiological and psychological factors in the latter that it is no longer considered to be a modified manic-depressive reaction occurring at a particular physiological epoch. Both conditions, as well as the neurotic depressions, share with the healthy grief reactions their precipitation through the perception by the sufferer of a loss. That loss may be the death of or separation from some loved person or the disruption of an important bodily function, a desired social or economic status, or even a cherished ideal or hope for the future. Such a precipitating loss may be discovered in an actual event or apprehended in fantasy. While often obscure on casual examination, the existence of the precipitant in some interpersonal incident or its apprehension in fantasy may be discovered on closer and more penetrating study.

Loss as it pertains to those with involutional psychotic reactions is discussed later in this chapter in the section entitled Predisposing Factors. Its general and psychodynamic consequences are subjects of comment in both this and succeeding chapters concerned with varieties of depressive reactions.

Psychodynamics

Various psychoanalytic studies have suggested that the pathologic affects of the depressive state associated with helpless anxiety occur in those who must compulsively maintain goals or personal attachments (object-relations) in order to maintain a sense of security. Unlike those who are capable of passing through a healthy mourning process as the result of realistic perception of a loss, the psychotic depressive is unable to give up his wishes even though they are beyond attainment. Thus Bibring identifies three sets of aspirations and hopes which must be maintained and are not necessarily exclusive. They are the wish to be worthy and therefore loved and respected—and thus not to be inferior and disrespected; the wish to be strong, superior, and secure —and not to be weak and insecure; and the wish to be good and to love—and not to be aggressive, hateful, or destructive. It is in the conflict and tensions between these hopes and aspirations and their opposite potentials in reality or fantasy that the depressive complex arises.

There is now a recognition that the helpless anxiety of the psychotic depressive reactions is of a different kind from that which occurs in the psychoneurosis. The repetitive and constant demands for support, the clinging, and the response to consistent availability have suggested that the anxiety of involutional melancholia and other psychotic depressions is less differentiated and more primitive than that observed in the healthy or psychoneurotic. It suggests the dependent infant; thus depressive behavior and its associated affects are considered by many psychoanalysts as regressive to behaviors characteristic of the infantile state. They take place in those who have failed to develop the necessary defenses against the affective states induced in early life through the stress of partial separations or limited experiences of affect deprivations and in those who through the persistence of the infantile defenses of denial, projection, or obsessive reaction formations have warded off the socially maturing capacities of response to loss.

These views are in contrast to the early psychodynamic explanations of the depressive states wherein the central pathology was considered a sense of pathological guilt derived from a distorted development of the superego through excessive internalization of critical and punishing attitudes. Thus fearful of expressing rage toward loved objects, the depressed patient turned this emotion upon himself as a means of atoning for his guilt.

It would seem that in the psychotic depression one may discern in varying degrees in different patients both the regressive move to states of anxious infantile dependency and its associated physiological concomitants in sleep and eating disturbances as well as evidence in the thought disturbances of internally directed rage expressed in the atoning delusions of guilt, shame, and self-punishment.

INVOLUTIONAL DEPRESSIVE REACTION

The incidence of the depressive type of involutional psychosis is two to three times greater in women than in men. Among first admissions to hospitals for mental diseases it is exceeded in frequency only by schizophrenia, senile dementia, and syndromes associated with cerebral arteriosclerosis.

Age Factors

Although subject to considerable individual variation in the age of incidence, the involutional psychoses occur most frequently in women during the late 40's and in men during the late 50's. It will be noted that this is the period when the endocrine and reproductive glands begin to suffer a decrease in functional activity —the age generally known as the involutional period. As the activity of these glands declines, there are extensive changes in the metabolic and vegetative activities of the body. With the cessation of ovarian activity there may be a change in functioning of other parts of the endocrine system, involving an increased irritability of the sympathetic nervous system. Just what part these changes in essential physiological functions play in the genesis of the psychosis is uncertain, but there is much to suggest that they are not so important per se as are their psychological implications. The threat to the personality through the loss of prized biological functions and the imminence of the aging process with all it connotes may be more disturbing to the personality than endocrinological changes. The period is one of psychophysiological stress and one in which increasing threats to an insecure personality are likely to elicit anxiety, depression, and paranoid reactions or all of these, a period that threatens the security that has been established at a time when the individual can least afford to lose it. It is a period that, in women, has often been anticipated with exaggerated fear.

Prepsychotic Personality

In a significant number of cases of the involutional depressive reaction, there is found a certain general type of personality makeup and of habits of life. Usually the patient was an anxious child with a background of early fundamental insecurity. A review of the patient's previous personality and temperament often shows that she has been a compulsive, inhibited type of individual with a tendency to be quiet, unobtrusive, serious, chronically worrisome, intolerant, reticent, sensitive, scrupulously honest, frugal, and even penurious. Usually, too, she has been of exacting and inflexible standards, lacking in humor, overconscientious, and given to self-punishment. Such persons have been mild, submissive, and sensitive to the moods and feelings of others. They have never been boastful but have depreciated their own worth, which often has actually been high. Not rarely they have been exploited by the selfish. The prepsychotic personality has been marked by a rigidity that represented a neurotic defense, and the patient has been perfectionistic, prudish, and prone to feelings of guilt. The personality has been superego dominated. Many involutional patients have been self-effacing and self-sacrificing and have had an exaggerated need for, and dependency upon, the approval of others.

Undoubtedly involutional depression evolves out of a masked neurosis of earlier life. In some instances, hostile and aggressive impulses have been repressed with difficulty. Many psychiatrists consider, in fact, that the prepsychotic personality of the involutional depressive type has been developed as a reaction-formation against aggression. Often the patient's sex life has been suppressed or unsatisfactory. Her interests have been narrow and her habits stereotyped; she has cared little for recreation, has not sought pleasure, and has had but few close friends. Frequently the patient has been a loyal subordinate, meticulous as to detail, rather than an aggressive, confident leader. Many have been fidgety, fretful, apprehensive persons. Others have been characterized by caution or indecision.

Predisposing Factors

The age at which the psychosis develops is one at which adjustments to new situations and circumstances are no longer easily made. Perhaps life has not brought either the success or satisfaction that hope had cherished. At this period there is a more or less conscious recognition that early dreams and desires cannot now be fulfilled, that the zenith of life has been passed, and that ambition and life's forces are waning. The fact that opportunity no longer exists for repairing old errors or achieving new success creates a sense of frustration and increases the feeling of insecurity. In women, loneliness or fear of a loss of physical attractiveness may be a contributing factor. The high value placed upon youth, beauty, and sex in our culture contributes to the drastic reorientation that must be made. The patient

may feel that she is no longer attractive and feminine. At this period of life, some women have a deeply seated resentment, which may be expressed in depression and self-hate.

A rebellion against aging may also tend to promote depression. The transition to another stage of life with its new and difficult problems, both psychological and biological, is not easy. Regrets and a sense of failure contribute to the prevailing mood. Perhaps friends are beginning to die, or children to whom the patient has devoted her life are leaving home and becoming preoccupied with their own lives and families. The patient may feel that she is no longer needed. In some cases, aged parents who formerly represented security but are now dependent on the patient constitute a problem.

An ebbing potency in the male and the realization by the woman that her most highly prized biological possession, that of childbearing, perhaps long frustrated, is now a lost capacity, is for the patient more than the loss of one of the most fundamental of functions—it is a symbol that both the sources and ends of energy have failed. Sometimes sexual desires, which have previously been suppressed, are perturbingly aroused. Previous reaction-formations prove inadequate, and acquired compensations and other protective mechanisms begin to fail.

As the flush of maturity fades, thoughts of death are suggested and contribute to the anxiety so common in the disorder. With the decrease of physical strength, unconscious forces and old conflicts become relatively stronger and return to threaten and torment. This threat to the ego is ceaseless, and since the source of the danger is hidden and within, any escape from it is impossible. As a result, the apprehension, tension, and unrest of anxiety are intensified. In a certain number of cases, retirement from business means the renunciation of long-cherished interests and a withdrawal of psychic energy. Sometimes a real economic stress or the possibility of becoming dependent upon someone is added to other problems.

It is not surprising, therefore, that in the event of some disturbing experience, such as the breaking up of the home or other threatening change in the life situation, the loss of position, or the death of one upon whom dependence was felt, the psychosis, with its pathological depression, apprehension, ideas of death, and nihilistic and hypochondriacal delusions, is precipitated.

Symptoms

As with all the depressive reactions, the major component in the disturbance is the development of an unpleasant affective state. This state is compounded of a number of subjective components, of which grief and sadness represent only a part. Those others are varying degrees and combinations of intense anxiety, shame, and guilt. To these affects there are added as major components of the state ego attitudes of profound helplessness and diminution of self-esteem, with severe inhibitions of previous personality functioning.

The manifest symptoms of the psychosis are often preceded by a period of several weeks or a few months during which the patient exhibits hypochondriacal trends, becomes irritable, peevish, pessimistic, suffers from insomnia, is perhaps suspicious, shows a disinclination for effort, and may be given to spells of weeping. She is unable to concentrate and shows doubt and indecision. Frequently there are a narrowing of interests and a shrinking from the environment. The patient complains of distressing sensations in the head, eats poorly, loses weight, worries about health or finance, and becomes apprehensive and restless. In a more or less typical case, the most conspicuous symptoms are profound depression, anxiety, agitation, hypochondriasis, and guilty delusions of sin, unworthiness, disease, and impending death.

The patient's appearance becomes one of extreme emotional pain and misery. The fear, apprehension, and agitation increase; the patient wrings her hands, paces back and forth, weeps, may beat her head against the wall, picks at her face, bites her nails, and tears at her handkerchief or clothing. She moans, and in a whining voice constantly repeats, "Why did I do it?" "Oh, God, what will become of me?" or some other stereotyped expression indicating hopelessness and affective distress. The patient may constantly besiege doctors and nurses with inquiries, complaints, or requests for reassurance, literally clinging to them and reiterating the demand that they help her or that they not abandon her.

Some patients present a morose depression or a depressive hostility. Misinterpretations and delusions are almost constantly present. Feelings of guilt explain in part both the great emotional depression and many of the delusions. Trifling indiscretions of youth or unformulated sins become the "unpardonable sin." The patient holds herself responsible for the fate of others. She has infected, disgraced, or harmed her family. She is about to be horribly butchered, a fate that she says she deserves, but awaits with intense fear and with pleas for mercy—indicating her ambivalent desire both for death and for life.

The delusion that she is about to be destroyed may be the patient's rationalization of her sense that life forces are declining. Inner distresses and dissatisfactions are rationalized as physical disease and thus produce the hypochondriasis so frequently observed. In this way the patient comes to believe that her intestines are obstructed, that she has no stomach, or that her brain is "dried up." Hallucinations, although less frequent than illusions, may occur. She hears preparations for her torture. Consciousness remains clear, and the patient is oriented, although in some cases the subjective absorption of attention is so great that she may appear to be confused and not thoroughly in touch with her environment.

Some patients are perplexed and bewildered. Depersonalization with feelings of unreality may exist. Food is often refused, sometimes because of a desire for death; at other times this occurs when, because of self-accusatory ideas, the patient believes she does not deserve food; again, refusal may be caused by a belief that the food is poisoned, or by nihilistic ideas that she has no stomach or no intestines. There is no other mental disorder in which suicidal attempts are so common. There is great danger that previous unsuccessful suicidal attempts will be repeated.

Although the patient never has a discriminating insight, she nevertheless usually realizes that matters are not as usual with her mentally. Early in the disorder the poorly understood sense of apprehension and the affective distress are so great, and are recognized as constituting such a contrast to her previous feeling-state, that the patient often expresses the fear she is going to lose her mind. She remains, nevertheless, thoroughly convinced as to the correctness of the idea she expresses.

Most patients lose weight and in severe cases become seriously dehydrated. The hands are usually cold and cyanotic. The pulse is rapid and the respirations are shallow. The bowels are constipated and the urine scanty.

Another group of middle-aged patients are less disturbed yet appear dismal and hopeless and suffer as well from a loss of self-esteem. Behaviorally they appear withdrawn and apathetic and are isolated in social groups due to their attendant retardation in speech and thought. Such patients, too, may suffer delusions reflecting their sense of guilt and shame. But the clinging helplessness, agitation, hypochondriacal complaining, and somatic symptoms of insomnia, anorexia, and constipation are absent or much less conspicuous than in the most seriously disturbed group. Premorbid adaptation has usually been that of a well-adapted compulsive personality with the depressive state coming on as the result of physical illness and aging.

The following summary illustrates many of the common features of involutional melancholia.

E. M., a single woman in her early 50's, was admitted to a hospital following a suicidal attempt. She was described as having been a shy, sensitive, and affectionate child. Although in early life she attended dances, she was never known to have had any male friends. She always said she wished to "live alone and not be bothered by a man's company." After coming to America from Ireland at age 23, she secured employment as a domestic. She apparently was well regarded by her employers, to whom she became quite attached and with whom she usually remained for many years of continuous service. She was described as always using all her spare time in "doing little things about the house, darning stockings, cleaning something, and doing ironing." She was conscientious, likeable, ambitious, and affectionate, but stubborn and difficult to convince. She was carefully observant of what she considered to be her religious duties and attended church regularly.

On arrival at the hospital, her facies denoted fear and apprehension. Although agitated, she supplied the usual admission data, and when asked if she was married, she at first replied in the affirmative, but a moment later stated that she was not married. Shortly afterward, when seen in the ward, she repeatedly inquired if the place was a jail. Upon being asked the reason for such a question, she replied, "Because jail is the safest place. I hope I don't be killed." She became increasingly anxious, agitated, and apprehensive, and on the day following her admission, she attempted to thrust her head through a closed window. Whenever a physician entered the ward, she approached him and with but little variation constantly repeated: "I am afraid, Doctor. Oh, my God! I am afraid of those men upstairs!" (There were no men in that section of the building.) "Look at those big snakes! Look at those big dogs!"

The patient had always lived frugally and had methodically deposited her savings in a bank, where she had accumulated several thousand dollars. She maintained, however, that her money was all lost and that she was destitute. Several days after her admission the patient was brought before the staff for diagnosis. At that time she showed the same anxious depression and agitation that had characterized her entire hospital residence. Soon after entering the staff room, she asked if the door leading to an anteroom where patients of both sexes were waiting was locked. When asked the occasion for the question, she replied, "I am afraid of the men."

Many of the factors that resulted in this woman's psychosis are comparatively simple and evident. The rigid environment in which she had been reared discouraged a normal interest in those of the opposite sex. That she had repressed any instinctive interest in men was betrayed by her statement that she did not want to be "bothered by a man's company." She became a faithful, conscientious servant, scrupulous as to detail but with an increasing limitation of external interests. Matters continued in this simple but hardly satisfying manner until physical capacity began to decline. The fact that life had not brought all that was desired became more or less vaguely realized; she was also aware that strength was waning and that whatever life had not already brought could never be attained. As physical energy declined with the involutional changes, the repression of material that had formerly been maintained, although with difficulty, began to fail. With their repression weakened, instinctive tendencies that had always been scrupulously denied any conscious recognition began to threaten from within.

With no escape possible, anxiety, depression, fear, and apprehension followed. This fear was projected as one of men, since it was the patient's repressed interest in them which she feared. This sense of danger was rationalized as one of threat to life, while affective and subjective material came to possess the vividness the patient had always associated with sensory experiences, with the result that she heard voices saying she was to be killed. Doubtless the patient's anxiety and depression represented much more than a weakening in the repression of instinctive tendencies of a psychosexual nature; the approach of an age when physical vigor and means of livelihood were declining, a sense of isolation, and vague feelings of disappointment and failure and perhaps of guilt all contributed to a sense of insecurity that added to the affective tension and apprehension.

Prognosis

Before the introduction of electric shock treatment, about 40 per cent of the patients with involutional melancholia recovered. Convalescence, however, was slow, and those who recovered were frequently ill for two or three years. With the use of electric shock, more than 50 per cent of the involutional melancholia patients showed prompt recovery. Now greater numbers are restored to health as the antidepressant pharmacologies have come into use. The more nearly the general manifestations of the reaction approach those usually seen in the depressive phase of manic-depressive psychosis, the better the prognosis. The greater the deterioration of personal habits the more grotesque the delusions or the hypochondriacal ideas, the greater the occurrence of hallucinations, the more marked the poverty of thought and the tendency to aversion, depersonalization, or rut-formation with its meager affect reaction, the worse is the prognosis. Whining, surliness, and seclusiveness are not favorable symptoms. The more narrow and rigid the prepsychotic personality, the poorer the prognosis.

Diagnosis

Psychiatric disorders that may present features requiring a consideration of differential diagnosis from involutional melancholia are manic-depressive psychosis, cerebral arteriosclerosis, and anxiety-depressive states occurring in the psychoneuroses. In *manic-depressive psychosis,* the question of involutional melancholia need not be considered unless the age of the patient is compatible with the latter diagnosis. In that case, there is usually a history of previous attacks either of excitement or of depression. Frequently the manic-depressive has been of a cyclothymic temperament, whereas the involutional depressive has a compulsive type of personality. In the depression of a purely affective psychosis, there is typically a retardation in the flow of thought and in activity. The presence of agitation, hypochondriacal and nihilistic ideas, peevishness, and hallucinations points toward an involutional depressive reaction. In this, fear, apprehension, and ideas of impending destruction are more marked. Stereotypes of behavior or speech and admixtures of other schizophrenic symptoms are more consistent with involutional melancholia.

Occasionally the *arteriosclerotic* patient is apprehensive and agitated, but he lacks profound and sustained fear. If the involvement is principally in the smaller vessels, the headaches and unpleasant cephalic sensations may suggest the hypochondriacal ideas of involutional melancholia, but the easy mental fatigability, occurrence of confused periods, slight delay in comprehension, a lessening of initiative rather than a preoccupation, and a slight memory loss should indicate the organic source of the mental disorder.

Among the psychoneuroses, the anxiety and depressive reactions must be differentiated occasionally from the involutional psychotic reactions. While a sustained apprehensiveness associated with phobias occurs with the anxiety neuroses and may be confused with the agitation and the obsessive delusional state in the involutional state, the episodic attacks of acute anxiety with hyperventilation and its physiological concomitants of breathlessness, palpitation, sweating, and paresthesias characteristic of the former condition are not seen in the psychotic state. The patient with an anxiety neurosis contacts others easily, and is voluble and capable of speaking at length of his life problems. There is no psychomotor retardation nor does he suffer from the somatic symptoms of insomnia, anorexia, or constipation.

The history of depressive affect immediately reactive to an evident loss, without significant impairment of capacity for interpersonal transactions, motor retardation, anorexia, or disturbance of libido, but with some degree of intermittent insomnia, distinguishes the neurotic depressive. The latter may also manifest acute anxiety attacks with hyperventilation. In these conditions there is no general inhibition of personality functioning.

Treatment

The patient suffering from an involutional depressive reaction should usually be cared for in a hospital, particularly since there is no other type of mental disorder in which so large a percentage of patients attempt suicide. The general lines of treatment are the same as those employed in the depressive phase of manic-depressive psychosis, but with particular stress on improving the physical state of the patient, which frequently becomes weakened and impaired. On arrival at the hospital, many patients are badly dehydrated and nearly always undernourished. There must be assurance, therefore, that the patient receives an abundance of liquid and food. If the patient is undernourished, it is often helpful to give her 20 units of insulin 30 minutes before meals. Because of their fear and apprehension, the purpose of any procedure or change from routine should be carefully explained to these patients.

Electroshock therapy is the most effective measure in the treatment of involutional depression. The technique of its application is discussed in Chapter 33. Although there are usually few contraindications to its use, the patient should first receive a careful physical examination. It should not be employed in case of cardiac decompensation. Except for recent fractures, bone disease is not a frequent contraindication. The patient should usually receive from 12 to 20 treatments. Most physicians find it desirable to "soften" the seizure by means of succinylcholine dichloride (Anectine). If the patient is greatly agitated, chlorpromazine may be used for its tranquilizing effect.

The antidepressive agents also are now used, perhaps most effectively as maintenance medication after electroshock therapy. Lobotomy is performed today only rarely for this condition.

While estrogenic hormones help to relieve menopausal symptoms such as hot flashes, sweats, tensions, uneasiness, and headaches, they are of little or no value in true involutional melancholia. The convalescent patient will frequently be deeply grateful for reassurance and support.

INVOLUTIONAL PARANOID REACTION

A certain number of persons develop a paranoid psychosis during the involutional period. Although never previously psychotic, nearly all such patients are found to have been persons whose prepsychotic personality was characterized by projective defensive patterns. Usually it will be found that she has been critical and inclined to blame others for her failures and has seen slights where none were intended. By her associates she was probably regarded as obstinate in opinion, jealous, unforgiving, secretive, unhappy, dissatisfied, given to nursing of grievances, resentful, and suspicious. These defensive character traits prove sufficient support for the personality until the involutional period when, with the added physiological and psychological burdens previously mentioned, they are no longer adequate, and resort is made to the more extreme defensive and compensatory measures provided by the paranoid psychosis with its delusions and misinterpretations. The delusions usually revolve around ideas of persecution and are well organized, but they lack the fantastic content observed in schizophrenia. Many patients show much bitterness and hostility. The prognosis is less favorable than in melancholia. Electroshock treatment is of limited benefit. The aggressive and disturbed patient may be helped by chlorpromazine.

The following case illustrates many of the features often seen in paranoid involutional psychosis.

A. S. was admitted to the hospital at the age of 59. The patient was born in Latvia. Little is known concerning her childhood experiences and the emotional climate of the home. She came to the United States at the age of 19 to marry a man who had preceded her to this country. She and her husband returned to Latvia, where the husband took over his father's farm and attained considerable success and status. At this point the farm buildings were destroyed by fire, and the patient was so seriously burned that she required hospital care for three months. They returned to the United States and the husband established an upholstering business in which the patient assisted until this business failed. The husband then began to drink, and he committed suicide by hanging, a casualty discovered by the patient.

When she was approximately 54 years of age, the patient began to complain that people were talking about her, that her son-in-law was maritally unfaithful, that nearly all persons, especially the clergy of a different religious faith, were sexually immoral. She expressed a fear that she would be "signed away for experimental purposes." She stated that a physician who had treated her at the menopause had given her cancer. Finally, after having complained to the police on several occasions that her food was being drugged and that a "society of science" was plotting against her, she was committed.

Following the patient's admission to the hospital, her daughter, in describing her mother's personality pattern, reported that she had always been a meticulous, hard-working person who was critical, suspicious, stubborn, uncompromising and domineering. The daughter described her mother as an immaculate housekeeper who also did "beautiful sewing."

On arrival at the hospital, her sensorium was clear, and she was fully oriented. She was suspicious, and when her abdominal reflexes were tested, she asked if the physician was going to operate on her. At times she became quite agitated and hostile and insisted that she be permitted to leave. Someone, she said, was trying to secure possession of her home and to kill her; she must therefore appeal to the police to help her. She complained that the nurses were trying to compel her to perform unpleasant tasks because they were members of a religious organization that was persecuting her.

Because of an electrocardiogram suggestive of coronary involvement and myocardial damage, it was decided not to give the patient electroshock treatment. After seven months of hospital residence, the patient became much less tense, was pleasant and coöperative, and was regarded as one of the most faithful and capable workers in the hospital cafeteria. Within a year after her admission, she was given freedom of the hospital grounds and was to spend weekends with friends. Unless questioned, she expressed no delusional ideas. Upon inquiry, however, it was found that there had been no fundamental change in her paranoid ideation. Fifteen months after her admission the patient was permitted to leave the hospital. A year later her employer wrote: "Mrs. S. is cheerful and pleasant and I am very satisfied with her work."

So little is known about this woman's emotional relations with parents and siblings during childhood and any early traumatizing experiences that it is not easy to construct a desirably complete genetic-dynamic formulation of her psychotic personality disturbance. Her daughter's report that the patient was a meticulous, critical, suspicious, stubborn, dominating, and uncompromising person suggests that, because of a basic feeling of insecurity, she had developed these personality characteristics to serve as defenses. In spite of a long series of threats, these defenses proved adequate for many years until the involutional period, with its various accompanying psychological factors, became so menacing that life-long traits were no longer able to control anxiety-producing threats. As a further defense, therefore, the patient resorted to projection to a reality-sacrificing, or psychotic, degree.

Although the problems that the patient had found too difficult to meet must remain a matter of speculation, one suspects, in view of the nature of her personality traits and the character of her delusions, that a deeply seated hostility, the fear of economic insecurity, and a weakening in the repression of instinctive sex drives may have been important ones.

MANIC-DEPRESSIVE PSYCHOTIC REACTION

Although the contrasting affective states, depression and elation, had been recognized for many years to occur in the same patient, it was not until 1896 that Emil Kraepelin designated the condition as manic-depressive insanity. He observed the periodicity and favorable outcome of the seemingly opposite stages of disordered affect and concluded they were variations of a single morbid process based upon physiological determinants.

Today, it is known that many patients may have only recurrent depressive reactions without elation; few present the alternation between the two affects. For these reasons, these conditions are subclassified in the nomenclature as manic-depressive reaction, "manic type," or "depressive type," or manic-depressive "circular." In the "circular," existence of one or another state is denoted as manic-depressive, circular, or manic-depressive, depressed.

Genetic, clinical, and therapeutic studies of recent years challenge the current nosological classification of manic-depressive illness as a single entity. They suggest that there is a need to discriminate the bipolar (patients exhibiting both manic and depressive phases of behavior) from the unipolar states (those exhibiting only recurrent depressions). Now it is reported that bipolar illness is apparently discoverable only in descendants of families in which there is a record of its occurrence in previous generations. Parental deprivations by death or divorce also characterize this group, suggesting that manic episodes are destructive to the family relationship. Phenomenologically, the bipolar patients exhibit lesser levels of physical activity and overt expressions of physical complaints than the unipolar group.

Prevalence

There are striking differences in the reporting of manic-depressive psychoses in various countries. Thus Kramer has stated that the admission rate of manic-depressives to hospitals in England and Wales exceeds that for the public mental hospitals in the United States by 18 times (36 per 100,000 population versus 2 per 100,000 population) and by 9 times when admissions in the United States are computed for both public and private mental hospitals. The recorded rate of first admissions of those with manic-depressive psychoses in New York state fell steadily from 1930 to 1950. They were as follows: 177 per 100,000 in 1920; 174 in 1930; 111 in 1940; and 71 in 1950. The explanations for these variations are numerous. It has been suggested that constitutional or genetic differences determine higher rates in northern European countries; that increasing immigration of southern Europeans to the United States has led to dilution of the older northern European population, with the diminished frequency of illnesses characteristic of northern populations; and that the diagnostic criteria vary from country to country and generation to generation. Also, the admission rates of the manic-depressive to the private psychiatric hospitals in the United States, which cater largely to the wealthier families of older stock, greatly exceed rates for the public mental hospitals serving the more deprived economically and representing largely waves of immigrants from southern

Europe. Another reason for the decline in hospital admissions of this group perhaps rests in their increasingly successful treatment through clinic or office therapy.

Genetics

The not uncommon occurrence of manic-depressive psychoses in the same family suggests that a biogenetic factor may be at least a contributory cause, but this can scarcely be proved or denied. Rüdin has stated that the incidence of manic-depressive psychosis is 25 times as high among the siblings of manic-depressive patients as in the average population. If it occurs in monozygotic twins, both of them will be affected in more than half of the cases. In a German psychiatric clinic to which patients are admitted irrespective of social position, Luxemberger found manic-depressive psychoses to be nearly three times as frequent in the highest social class and four times as frequent in the professional classes as in the general population. This distribution of incidence seems to be similar to that observed by American psychiatrists. In World War II, manic-depressive psychoses were three times as frequent among officers of the American army as among enlisted men.

Winokur and his colleagues are of the opinion that the manic-depressive reaction differs from other affective psychoses based on their studies of familial and genetic patterns. They suggest that a dominant x-linked factor is primary for the transmission of manic-depressive illness when one limits the definition to families in which one or more have had manic episodes as well as depressions. Thus they found maternal relatives in their families with affective illness twice as frequently as paternal. So, too, they are in pursuit of association of color blindness as a sex-linked genetic marker with manic-depressive illness and have discovered this association in two families. Others are now attempting verification of the Winokur findings.

Certainly, until there has been established international agreement on diagnostic criteria for all the psychoses and evidence has accumulated that clinical observations and diagnosis in differing geographic areas are highly reliable, the differences in prevalence rates and their interpretations offer dubious support to any theories on etiology.

They occur about twice as frequently in women as in men, and the average age of onset in women is younger. The aggressive woman with masculine strivings seems to be especially predisposed. Although these reactions are most frequently recognized during early maturity, more recent clinical observations have shown initial periods of depression with crying commencing in early childhood. The nuclear facets of the personality characteristics defined in the adult patients are then already evident.

Pathophysiology

That genetic and/or constitutional factors play a significant role in the manic-depressive psychosis has been argued upon the basis of selective response to electroshock therapy and the aminodibenzol antidepressants. Thus those with so-called endogenous depressions respond much more favorably to electroshock and the antidepressant pharmaceuticals than those classified as suffering reactive or neurotic depressions. Again the clinical observation that certain patients in the depressed phase of this reaction shortly become manic after administration of imipramine and its analogs suggests that biological processes play an important role in the occurrence of the psychotic affective states.

From the accumulation of evidence on the action of drugs which influence the affective states and the growing understanding of their pharmacological effects, there has emerged a hypothesis relating changes in catecholamine metabolism to states of depression or elation. Those drugs which potentiate the action of brain norepinephrine also stimulate overt behavioral expressions, including excitement, and function in man as antidepressants, while those which inactivate or deplete norepinephrine centrally predispose to sedation and depressions. It has been suggested then that some depressions, and perhaps all, are associated with a deficiency of catecholamines, and especially norepinephrine, at the significant adrenergic receptor sites in the brain, while an excess of these amines exists with behavioral states of elation. This hypothesis is based on indirect evidence, reviewed by Schildkraut.

However, in the light of other data the catecholamine hypothesis is now recognized as too simplified. Other biogenic amines are concerned in synaptic transmission, and perhaps their relative participation in this or that brain subsystem determines the effective integrative fusing within the brain. Thus Murphy and his colleagues have reported the regular induction of hypomania by L-dopa in "bipolar" manic-depressive patients. Coppen has found that the average urinary excretion of tryptamine during depression is half that of the normal, and other studies have shown that the concentration of 5-hydroxyindoles in the cerebrospinal fluid is lower than in the nondepressed. Glassman points out that the indoleamines (tryptamine and serotonin) are involved as well. Much additional research is required before a clear comprehension is achieved of the relationship of biogenic amine metabolism to manic-depressive illness. Nevertheless, the evidence for such a relationship is very powerful.

Rosenblatt and Chenley have found that infused norepinephrine appears to be metabolized differently in manic-depressive patients from in the involutional psychotic states and in the healthy. They report an increase in the proportion of urinary metabolites of norepinephrine that retain an amino group as compared to those which undergo deamination. If such metabolic differences are confirmed by others, substantial support will be gained for the hypothesis that the catecholamines are a major contributing factor in the genesis of the manic-depressive reaction.

So, too, it appears that electrolytic metabolism is damaged in the manic-depressive psychosis. During depression sodium retention occurs and its distribution may be altered. Potassium and water excretion varies with the mood, being increased during depression and decreased during elation. This assumption gains support from the fact that lithium salts effectively inhibit the manic phase of the illness.

Others have reported changes in adrenocortical function judged from studies of the circadian variations of excretion of plasma and urinary steroids and high plasmin lipid values in manic-depressives.

Hartmann has found that the sleep dream cycle of manic-depressive patients, examined electroencephalographically, differs from that in health. Total sleep time is always lower during manic phases, but varies in depression from unchanged to increased. Total rapid eye movement (REM) and dream time (D-time) are also less in the manic phases and tend to be higher during the depressions. So, too, D% is low in the manic stage and high during the depressions, but less so in the absolute D-time. D latency (amount of sleep before the first D period) varies with manic phases but is low during depressions. The findings differ from those of other depressed patients. They suggest that the manic-depressives have a need or pressure for dreaming time. Hartmann suggests that the shifts in the physiological stages of sleep may be related to catecholamine metabolism.

Strongin and Hinsie's finding that the rate of salivary secretion is lowered in depression has been confirmed repeatedly. This diminution of salivary secretion has not been correlated with the clinical degree of depression and may persist after improvement. Salivary secretion is easily measured by the methods described by Busfield.

The "sedation threshold," defined by Shagass as the amount of amobarbital sodium in milligrams per kilogram of body weight required to produce a specific inflection in the amplitude of frontal lobe electroencephalographic activity during intravenous injection, is lowered in those with psychotic depressive reactions, again in contrast with other types of psychosis. The threshold for each individual is reproducible over time, and it is not modified greatly by moderate doses of phenothiazines.

Shagass and Schwartz also report a significant increase in the mean recovery time of the cycle of cerebral cortical potentials following stimulation of the ulnar nerve in the psychotic depressive, the schizophrenic, and those with personality disorders. The techniques of defining and measuring the sedation threshold and the cycle of cortical excitability are given in various papers cited by Shagass and his co-workers.

Psychopathology

There are two well-defined types or phases of the manic-depressive psychoses: a manic or hyperactive phase, and a depressive phase.

Although the disorder typically assumes the form of psychotic episodes separated by intervals of mental health, a person may suffer only from one episode, or, again, the disorder may become continuous. These episodes may be in the nature of a manic or of a depressive reaction; there is no constant sequence or alternation of these reactions. The swings from one phase to another seem to prove the homogeneity of the manic-depressive psychoses.

MANIC PHASE. In his personality make-up the patient whose episodes are of a manic type has usually been a self-satisfied, confident, aggressive, effervescing extrovert, at ease with other people. He has been inclined to scatter his energy over a wide field of interests. His affective attitude has been one of emotional expression and responsiveness. The manic phase or reaction is usually preceded by a simple depression. This depression is of brief duration and mild in degree, often lasting for only a few days and either not noted by the patient's family or not considered significant. This brief period is followed by exhilaration or mild excitement.

Sometimes the attack remains in this attenuated form known as *hypomania*. In this hypomanic state there are increased assertiveness, an air of self-assurance, careless gaiety, breezy affability, self-satisfaction, buoyant self-confidence, and boundless energy. No matter how inhibited the patient may normally have been, he is now irrepressible, demanding, uninhibited, effusive, and often astonishingly unconventional in speech and manner. He is narcissistic, childishly proud, and quite intolerant of criticism. Glib of tongue and genial of hand, the patient is socially aggressive, witty, boastful, flippant, argumentative, spends his money extravagantly, pawns his belongings, is full of ambitious schemes and starts enterprises that soon fail or that he soon abandons. Excessive indulgence in alcohol colors and confuses his behavior.

Often striking is the frequency of use of direct and indirect quotations, particularized references, and adverbs of degree ("absolutely," "much," "never"). His conversation is directed principally to a recital of events, circumstances, and meetings with others, but it seldom contains statements as to their inner affective meaning to him or as to his personal evaluation of the interactions between himself and others. Thus there is little evidence of introspection but more that of comparing, weighing, and evaluating the performances of others and himself. From this trend, coupled with the many indications of denial and overcompensatory self-references, there emerges a self-image toward which the patient appears to be striving.

His excuses and arguments contain a superficial but specious plausibility. His disregard for the truth may carry great conviction to those not previously acquainted with him. The patient is bored with routine, lacks a sustained interest in any activity, and is too busy to submit his impressions to critical examination. Attention is often easily distracted, thought processes are accelerated, and the stream of thought is prone to wander. His manner of speaking has an undertone of emphasis and exaggeration.

Many hypomanic patients are mischievous, boisterous, and full of pranks, indulge in risqué remarks and coarse and unseemly jokes, and make facetious comments about some object, or especially some person, in the environment. They are superficial in their relationships with other persons and insensitive to the latters' needs and feelings. Some hypomanic individuals delight in joking efforts to tease the physician. Unbridled criticism and bluntness of speech, even to the point of impudence, are common. Without constraint, the manic patient blurts out what he has doubtless long wished to say but has previously been afraid to express.

The usual good humor, which is often infectious in nature, frequently continues as long as every whim of the patient is gratified, but it tends to be replaced with anger, caustic speech, and verbal abuse if anyone questions his opinion or thwarts his wishes. In place of this good humor, one occasionally meets with a sustained anger, argumentativeness, irritability, haughtiness, arrogance, sarcasm, and querulousness. Open hostility to members of the family is common. After her recovery, one woman whose hypomanic attacks were characterized by a great outburst of hostility described her psychotic episodes as seeming "like a prolonged spell of anger." In her normal periods, she was a friendly person, anxious to help others, and took great pride in her love for them. (One suspects that this desirable personality characteristic was a reaction formation that served as a defense against a deep-seated hostility.)

Sudden oscillations of emotion are common. In the midst of an exuberance of manner and spirits, the patient may suddenly burst into tears and give expression to some depressive idea, but after a moment be as cheerful as ever. He may likewise change rapidly from irritability to affability. The hypomanic patient may work with great, but capricious, enthusiasm and energy, but his stimulation and expansiveness impair his judgment. He is often so officious and meddlesome that he becomes an annoyance to those about him. He declares that he needs no rest. Although under a constant pressure of activity, he feels no sense of fatigue. He writes numerous letters in which he underscores many words and passages and introduces various parenthetical remarks. The style of composition may be flowery and witty and the script large, flowing, and perhaps graceful. No sooner, perhaps, has he posted a letter than he decides that the mail is too slow for his urgent business so he dispatches a telegram to his correspondent. He discusses with strangers and without reserve matters of an intimate, private nature. The hypomanic is often erotic and, if a man, may indulge in sexual excesses, while a previously chaste and modest young woman may become sexually promiscuous. Although from custom and convenience the symptoms just described are designated as hypomanic, any attempt to divide the imperceptible gradations of hyperactivity occurring in manic-depressive psychosis into clinical groups is entirely arbitrary.

In a well-developed picture of mania the *affective tonality* is one of eagerness, exaltation, and joyous excitement. The tempo of the whole personality is quickened. The patient's patterns of thinking and behavior reflect his mood. He sings, dances about, whistles, and may be exhilarated to the point of noisy hilarity. He shows an unrestrained playfulness and mischievousness. His elation stimulates ideas of grandeur and perhaps fleeting delusions of wealth and power. The exhilaration may be punctuated with anger, irritability, and even with combativeness if the patient is denied some request or privilege, a granting of which his disturbed state forbids. Again, a well-developed *paranoid trend* may exist, and the patient may be verbally abusive to the person toward whom, for the moment, he may feel most resentful. Patients with this impure affect are often haughty, demanding, revengeful, sarcastic, and arrogant. They may seem to delight in an unbounded expression of aggressiveness and hostility.

The *stream of thought* is characterized by loquaciousness and rapid association of ideas. Frequently the patient speaks with a crispness and vigor of articulation, with emphatic accents and frequent changes of pitch. His style of phrasing may be pompous, and his speech may assume the character of theatrical declamation. As the hypomanic state passes into acute mania, the pressure of speech develops into a flight of ideas with rhyming, play upon words, and "clang" associations of words having similar sounds but no relation in meaning. Superficially the therapist receives the impression of a great variety of ideas, but if he carefully observes the manic patient's associational products, he discovers that their range is really limited. As a matter of fact, the manic individual evades thinking and is occupied with phonetics rather than meaning. Associations that remind the patient of some overvalued idea or egocentric interest are particularly apt to divert the stream of thought. Although the patient's racing flow of ideas appears illogical and directed by such stimuli as similarity of sound and environmental objects and events, beneath these superficial associations may often be discovered an underlying but limited range of topics toward which associations tend to flow. Without realizing their significance, the patient often makes remarks that afford a hint as to the unconscious motivation of his ideas, since, although apparently devoid of motivation, they are not so in fact. In both sequence and significance, they approach the character of free associations and therefore, like them, are prompted by unconscious and instinctive agencies.

The third of the mental fields in which it has been customary to describe disturbances as taking place is that of *psychomotor activity*. There is an overactivity, ranging from the pressure of occupation described in hypomania to the violent motor excitement of acute mania. In the hospital the patient meddles with ward activities and with other patients; he has numerous suggestions as to how the institution should be conducted. He decorates himself with trinkets and improvised badges and medals. In more excited states, he tears his clothing into ribbons with which he decorates himself in a grotesque manner. He sings, shouts, and assumes dramatic attitudes. He may destroy bed and personal clothing, an activity usually prompted not by malice but by an urge to be busy. A woman ordinarily refined and modest may disregard all former sense of propriety, make indecent sexual proposals, and be obscene in speech. The overactive manic sleeps little and yet does not appear fatigued. He sustains cuts and abrasions to which he pays no attention and for which he will permit no treatment. Infections may occur and complicate the clinical picture. Rarely the patient shows such a pressure of activity that he does not eat and requires tube feeding, although in the usual degree of excitement the patient may bolt large quantities of food with complete disregard of manners.

The attention of the manic is usually much disturbed, the disorder being caused not by any defect in vigility but by lack of tenacity, as a result of which attention is easily distracted. Environmental noises and activities constantly divert his attention. Not rarely he misidentifies persons, being particularly prone to identify a stranger as a former acquaintance because of the fact that he discovers some slight point of similarity but fails to scrutinize the points of dissimilarity. The patient usually remains well oriented, but at times his grasp of his environment may be faulty because of an absence of sustained and discriminating attention.

Hallucinations may occur in manic excitement but are not common and are usually more in the nature of illusions.

Although delusions are not conspicuous symptoms, they often occur, are usually expansive or wish-fulfilling in nature, are fleeting, and not systematized. Ideas of persecution are not rare.

As may be implied from the foregoing description of overt behavior, judgment is markedly impaired. As Platman and his colleagues have found, while manic, the individual regards himself as sociable, trusting, pleasant, and unaggressive. Those whom he contacts perceive him as barely acceptable socially, impulsive, rebellious, and aggressive. On recovery from the manic state, the same individual assesses his ill behavior much as do those who have contacted him while ill.

Physically the patients classed as milder cases appear in excellent health. The eyes are bright, the face flushed, the head erect, the step quick, and weight may be gained. In extreme excitement the patient may lose weight because of great expenditure of energy. In greatly overactive states, the patient is usually dehydrated. Pneumonia, acute nephritis, and other infections may be unrecognized because of the difficulty in making a physical examination of a patient so extremely excited. In such cases, the real nature of a superimposed delirioid state may escape recognition. Any real clouding of consciousness in a patient who has been greatly excited should suggest the possibility of a complicating infection.

The following taken from the records of a man who first entered a public institution for mental diseases when 54 years of age illustrates many of the typical behavior reactions of manic excitement:

At ages 35, 41, and 47, the patient suffered from depressed episodes, each attack being from four to six months in duration. In January he became restless and talkative. Early in February he began to send checks to friends, sometimes even to strangers who, he said, might be in need. Ten days later he was sent home from the office where he was employed with the explanation that he was becoming overwrought. A few days after his suspension from work he was admitted to a private institution for mental disorders where he pretended to commit suicide by mercury poisoning. He then drew a skull and cross bones on the wall of his room. After three weeks he was taken home, but a few days later he was committed to a public institution where he bustled about the ward, giving the impression that he had important business to which he must attend.

Occasionally he was seen lying on a bench, pretending to sleep, but in a few minutes he resumed his usual activity. He talked quickly, loudly, and nearly constantly. He was interested in everything and everyone around him. He talked familiarly to patients, attendants, nurses, and physicians. He took a fancy to the woman physician on duty in the admission building, calling her by her first name and annoying her with letters and with his familiar, ill-mannered, and obtrusive attentions. On his arrival he gave five dollars to one patient and one dollar to another. He made many comments and asked many questions about other patients and promised that he would secure their discharge. He interfered with their affairs and soon received a blow on the jaw from one patient and a black eye from another. He wrote letters demanding his release, also letters to friends describing in a circumstantial, inaccurate, and facetious way conditions in the hospital. His letters were interlarded with trite Latin phrases. He drew caricatures of the physicians and the nurses and wrote music on toilet paper. He drew pictures on his arms; on one occasion he secured a bottle of mercurochrome and painted the face of another manic patient. When permitted to play the ward piano, he played piece after piece without stopping, improvising a great deal. A doctor rarely passed through the ward without being called by the patient, who would slap the physician on the back or shake hands effusively and talk until the door closed. At times during an interview his voice became tremulous, tears came to his eyes, and he sobbed audibly with his face buried in his arms. A moment later, however, he was laughing—a manifestation of the bipolarity of emotion so markedly illustrated in this disease.

DEPRESSIVE PHASE. Although a larger percentage of the episodic depressions of this disorder occur in persons who have also a history of manic episodes, in some manic-depressives the psychotic episodes are confined to those of a depressive type. In such cases one often finds a rather characteristic type of prepsychotic personality. Many of these individuals whose psychotic episodes are limited to depressive reactions have always been friendly, unobtrusive, timid persons with an underlying sense of insecurity and overdependency. Not a few have manifested sensitive and appreciative emotional responses. Many have been scrupulous persons of rigid ethical and moral standards, meticulous, self-demanding, perfectionistic, self-depreciatory, prudish, given to self-reproach, and sensitive to criticism. Their obsessive-compulsive tendencies have doubtless been defensive mechanisms for handling hostility, which characteristically they cannot express externally. Frequently they have had fixed opinions and set ways of doing things and are habitually apprehensive and fearful. Many have been hesitant and without courage, yet have sought and achieved worthwhile accomplishments. Frequently their greatest emotional need seems to have been love, respect, and belonging.

Just as in the manic type of manic-depressive psychosis all degrees of overactivity are found, so in the depressive type one meets with varying degrees of depression. If arbitrarily we describe three degrees of activity—hypomania, acute mania, and delirious mania—in the excited phase, so mild depression, acute depression, and stupor may be said to represent the different degrees of depression. One should remember, however, that these arbitrary divisions merge imperceptibly one into the other.

Because of the absence of striking disturbances, the real nature of *mild depression* is frequently not recognized. In fact, it should be borne in mind that various moods that are called normal pass imperceptibly into the different forms of manic-depressive psychosis. Mild depressive phases tend, roughly speaking, to assume one of two general forms: either a period of fatigue, staleness, and inertia, or one during which the patient has physical complaints for which no organic basis can be discovered. Affective depression exists in both forms but does not constitute the chief complaint and consists in a mild downheartedness. Occasionally the onset is characterized by obsessive features. If the depression stands a bit to the fore, the patient's friends may speak of his episodes as "blue spells." The patient lacks confidence in himself, loses his zest for living, feels inadequate and tired, shows a growing aversion to activity, likes to be left alone, and finds it difficult to perform his ordinary duties. Color and joy are gone out of life. Every task seems a burden, and in many cases the patient gives up any attempt to continue his employment. He has doubts and fears, is frequently overanxious about his family, states he has not provided amply for their future welfare, and has mild ideas of unworthiness. Thinking may be difficult, ideational content becomes confined to a few topics, spontaneous speech is limited, replies to questions are delayed and condensed as much as possible, and the patient is disinclined to reveal his private thoughts. Social contacts are not sought, and the patient may even show an obstinate unwillingness to meet people. Many show a marked indecisiveness, probably indicative of their apprehension of further failure, rejection, and retaliation.

Less frequently encountered are those that tend to be morose, gloomily irritable and sensitive, often stubborn and inconsiderate of others, and inclined to project in the form of dissatisfaction or fault finding. Sadness is little evidenced. Others are openly hostile, angry, and punitive. They resent efforts to assist them and deny the existence of their illness. These persons usually have manifested domineering and outwardly aggressive personality traits prior to their illness and they become depressed when their sense of self-sufficiency and ability to control their environment is frustrated.

In the second group of mild depressions, physical complaints are among the most conspicuous symptoms and may mask the depression. There is not merely the loss of weight, coated tongue, disturbed and unrefreshing sleep, and poor appetite observed in depressive states, but the patient has various hypochondriacal ideas. He feels weak and fatigued, worries over trifles, and suffers from insomnia, headache, and debility and perhaps from precordial or epigastric distress. Any bodily sensations that may arise on a physical, tension, or anxiety basis become the principal object of the patient's attention. He therefore believes, as often do his friends, that the real disorder is physical and that his downheartedness is the natural result of ill health, whereas the physical complaints are really but the rationalization of a primary affective distress. To the inexperienced practitioner, these depressive episodes may appear to be neurasthenic. Occasionally there is a history of laparotomy or pelvic surgery without a discoverable pathologic condition having been revealed.

The onset of a *severe depression* may resemble the mild depressive states just described, but the initial downheartedness soon passes into a profound affective distress. Posture, muscle tensions, and various physical signs and symptoms present a composite picture indicating depression. The body is stooped, the head flexed, the facies immobile, the forehead furrowed, and the patient looks fixedly downward. Deep vertical wrinkles appear between the eyebrows, the nasolabial folds are marked, and the down-turned angles of the mouth constitute a picture of dejection. The face may have a troubled, perplexed expression. The patient loses weight and appears ill. Perspiration and other secretions are decreased. Muscle tone is decreased, the bowels are constipated, sexual desire is decreased, and the male patient is usually impotent. The sleeping pattern is disturbed in a characteristic way. Although there is usually little delay in falling asleep, the patient awakens much earlier than when he is well. The diurnal severity of his depressive affect also varies in a customary way in that it is usually most severe in the morning and relents as the day wears on. As the depression becomes more profound, everything is interpreted in terms of hopelessness and despondency.

Occasionally a patient says he has no feeling. Others complain that things seem strange and unnatural—feelings of unreality. They usually recognize that the change, caused by the influence of depressed feeling-tone on perceptions, by the loss of interest in external phenomena, and by the altered affective relationship to them, is in themselves and not in the fundamental nature of environmental objects. Many patients have an indefinite dread or a sense of impending disaster, frequently accompanied by an attitude of submission to their fate. Efforts at reassurance make no impression, and the patient

shows no response to appreciative and sympathetic counsel. A sense of fear is not uncommon and, if it is intense, consciousness may be clouded and the patient may be confused.

In the *retarded depression* there is an inhibition of the stream of thought and of psychomotor activity. The retarded patient speaks slowly and seems at a loss for words. His replies are brief, frequently monosyllabic, and expressed in a low tone. Not rarely he begins, but never completes, the reply to some inquiry, or else he finishes it only as the examiner moves away. Perhaps he may merely move his lips but fail to utter any intelligible response. Efforts to make decisions result in vacillation or perplexity.

In the psychomotor field, externally directed behavior becomes progressively retarded and inhibited. There is slowness both in initiation and in execution. The patient complains of an inability to carry out suggested activities, and every attempt requires great exertion. Retardation may be so pronounced as to amount to stupor.

In depressive states the patient's ideas tend to represent a projected expression of his inner feelings and a rationalization of his affects. The delusions of both manic and depressive patients seem to be more the reflections of their mood than true delusional experiences, as in schizophrenia. The delusional content of the depressive patient is therefore characterized by self-depreciation, ideas of guilt, remorse, self-accusation, and hypochondriasis. Not infrequently there is a suspicious, paranoid, complaining, and persecutory trend to the patient's ideas. This is particularly the case when the patient's prepsychotic personality was characterized by sensitiveness and feelings of inferiority.

Hallucinations are not conspicuous symptoms in the depression of manic-depressive psychosis, and although they may occur, a persistent falsification of reality in this way should raise the question of a more malignant psychosis, particularly if the hallucinations do not clearly represent the projection of affective distress. Illusionary misinterpretations are frequent—a pounding in the basement is that of workmen constructing the patient's coffin.

Dream life of the depressive tends to change as he moves from the phase of severest suffering to that of recovery. During the former period, as Miller has found, dreams tend to be bland and pleasant, denying the anguish of the illness. As recovery ensues, the dream content shifts to reveal concern over being hurt by others; that hurt is delivered largely through coercive interaction. Coercion by others plus the personal inability to cope effectively with it may be a central problem in depression. It deserves much study.

The patient usually remains well oriented unless from his affective distress he becomes so preoccupied that attention is impaired. As already indicated, he may be confused if his fear is intense. Depressed patients usually have little or no appetite, and some would starve if not encouraged or forced to eat. Spoon or tube feeding is sometimes necessary. This failure to eat may result from the profound psychomotor inhibition, or from the patient's belief that he is unworthy to receive the food, or from a desire to die. This feeling of unworthiness and the desire for self-punishment often lead to suicidal attempts and occasionally to mutilation of self.

The most intense form of the depressive phase is depressive *stupor*. It was probably this type of stupor to which Esquirol gave the name "acute dementia." In this profoundly inhibited state, there is practically no spontaneous motor activity. There is a complete, or almost complete, immobility, with a minimal response to external stimuli. The patient is mute, his sensorium is clouded, and he is intensely preoccupied, often with ideas of death and with dream-like hallucinations. The face is either mask-like or rigidly anxious. Many have to be tube-fed; some soil and wet themselves.

Elderly depressed patients may manifest organic mental symptoms such as confusion, disorientation, and memory defects, which are alleviated or may even disappear with recovery from depression. Not rarely, a depression terminates with a brief hypomanic reaction.

Crimes of violence may occur with the manic-depressive psychoses. Such crimes are more frequent in depressed than in manic states, probably because depression may be a result of a weakening in the repression of hate and aggressive strivings. It is reported that, of 90 patients confined to the Broadmoor, England, Criminal Lunatic Asylum because of murder committed during affective psychoses, 62 were suffering from depression and 28 from mania at the time the homicides took place. More homicides are committed by depressed women than by depressed men. Usually the victim is not only a member of the patient's family but the one who has apparently been the most loved. It has been suggested that the homicide may be regarded as an extension of the suicidal impulse. As suicide is an act of aggression against self, then the homicide (in depressive patients) might be considered an extension of aggression to include not only the self but those nearest the self, the victim being almost a part of the self. An example of this psychopathology is manifested when a depressed mother kills both herself and her child.

The following case report is that of a severe depression unaltered by modern therapeutic measures. It is presented because such pathology continues to be seen.

E. D., aged 60, was admitted to the hospital because he was depressed, ate insufficiently, and believed that his stomach was "rotting away." The patient was described as a friendly, sociable individual, not quarrelsome, jealous, or critical, and with a sense of humor. He was considered even-tempered, slow to anger, tenderhearted, and emotional.

At 51 the patient suffered from a depression and was obliged to resign his position. This depression continued for about nine months, after which he apparently fully recovered. He resumed his work but after two years suffered from a second depression. Again he recovered after several months and returned to a similar position and held it until two months before his admission. At this time he began to worry lest he was not doing his work well, talked much of his lack of fitness for his duties, and finally resigned. He spent Thanksgiving Day at his son's in a neighboring city, but while there he was sure that the water pipes in his own house would freeze during his absence and that he and his family would be "turned out into the street." A few days later he was found standing by a pond, evidently contemplating suicide. He soon began to remain in bed and sometimes wrapped his head in the bed clothing to shut out the external world. He declared that he was "rotting away inside" and that if he ate, the food would kill him. He urged the family not to touch the glasses or towels he used lest they become contaminated.

On arrival at the hospital, he appeared older than his years. He was pale, poorly nourished, and dehydrated, with his lips dry, cracked, and covered with sordes. His facial expression and general bearing suggested a feeling of utter hopelessness. He was self-absorbed and manifested no interest in his environment. When urged to answer questions, there was a long delay before he attempted to reply, but he finally spoke briefly, hesitatingly, and in a low tone. He occasionally became agitated and repeatedly said, "Oh, doctor, why did I ever get into anything like this? Doctor, I am all filled up! I can't get anything through me—what am I going to do? Oh, dear! Oh, dear!" In explaining his presence in the hospital, he said he realized he had been sent by his family because they believed he would be benefited by the treatment, but added, "I don't know how they sent me here when they had not the means. My wife cannot pay for me, and by this time she must have been put out of the house."

After several months the patient began to improve, although hypochondriacal ideas persisted for a considerable period. Finally, when the matter of freedom of the hospital grounds was considered, he seemed in a normal mood and indicated that he was beginning to think somewhat differently concerning his gastrointestinal tract. At that time he commented, "There's a good deal of life in the old horse yet." A month later he passed into a mildly hypomanic state. He became alert, animated, talkative, exuberant in spirits, and confident in manner. This mildly excited state continued for about two months, when he settled down into what seemed to be his normal mood and state of activity. After a few weeks he was discharged, but several months later he again showed signs of depression and hanged himself before arrangements for readmission had been made.

CYCLIC TYPE.   Although the episodes suffered by some patients are always manic or always depressive, those of others may be of irregular sequence in respect to the mood disturbance. Again, the episodes of still other patients may be characterized by an alternation of manic and depressive reactions. In some patients there may be no appreciable interval of normality between the alternations; in other cases there may be variable periods free from symptoms.

The following case illustrates the cyclic tendency and its influence in preventing successful adjustment during a large part of the patient's adult life.

M. M. was first admitted to a state hospital at the age of 38, although since childhood she had been characterized by swings of mood, some of which had been so extreme that they had been psychotic in degree. At 17 she suffered from a depression that rendered her unable to work for several months, although she was not hospitalized. At 33, shortly before the birth of her first child, the patient was greatly depressed. For a period of four days she appeared in coma. About a month after the birth of the baby she "became excited" and was entered as a patient in an institution for neurotic and mildly psychotic patients. As she began to improve, she was sent to a shore hotel for a brief vacation. The patient remained at the hotel for one night and on the following day signed a year's lease on an apartment, bought furniture, and became heavily involved in debt. Shortly thereafter Mrs. M. became depressed and returned to the hospital in which she had previously been a patient. After several months she recovered and, except for relatively mild fluctuations of mood, remained well for approximately two years.

She then became overactive and exuberant in spirits and visited her friends, to whom she outlined her plans for reëstablishing different forms of lucrative business. She purchased many clothes, bought furniture, pawned her rings, and wrote checks without funds. She was returned to a hospital. Gradually her manic symptoms subsided, and after four months she was discharged. For a period thereafter she was mildly depressed. In a little less than a year Mrs. M. again became overactive, played her radio until late in the night, smoked excessively, took out insurance on a car that she had not yet bought. Contrary to her usual habits, she swore frequently and loudly, created a disturbance in a club to which she did not belong, and instituted divorce proceedings. On the day prior to her second admission to the hospital, she purchased 57 hats.

During the past 18 years this patient has been admitted and dismissed from the hospital on many occasions. At times, with the onset of a depressed period, she has returned to the hospital seeking admission. At such times she complained that her "brain just won't work." She would say, "I have no energy, am unable to do my housework; I have let my family down; I am living from day to day. There is no one to blame but myself." During one of her manic periods, she sent the following telegram to a physician of whom she had become much enamored: "To: You; Street and No.: Every-where; Place: the remains at peace! We did our best, but God's will be done! I am so very sorry for all of us. To brave it through thus far. Yes, Darling —from Hello Handsome. Handsome is as Hand-some does, thinks, lives and breathes. It takes clear air, Brother of Mine, in a girl's hour of need. All my love to the Best Inspiration one ever had."

In the last year Mrs. M., now 59, has been making an excellent home and community ad-justment. Her husband has had several cerebro-vascular accidents and has required considerable nursing and assistance. She has efficiently met the various responsibilities and family emergencies that have befallen her and has supplemented her husband's pension by baby-sitting. It is altogether probable, however, that she will experience re-turns either of excitement or of depression.

MIXED TYPES. Psychomotor activity, flow of thought, and affectivity were formerly thought of as independent and more or less separable functions of the mind, which in their positive or negative variations could be combined in various ways as may the letters of the alphabet. Basing his ideas on this conception of a coexistence of manic and depressive ele-ments, Kraepelin described special clin-ical forms. These he designated as the "mixed" types of manic-depressive psy-chosis. He described such "mixed" forms as agitated depression, manic stupor, un-productive mania, depressive mania, de-pression with flight, and inhibited mania. The present tendency is to discontinue such artificial classifications.

Of these groups, *agitated depression* most nearly deserves a special recognition, yet this group is really a depressive reac-tion in which the agitation is simply an expression of anxiety—a persistent ex-pression of the apprehension, tension, and feeling of prospective harm arising from threatening factors deep in the mental life. The great internal uneasiness pro-duces a psychomotor agitation.

Psychodynamics

The manic-depressive state has certain psychopathology in common with other depressive reactions. There is the depres-sive complex itself, composed of various combinations and intensities of the affects of sadness, anxiety, rage, shame, and guilt. To these affects are added a profound sense of helplessness associated with a diminished self-esteem and the general inhibition of personality functioning.

As described earlier in this chapter for the involutional psychotic reactions, it is considered now by various psychoanalysts that the state of helplessness expressive of the sense of loss and attendant anxiety so conspicuously evident in the psychotically depressed is different from that seen in healthy or neurotic personalities. It is primary in that it is equated with the helpless infantile response to separation which exists before or shortly after per-sonal differentiation has taken place. This anxious helplessness or its clinging repre-sentation in some patients, then, is recog-nized as a profound affective regression. The failure of the ordinary personality defenses, occurring in a person perhaps genetically or constitutionally predis-posed, leads to the reëmergence of this infantile state of helplessness and en-genders as well much of the loss of self-esteem.

The capacity for warm and responsive social relationships which exists in the manic-depressive perhaps rests on a satis-fying early infantile mothering contact during which the child commences to evolve the early nucleus of personal iden-tity and sense of security. Yet for reasons poorly understood, the capacity to accept separation, with the limitations it imposes thereby and the attendant affective arousal, is not fully mastered. Those who respond with pathologic depression main-tain, as Bibring has emphasized, a pre-senting and often compulsive fixation on the significant and wished-for object rela-tionship or its symbolic representation in some goal which will assure love, respect, or power and which will provide escape from isolation, humiliation, and a sense of weakness. Thus even in the depressive there is a persistent denial of loss, and projection may be utilized as a defense to escape the realization of personal limi-tations imposed as the consequence of the loss, whether actual or fantasied. Such denial is conspicuously present in the manic and hypomanic states.

These psychodynamic theories, relevant to all depressive reactions, add to the earlier theories which emphasized that depression should be regarded as a result of anxiety in a person who experienced severe loss, real or fantasied, at an early stage of development. The loss is perceived as rejection, which precipitates anger. Since the feeling of anger cannot be tolerated, it is repressed and turned inward on the self. Although these feelings of anger and hostility are repressed, they cause the individual to feel guilty, unworthy, and depressed.

There remains to be formulated a psychodynamic explanation for the recurrent episodes of affective disturbance and the cyclic shifts from depression to mania which give this psychosis its nominal designation. It well may be that the shift from depression to elation takes place in association with vacillating processes of identification with parental figures. During depression the patient identifies with the maternal figure in a submissive role. At the initiation of the period of elation, he denies the submissive, maternal identification and acts out an intense, acquisitive, sadistic drive with fantasies of strength in which he becomes emancipated, elated, and overaggressive, in imitation of the paternal figure, with whom he is now identified. With the failure of his aggressiveness to accomplish the fantasied aim of revenge, the patient again has to renounce the paternal identification and to deny his aggressiveness, and so he becomes depressed and helpless. These aggressive and assured personality characteristics of the manic are not necessarily related to the parental sex, as in some instances the mother is identified as the striving person who provided for the child the ideal of strength in times of family stress. As one woman manic patient expressed it, "When our family and its fortune was falling apart during the depression, my mother laughed and made light of it—my father withdrew. I have always admired her and sought to be like her when things were bad."

The manic's behavior is essentially a defense of massive denial against the underlying depression. Although he may appear confident and occupy the role of a leader, the manic is basically overdependent. Although he appears outgoing and friendly, he is self-centered, actively controlling, and manipulating. These attitudes are based on an emotional need for a dependency relationship. When his demands are frustrated, hostility is generated, which must be repressed so that it does not further imperil the dependency relationship. The imperfectly repressed hostility may, in turn, produce depression.

To interpret his behavior in a psychosocial or transactional sense, the manic would seem to perceive threat and danger in accepting his dependent needs to be cared for by others. To maintain his self-esteem and to defend himself, to maintain his key perception of power and strength, he appears to use those transactions which control others to whom he looks for emotional support. His repertoire of behaviors requires that he must appear extraordinarily independent, needing no one. He thus develops a repertoire of behaviors in which he suggests that he will care for others—his grandiose schemes. He repeatedly attempts to test, manipulate, and overcommit others so that he involves others around him to care for him. As Janowsky and his colleagues interpret this behavior, he obtains the needed dependent role while challenging external constraints under the guise of an aggressive pseudoindependence.

Sometimes an important source of conflict for the manic-depressive patient seems to be strong hostility connected with envy which is repressed and avoided. He is often the best-endowed member of the family and has been expected to provide the prestige for the group. This position places great responsibility on him, yet exposes him to the envy of his siblings, or even to envious competition with his parents. The future manic-depressive has grown sensitive to envy and competition, and to counteract the potentiality of suffering the hostility of envy due to his own abilities, he has unconsciously developed the pattern of disparaging himself in order to conceal his full capacity.

Feelings of guilt and reflected depression springing from them arise in various ways. Some repressed wish, for example, is occasionally granted by accident, such as by the death of a parent whose continued existence had prevented the fulfillment of a greatly desired wish. In such a case, a depression may sometimes result because of the feeling of guilt that follows the gratification of the consciously repudiated desire. In general, as already indicated, feelings of guilt giving rise to depression arise not so much from what one has done as from what one has unconsciously wished to do. Depression represents a penance for repressed hatred, aggressiveness, and other repudiated tendencies and impulses that have given rise to feelings of guilt. Guilt, too, may be expressed in terms of self-punishment. There is much to suggest that hostility is the denominator common to both manic and depressive phases. Because of his rigid superego, the depressed patient does not permit himself to live out his hostile, aggressive tendencies against others but redirects them against himself or expresses them in projected form. The influence of pathological feelings of guilt and of hostile impulses turned against the self may therefore find expression in suicide. The fact that feelings of guilt and self-accusation may be assuaged by attaching to others the motives that created them contributes to the paranoid features that may accompany depression. If the release of repressed impulses is particularly threatening, the depression may be accompanied by manifest expressions of anxiety.

The easiest and most natural way by which an ill-defined sense of guilt or of remorse may be rationalized and thereby find the required sense of reality in the consciousness of the patient is by linking it up with some trifling indiscretion of earlier life. This indiscretion is usually found to have been really trivial, although it never enjoyed full approval of the individual's socially determined conscience. All the energy of the affect, tied up with the repudiated wishes and material that have been repressed, usually with difficulty and for a long period, is displaced to this lapse and its ideational representation. This idea receives the displaced affect that both rationalizes and renders concrete the vague feeling of guilt arising from disowned strivings and desires.

Differential Diagnosis

The most difficult problem in the differential diagnosis of manic-depressive psychosis is its distinction from *schizophrenia*. In the typical case, this presents no difficulty, but in many cases there is doubt as to how symptoms should be interpreted. In general the disturbance in personality in manic-depressive psychoses seems to be a quantitative one, a matter of "too much" or "too little," rather than a lack of organization of personality, as in schizophrenia. There is not, moreover, complete agreement among psychiatrists as to how much temporary disorganization of the personality may be considered consistent with the diagnosis of manic-depressive psychosis, or as to how much diagnostic weight should be assigned different symptoms. Behavior may be equally disturbed in the manic excitement of an affective psychosis and in the catatonic excitement of schizophrenia.

In approaching the problem of differentiation, it is necessary first to secure as full a knowledge as possible as to the prepsychotic personality of the patient, to determine whether cyclothymic or schizoid characteristics have predominated, and whether energy has been directed into extroverted channels and marked by objectivity and realism, or whether it has been introverted and characterized by subjectivity.

In general, the interpersonal contact with the manic or depressive is more conventional and initially is perceived as a close one by the psychiatrist. With the schizophrenic, the interview is felt to be an uneasy one of distance, unfamiliarity, and suspicion. The presence of flight of ideas and of psychomotor activity in the early phases of a mental disorder may not constitute unequivocal diagnostic criteria, since both may exist in reactions that eventuate as schizophrenia. In schizophrenia, there tend to be more incoherence and greater poverty of ideas. The excitement of the schizophrenic lacks the depth of emotional expression that is usually observed in the excitement of the manic-depressive, is less influenced by the reality of the environment, is more episodic and impulsive, and tends to be undirected, stereotyped, confined to a limited space, and determined more by hallucinations, delusions, and autistic processes. The more grotesque, and therefore the more primitive or highly symbolized, the ideas, the more are they to be looked upon as schizophrenic.

The mood of the schizophrenic lacks both an infectious element and that component causing one to feel empathy with the patient, who, in general, is less accessible than the manic-depressive. The greater the harmony between mood, ideational content, and behavior, the more is a manic-depressive psychosis suggested, while the less the mental processes remain integrated, the more is schizophrenia denoted. Even though it may at first be temporary, the greater the disorganization of the personality, as shown by absence or inappropriateness of affect, by hallucinations, soiling, and apparent noninterpretability of behavior, the more does one expect an ultimate, and for the most part permanent, schizophrenic disorganization. The clinical picture of some young patients initially considered to be suffering from a manic phase of a manic-depressive psychosis changes to one that is clearly schizophrenic in nature.

Many hypomanics in whom the emotional exaltation is replaced by anger, resentment, irritability, irascibility, litigious tendencies, and perhaps paranoid delusions were formerly diagnosed as having acute *paranoia*. Such hypomanics lack the solitary and asocial tendency usually exhibited by the true paranoid, who presents a more sustained, brooding, sensitive, suspicious reaction pattern. Persons in whom these impure affects replace an exaltation are ones who, prior to their psychosis, were characterized by a tendency to defensive projections.

The sense of inadequacy, abnormal fatigability, depressive ideas, and apprehension that may accompany mild forms of the depressive or mixed types, particularly in the early stages, are often misinterpreted as symptoms of *neurasthenia,* of a *compulsion neurosis,* or of an *anxiety state.* In manic-depressive psychosis, sluggishness of thought and action is more common, the patient is more reticent as to his feelings, and he does not show the eagerness to interview the physician usually seen in the psychoneuroses. Also, the severe disturbance or inhibition of physiologic functions in areas of sleep, alimentation, and sexual functioning do not occur. Psychogenic causes and processes are usually more easily ascertained in psychoneuroses. Mild but often unrecognized forms of the depressive type are of frequent occurrence, with the result that the number of manic-depressives in extrainstitutional life probably exceeds those under treatment in hospitals for mental disorders. "Masked depressions" often present in the form of episodic alcoholism, drug addiction and drug abuse, or "acting-out" behavior, including antisocial behavior.

In the depressive phase, there occurs the customary disturbance of the sleep pattern, with early morning awakening and the morning aggravation of depressive affect, anorexia, weight loss, amenorrhea, and impotence. The physiological diminution of the rate of salivation and the low sedation threshold may be used as differential points.

In early *syphilitic meningoencephalitis,* the presenting symptoms may reflect previous personality trends and therefore suggest a manic-depressive psychosis. Neurological signs and serological tests will at once make a diagnosis possible.

Prognosis and Course

It has already been indicated that the prognosis for a single affective episode is usually to be regarded as good but that recurrences are not uncommon. That for the illness over time is also favorable, as several recent reports have confirmed. Only one-fifth did not recover fully, and less than one-tenth became chronically ill. Women did less well than men, both those with mania alone and those with the "bipolar" form.

Perhaps there has been too great a tendency to stress the frequency of recurrence. Of admissions to state hospitals because of manic-depressive reactions, 55 per cent are first admissions, about 25 per cent second admissions, and 9 per cent third; 5 per cent of the patients have had more than three admissions.

Another important feature of manic-depressive psychosis is the fact that even repeated episodes usually leave the mind unchanged in its intellectual, affective, and conative aspects, and that a disorganization of the personality does not follow. Many highly productive and socially respected individuals have suffered this personality disorder. Not a little of Ruskin's best work was done during his hypomanic states. Occasionally, after a series of attacks, the patient shows impairment of initiative and of judgment and becomes less able to deal with everyday affairs of life.

The most frequent age for the first manic episode is between 20 and 25 years. The average age of onset for first depressive attacks is about 10 years later. The earlier the onset of either type, the worse the prognosis for the occurrence of further episodes. If the first attack be manic in type, it almost certainly will not be the only one; if it be of a depressed type, it may not be followed by a recurrence. Some recent studies give indication that the prognosis is worse when the precipitation of illness is related directly to an actual loss (exogenous cause) than when it is due to covert experiences or factors (endogenous). This information is contrary to previous viewpoints and differs from data on the outcome of schizophrenic psychoses.

The patient's prepsychotic personality traits influence the prognosis as to both duration and outcome. If he has shown himself to be flexible, tolerant, conciliatory, without defensive or compensatory traits or other signs of a deep sense of insecurity, and has had varied and wholesome interests, the prognosis is more favorable than if his personality patterns have been of the opposite type. As age increases, there is some tendency for attacks to be depressive rather than manic, perhaps because of the changing outlook on life. (See discussion of etiological factors in involutional psychotic reactions.)

The duration of manic-depressive episodes is extremely variable. The average duration of untreated manic attacks may be estimated at six months and of depressive episodes at nine months. There is a tendency for depressions to increase in length with advancing age. Many depressions terminate with a brief hypomanic elation. The duration in individual cases may be either much shorter or much longer. One is never safe in predicting the probable duration of a given episode. Some patients may never have more than a single episode; in others a large part of the time may be occupied with recurring psychotic periods. The more frequent the attacks, the poorer the prognosis. The more chronic the illness, the less severe the symptoms. Depression is much more likely to become chronic than is mania. Chronic mania is uncommon before the age of 40. The prognosis is considered less favorable in depressions manifesting a nihilistic hypochondriasis, particularly if accompanied by anxiety or when associated with paranoidal trends.

Treatment

Depending upon the severity of the depressive or manic reaction and its influence upon the patient's capacity to function in his accustomed vocational and social life, initial therapeutic judgments must be made as to the wisdom of urging continuation of work or advising withdrawal, and whether to provide treatment at home or in a hospital environment.

DEPRESSION. The treatment of mild depressions may, in certain respects, constitute a greater problem than does the treatment of the deep depressions. The friends of the patient suffering from a mild episode of a manic-depressive nature often refuse to believe that he is suffering from a major mental disorder or that he may have suicidal tendencies.

Today, the mildly depressed preferably should commence pharmacological treatment with an antidepressant agent and usually with one of the aminodibenzol derivatives. Of those available, imipramine (Tofranil) has proved to have the widest and most effective application. Given orally in divided doses of 75 to 300 mg. daily and supplemented with appropriate sedation for insomnia, it produces an effective response usually from 3 to 14 days after its initial administration. In those patients who fail to respond to the usual dosage range, one may try an elevated dosage level or simultaneous use of methylphenidate in either sex or thyroid extract in women as a means to elevate the levels of circulating drug. Many patients have responded by this modification of the pharmaceutical management. In other instances, one of the monamine oxidase inhibitors may be tried. The use of these agents and the complications attending their administration are described more fully in Chapter 32. With office or outpatient treatment, the patient should be seen on a schedule of fixed appointments at frequent intervals. A favorable response presents itself usually in a lessening of self-deprecatory and accusatory statements and hypochondriacal complaints, improvement in the sleeping pattern, increased activity, and interest in socialization. Many patients with mild depression may continue at work with treatment by the antidepressant pharmaceuticals.

If a significant change is not evident within two weeks of institution of phar-macologic therapy, another agent, perhaps one of the monamine oxidase inhibitors, should be administered or consideration should be given to initiating electroshock without further delay.

In more severe cases, in which psychomotor retardation is of such a degree as to impair or make impossible the patient's usual vocational activities, the issue of hospitalization becomes immediately primary. Many families may be unwilling to accept the physician's opinion and advice; this should usually include a recommendation for the use of electroshock therapy. Although most physicians prefer that the patient be hospitalized during this form of therapy, some give treatments either at the patient's home or in the physician's office in the case of mild depressions. If there is little danger of suicide and the family is coöperative, treatment may be attempted at home. However, with the more severely ill, treatment at home is inadvisable unless skilled nursing services are available. An attempt on the part of the relatives to care for the patient is generally unwise, if for no other reason than that they usually either argue with him concerning his fears, constantly attempt to distract him, or urge the patient to rouse himself. With such patients, an organized program that fills the patient's day is desirable. This should be of a type which will not require spontaneity, close concentration, or strenuous activity. The program may include handicraft, walks, reading, games, social and recreational activities, and the encouragement of special aptitudes and interests. Although the patient should not be idle lest he become unduly preoccupied with his problems and with self-examination, it should be borne in mind that a depressed patient, prompted by his lifelong rigid requirements of self, may undertake too much and become more depressed when he finds he falls short of expected accomplishment. Many depressed patients complain of fatigue, but since this type of fatigue is really an expression of mood, it is not relieved by rest. One should remember that the depressed patient's tendency to hypochondriasis has at times led to unnecessary surgical operations. Unless carefully supervised, the depressed patient may not receive sufficient food.

In case of severe depression, treatment in a hospital is wise. In nearly all cases, the use of electroshock therapy is accompanied by a gratifying improvement. Treatments are usually given three times a week. With many patients, 10 or 12 treatments are effective; others require 20. Approximately 90 per cent of the depressed patients recover with this form of treatment.

If the patient is greatly agitated, chlorpromazine may be employed, either alone or in conjunction with other antidepressants or electroshock therapy, for its tranquilizing effect. He should not receive reserpine, since this drug frequently aggravates depressions.

It is highly important that the depressed patient receive a diet of high caloric content. Usually it is desirable that he receive milk or additional food between meals. Refusal of food should not be permitted for long. Sometimes after one feeding the patient will, with a little assistance, eat voluntarily.

Occasionally the hospital physician finds that for a considerable period before admission a patient has not been receiving sufficient food or water. His tongue is dry and leathery, his breath is foul, he appears dehydrated and has a slight tendency to acidosis. In these patients, special effort must be made to have them receive an abundance of fluid. In depressive stupors, attention should be paid to the condition of the bladder and the bowels.

The danger of suicide must be constantly borne in mind, a fact that should be impressed upon both nurse and family. Suicide is more frequent in patients who have shown tension and anxiety. The history of a suicide in the family increases the possibility that the depressed patient may end his life. It is not unusual for a patient to repeat a previous unsuccessful suicidal attempt.

Among the early signs of recovery are a return of interest in eating, increase in weight, bowel function, and restful sleep. Interest in others, initiative, and self-confidence follow. As convalescence proceeds, there should be a gradually increasing participation in occupational and recreational activities. The patient should be relieved of the necessity for making decisions until he is well on the road to recovery. An early resumption of usual duties and responsibilities is to be discouraged. The question as to when the convalescing depressed patient may be dismissed from the hospital is not always easy. The usual opinion is that he should remain in an institution with its simple routine until convalescence is well established. It must be remembered, too, that, because of the increased danger of suicide during convalescence, the patient may require closer supervision during that period than is possible at home. On the other hand, a return home before the depression is entirely cured may sometimes hasten the patient's recovery. He should not resume full duties for several weeks.

MANIA. The question whether the mild forms of excitement or hypomania should be treated in a hospital is not always easy. In the case of the hypomanic, it is often evident to the psychiatrist that prudence requires more control of the patient's activities than is possible in the home. Since, however, there is nothing "unpsychological" in his behavior, the patient's relatives frequently fail either to accept the statement that his exuberance of spirits, pressure of activity, and volubility are evidence of mental disorder, or to appreciate the embarrassment to themselves and the aggravation of the psychosis that may result from the absence of restraining measures. For these reasons, they are frequently averse to the patient's admission to a mental hospital. They often believe that the only required treatment is a change of scenery or an urging of the patient to rouse himself.

The apparently inexhaustible energy of the hypomanic may suggest that an outlet for it should be provided. The physician should remember, however, that fatigue produces not tranquility but excitement. The usual desire for almost constant activity must therefore be curbed, although with the production of as little irritation as possible. The hypomanic patient must be protected from his tendency to enter into unwise business or financial schemes. Careful supervision of the patient who is not hospitalized may be necessary lest an increase in sex drive lead to regrettable indulgences. Frequently the prepsychotic personality of the manic has been characterized by a sensitive pride. The physician will therefore carefully guard against the contradictions and arguments that the hypomanic's irritability, unrestrained speech, activity, and resentment at interference with his wishes are prone to provoke.

Pharmacological control of the manic overactive is best initiated with a phenothiazine, preferably chlorpromazine (see Chapter 32). If the manic patient shows extreme psychomotor activity, he may be given electroshock treatments twice a day for three or four days. This results in considerable confusion, and the frequency of treatments should soon be reduced to three per week. Episodic recurrences of the manic-depressive psychoses are not prevented by electroshock therapy, and the duration of symptom-free intervals is not made shorter by reason of its use.

Highly effective control of chronic and recurrent mania may be obtained by the oral administration of lithium carbonate. The serum lithium concentration must be maintained below levels of 2 mEq. per liter, which may be measured with the use of a flame photometer. Lithium therapy is reported to be effective in patients not responding to the phenothiazines and electroshock and also to have value, if given continuously, in damping the depressive phase of the cyclic reaction. Although Baastrup et al. state that continuous lithium treatment will prevent recurrent depressions, their findings are not confirmed by others. Due to its high toxicity for kidney function, it is contraindicated when the function of this organ is impaired, or in heart disease, epilepsy, and the elderly.

The most common minor toxic symptom is a fine tremor of the hands. The drug should be withdrawn if diarrhea or vomiting ensues or if tremulousness is very severe and associated with drowsiness, ataxia, or dizziness. Other symptoms of intoxication are thirst and a large output of urine. A further discussion of lithium and its pharmacologic properties is given in Chapter 32.

Those manic patients who respond poorly to lithium treatment are those in whom there existed continuing anxiety-provoking situations in their lives—particularly conflict. In reviewing the manic defense, Aranoff and Epstein suggest that in some poor responders a psychologic shift occurs that may affect metabolic processes adversely. Good response in an early phase of lithium treatment is not always correlated with similar response during prolonged treatment, in which adverse emotional reactions to interpersonal events may not be avoided.

PSYCHOTHERAPY. This form of treatment has been employed successfully in the treatment of the mild depressive and hypomanic states; some physicians are attempting to examine its usefulness as a preventive for recurrent or cyclic attacks. Efforts have been made to treat the manic-depressive patient by classic psychoanalytical techniques. It has usually been found that neither the retarded nor the hyperactive patient lends himself to the rigid routine of the customary psychoanalytical process. New efforts have made it evident, however, that modified, analytically oriented psychotherapy is possible for some patients and seems to be beneficial.

Experience indicates that it is not advisable for the psychotherapeutic interviews with the depressed patient to be held four or five times a week, as is frequently to be recommended in the case of the schizophrenic or often with the neurotic. Interviews, with their implied insistence that the patient be productive, if held more frequently than once or twice a week seem to cause him to exaggerate his shame and guilt. Because of the high personal standards that the depressive requires of himself, and because of his feelings of impotence and incapacity, therapy may be very difficult if the psychiatrist urges productiveness. Because of his feelings of guilt and shame, the patient is unable to express his underlying sadness and rage. Since he is unable to meet the demands that he feels the therapist exerts, pressure by the latter arouses additional feelings of hatred and shame. The therapist does not, however, adopt the passive role usually followed in a more classic form of psychoanalysis.

Other features of this modified analysis are a constant reassurance of the patient that he will recover and a certain directness and openness in dealing with his problems. It will be remembered that in his depression the patient is overreacting emotionally to an actual or fantasied loss of a love object. He is therefore seeking another, or substitute, love object. The process of calm reassurance fits this need symbolically. The patient has also a need to escape from the feelings of guilt caused by his repressed rage in his depression. If, therefore, he reports events that seem to be conducive to the production of rage and anger within himself but has not expressed their emotional connotation, the therapist may verbalize such feelings and state their relationship to other persons involved in the patient's situation. In this way the patient is relieved of the burden of stating his rage or anger and is not exposed to subsequent feelings of guilt for expressing the forbidden emotions. With this elastic, nondemanding, and at the same time, active, interpretive approach, it is at times possible to abort depressions. Some therapists suggest it is better initially to have the depressed patient focus on an experience of recent loss rather than to encourage him to recall the earlier events and interpersonal experiences in his life that determined or reinforced his depressive symptomatology. Dream productions in the depressed patient are often helpful in breaking through to deep-seated associations that give a clearer understanding of his basic longings and conflicts.

Psychotherapy with the hypomanic or manic is difficult. Since such a patient usually identifies with a covertly aggressive, sadistic, and successful member of the family, the therapist must constantly guard against the provocation of rejecting a patient whose behavior seems designed for such a purpose, i.e., of embarrassing significant object relations. It is generally agreed that the conversion of manic or hypomanic symptoms to depressive ones is desirable. Sometimes this is effected by the therapist's simply indicating his doubts as to the soundness of the patient's presumption that he has reason to behave as if he were successful or in control of the situation.

Psychotherapeutically the aim of treatment of patients with the manic-depressive syndrome is to bring them to the point where they can consciously face periodic loneliness and separation without resorting to either submissive depression or revengeful overactivity.

PSYCHOTIC DEPRESSIVE REACTION

Not all psychotic depressive reactions should be included among those of a manic-depressive type. In the latter type of depressions, there is usually the history either of previous, perhaps repeated, depressions or of cyclothymic mood swings in which periods of elation as well as of depression may have been of psychotic degree. Occasionally one meets with depressions which lack the distinctive features of a manic-depressive reaction. Such depressions arise when the patient has been confronted with a personal situation of great stress. Environmental factors and personal experiences have been cruelly frustrating, have aroused intense feelings of guilt or remorse, or have painfully wounded pride. In these disorders, the reaction to the current situation is a definitely pathological depression, at times associated with gross misinterpretation of reality in the form of delusions, frequently, but not always, somatic, suicidal ruminations or attempts, intense feelings of guilt, and retardation of thought and of psychomotor activity.

In four-fifths of manic-depressive life histories definite disturbing events are discoverable which may be assumed through psychodynamic forces activated in the personality to precipitate the emotional disturbance. This, in turn, mediates the related psychophysiologic disturbances through aroused mechanisms within the central nervous system. In middle or late life one finds, in addition to loss of significant personal relationships, the threats to social, economic, and physical security as precipitants to the recurrent episodes of the illness.

BIBLIOGRAPHY

Adelstein, A. M., Downham, D. Y., Stein, Z., and Susser, M. W.: The epidemiology of mental illness in an English city. Social Psychiat., 3:47–59, 1968.

Aranoff, M. S., and Epstein, R. S.: Factors associated with poor response to lithium carbonate: A clinical study. Amer. J. Psychiat., 127:472–480, 1970.

Baastrup, P. C., Poulsen, J. C., and Schou, M.: Prophylactic lithium: Double blind discontinuation in manic-depressive and recurrent depressive disorders. Lancet, 2:326–329, 1970.

Baer, L., Platman, S. R., and Fieve, R. R.: The role of electrolytes in affective disorders. Arch. Gen. Psychiat., 22:108–113, 1970.

Biegel A., and Murphy, D. L.: Unipolar and bipolar affective illness. Arch. Gen. Psychiat., 24:215–220, 1970.

Birthnell, J.: Depression in relation to early and recent parent death. Brit. J. Psychiat., 116:299–306, 1970.

Brandrup, E.: A controlled investigation of plasma lipids in manic depressives. Brit. J. Psychiat., 113:987–992, 1967.

Bratfos, O., and Havy, J. O.: The course of manic-depressive illness. Acta Psychiat. Scand., 44:89–112, 1968.

Brodie, H. K., and Leff, M. J.: Bipolar depression —a comparative study of patient characteristics. Amer. J. Psychiat., 127:1086–1090, 1971.

Cookson, B. A., Huszka, L., Quarrington, B., and Stancer, H.: Longitudinal studies of diurnal excretion patterns in two cases of cyclical affective disorder. J. Psychiat. Res., 7:63–81, 1969.

Coppen, A.: Defects in monamine metabolism and their possible importance in the pathogenesis of depressive syndromes. Psychiat. Neurol. Neurochis., 72:173–180, 1969.

Fieve, R. R.: Lithium in psychiatry. Int. J. Psychiat., 9:375–412, 1970.

Gibson, R. W., Cohen, M. B., and Cohen, R. A.: On the dynamics of the manic-depressive personality. Amer. J. Psychiat., 115:1101–1107, 1959.

Glassman, A.: Indoleamines and affective disorders. Psychosom. Med., 31:107–114, 1969.

Hartmann, E.: Longitudinal studies of sleep and dream patterns in manic-depressive patients. Arch. Gen. Psychiat., 19:311–329, 1968.

Janowsky, D. J., Leff, M., and Epstein, R. S.: Playing the manic game. Arch. Gen. Psychiat., 22:252–261, 1970.

Kraepelin, E.: Manic-Depressive Insanity and Paranoia. Translated by E. Barclay. Edinburgh, E. and S. Livingstone Ltd., 1921.

Kramer, M., Baldridge, B. A., Whitman, R. W., Ornstein, P. H., and Smith, P. C.: An exploration of the manifest dream in schizophrenic and depressed patients. Dis. Nerv. Syst., 30:126–130, 1969.

Lewin, B. D.: The Psychoanalyses of Elation. New York, W. W. Norton & Co., Inc., 1950.

Maddison, D., and Duncan, G. M. (eds.): Aspects of Depressive Illness—a Symposium. Edinburgh and London, E. & S. Livingstone Ltd., 1965.

Mayfield, D. G., and Coleman, L. L.: Alcohol use and affective disorder. Dis. Nerv. Syst., 29:467–474, 1968.

Miller, J. B.: Dreams during varying stages of depression. Arch. Gen. Psychiat., 20:560–565, 1969.

Murphy, D. L.: Regular induction of hypomania by L-dopa in "bipolar" manic-depressive patients. Nature, 229:135–136, 1971.

Platman, S. R., Plutchik, R., Fieve, R. R., and Lawlor, W. G.: Emotional profiles associated with mania and depression. Arch. Gen. Psychiat., 20:210–214, 1969.

Rosenblatt, S., and Chenley, J. D.: Differences in the metabolism of norepinephrine in depressions. Arch. Gen. Psychiat., 13:495–502, 1965.

Schildkraut, J. J.: The catecholamine hypothesis of affective disorders: A review of supporting evidence. Amer. J. Psychiat., 22:507–522, 1965.

Shagass, C., et al.: An objective test which differentiates between neurotic and psychotic depression. A.M.A. Arch. Neurol. & Psychiat., 75:461–471, 1956.

Shagass, C., and Schwartz, M.: Cerebral cortical reactivity in psychotic depressions. Arch. Gen. Psychiat., 6:235–242, 1962.

Shobe, F. O., and Brion, P.: Long term prognosis in manic-depressive illness. Arch. Gen. Psychiat., 24:334–337, 1971.

Spiegel, R.: Communications with depressive patients. Contemporary Psychoanal., 2:30–35, 1965.

Stancer, H. C., Furlong, F. W., and Godse, D. D.: A longitudinal investigation of lithium as a prophylactic agent for recurrent depressions. Canad. Psychiat. Assn. J., 15:29–40, 1970.

Winokur, G., Clayton, R. J., and Reich, T.: Manic-Depressive Illness. St. Louis, C. V. Mosby Co., 1969.

Zetzel, E. R.: The predisposition to depression. Canad. Psychiat. Assn. J., 11 (Suppl.): S 236–S 249, 1966.

Chapter 23

Paranoid Psychoses

PARANOID REACTIONS (PARANOIA AND PARANOID CONDITIONS)

Paranoia is a chronic mental disorder of insidious development characterized by persistent, unalterable, systematized, logically reasoned delusions. General demeanor, talk, and emotional and behavior reactions remain unaltered except as they are influenced by delusional beliefs, which become the uppermost and guiding theme of the patient's life and may therefore seriously impair discretion and judgment. The term was first used in 1863 by Kahlbaum to designate various persecutory and grandiose states. That the most conspicuous symptom is in the field of thought is indicated by the etymology of the name applied to mental disorders of this type (παρά, beside, in the sense of altered or changed, and νοῦς, intellect or reason).

Etiology

There seems to be convincing evidence that the causes of paranoia and paranoid conditions are psychological. Among these psychological causes may be ambitious but frustrated strivings; a need for defense of the personality against undesirable tendencies and repudiated impulses; feelings of insecurity, guilt, or other anxiety-producing factors; a continued failure to achieve overvalued goals; or a need for enhancing prestige or self-esteem. Specific traumatic life experiences may serve as contributory factors. In a significant number of cases it will be found that the paranoiac comes from a family that has been severely authoritarian, harsh, and cruel. Frequently a parent, usually of the same sex, has been a hostile, controlling person who rejects the child and, through accusations, produces fear, anxiety, feelings of inadequacy, and a self-image of the "bad" child, which, however, he does not accept. In many, perhaps in most, cases there has been an early overidentification with the parent of the opposite sex. As a result of his emotional experiences and frustrations, patterns of hatred and aggression are frequently established; these, however, the child must endeavor to repress because of fear of his parent.

As is frequently observed, parents whose personalities were warped through unwholesome attitudes and relationships with their parents may affectively distort those of their own children. Often the child has been involved in, observed, or come to knowledge of parental or family transgressions which, if revealed, would have seriously damaging social consequences for him or the significant person. On occasions the parent or other person may deny the act and threaten the child, insisting that he hold the secret. Thus the use of denial and rationalization is enhanced by the child. Simultaneously the child must repress his own rage toward the parental figure with whom he is involved. In other instances fantasies of parental or family transgressions function in the same manner. The nature of the behavior then may lead the child or young adult to withdraw from social contacts and thus come to feel rejected. This may

387

stimulate resentment and contribute a
paranoid element to the developing personality that may finally culminate in the
paranoid psychosis. Sometimes self-pity or
sibling rivalry seems to facilitate the establishment of paranoid tendencies.

Another train of events has been suggested by Artiss as means of development
of the paranoid personality. Thus when
high expectations for outstanding achievement are fostered by the parent, the
doubtful child may develop secret longings
and also subterfuges to attain the desired
goals. When these secretly elaborated fantasies which are resorted to as a means of
maintaining respect within the family
group are frustrated, there follow a sudden and terrifying anxiety and depression
compensated for by the erection of the
defensive internalization and projections
so characteristic of the paranoiac.

Even as a child, the future paranoid
individual usually shows troublesome
trends that make it difficult for him to
participate in congenial play with other
children for more than brief periods. He
is often a lonely, unhappy, brooding, insecure child, lacking friends with whom
he can share confidences and exchange
perspectives. Frequently he is suspicious,
stubborn, secretive, obstinate, and resentful of discipline. When crossed, he is apt
to be sullen, morose, peevish, and irritable. As adult life is approached, the
early personality characteristics become
accentuated. The future patient becomes
increasingly sensitive about the attitude
and behavior of others, "builds moun-
tains out of molehills," and may believe
that others wish to do him injury. He is
lacking in a sense of humor and impresses
others as egotistic, sarcastic, derogatory,
querulous, embittered, and resentful.
Usually the paranoid person has always
been demanding, inflexible, biased, mistrustful, impatient, and often defiant of
conventions. Characteristically he has
been argumentative, uncompromising, and
aggressive. Interpersonal relationships are
difficult. He approaches others with a
"chip-on-the-shoulder" attitude. The drive
for achievement may be intense and may

impel him to seek goals that are beyond
his capacity. Intolerant of criticism and
unable to accept suggestions, he readily
criticizes and belittles others. Meticulous
and precise, he is in some respects highly
efficient but is jealous and unadaptable.
He needs to demonstrate his superiority.
If in a position of authority, he may be a
petty tyrant.

At times one meets persons handicapped
by such *paranoid personality* characteristics that, however, never develop further. In others these characteristics become
gradually and insidiously intensified until
the patient is clearly psychotic. In the
same problems and factors are to be found
the sources of both the paranoid personality and the paranoid psychosis. The
latter represents a progressive, developing
continuance of the former. In some instances, as in other paranoid reactions,
repressed homosexual impulses seem to
be the source of the psychopathology.

The mental mechanisms and reactions
observed in paranoia are but exaggerations of ones noted constantly among persons who are not thought of as psychotic.
In everyday life, fear and insecurity are
expressed in such disguises as pettiness,
oversensitiveness, irascibility, never-ending
bickering, overcompensation, seclusiveness, selfishness, or cynicism. Even caution
may develop into suspiciousness. Many
people are at times inclined to feel
slighted, to think that their merits are
unrecognized, to blame their environment
for what are really dissatisfactions with
self, or perhaps in part to fulfill their
wishes in fantasy. Daily we meet those
who are unable to recognize and admit
their faults and defects. Real or imagined
injuries to pride tend to result in feelings
of resentment and bitterness of variable
duration. The well-defined paranoid personality often seems to display a remarkable genius for detecting in the ordinary
run-of-life situations just those tiny
slights, inadvertencies, or trifling dispar-
agements that others overlook but that he
builds up into crucial issues, not altogether imaginary but vastly overemphasized.

One must agree with the English psychiatrist, Crichton-Miller: "For every fully developed case of paranoia in our mental hospitals there must be hundreds, if not thousands, who suffer from minor degrees of suspicion and mistrust; whose lives are blighted by this barrier to human harmony; and who poison the springs of social life for the community."

The paranoid personality may be over-aggressive as he sees an aggressor in everyone around him. This makes him feel that his war against the world is waged in self-defense. A rebellious, superior attitude may serve to bolster self-esteem and prevent a realistic but intolerable self-evaluation. Thus the paranoid individual treats others as projections of certain of his own unconscious trends. As a result, his statements, manner, and behavior alienate friends and create enemies. The fact that he thereby incurs the hostility of others and is therefore often rejected and isolated adds more fuel to the psychopathogenic fire.

In the paranoid personality, we meet with an exaggeration of the common tendency to ascribe responsibility to others, to repudiate aspects of the personality that do not measure up to the standards the individual has set for himself, to obtain satisfaction through compensatory strivings, to maintain self-esteem by constructing emotionally satisfying but irrational explanations for his own failures, and to attribute hostile or aggressive motives to others. Disappointments, humiliation, or injuries sustained may accentuate a paranoid tendency and even appear to precipitate a paranoid psychosis. The causes of paranoia are, then, to be sought in the need for protecting particularly vulnerable aspects of the personality, in the craving for a recognition greater than attainment can command, in the particular mental conflicts of the individual, in frustrations and vague fears, and in a need for relieving one's own anxiety over guilt by blaming someone else. Many cases of paranoid psychoses seem to derive from the mechanism whereby guilt-inspiring impulses are repudiated by projection to

a persecutor.

As we study the behavior of individuals and the methods by which they meet conflicts within and blows from without, we often find it difficult to say when the expressions of a paranoid personality become the symptoms of a paranoid psychosis. Anomalies of character become continuous with the psychosis, both, to a large degree, going back to the needs and problems of the personality and to the habitual techniques or patterns that the individual has adopted in attempting to meet such irregularities.

Formerly there was a tendency to subdivide the permanent paranoid reactions into definite disease entities. Kraepelin looked upon paranoia as a fixed type of disease resulting exclusively from internal causes and characterized by persistent, systematized delusions, the preservation of clear and orderly thinking and acting, and the absence of hallucinations. Intermediate between paranoia and paranoid schizophrenia he recognized an entity he called *paraphrenia,* differing principally from paranoia by the fact that the delusions lack the logical systematization of the latter disorder. The delusions are more apt to be extravagant and, in addition, hallucinations are present at times. Not for many years, if at all, is there any deterioration of general interest or of personality.

Psychopathology

As previously noted, there is no clearly defined point at which the personality marked by the characteristics previously described should be called psychotic. The paranoid tendencies rarely become so extreme as to justify a diagnosis of paranoia before the age of 30. The disorder is more common in men. As already indicated, the presenting symptom of paranoia and of paranoid states is a rigid, persistent system of delusions. At times the patient's delusions may take their origin in some actual fact. On cross section, his behavior and thought content may be deceptive, and a severe disorder be camouflaged by a seemingly normal surface. On longitudinal section, however, the paranoid theme is discovered. The content of paranoid ideas varies widely and is determined primarily by the particular psychological needs they are created to fulfill, and secondarily by the type of rationalization that will appeal to the ideas and beliefs current in the patient's environment.

The patient's own inclinations are mirrored in the particular motives and intentions attributed to others. His rationalizations are vigorously defended, and he exhibits a convincing earnestness in his efforts to win others to his delusional beliefs. The patient may rationalize so plausibly that his friends accept his allegation that specific individuals, rather than himself, are responsible for his difficulties. His superior intellectual endowment may remain unimpaired. Some paranoiacs become aware that the credibility of their delusions is questioned and therefore attempt to hide them. The patient's judgment may be defective only in relation to his delusional system, which often develops slowly and ultimately becomes intricate and complex. The dominating ideas tend to be those of persecution, of expansive grandiosity, or of both themes.

As *persecutory* trends develop, the patient attributes hostile or aggressive motives to others, nurses his grievances, and becomes increasingly secretive. In the earlier period of his psychosis, he may be hypochondriacal and uneasy. He may become depressed, gloomy, spiteful, vindictive, and given to morose rumination. Frequently he manifests a self-righteous resentment against others. Misunderstandings and misinterpretations develop into delusions of persecution.

The tendency of the paranoiac to seek for ulterior motives on the part of others or to misinterpret events is illustrated by the case of a woman who, soon after graduation from a law school, the faculty of which had awarded her the annual prize for the greatest improvement in scholastic work during her professional course, sued the school for damages, alleging that the awarding of such a prize was for the purpose of representing her as having been more poorly fitted than her associates for the study of law. (Doubtless the same sense of insecurity that led to her psychosis determined also her choice of law as a profession.)

In his effort to control his hostile impulses in which the genesis of his paranoid reaction is often to be found, the patient projects them and experiences them as being directed against himself. Filled with hate, he feels and believes that he is the victim of persecutors, who, in fact, are but the objects upon whom he has projected his own hate.

The mood of many paranoiacs is one of sustained sullenness. Ideas of reference appear: there is a hidden meaning in what is taking place in his environment; cryptic significances are read into casual remarks and events; slights and indignities are imagined; far-reaching significance is attached to trivial details in the behavior of others. Vague feelings of fear tend to increase suspicion and the patient's malevolent trend of thought. Although in the case of the "normal" person incredulity, indignation, and danger often help to prevent the individual from becoming aware of qualities, strivings, and tendencies that offend self-esteem, these defensive reactions are used much more by the paranoid patient.

Delusional ideas extend: the patient believes that people spread lies about him; persons tamper with his mail; accusing remarks are overheard; hostility and jealousy are observed on every hand; business plans are thwarted; he is the victim of a conspiracy, and the agents of malevolent social organizations pursue him, persecutors who seek to conceal their identity by various disguises. He may become depressed and even suicidal because he feels overwhelmed by an environment with which he cannot cope.

In the persecutory as well as in other forms of paranoia, there is a central delusional theme that pervades the whole life of the patient, who is quite incapable of criticizing the pseudologic he employs in supporting this dominant idea. His premises are not scrutinized, and present events, regardless of their relevancy to the prevailing idea, are interpreted wholly with reference to it. Affect determines the patient's logic. Incidents of the past receive a new interpretation and are fitted into the framework of present persecution —a process known as retrospective falsification. As a result, the delusional system constantly extends, and the most commonplace incidents, because of their affective interpretation with reference to the prevailing idea, become events of the greatest importance. In all paranoid reactions, the patient, always confident that he is right, clings obstinately to his opinions, since his inner sense of insecurity cannot permit him to feel otherwise. He maintains his delusional misinterpretations, too, by continually overemphasizing the inferred or implied meaning and by discarding the obvious and real content of a statement or action.

A common form of paranoia is the *litigious* type. Although it will usually be found that this type of paranoiac individual was always stubborn and insistent upon his "rights," with many defensive mechanisms, the litigious activities frequently do not appear until after some legal experience that eventuated less satisfactorily than the patient desired. Because of his dissatisfaction, the patient initiates further but ill-advised legal action. He always fails to see that he has not proved his case. Every new litigation brings further controversies and new grievances for which the patient feels prompted to seek redress. His attempts to secure it, however, result in fresh feelings of injustice. Fundamentally, it is often not a question of law and justice, as the patient insists, but of attempts to put others in the wrong, to show that he was right, that he is superior, in order that thereby his sensitive insecurity may be strengthened and the weak points of his personality may be protected.

In the *exalted* type of paranoia, the ideas of grandeur may appear after a long preceding stage of persecution, or at times the grandiosity may be present practically from the beginning of the psychosis. Ideas of invention constitute a frequent form of grandiosity. Patients with such beliefs usually neglect their usual method of livelihood and devote their time to the drawing of plans and the construction of models. At times the patient claims that models are completed but that enemies prevent him from securing a patent; again, he is on the point of perfecting the machine. In either case, the patient frequently claims to utilize some force or to attain some objective contrary to the accepted laws of science. In this type of disorder, the patient may have a sense of mission and pursue his impracticable goal with more zeal than discretion. Others have expansive ideas of noble birth. Frequently the grandiose patient attempts to play the role that his ideas have assigned him. If, for example, he believes he is a religious leader, he may wear long hair and a beard and affect an air of humility —an air that often disguises but poorly a repressed hatred.

The exalted beliefs in some paranoid states are of a religious nature. The patient is the chosen one of God, is Christ, prophesied the war, has supernatural powers. Some establish new religious sects and secure adherents; others proclaim themselves leaders of a new order but are so bizarre in belief and behavior that they fail to secure followers.

Occasionally paranoia assumes an *erotic* form. The patient believes that some woman of title or wealth whom he may have casually seen or met is in love with him. He writes her affectionate letters and perhaps poems. Her failure to reply to them is intended solely to test his love. Items in the newspapers, the flight of the birds, and various events are disguised recognitions of her presence and acknowledgments of her love. Such patients may become annoyingly persistent in their attentions and threatening in their manner.

The paranoid psychoses have been studied in much more detail among men than women. Modlin describes a group of premenopausal married women between 30 and 45 years of age who had established adequate sexual relations within marriage but became acutely psychotic with paranoid ideation. None had extramarital relations, and all had exhibited stability and considerable ego strength before the illness. Precipitating the illness in each instance was a change in the husband-wife relationship which led to a reduction in frequency of or cessation of sexual intercourse. In some instances other family members moved into the home; in others the husband became ill or overly preoccupied with the demands of his employment, thus expending less energy and time with the future patient. In some illnesses the initial phase of the psychosis was marked by depression in which the patients feared they were losing their husbands. Suspicious attitudes and ideas of reference were followed by a florid paranoidal delusional system. In this series the illness had lasted, with remissions, from over one to seven years.

More recently Freedman and his colleagues have suggested from their clinical studies that one may separate paranoid patients into two groups: those who are socially isolated, nonbelligerent, and with an undifferentiated cognitive function, the latter defined according to various responses to the Rorschach tests and human figure drawings; and those who are socially active, aggressive, and demonstrate in psychological test behavior a differentiated cognitive style. The two groups respond variously to treatment; those in the first are likely to remit, whereas those in the second are unlikely to do so.

Among common causes for the commitment of paranoid patients are homicidal or suicidal attempts, the writing of anonymous letters to persons in authority, litigation, or persistent statements that they are the victims of a conspiracy.

Psychodynamics

Although disparity between achievement and ambition, early experience heavily loaded with affect, vague or subconscious feelings of dissatisfaction or irritation with self, and injuries to self-evalua-

tion, as well as various other needs for defense, may act as dynamic agents and lead or contribute to a fixed paranoid reaction type, there is much to suggest that repressed homosexual impulses may be a genetic factor. The persistence of homosexual impulses, unrecognized consciously, may doubtless be caused by more than one factor, but, characterized as the homosexual is by his infantile survivals and mother imprint, there seems good reason to believe that if, at puberty, an inhibitive maternal overpossessiveness impedes the maturation of the psychosexual aspects of her son's personality, these may remain fixated and never attain a mature heterosexual development.

Criticisms of the theory that repressed homosexual drives contribute to the genesis of paranoid elusions are the clinical observations that in many instances the paranoid symptomatology does not reflect a homosexual reference and also in some cases patients appear to accept an existing overt homosexuality without conflict. From the standpoint of psychoanalytic theory it is pointed out that manifest and latent homosexuality are dissimilar in that they occupy different levels in the psychic apparatus and operate independently. Thus, as Carr indicates, a patient may consciously accept and engage in homosexual practice but deny the unrecognized and unconscious murderous and sadistic homosexual fixations derived from his early infantile and childhood attachment to a punitive and aggressive parent. What is overlooked commonly in the paranoid homosexual fixation is the competitive and hostile aggressive component of the attachment, with overemphasis placed on the libidinous attachment to a member of the same sex. What is overlooked according to Ovesey and many other recent theorists is the "power anxiety" of the paranoid, which essentially should be regarded as the primary motivating force in the development of his pathological defenses. Consciously and unconsciously perceiving himself as weak, defective, or inadequate, whether he evaluates his performance socially, vocationally, or sexually he builds up a structure of projective defense—the paranoid system.

Assuming that there is a relation between this fixation, or incomplete evolution of the personality, and homosexuality, how does the latter lead to paranoia? According to Freud, it is through the mechanism of projection by which the original but repressed and therefore consciously rejected affect is reversed and transferred to the homosexual object. Because it is consciously inadmissible, the patient's "I love him" is changed to "I do not love him; I hate him," which, to be acceptable, requires projection as "He hates me" and is elaborated into "I am persecuted by him."

An abnormally high percentage of paranoids do not marry, while many others are divorced. This is not only because of a basic homosexual orientation but also because of the fact that their chronic hostility and anger make them undesirable as partners. If the paranoiac does marry, the marital life is so full of discord that it frequently ends in divorce.

The "true" paranoiac is often a person of superior intellectual endowment, but his energy is so largely expended in repudiating desires that do not wish to be recognized as such, in compensatory efforts whereby self-esteem may be enhanced, and in striving for satisfactions that life has not supplied, that social relations become disturbed and constructive achievements are nil. The fact that life has failed to bring the success and satisfactions to which the native intelligence of the patient would ordinarily have entitled him undoubtedly tends to aggravate his defensive reactions. Another reason why a large percentage of cases of paranoia occur among people of superior intelligence is perhaps that the person of superior intellectual endowment finds rationalization and projection to be readily available and satisfactory mechanisms of defense. The more promptly and passively the individual gives up the struggle for self-esteem and for recognition, the more nearly will the reaction approach the schizophrenic, regardless of the native intelligence, while the more active and sustained the struggle, the more likely is the result to approach paranoia.

The following case presents, in some respects, many of the characteristic features of paranoia:

P. G. was committed to a hospital for mental diseases because of his peculiar religious ideas and rites, one of them being the practice of going about nude. The patient's parents were strict in their moral principles and rigid in discipline. All the paternal siblings were teachers except the patient's father, who was a farmer and who was always dissatisfied with his lot, often expressing the wish that he could "get away where he could read and study and reform the world." The patient had one sister, also a brother who was older and stronger and who used to "lord it over" the patient. His association with his sister was close, and shortly before leaving home as a young man he suggested to her that if she would not get married, he would not do so either, and they would live together.

As a child he was described as sensitive and fearing criticism. "Because he was not strong, he was somewhat of a sissy," the sister stated. At school he was a ready scholar and completed the equivalent of two years of high school work. If he received less than 90 in his grades, he felt disgraced. Prior to his marriage at age 26 he had paid little attention to persons of the opposite sex. At that age he married his landlady, a woman of 66, "as a humane act"; this was his characterization of the match when he entered the hospital. When questioned concerning his sex life, he stated that men had aroused him sexually more than women, for whom he had no sexual desire. He took part in homosexual practices on only a few occasions. When asked if he thought his religion had helped him in repressing his homosexual tendencies, he replied, "I do not think so, I know it." He acknowledged that he derived pleasure from exposing himself to other men, although he claimed that his practice of going about nude was a health measure permitted by his religion and not for the purpose of satisfying exhibitionistic impulses—doubtless a rationalization of socially prohibited inclinations. When questioned concerning his social life, he had, he said, "a distinct aversion to secret organizations"—perhaps an unconscious defense against his homosexual tendencies, since such organizations, made up as they usually are of individuals of one sex, serve to provide a sublimated and socialized outlet for homosexual trends, although the psychological basis of these bodies is also one of narcissism and compensation.

During his early adult life, the patient became interested in various unusual religious cults (probably an effort to obtain a feeling of security), although this striving did not result in such a serious disturbance in thought and behavior as to lead to his being considered psychotic until after he was 40 years of age. He described himself as suffering at about that period from "lack of initiative, inability to concentrate, general weakness, anxiety about the future, irritability, and hypopotency of the heart." Doubtless this represented a stage of subjective analysis often occurring in the disease. He addressed a prayer to the "Deity" asking for aid and threatening to commit suicide if it were not forthcoming. Almost immediately it was "revealed" to him, not through a voice or visible signs but "simply through thought process," that he was to establish a new religion to take the place of Christianity, one that would be more comforting and satisfactory. He called his new religion "Omnivitism" and spent day after day writing "a set of mottoes instead of commandments, a set of actions and ideals, prayers, verse, comment on principles, affirmations and denials, suggestions regarding services, and miscellaneous dissertations." When questioned as to the specific teachings of his religion, little but vague generalities was to be secured. "It teaches," he said, "that all forms and phases of existence are essential factors of one all-sufficient existence that is called 'Omniad.'" He had tracts printed and distributed them widely, setting forth "the rule of Omnivitism, which is to teach according to his needs."

About this time he began to go to isolated spots and to walk about nude, explaining that he was taking "sun baths." Gradually he made fewer attempts to retire from sight when taking his "sun baths," particularly after he derived considerable enjoyment from the fact that he was seen by the occupants of two automobiles that passed while he was unclothed. Finally, after having been warned on repeated occasions by the local constable that he must not continue his exhibitionistic practices, the patient was committed to a hospital for mental disorders.

On arrival at the hospital, the patient was pleasant and smiling but obviously exalted, with an air of self-satisfaction and superiority. He was a small man of rather effeminate physique. His hair reached nearly to his shoulders, and his beard was long, his appearance strongly resembling the traditional picture of Christ. He accepted his detention philosophically, expressing the opinion that it was what one in his position must expect—a sort of martyrdom in a worthy cause. He had, he said, founded a religion "more up to date" than Christianity and one that would supplant the latter and dominate the world; it had been revealed to him that by 1940 it would have been substantially established. Further, the patient was to have been President of the United States. This, he added, was in accordance with the prophecy of Sir William Hope made on the day of Washington's birth. On that day he foretold that a new nation would arise in America and the part that would be played by Washington, and that finally there would come a ruler whom he characterized as "six plus added six—great, good and wise," at the same time referring to "a star that on his way shall shine." This prophecy, the patient said, referred to him, since

there were six letters in each of his names, while his sister was the star, since it was she who had invited him to come to their old home. In an old novel, too, the patient claimed he had found the following: "There will come in the western continent a greater man than this world has seen since this civilization began. It will not be through the ignorance of the people that this man will be carried into the White House. In some respects this man will be the intellectual and philosophical leader. He will be to the world what Mohammed was to Arabia, Columbus to the New World, Moses to the Jews, Plato to the Greeks, et cetera—yet he will be greater than all and more powerful for good." This, the patient said, referred to him.

On psychometric examination by the Stanford-Binet scale, the patient was found to have an I.Q. of 115. It is interesting to note that in ability to see logical relationships, language ability, and constructive visual imagery he attained an 18-year level, but on practical judgment in social situations he graded at a 9-year-and-1-month level. In describing his attitude toward the examination, the psychologist recorded that the patient seemed to enjoy the opportunity of demonstrating his intellectual endowment, that he frequently laughed in a superior manner, that he exhibited great precision of speech, and delighted in showing off his large and unusual vocabulary. On several occasions, in a tolerant and somewhat condescending manner, he criticized the examiner for her use of words.

The patient's paranoid system was associated with too great disorganization of personality and disturbance of reality evaluation to permit the diagnosis of paranoia, but may properly, we believe, be regarded as a paranoid state rather than paranoid schizophrenia. The patient was unable to secure a satisfying adjustment to a sense of biological and social inadequacy, to a fundamental homosexuality, and doubtless to other conflicts. However, instead of investing the external world with his own unrecognized but repudiated trends and feelings, he organized his emotional constellations into ideational systems that afforded a satisfying but unsocialized adjustment. The compensatory feelings of superiority developed to meet the subconscious feelings of inferiority and doubtless of guilt (arising from an imperfectly repressed homosexuality) were rationalized into grandiose delusions.

Other factors, too, presumably contributed to the life pattern of the patient's personality and his desire for high personal value. It may well have been that the dissatisfactions with self and the vaguely defined strivings owed their origin in part to absorption from the early family life, since we learned that his father was dissatisfied with his lot and wished to "study and reform the world." The fact that he was "lorded over" by a stronger brother presumably led to feelings of inadequacy and contributed to the psychological need for the artificially obtained feeling of security and self-esteem. To have been taught that school grades below an unreasonably high standard constituted a disgrace tended to lead the boy to form ambitions that, with his limitations of personality and opportunities for training, inevitably resulted in wounds to pride and vanity.

Among the traits of childhood were sensitiveness and fear of criticism. His slightness of physique called for compensation, and a certain degree of biological deviation and the failure to emancipate himself emotionally from his older sister, who perhaps served as a mother surrogate, served to fix the development of his personality at a homosexual level. His exhibitionistic practices are doubtless also to be explained on the basis of arrest in psychosexual evolution. His egotistic wishes prejudiced his judgment and led it to disregard the usual criteria of reality, thereby both preventing a correct perspective and destroying the capacity for self-criticism.

Folie à Deux

Inasmuch as the clinical features are nearly always paranoid in nature, mention may be made at this point of an induced or communicated form of psychosis described by Lasèque and Falret in 1877 to which they gave the name *"folie à deux."* Identification is usually an important mechanism in its production. This is a mental disorder in which mental symptoms, particularly paranoid delusions, from which one of two persons intimately

associated with each other, usually for years, is suffering are communicated to and accepted by the other. Most frequently such a dual psychosis involves mother and daughter, two sisters, or husband and wife. The person suffering from the primary psychosis is usually the dominant individual, while the one who develops the secondary or induced psychosis is of a submissive and suggestible type, dependent upon and having a close emotional attachment to the infector. As misinterpretations, illusions, and ideas of persecution increasingly disturb the infector, he persuasively relates his convictions and psychotic experiences to the weaker person or infectee, who comes to accept and react to the systematized delusional ideas of the first.

It will often be found that both persons have been poorly adjusted individuals having a narrow range of interests, of the same general background and environment, and facing perhaps the same situation. The induced ideas must be acceptable and usually offer some satisfaction to the person infected. In nearly every instance the delusional ideas are dropped by the recipient if he is removed from association with the dominant person.

The usual setting of the disorder is one in which the two persons concerned live in comparative seclusion. It is more frequently found among women. This is probably because they tend to be more isolated within the domestic circle, and their outside interests and ambitions are more likely to be restricted or frustrated.

Diagnosis

At times psychiatric literature contains references to "acute paranoia." Although descriptively this is a good term, it is somewhat misleading, since it will be found that the episodes thus classified are fundamentally affective in nature, being hypomanic attacks of manic-depressive psychosis in which the usual emotional exaltation is replaced by irritability and anger. The patient is aggressive, haughty, hostile, and complaining. In paranoia there is a greater tendency to project and to rationalize one's affective state than in the usual manic episode. The true paranoiac is more restrained both in behavior and in speech, and his ideational content is characterized by a more sustained and dominant idea than is the more excited manic with his fleeting charges. As the affect subsides, the delusional ideas of the acute paranoid episode are dropped, but they are not corrected, and the manic patient remains without insight as to the beliefs he formerly expressed with great conviction and feeling.

Concealed behind the symptoms of anxiety, sometimes erythrophobia, and a history of frequent spoiling of occupational success, there often exist the essential components of the paranoid. These patients, too, have overwhelming aspirations for success and desire for recognition coupled with an intense but repressed capacity for guilt due to the association of success with aggression symbolized as a murderous hostility. Among patients with this symptom complex and personality organization will be found some with a capacity for paranoid hallucinatory decompensation. Their discrimination from those with psychoneurotic personality is important before undertaking dynamic psychotherapy, as the course may be interrupted by sudden decompensation. The greater the logical systematization of delusions and the less the patient's relations with reality are disturbed, the more nearly does the psychosis approach traditional paranoia. The greater the extent to which repressed material comes through to consciousness in the form of hallucinations, the more bizarre the delusional system, and the more regressive and disorganized the form of adjustment, the more nearly does it approach paranoid schizophrenia. Although anger and hatred are common in all the paranoid disorders, as time progresses there is an increasing tendency for the schizophrenic patient's affect to "burn out." The paranoid schizophrenic patient lacks the intensive drive for achievement usually seen in paranoia.

Often there is difficulty in deciding whether a person whose behavior is governed by, and indicates a thorough contact with, reality, who has suffered no dilapidation of affect or of personality, and who is not hallucinated, but who constantly employs projection and other defensive measures, should be considered as suffering from paranoia or as a paranoid, but not psychotic, personality. In general, if the exaggerated reaction is continuous, if the beliefs through which it manifests itself cannot be corrected, if they disclose an inadequacy of logic, and particularly if they tend to spread and to reveal that the affective and conative forces are sustained and have great energy, then the reaction must be looked upon as psychotic. The psychiatrist will not forget that paranoid tendencies may be channeled and expressed in many eccentricities and fanatical ways.

West suggests that one must separate reactions of severe pathological jealousy from the group of chronic psychotic reactions. In discussing the "Othello syndrome," he emphasizes the fact that cultural factors, including racial prejudice, feed into and contribute to the development of such states.

Prognosis

It is doubtful if a patient with traditional paranoia ever fully recovers. In those cases in the paranoid series that most nearly approach paranoid schizophrenia, a remission may rarely occur, but in these, also, the ultimate prognosis is poor. In true paranoia there is little or no general personality disorganization, and the patient's conduct usually remains within the bounds that society will tolerate. For this reason, a large proportion of such patients do not enter a hospital for mental disorders. In the community the individuals are often looked upon as "cranks," but, as they usually do not act without reflection, show a certain amount of self-control, and limit themselves to legal means of redress, they avoid commitment much more frequently than do those with paranoid conditions that approach the schizophrenic pole of the series. The latter are less sociable, less industrious, and less restrained by social custom and law.

An analysis of the causes of death in the psychoses shows that a larger percentage of paranoid patients than of any other group with biogenetic psychoses die of degenerative circulatory disease.

Treatment

Unless his behavior is too disturbing socially, it is well for the patient with paranoia to remain in the community, since interference and restraint embitter him and lead to an extension of his delusional system and to a stimulation of his hatred. If the paranoiac is considered dangerous, commitment, of course, becomes imperative.

To determine when he has become dangerous is not always easy. A careful evaluation of the patient's history will usually indicate the extent to which delusions may be expected to control behavior. If delusions have exerted an important influence on behavior and if they are directed toward particular individuals, this estimate should be made. The willingness and the degree of objectivity with which the patient will discuss his delusions are important. The character and intensity of his emotional reaction will greatly aid in deciding the questions as to the hazard entailed in the patient's liberty; the greater the overt hostility, the more imperative is his removal from society. Many times the patient will discuss the extent to which he believes he is justified in protecting himself or his interests or in securing redress. An indication can thus be obtained as to the probability of acts of violence.

Whether the patient is to be treated as an inpatient or outpatient, the therapist must keep clearly in mind certain expectations relative to the transference. The paranoid is generally suspicious and distrustful, considers himself unloved and incapable of giving affection, and has usually come to believe through long experience that what is conveyed by the spoken word does not reflect the actual intent of those with whom he has been closely related. He has a need to see himself as a center of interest and activity as a means to sustain a façade of importance that protects him from suffering hurt by his deep sense of personal inadequacy, shame, or humiliation.

Treatment, then, should initially be as permissive as possible. The physician should maintain an open, courteous, considerate attitude, coupled with scrupulous truthfulness and good faith. Recalling the essential pathology, attention should be paid to the patient's delusions, but no attempt should be made to criticize or convince the patient that he is in error as to his conclusions. Such efforts only produce a further lowering of self-esteem and arouse greater compensatory deficiencies or outright acts of destructive hatefulness. Nor should any efforts be made to convince him that he is among friends who are kindly disposed to him, or that he has a warm and attractive personality himself. All forms of ingratiation should be avoided, as they will be interpreted as evidence that the patient is again dealing with persons similar to those whom he believes have betrayed him in the past. The physician's attitude to the delusions will not imply agreement, however. It will imply rather, "I can understand how you feel, but it does not seem so to me." The physician will make his role and his position clear and hold them firmly.

The patient's anxiety and tension should be relieved by the administration of a phenothiazine as described in Chapter 32. With these measures, many paranoid patients will, if allowed the opportunity, commence exploration of their problems in psychotherapy. Such a patient should be allowed to follow his own leads, and, when occasions arise, the physician may offer tentative and alternative hypotheses as to the determining factors that the patient provides to explain his delusional interpretations of his relations to others, his failures and successes. By such means, creation of doubt may be created in the patient's concept of his relations with others. Later, more direct confrontations may be used, and realistic appraisal of his interpretations may be provided.

As for the homosexual trends, oftentimes these are regressive fantasies due to fear of rejection or lack of success in relating to women. Sometimes they are representative of impotency, which is the outcome of the deep lack of security of the patient. Sexual fears will be dealt with, then, in terms of the patient's anxieties in relation to those of the opposite sex rather than by humiliating remarks or interpretations concerning homosexuality. The patient should be advised that from time to time he is likely to become suspicious or distrustful of the psychotherapist and also advised he should speak of it when he has this experience so that the underlying reasons may be clarified.

This therapeutic approach, which consistently allows a deeper examination of reality without exposing the patient to shame and, at the same time, strengthens the patient's satisfaction in achievements within the limits of his capacities, has been of aid in bringing about satisfactory social adaptation.

As for the women, described by Modlin, who become paranoid when their sense of strength and power is undercut by the lessening sexual activity of their husbands, he recommends a treatment regimen of firm, authoritative control of the patient's behavior while in hospital, to cut through her tendency to misinterpret and react to the environment on the basis of her abnormal perceptions. He also emphasizes the usefulness of focusing on current realities and of avoiding expressive or supportive psychotherapeutic positions. Her delusional expressions should be accepted with little if any comment, except when she herself expresses some doubts as to her interpretations. At such times opportunity should be seized to provoke by questions further dubiousness of the abnormal ideation. The husband should be drawn into the treatment program, as well as any important family members.

BIBLIOGRAPHY

Artiss, K. L.: Paranoid thinking in everyday life. Arch. Gen. Psychiat., 14:89–93, 1966.

Carr, A. C.: Observations on paranoia and their relationship to the Schreiber case. Int. J. Psychoanal., 44:195–200, 1963.

Freedman, N., Cutler, R., Engelhardt, D. M., and Reuber, M.: On the modification of paranoid symptomatology. J. Nerv. & Ment. Dis., 144:29–36, 1967.

Freud, S.: Certain neurotic mechanisms in jealousy, paranoia and homosexuality. Internat. J. Psycho-Analysis, 4:1–10, 1923.

Freud, S.: Psychoanalytic Notes upon an Autobiographical Account of a Case of Paranoia. In Collected Papers, Vol. 3, London, Hogarth, 1925.

May, R.: Paranoia and power anxiety. J. Proj. Tech. & Person. Assess., 34:412–418, 1970.

Michaud, R.: La folie à deux (ou folie communiqué). Lasèque, C., et Falret, J. Ann. Med. Psychol., 18:321–355, 1877. English translation and bibliography. Amer. J. Psychiat. (Suppl.), 121:1–23, 1964.

Modlin, H. C.: Psychodynamics and management of paranoid states in women. Arch. Gen. Psychiat., 8:263–268, 1963.

Novey, S.: The outpatient treatment of borderline paranoid states. Psychiatry, 23:357–364, 1960.

Ovesey, L.: Fear of vocational success: a phobic extension of the paranoid reaction. Arch. Gen. Psychiat., 7:88–92, 1962.

West, L. J.: The "Othello Syndrome." Contemporary Psychoanal., 4:103–110, 1968.

Wolowitz, H. B., and Shorkey, C. T.: Power motivation in male paranoid children. Psychiatry, 32:459–466, 1969.

Chapter 24

"The fears we know are of not knowing"

W. H. Auden

The Neuroses

The psychoneuroses comprise a group of personality disturbances that are often described as being intermediate, or as forming a connecting link, between the various adaptive devices unconsciously utilized by the average mind on the one hand and the extreme, often disorganizing, methods observed in the psychotic on the other.

Psychoneurotic personality disorders arise from an effort to deal with specific, private, internal psychological problems and stressful situations that the patient is unable to master without tension or disturbing psychological devices caused by the anxiety aroused. Many regard the affect of anxiety as the common dynamic source of the neuroses. The symptoms of these disorders consist either of a manifestation of anxiety as it is directly felt and expressed or of automatic efforts to control it by such defenses as conversion, dissociation, displacement, phobia formation, or repetitive thoughts and acts. Ordinarily repression, frequently aided by socially acceptable and useful reaction formations, enables the individual to deal comfortably with feelings and situations that tend to create anxiety. In the psychoneuroses, however, repression is never complete enough to prevent both the feeling and manifestation of anxiety and the formation of unconscious, repetitive techniques designed to control it. These feelings and manifestations of anxiety or the methods of adaptation (defenses) to it constitute the symptoms of the neurosis.

The methods of adaptation utilized by those with a psychoneurosis, in addition to their repetitive and unchanging character, are considered to represent behavioral, affective, or psychological traits that proved satisfying at an earlier stage of development. In short, they represent either a regression to an earlier, more gratifying type of behavior, or a failure to develop beyond a fixation at a developmental level that proves inappropriate and inadequate in the face of the responsibilities of later life. Neurotic adaptations are never fully satisfying, since secondarily they lead to feelings of inadequacy, shame, and guilt. In the psychoneuroses, therefore, the symptomatic clinical phenomena are usually not significant in and of themselves but merely indicate that anxiety-producing meaningful situations are perturbing to the individual. Although symptoms observed in the psychoneuroses are described in this chapter, these mental disorders should be studied from a functional rather than from a symptomatic standpoint. Many times, it is true, the symptom may afford a clue to the nature of the underlying problem, but the understanding of a neurosis depends on a recognition of the unconscious, neurotic purpose it serves.

The form of the neurosis is determined largely by the type of defensive measure that the patient employs to control anxiety. Relatively few patients confine themselves to a single type of measure. Many psychoneurotics, therefore, show mixed features. The patient's symptoms represent his defense reaction to an anxiety-producing situation that he finds unmanageable by other means. Regardless of the form that they may assume, it is now realized that the neurotic patient's symptoms are intelligible only in psychological, or rather psychobiological, terms.

The relationship between his emotional conflicts and perturbing situations, on the one hand, and his disturbed personality functioning, on the other, is not recognized by the patient. For example, he may, without any apparent reason and without ideational content, develop an attack of anxiety, or without apparent reason develop a panic-like reaction in a crowd or in an open place. Again, without any recognition of its face-saving function, the patient may develop an invalidism that provides escape from a difficult situation. Another patient may experience the persistent recurrence of an appalling or disgusting thought, or feel an overpowering urge for the repeated, ritual-like performance of some act that serves to ward off anxiety. Aggressive, hostile wishes may become so threatening that the patient has to employ some neurotic mechanism for handling them. These defenses are often so ego-hampering that they are quite burdensome to the patient. Many persons presenting a variety of symptoms and known to the laity by such terms as "nervous invalids" are suffering from psychoneurotic disorders. The term "nervous" is euphemistic and evasive, since there is in fact no physiological disturbance of the nervous system. Each case is a problem of emotional dynamics.

Psychoneuroses Versus Psychoses

Many criteria have been suggested to differentiate between psychoses and psychoneuroses. The great variations in those proposed suggest that the distinctions are superficial. Some designate the psychoses as "major reactions" and the psychoneuroses as "minor reactions," the distinction being made on the extent of the involvement of the personality.

In general, the diagnosis of psychosis implies a greater severity of personality disturbance than occurs in psychoneurosis. The psychoneurotic's defenses against anxiety are largely substitutive or symbolic; the psychotic's defenses are more extreme, regressive, and disregardful of reality. In many instances, there is a difference in their outcome as regards the integrity of the personality. In the psychoses, the distortion or disorganization of personality is often great, and its social functioning is greatly disturbed, whereas in the psychoneuroses the personality usually remains socially organized. In the psychoneuroses, inner experiences do not upset external behavior to the extent or in the abnormal manner that occurs in the psychoses. In the psychotic individual, the capacity for discriminating between subjective experiences and reality may be greatly impaired. In the psychoneurotic individual, there is no grave interference with reality-testing; the ego remains sound. Any evasion of reality is partial and at comparatively little expense to the personality. As Freud put it: "Neurosis does not deny the existence of reality, it merely tries to ignore it; psychosis denies it and tries to substitute something else for it."

The psychotic creates a new environment to which he imputes the forces and properties of reality. He may distort or falsify reality in the form of delusions or hallucinations. The environment of the psychoneurotic remains unchanged, although certain elements may be invested with abnormal affective values. The thinking of the psychotic may be dereistic, a type of thinking not occurring in the psychoneurotic. The content of thought in the psychoneurotic may be temporarily restricted by overvalued ideas, yet true delusional formation does not occur. Associations are frequently disturbed in the psychotic but remain unimpaired in the psychoneurotic. Desires and motives are often projected in the psychotic, but they are never so externalized in the psychoneurotic, at least not to the extent of producing delusions. In the psychotic, repression may be destroyed, the ego being so changed that it will tolerate repressed impulses or fantasies uncritically, or will fail to recognize that they arise from itself. In the psychoneuroses, repression appears to be maintained, but nevertheless the repressed material returns, although in such a distorted form that it is acceptable to the ego.

Conation may be profoundly disturbed in the psychotic, but only to a slight degree does it suffer in the psychoneuroses. In the psychotic the changes in affect may be great, and affective lability is often decreased, while the psychoneurotic affective changes are slight and lability is maintained. Any depression in the psychoneuroses is determined more by evident environmental factors than is the case in psychoses and is accompanied by a greater degree of insight and by an absence of retardation. The psychoneurotic usually retains well his interest in the outer world and he remains sensitive to changes in the social atmosphere; the interest of the psychotic may be lost. The psychoneurotic conforms more nearly to the social norm in his relationships, while the regression of the psychotic may be extreme, but it is not an important mechanism in the psychoneurotic who never, if consciousness is clear, regresses to an infantile level with its excretory soiling.

Generally speaking, the psychotic does not recognize that he is ill and therefore has no desire for change in his subjective status. The psychoneurotic, on the contrary, usually feels keenly his subjective suffering and consciously wants to get well, although it is known that his more powerful unconscious desire is to the contrary.

The psychoneurotic, especially the hysteric, often exploits his symptom for *secondary gain,* whereas the psychotic patient acquires no secondary gain from his illness.

There is no sharp line between the psychoneuroses and the major psychoses. They merge one into the other by intermediate, scarcely perceptible stages. The differences are largely descriptive and ones of degree. Given psychogenic factors may in one individual lead to defenses and reactions characterized as psychoneurotic and in another person to those classified as psychotic. Frequently a reaction that would be classified as neurotic will later assume a form descriptively classified as psychotic. This does not mean that one type of mental illness is being superseded by another form fundamentally different in nature. It is, in fact, the opinion of some psychiatrists that if the life history of a patient suffering from a psychosis not associated with toxic or organic factors is fully known, evidence will always be found of an untreated or inadequately treated preëxisting neurotic-like syndrome out of which the psychosis grew.

In the so-called borderline cases, both neurotic and psychotic mechanisms may be noted.

Here, Kubie suggests that the neurotic process evolves as a chain of progressive distortions in which the sufferer has become enmeshed and trapped in conflicting and unattainable drives. When that process moves farther and to it are added symptoms that are also conflicting and irreconcilable, the individual becomes vulnerable to ego disorganization or psychoses. Thus one may be caught in a conflict over ambitious drives to succeed and the wish to be cared for. Gratified in neither area, and attempting to repress secondary rage, the patient may then elaborate, be overpowered by anxiety, and successively develop contradictory phobias which defeat both the original wishes. It is at this point that psychotic regression may ensue.

Classification of Psychoneurotic Disorders

The psychoneurotic disorders are now classified as follows:

Anxiety
Hysterical
   Conversion type
   Dissociative type
Phobic
Obsessive compulsive
Depressive
Depersonalization
Hypochondriacal
Other

The so-called "types" are not disease entities in genesis, mechanisms, or manifestations. The psychoneuroses should be regarded as a series of varying types of reaction brought about by multiple causative factors that vary from case to case. The more carefully the reactions of the neurotic are examined, the more frequently it will be found that there are no sharply defined lines among the various types of neuroses. It is rare, for example, to find a "pure" hysteria or "pure" obsessional neurosis. Frequently the neurotic will, in varying degrees, show hysterical, obsessional, anxiety, and even psychosomatic manifestations. Thus definite assignment to a certain type may be difficult or arbitrary. Overt anxiety, for example, although the most conspicuous and characteristic symptom in anxiety states, is frequently an important picture in other forms. Also, just as the distinction between the psychoneuroses and the psychoses often is not sharply defined, neither is that between the psychoneuroses and many character traits of the so-called "normal" person who consistently uses the "neurotic process" to fend off anxiety. Far more frequently than is realized, outstanding character traits are really neurotic reaction formations that serve as defenses. Neurotic syndromes fit into the personality pattern of the individual and are allied to the techniques he has employed all his life in handling situations.

Causes

When we seek for the causes of the psychoneuroses, we must conclude that emotional, meaningful factors play a predominant and, in a broad sense, perhaps an exclusive role. Usually from early life the psychoneurotic has shown personality traits that are so deeply rooted in the make-up of the individual that some refer to them as constitutional. Probably, however, these traits are acquired during impressionable years through close association with, dependence upon, and transactions with various members of the family. Most major neurotic patterns are basically dependent on conflicts and feeling-attitudes that arose in childhood; thus in order to understand a patient's neurosis, an attempt should be made to connect the patient's present symptoms with some unliquidated childhood situation. One will therefore agree with Freud's statement that the analyst deals more with scars than with bleeding wounds.

Often the childhood of the psychoneurotic was characterized by such disturbances as sleepwalking, crying out in sleep, enuresis, disturbances of speech, food idiosyncrasies, delirium accompanying slight rises in temperature, destructiveness, emotional excitability, temper tantrums, phobias, compulsions, shyness, nail-biting, and other disguises looked upon as constituting personality and behavior problems. These childhood symptoms should be regarded as evidence that specific conflicts and situational factors produced anxiety and led to neurotic symptoms or character traits. It is necessary, however, not only to examine the childhood background for scars that the special circumstances of early life have left, but to be alert for feelings of guilt, conflicts over unconscious needs, meaningful life-events, recurrent, cumulative stresses and tensions of interpersonal relationship difficulties, and the everyday stresses of family living, including marital or sexual problems. The role that each plays in establishing the primary distortions in the neurotic process, the secondary affects of anxiety, guilt, and shame, and the tertiary defenses in denials in the style of life or in symptomatic defenses are only understandable in careful and detailed study of conscious and unconscious processes in the life of the individual patient.

It is also important to consider that immediate reality factors are not always fundamental etiologic factors but rather precipitating causes. Often it will be found that an apparently smooth adjustment has been a cover for stormy problems that have long existed beneath the surface.

This is the reason that a neurotic reaction may become manifest suddenly even in middle or late life. Thus the seemingly successful compulsive worker in our Western culture may become anxiety-ridden and depressed in the face of a mandatory retirement or the loss of those skills required to maintain his driven performance.

Whatever determined their personalities, there seem to be individuals who are unusually sensitive to tension and conflicts of life, persons who have never really faced its problems and are especially prone to deal with its tensions, wishes, and conflicts by the faulty reactions designated as neurotic. Although the efficiency of most persons is impaired by psychoneurotic tendencies, much of the best work of the world is done as an expression of neurotic disorder. This has been particularly apparent in the case of art and literature.

Of the immediate causes for the development of the psychoneuroses, it may be said they are frequently to be found in the necessity to repress, distort, or displace emotions of hostility or rage or the drives of sexuality and dependency as they emerge and conflict with order and peace in the patient's personality. These and similar factors, often of a conflict-producing nature, create *anxiety,* which is the commonest and most important source of psychoneurotic disorders. Anxiety, engendered by a too severe and exacting superego but perhaps stimulated by an external situation, mobilizes the defenses of the personality.

As already indicated, the manner in which the patient adapts to this anxiety, which is sometimes characterized as the most unpleasant of subjective emotional states, and tries to mobilize the defenses of the personality against it, determines the type of the psychoneurotic reaction. If the anxiety is felt and expressed directly, is "free-floating," and is not confined to definite situations or objects, the neurosis is spoken of as an anxiety state or anxiety neurosis. If the repressed wish or impulse causing the anxiety is "converted" into functional symptoms in organs or parts of the body, the clinical picture is that of conversion hysteria. If the anxiety overwhelms and temporarily controls the individual, the clinical picture is that of hysterical dissociation as in hysterical stupor, fugue, or amnesia. In compulsion neurosis, the patient controls his anxiety by a repetitive activity. This activity or ritual protects the patient against the threat of repressed impulses. In phobias, anxiety is controlled by detaching it from some idea or situation and, by displacement, attaching the fear to some specific object or situation that serves as a symbol.

The psychoneuroses are more frequently diagnosed in women than in men, partly because of the fact that a more rigid repression of basic biological needs and instincts is required of women, with the result that anxiety defenses in the form of neurotic symptoms are more frequently required than in men. The psychosexual life, with its many taboos and social restrictions, is by no means, however, the only factor, since any fundamental urge or desire against the expression of which a defensive barrier must be constructed, or the gratification of which must be vicarious, may give rise to neurotic symptoms. Feelings of guilt, social situations, or irritating relationships that strain the ability to adjust, or marriage with its new responsibilities are examples of the many factors that may contribute to a neurosis. In a married woman, a chronic marital dissatisfaction and disappointment may contribute to the development of a psychoneurosis. The husband may not have proved to be the ideal mate that was expected, desired demonstrations of affection may have been lacking, or marriage may have failed to be the sustained romance that the wife had dreamed it would be. She may deny any dissatisfaction that may be consciously acknowledged only if she frankly faces her feelings. Other women, interested in a business or professional career, or hesitant to exhibit any interest in, or behavior toward, the opposite sex that would lead to marriage, may put it off until they reach an age when opportunities for marriage are infrequent. The sense of frustration and of a certain emptiness of life may lead to a neurotic reaction. Again, the involutional period, with its reluctantly acknowledged psychological implications, may be accompanied by anxiety, depression, or irritability that is readily converted into functional symptoms.

At times a psychoneurosis may develop as an indirect result of long-continued physical illness. In such a case, the prolonged and perhaps severe illness may threaten the patient's sense of security, compel him to give up activities and interests that have been highly prized, or jeopardize his ability to function at his previous level. Such factors may stimulate an anxiety that had previously been handled without difficulty.

Most neuroses of adults develop between late adolescence and 35 years of age. This is the period when the individual becomes confronted with the problems of adult adjustments and responsibilities. It is the period when satisfying social, economic, and sexual situations should be established. Frustrations in these critically important fields may lead to conflict and anxiety that can be met only by neurotic mechanisms.

Elaborate disguises, including fears which have no obvious connections with immediate realities and make the neurotic's behavior more or less incomprehensible both to himself and others, are among the conspicuous features of neurotic behavior. A rational explanation for the apparently unintelligible behavior will be found, however, when its psychodynamics is studied. It will be observed, too, that neurotic syndromes tend to fit into the established personality pattern of the individual and are allied to the techniques he has employed all his life in handling difficult situations.

In some psychoneurotic reactions, particularly in anxiety states, the patient often fears the existence of some serious physical disease, whereas the causes of the symptoms are in fact purely psychogenic. In such cases, the patient will usually not accept the psychiatrist's assurance of good physical health unless the physician has first made such a painstaking physical examination and has shown such open-mindedness and true interest concerning the possible existence of physical disease as will make the patient willing to accept the physician's statement that he has no organic basis for the symptoms. It should be emphasized, however, that a diagnosis of psychoneurosis cannot be made merely by the exclusion of organic factors. It can be made only on the discovery of positive factors in the psychological sphere sufficiently pertinent to offer a logical explanation for the symptoms. This evidence is to be found in a study of the patient's personality aimed both at an analysis of the present picture and at a reconstruction of the sequences of psychological experiences that have influenced personality development and structure. It will frequently be found that as time passes a neurosis becomes more complex and irradiates into more aspects of life.

Prevalence

Certainly the psychoneuroses are the most ubiquitous of the disorders that afflict man. The exact prevalence is uncertain, owing largely to the differences in definition which exist among psychiatrists, the varying cultural attitudes to certain psychoneurotic character traits and symptoms, and the variable methods used to collect the data. A recent study by Taylor and Chaves of an English town found neurotic symptoms insufficient to bring the sufferer to medical attention in 330 per 1000 residents. Eighty-one per 1000 sought help for such symptoms from a general practitioner, 44 per 1000 attended a psychiatric outpatient department, and 1.9 per 1000 were admitted to a hospital for a period of treatment. In various surveys of general hospital services and clinics as well as practice of general physicians, upwards of 30 to 40 per cent of patients who come for treatment have been considered to have a psychoneurosis, either as the primary diagnosis or in conjunction with and complicating other illnesses. A recent study of the practice of internists in New York City found that approximately 10 per cent of patients examined on the first visit on referral from general practitioners had mental, psychoneurotic, or personality disorders; probably the vast majority were psychoneurotic.

CHARACTER NEUROSES

While the official schemes of classification of the neuroses designate the subvarieties in terms of the predominant psychological defenses, it is generally recognized by practicing psychiatrists that each psychoneurotic patient has a distinctive character structure. This character structure, usually referred to now as the *character neurosis,* has served as a means of containing anxiety, of repressing it in the individual's ongoing interpersonal transaction. It is betrayed by his more or less fixed attitudes, affectations, and mannerisms, a variegated host of traits of relating himself to others, as well as by deeply rooted and persisting affects held over from infancy and childhood. These characterologic manifestations of the neuroses are perceived with difficulty unless one has the opportunity of relating to the patient closely over prolonged periods. They are rarely the subject of complaint at the time the psychoneurotic presents himself for examination; he is most likely then to state his problem in terms of symptoms expressive of anxiety or the psychological defenses against it. His family, close friends and others, whom he sees frequently and regularly, usually have some recognition of the rigidities and peculiarities of his behavior that constitute the neurotic façade or character. Some character traits serve to discharge drives or impulses while others are reactive. The latter are sometimes referred to as "character armor" protecting the individual from arousal of conflict through attitudes of avoidance or opposition.

Environmental situations which face the personality with unusual intensity or duration or unexpected expressions of stress are those that break through the ego "character armor." It is then that the personality responds with the open expression of symptoms recognized in the well-known varieties of neuroses.

Certain of the neurotic personalities and their expressions in characteristic attitudes and traits are described in Chapter 6, e.g., the hysterical and obsessive personality. In some the neurotic character fixations are seen in actions typifying excessive dependency or submission to others and often arise from a continuing feeling of personal insignificance which leads to overvaluation of others. Ingratiating and self-effacing behavior coupled sometimes with demanding requests for affection and appreciation represents one form of this character. Others may demonstrate their character defense in repetitive and persistent tendencies to mistrust or dominate their fellows, or to insist on their self-sufficiency; thus they become detached. Still others are masochistically self-sacrificing, constrained or inhibited in asserting their talents, or insistent on rigid ways of behavior under the guise of seeking an unrealistic or idealistic goal. Some are compulsively driven to activity, others to a repetitive search for relief from anxiety through sensual means in long series of sexual or oral efforts. The need to dominate in order to suppress the anxiety of insecurity may be expressed in the drive to accumulate wealth or position, to excel others in giving or in spending, or to overvalue collections of facts and ideas.

Today in centers where knowledge of dynamic psychiatry is widespread and numerous psychoanalysts are available, increasing numbers of those with psychoneuroses present themselves for treatment of the character disturbances prior to dissolution of this ego defense and emergence of frank psychoneurotic symptoms.

ANXIETY REACTIONS

As previously indicated, anxiety may be described as a painful uneasiness of mind, a state of heightened tension accompanied by an inexpressible dread, a feeling of apprehensive expectation. It may arise with any situation that constitutes a threat to the personality. The emergence of repressed material is particularly apt to be anxiety-producing. Anxiety may arise, for example, when self-requirements and the security of the personality are threatened by the danger of a breakdown in the repression of forbidden sexual desires or of attempts to ward off loneliness through dependency or of unconscious hostile and aggressive feelings. Again, anxiety with its obsessive apprehensiveness may arise in association with frustrations or dilemmas occuring in some major life problem related to such topics as vocational, sexual, or marital adjustment.

In the other psychoneurotic reactions, some specific, auxiliary form of psychological defense mechanism is devised to control anxiety. In anxiety reactions, however, there is no such specific method of defense. Repression alone is insufficient to control the anxiety. As a result the anxiety, not being displaced as in phobic reactions, not being "converted" into functional symptoms as in hysteria, not being discharged by some gross personality disorganization such as dissociation, fugue, or amnesia, and not being automatically controlled by some repetitive thought or act, remains diffuse and uncontrolled, with the result that the patient is in a state of constant anxious expectation. Anxiety reaction is therefore sometimes spoken of as the simplest form of neurosis.

If the diffuse anxiety is not too painful, it may be expressed or controlled through certain personality traits. Individuals who are constantly beset by pervading anxiety are characteristically tense, timid, apprehensive, sensitive to the opinions of others, easily embarrassed, and tend to worry. Many persons with such a constant sense of anxiety are self-distant, given to inferiority feelings, experience difficulty in making decisions, and are afraid of making mistakes. Usually they are scrupulous, overconscientious, ambitious, and feel that they must live up to self-imposed high standards. Although such a person suffers moderate distress through apprehension and other tendencies previously noted, the tension is not usually intolerable. If, however, the anxiety becomes more disturbing, it may be expressed in such symptoms as depression, sleeplessness, irritability, restlessness, a paralyzing indecision, psychosomatic disturbances, outbursts of aggressiveness, attacks of weeping, and feelings of inadequacy and inferiority accompanied, perhaps, by a paranoid attitude. Usually the patient with an anxiety reaction feels chronically fatigued and complains of inability to concentrate. Some express the fear that they are "becoming insane."

Anxiety Attacks

In addition to a chronic state of tension and mild anxiety, the patient with anxiety neurosis may be subject to acute, terrifying, panic-like exacerbations lasting from a few moments to an hour. The patient suffers from rapid heartbeat, palpitation, precordial discomfort, nausea, diarrhea, desire to urinate, dyspnea, and a feeling of choking or suffocation. The pupils are dilated, the face is flushed, and the skin perspires; the patient suffers from paresthesias and tremulousness, feels dizzy or faint, and often has a sense of weakness and of impending death. Restlessness is acute, and tremulousness, feels dizzy or faint, and often has a sense of weakness and of the psychophysiological mechanism of hyperventilation is described; this is the mechanism that causes these symptoms in perhaps the majority of acute anxiety attacks. Other physiological expressions of acute anxiety perhaps occur through activation of various segments of the autonomic nervous system and the adrenal medulla and its secretions. In an acute reactive anxiety attack, the clinical picture may be colored by a traumatic situation. This is well illustrated in the anxiety attacks of combat neurosis.

The patient who is subject to acute anxiety attacks usually suffers also from a chronic anxiety state. He experiences difficulty in falling asleep, is disturbed by fearful dreams, suffers from coarse tremors or "trembling," and complains of a "band around the head" or of a "quivering in the stomach." He is absent-minded and seems worried without knowing about what or why. He complains that his mind is in a constant daze and that he is unable to control his thoughts. He is apprehensive and is afraid to be alone, yet he does not desire conversation. He feels too tired to attempt anything constructive and continually seeks a physical explanation for his distressing mental state.

Physicians lacking an appreciation of psychological factors in the production of symptoms have at times erred in failing to recognize that the precipitating factors which induce anxiety attacks are psychological, not physiological. They have diagnosed them as heart disease, thyrotoxicosis, hyperinsulinism, or dysinsulinism.

The anxiety reactions are most frequently associated with phobic defenses that are often overlooked. Untreated, the phobic anxiety state, often designated "anxiety hysteria," may extend with either the development of obsessive ideation and disappearance of the acute anxiety reactions or progressive withdrawal associated with phobic diffusion that leads to a state of helpless isolation simulating a psychotic regression.

A 27-year-old woman entered the hospital complaining of multiple fears. She was too frightened to get on streetcars or buses, to go to the movies, and to go out to supper. She was also afraid that she would not live up to the expectations of her mother, was dubious about her own capabilities, and indicated that her marriage was in difficult straits and that she had previously been separated from her husband for 18 months. She stated that their only son was a bed wetter. In addition, she presented the symptoms of acute anxiety with palpitation, perspiration, dizziness, and shortness of breath caused by the hyperventilation syndrome.

Brief questioning elicited the information that her mother had been a nagging, sadistic person, who unmercifully switched the patient and her brother whenever they failed to obey her command. The father, a mild, subservient individual, had seldom been at home. The patient was a quiet and obedient, though fearful, child, usually timid and retiring, who felt that she must always acquiesce to the wishes of others or be subject to their criticism and withdrawal of affection.

The diagnosis in this case was long-standing anxiety neurosis, associated with the hyperventilation syndrome and a phobic state. The anxiety attacks occurred regularly in situations in which the patient's husband, mother, or even the doctor did something or said something to arouse in her a fear of separation associated with a wish to retaliate angrily. She could not allow herself to express further criticism and rejections. Although the majority of anxiety attacks were relieved after several months of psychiatric treatment, she was not entirely free of her symptoms until a year of regular visits had elapsed.

Treatment

Two phases of an anxiety reaction require attention—one, the acute anxiety attack, the other, the anxiety neurosis. During the attack, the rapid pulse and pounding heart lead the patient to believe that only a heart attack could have produced his distress. After an examination of the heart and other organs has been made and no physical disorder discovered, the patient should be confidently assured that he has no heart disease. Frequently, the cause of the symptoms may be demonstrated easily by the simple medium of requesting the patient to overbreathe for a period of two minutes, as described in Chapter 25 under the hyperventilation syndrome. Further somatic complaints should be disregarded and the examination of the heart should not be repeated. The patient should not, through the use of drugs, be led to believe that his pathologic condition is physical rather than emotional, and rest should not be advised, nor should personal reassurance be repeated to a degree that the patient constantly feels the need for it.

Treatment of the basic neurosis may commence with an attempt to relieve symptomatic distress through the use of the hypnotics or minor tranquilizers. These alone are seldom sufficient unless the anxiety is produced by a transient social stress.

At the same time, attention should be

directed to uncovering the unrecognized sources of anxiety, to the action of psychodynamic factors, to their adjustment, and to reëducation. Less attention should be paid to the anxiety attacks than to a study of the patient's personality and to attitudes and situations that cause frustration and tension. Although a more formal analysis is desirable in severe anxiety neuroses, many patients with milder cases can be helped by a psychotherapy on the conscious level and by a face-to-face discussion. Consideration should be given to the meaning of symptoms, the role of emotions, the stress of present circumstances, and the effect of well-remembered past experience in molding present attitudes and habits of thinking and feelings. The demonstration of a correlation between the time when anxiety appeared and certain preceding events in the patient's life history may give insight sufficient to produce considerable relief. A desire to violate self-imposed rigid standards may at times be discovered. Troublesome sex problems, including any arising from faulty contraceptive technique, should be adjusted. The patient should be encouraged to continue physical exercise and recreation. If chronic tension states and associated muscular pains occur in neck and shoulders, physiotherapy is helpful.

Meprobamate, the various phenothiazines, and the barbiturates may be used to provide symptomatic relief from the chronic symptoms of anxiety.

In the chronic anxiety states associated with phobias, in addition to the dynamic psychotherapies described in brief above, trials have been made recently of the behavioral therapies. Both are described in later chapters of the book. Prolonged and permanently disabling anxiety states have been benefited by prefrontal lobotomy when all other measures have failed.

PHOBIC REACTION

While phobias are among the more common symptoms in populations of pa-

tients recognized to have a psychiatric disability, the phobic reaction *per se* is diagnosed relatively infrequently. A figure of approximately 3 per cent has been found in reports from psychiatric clinics in the United States. Perhaps the failure to report the phobic reaction more frequently is due to the common association of this symptom with anxiety, and also its occurrence in association with other psychoneurotic symptoms. Phobias, and their associated dynamisms and treatment, are discussed in the next section. Phobias are reported to be twice as common among women as among men.

As mentioned in the previous section of this chapter, phobias are present in a large number of the chronically apprehensive persons who suffer anxiety attacks. At one time this triad of symptoms, so well described by Freud in his original paper on the anxiety neurosis, was designated *anxiety hysteria*. It was his study of "little Hans," reported in his paper "Analysis of a Phobia in a Five-Year-Old Boy," upon which rests the psychodynamic understanding of phobic reactions. Freud interpreted the fear of Hans of going into the street because he was afraid that a horse would bite him as a displacement of the boy's fear of his father. That fear was inferred to have its origin in expected punishment for his unconscious hostility toward the father in his competition with him for his mother's affection. Thus the displacement of the fear to the horse avoided the exposure of his hostility and the fear of retaliation and permitted him to retain his love for his father.

Thus a phobic reaction is a defensive one in which the patient attempts to deal with his anxiety by detaching it from a specific idea, object, or situation in his daily life and displacing it to some associated object, situation, or idea in the form of a specific neurotic fear. Although the patient consciously recognizes that no actual danger exists, if exposed to the specific phobia-stimulating symbolic object or situation, he is powerless to keep from experiencing an intense sense of fear. The intensely distressing sense of apprehension associated with the consciously feared object or situation is actually derived from other sources—sources of which the patient is unaware. A defense against the anxiety arising from this unrecognized source is provided through the mechanisms of displacement and symbolization. By these means, the anxiety is detached from its real source—unconscious, forbidden tendencies and impulses, for example—and displaced to some situation or object that is usually symbolic of the threatening tendency or wish. A great variety of phobias have been described. Among them are fear of dirt, of bacteria, of certain animals, of travel by a certain type of vehicle. Many of them have Greek names attached to them, as agoraphobia, a fear of open places, or claustrophobia, a fear of confined spaces. A claustrophobia might, for example, prevent the occupancy of a Pullman berth.

When exposed to the specific situation that evokes his fear, the phobic experiences faintness, fatigue, palpitation, perspiration, nausea, and tremor. This is the typical acute anxiety attack, usually expressed in hyperventilation. He may be unable to continue with the duty at hand and be overwhelmed with panic. He can control his anxiety if he avoids the phobic object or situation. If the patient were to carry out the feared activity, it would unconsciously mean to him that he was performing the forbidden activity that arouses the dreaded anxiety. He also constantly punishes himself for his unconscious tendencies and impulses by the distressing restrictions and sufferings imposed by his phobia.

A major component of the phobic reaction is the avoidance pattern. While avoidance of the feared situation, person, or idea allows a partial control of anxiety and for a time allays the fears, very often the phobic avoidance fails and the sufferer has a distressing outbreak of anxiety under situations other than the feared one. Then the displacement is generalized to new situations and additional phobias evolve. In some the generalization of the phobic reaction is so widespread that their

activities eventually become circumscribed to a few rooms and they become socially isolated.

The maintenance of the phobia often depends upon the secondary gains obtained through the control the symptoms may exercise upon those with whom the patient lives. The phobic wife now leaves her home only in the company of her husband, and he may leave her alone only at the risk of a terrifying anxiety attack. It is this aspect of the phobic reaction that is so conspicuous in the school phobias of children, which require treatment for the participation of the family member or members engaged in the symbiotic perpetuation of the symptom.

The phobic sufferer oftentimes comes from a family in which the mother is fearful of her aggression, is herself phobic, and is unable to exact conforming behavior except through nagging insistence from the children and even the father. If the father overtly complies with the mother's phobic insistence, even through he appears firm, some of the children may become phobic as well, as this becomes the dominant adaptation for control. Simple association is considered by many to determine the choice of the phobic object to which displacement occurs. Psychoanalytic theory, however, suggests that the choice of phobic object is made on the basis of its symbolic meanings.

The success phobia is a subtle expression of this reaction. Unconsciously fearful of retaliation for aggressive aspirations, men or women with this phobia suffer outbreaks of anxiety at those times when they verge on some personal success. Later the partial avoidance of competitive success may be followed by periodic depressive reactions as a substitute for the anxiety which may occur when a desired position is achieved.

The *counterphobic defense,* while seemingly very different from the avoidance behavior of the usual phobic sufferer, nevertheless bears a dynamic relation. In this instance the sufferer attempts to master his anxiety by repetitive confrontation with the phobic object and may, if successful, evolve a drive to gratifying repetition. Its senseless and compulsive bravado distinguishes it from anxiety-free confrontation.

In terms of differential diagnosis, phobias may occur in association with many other psychiatric symptoms and syndromes. These are discriminated from obsessive thoughts by the associated affect. With phobias the affect is anxiety with obsessive guilt. Most adults suffer minor fears of an emotional nature which may transiently impede but not affect their social functioning. According to Marks, one may classify adult phobias into those related to external situations, of which the agoraphobic syndrome is the commonest and most distressing, or those of internal situations. The agoraphobic syndrome relates to irrational and repetitive states of apprehension and anxiety, commencing in adult life, related to entering into public places or going out alone. These states are amenable to treatment with the dynamic and behavioral psychotherapies. They are reported by some to be alleviated through use of antidepressant medications.

The phobias of internal stimuli, related to assumed illness such as cancer, heart disease, venereal disease, and the like, more frequently have an obsessive character and are discovered in the neurotic hypochondriacal states or as symptoms of incipient schizophrenia.

Animal phobias are usually uncommon monosymptomatic fears commencing in childhood before the age of eight. Marks states that patients with such phobias condition differently from adult phobic patients. The animal phobias often respond well to behavioral desensitization techniques, in contrast to the agoraphobic syndrome of adults.

HYSTERICAL NEUROSES

Dissociative Reactions

At times anxiety may so overwhelm and disorganize the personality that certain aspects or functions of it become disso-

ciated from each other. In some instances, the personality may be so disorganized that defense mechanisms govern consciousness, memory, and temporarily even the total individual, with little or no participation on the part of the conscious personality. In such a case the patient may appear psychotic. Formerly the dissociative reactions were classified as a type of conversion hysteria.

One of the commonest anxiety-stimulated and defensive dissociative reactions is *amnesia*. Forgetting is a simple expedient. It is therefore not surprising that amnesias obliterate recollections, particularly for definitely circumscribed periods of time. Dissociative amnesia is, however, not a mere forgetting. It is an active process, a blotting out of awareness of unpleasant features. Periods of stupor or of twilight state may precede such an amnesia, which then tends to become selective and limited to the particular element or experience that evoked it. Among experiences that suspend the ability to bring pertinent factual data to consciousness are those involving great terror, as in war, or covering periods and behavior with which shame, guilt, or other intense feeling-tone is connected. How satisfactorily an amnesia exercises its protective and escape purpose is shown by the unperturbed manner in which the patient accepts his loss of memory. Although most dissociative amnesias are of brief duration, they sometimes blot out long periods, sometimes even the patient's entire previous life. In some instances, there is a reversion to an earlier period of the patient's life, with retrograde amnesia for events subsequent to that period. In differentiating between an organic and a dissociative amnesia, it will be found that a sudden return of memory is indicative of its dissociative loss. The onset, also, of the dissociative amnesia will have been sudden.

Dissociative reactions are characterized by mental symptoms involving *disturbances of consciousness*. These may be in the form of stupor or of various forms of "twilight state." Frequently the latter suggests delirium. Such psychogenic delirious states are usually preceded by marked emotional experiences or displays and consist of dream states accompanied by more or less confusion, dramatic posturings and activities, and an excessive flow of speech appearing nonsensical, but in which occur references to strongly affective experiences. Dissociative delirium often represents the dream-like realization of a wish or the dramatic reliving in fantasy of an affectively traumatic experience. Its clouding of consciousness and the presence of illusions and hallucinations may exclude the reality of the outside world and falsify it in accordance with deep-seated motives and unsatisfied wishes. Occasionally the patient spins fantastic stories. Such instances usually represent an effort to supply romance and drama to a life devoid of emotional satisfactions.

To be differentiated from the dissociative deliria are those sudden disruptions of ego functioning which take place under severe emotional stress in those with hysterical personalities. These conditions, referred to as *hysterical psychoses,* are transient and seldom persist more than three or four weeks. Usually the outbreak of this acute delusional-hallucinatory experience takes place dramatically after a period of mounting frustration in some important personal relationship. Often the precipitating event for the anxiety occurred in perception of a threat or loss of the significant relationship, a death, or some act of aggression. On analysis the hallucinatory and delusionary experiences may be discovered as representing family themes, preoccupations, or persisting anxieties. They are, as Richman and White state, family syntonic. The condition resolves rapidly, particularly if the dynamic forces of the outbreak are brought into the open and the patient is led, through interpretation, to understand them. It is to be differentiated from acute schizophrenia; the personality of the hysterical psychotic is not schizoid, nor is the schizophrenic thought disorder evident.

At times a psychic escape may be in the form of a dissociative *fugue.* In this there is a sudden change in state of consciousness, during which the patient may be impelled by unconscious forces to perform complicated activities, perhaps involving travel over long distances. Throughout this period, the patient may appear quite normal to the casual observer. In some instances there is a loss of personal identity. In the fugue the patient indulges in acts or fantasies that are in conflict with his superego, and the function of the fugue is to permit the carrying out of these acts or fantasies. A further defense mechanism becomes necessary, however, and so the patient attempts to protect his ego by forgetting his name and past history, that is, by losing his identity. In other instances there is not a loss in personal identity but a change in it. In such a case the patient assumes a false name and identifies himself with the person whose name he takes. The assumption of the false name is associated with the unconscious fantasies responsible for the genesis of the fugue. O. Henry has presented a delightful picture of a dissociative fugue in his misnamed short story, "A Case of Aphasia." As Fisher[*] points out, the psychological formula is as if the patient says, "I did not commit this crime, because I am not I; I am somebody else."

After the termination of the fugue, the patient may have a complete amnesia for his journey until the memory of it is restored by hypnosis or other psychic means.

Examination of the patient either by sodium amytal narcosis or by other means of ascertaining subconscious mental content usually reveals the personal, emotional factors that prompted an escape mechanism in the form of an automatic, unconscious, uncontrollable withdrawal. In certain recent studies, it has been found that the fugue state is preceded by depression and may be regarded as an attempt to ward off this affect. The model for a number of fugue states apparently has

---

[*] Fisher, C.: Amnesic states in war neuroses. The psychogenesis of fugues. Psychoanalytic Quart., *14:*460, 1945.

been supplied by a previous head injury with a resulting amnesia, or amnesic states induced through alcohol, or identification with others who suffered dissociative reactions.

Ganser Syndrome

This rare syndrome, with its combination of instinctive, rational, purposeful, and deceptive elements and theatrical behavior, is an alteration of consciousness allied both to simulation and to dissociative dream states. In this syndrome, first described as occurring among prisoners under detention while awaiting trial, the patient, being in a situation that would be solved or mitigated by irresponsibility, desires, although not consciously so acknowledged, to appear irresponsible, and accordingly, without being aware of it, actually does develop mental disturbance. The conspicuous features of this disorder consist of a childish, ludicrous performance of simple acts, the correct procedure for which is fully known by the patient. The patient's responses to questions are wrong but are not far wrong and bear an obvious relation to the question. His replies show that he understood the meaning of the questions, but they are beside the point and are in the nature of approximate answers—a phenomenon known as paralogia, or "Vorbeireden." Thus, if asked how long he has been in the hospital, he might reply, "I could have come just now, couldn't I?" Or if asked the color of his shirt, he would reply giving a color other than the correct one. The purpose of the patient's behavior appears so obviously irresponsible that he may seem to be malingering. Since the circumstances under which the Ganser syndrome occurs are such that the advantages to be gained by a mental disability are greater than those obtained by physical disorders, the reaction takes place in terms of the former rather than of conversion hysteria. As in other dissociative reactions, the protection from a full realization of his situation affords the patient a relative freedom from

the anxiety that might otherwise be intolerable.

In Whitlock's recent review of the reported cases and a study of some six additional patients whom he considers to fit into the Ganser syndrome, he suggests that one should more properly regard the condition as psychotic. In many of the cases reported classic paralogia or "Vorbeireden" has followed acute cerebral trauma or appeared in the course of an acute psychosis of schizophrenic nature. Also, its occurrence has been noted often in those other than prisoners. Whitlock concludes that the basic element is disturbance of consciousness, which separates the condition from hysterical pseudodementia. He would restrict the diagnoses to patients who develop clouding of consciousness with paralogia following head trauma or with acute or psychotic reactions in which one may note a number of hallucinations and conversion symptoms. So, too, the condition must terminate abruptly.

CONVERSION REACTIONS

In a conversion reaction, anxiety, instead of being consciously experienced, either diffusely as in anxiety reactions, or displaced as in phobias, is "converted" into functional symptoms in organs or parts of the body innervated by the sensorimotor nervous system. The conversion symptoms serve to prevent or lessen any conscious, felt anxiety and usually symbolize the underlying mental conflict that is productive of anxiety. The reaction usually meets some need of the patient and therefore not merely serves as a defense against anxiety but also provides some more or less obvious "secondary gain," a phenomenon discussed in this chapter. Viewed a little differently, the hysterical symptoms may be regarded as expressing a conflict or an idea in symbolic form. It may, for example, "convert" a mental concept into a significant body symptom, as when hysterical paralysis of an arm expresses a wish to do a forbidden act, yet ambivalently prevents its accomplishment. The form of the conversion symptom is determined by some feature of the situation it was designed to meet.

If a person were consciously to counterfeit some physical sign or symptom of some mental disturbance for the purpose of attaining a particular objective, we would say that he was *malingering*. Conscious recognition of its intent is not necessary, however, in order that behavior may be purposive. In conversion hysteria, the symptoms, without awareness on part of the patient, provide some form and extent of solution for his problems and afford him a certain relief from the anxiety involved in the perturbing situation. Some hysterical phenomena are on the borderline between psychoneurotic reactions and simulation and therefore come close to malingering. Just where, as to awareness, the line between simulation and hysteria should be drawn is therefore arbitrary. In both there is a subtle interweaving of conscious factors. Both are related to some definite purpose, usually protective or wish-fulfilling in nature. It is not surprising that the difference in the hysteric's mind between reality and fantasy is often vague.

Causes

The immediate factor in the production of a conversion reaction is some anxiety-producing situation. With the frequent exception of the traumatic hysterias, we find that the conversion reactions of civilian life tend to develop on a certain personality background characterized by immaturity in the psychosexual and emotional fields. The most common personality type subject to expression of conversion symptoms is the hysterical, but those with passive-aggressive personality disorders, as well as certain obsessive and schizoid individuals, also are prone to such symptom development. Thus today, the diagnosis of "conversion reaction" is not thought synonymous with the designation of "hysterical personality," although the majority of sufferers of conversion symptoms have such a personality make-up.

Accepting conversion reactions as occurring in many other personality reactions than the hysterical and even applying diagnostic criteria as demanding in terms of symptom expression as those required by Woodruff, Clayton, and Guze to establish the diagnosis of hysteria, they found a prevalence of 2 per cent among a general female population.

Puberty is a favorite period for the appearance of conversion reactions. What may be called the normal psychic characteristics of that period are often found to persist in the mental life of the adult who is subject to conversion. Maturing drives, for example, may remain in an arrested or infantile state of development, a state to which a failure to attain an emotional independence from a parent sometimes contributes. Impulses, sentiments, and other bases of the personality are not integrated into a harmonious system. Some, with their immature personality development, are basically hostile and aggressive persons.

Although reference has already been made to the type of individual who seems predisposed to hysteria, further mention may be made of some of the personality characteristics frequently observed in the hysteric. It will often be found that evasions and mechanisms of retreat have been habitual since early life. The narcissism that tends to characterize her arrested personality development makes her prone to a self-display that if often expressed in childish and dramatic ways. Persons of the hysterical type of personality desire an immediate gratification of their wishes but avoid effort to gain their goal. They are self-engrossed, offended by trifles, and dependent in attitude; they bid for sympathy and attention and are given to suicidal "gestures." Such acts are not with intent to die. The threat or shock of the apparent attempt is used by the hysteric to control her environment, to gain attention, to arouse sympathy, or to frighten others into submission. Many seek to rule their environment by being sick, pitiful, and appealing. Such persons exaggerate any existing physical symptoms and even precipitately develop those of a critical or unique nature. Attention-getting, secondary-gain complaints are common. Craig called attention to the fact that hysterics, with their immature personalities, rarely react with awe, reverence, wonder, or pity; they may exhibit self-depreciation, remorse, or grief, but if so, it is because those emotions are the ones that gain them the greatest attention or best obtain a desired domination over their environment. These are the characteristics which often make such patients "special" in hospitals.

Hysterical patients are notoriously suggestible, and their symptoms tend to follow the fashion of their particular period. One now rarely sees the dramatic posturings that were common in Charcot's clinic or the astasia-abasia of Victorian women. They are frequently, however, imitations of actions or disabilities either seen or read about. If a hysterical patient, confronted with some difficult and unpleasant situation, observes the successful evasion of a similar situation by another person, that patient may develop the same symptoms as a means of escape. Such imitations of symptoms were so frequent in World Wars I and II that attempts were made to isolate from the observation of their associates those soldiers who had escaped combat service through hysterical disabilities.

In ordinary civil life, wishes, struggles, and disappointments associated with the sex life form, especially in women, one of the most important groups of experiences that produce the major forms of hysteria. The sexual impulse, although often active, may fail to develop toward a natural goal and is gratified in fantasy and autoerotic habits. A confused admixture of sexual desire and aversion, of erotic feelings and prudish attitudes often exists. Erotic fantasies often contrast with conscious expressions of fear and disgust in regard to sexuality. Among the problems that in women may give rise to hysteria are an unsuccessful love affair; jealousy, perhaps arising from the marriage of a sister; an undesired marriage; fear of pregnancy; difficulties in intercourse; or an unhappy marriage. Many such women are sexually frigid.

The developmental histories of such women make evident the sources for the disordered psychosexuality. In contrast to the earlier concept that the disorder resulted from disturbances in the Oedipal period, it often commences in the initial maternal relationship. In many instances the mother, of hysterical make-up herself, has been rejecting, arousing in the child retaliatory fantasies that have been repressed. The mother often has been recognized as hypocritical about sex, dependent herself, and subtly clinging to the child for whom she has special ambitions. The father of such patients is inadequate, repressing this through either alcoholism or passivity and usually derogated by the mother. This family situation forces the child to perceive her mother ambivalently —as "good" or "bad"—often "good" in the sense of offering concern during illness and as setting idealistic standards for repression of sexual and aggressive activity. She, however, is "bad" in lacking in tenderness, and her interest, even though denied, in the father and other siblings exaggerates feelings of jealous rivalry in the child. The latter, rejected herself, envies the father or male siblings, who she considers receive preferential treatment from the mother. Fixed to the mother, yet envying the father and brothers, she displays early tomboyishness, enuresis, difficulty with menstruation, and later difficulty in acceptance of the feminine role, which is shown in frigidity, vomiting in pregnancy, or hostile seductiveness with men. In all these reactions, the hysterical symptoms symbolically express her conflicts and confusion in regard to her sexual identification.

In men, threats to self-esteem, to economic success, or to self-preservation more frequently present situations from which escape is sought through the hysterical symptoms. Many men are of immature personality with a strong dependent attachment to a mother.

Striking forms of hysterical reactions, such as functional incapacities and symptoms with histrionic features, occur largely among young people. Such hysterical states rarely occur during or after middle age, by which time more permanent and less dramatic protective mechanisms have been established.

Frequently the factor or event that precipitated a conversion reaction may have been trivial but had some special meaning to the patient. Sometimes the precipitating situation may have some special similarity to a previous occurrence. It is therefore well to ascertain what the setting was at the time of appearance of the conversion reaction and also what the patient's emotional state was at the time. The nature of the earlier experiences that give special meaning to the precipitating event and the patient's predisposition to respond with a selective conversion mechanism may usually be determined only by psychoanalysis, although much recall may emerge in hypnotic or narcosynthetic states.

Symptoms

The nature of the hysterical symptoms is often determined by some need or feature of the situation that produced them and the type of disability that will be most useful in satisfying the subconscious purpose they are designed to meet. As a rule, the more turbulent the emotional undercurrents and the greater the disturbance of strong impulsive strivings, the more acute and striking the manifestations and the greater the evidence of anxiety.

Physical symptoms may be sensory or motor. The *motor disturbances* in hysteria are various. In all of them, function is disturbed without demonstrable physiological or anatomical change. Paralyses may be in the form of monoplegia, hemiplegia, or paraplegia and may be either flaccid or spastic. The deep reflexes are not lost in flaccid forms; they may be

exaggerated in the spastic forms, but there are no true clonus and no Babinski reaction. In hemiplegia the paralysis of the proximal muscles is greater than of the peripheral, being in this respect the contrary of that existing in organic hemiplegia. The forearm is extended instead of being somewhat flexed, as in organic hemiplegia; the leg is dragged instead of being swung in circumduction. There is no appreciable wasting of the paralyzed extremities. The maintenance of normal electrical reactions in flaccid paralysis is diagnostic, as is an absence of bladder symptoms or of tendency to bedsores in paraplegia. Contractures are not uncommon. A fairly frequent form is that of a tightly clenched fist. In hysterical paralyses, the muscles in question may be used in one voluntary movement and not in another. An attempt to exercise the paralyzed function is accompanied by a display of excessive effort. A not uncommon conversion symptom in women is that of urinary retention. Patients with this symptom are notoriously lacking in knowledge of urogenital anatomy and functions, have much guilt over early sexual exploration, and often have identified with other family members with urinary symptoms due to either a psychogenic or a physical cause.

Tics, tremors, usually coarse in nature, and choreiform and clonic movements occur. Aphonia, in which the patient cannot phonate speech but continues to cough as formerly, is not rare. Whereas in aphonia the patient finds no difficulty in communicating in whispers, the patient with hysterical mutism can utter no word, although he communicates freely and correctly in writing—a point of differentiation from aphasia. One patient who developed hysterical mutism in prison dreamed that the institution for mental diseases to which he had been transferred was on fire, whereupon he screamed and thereafter talked normally.

The occupational neuroses, such as writer's cramp, usually belong among hysterical reactions. The hysterical tic consists of a spasmodic, coördinated twitching movement of a small group of functionally related muscles. It may take the form of twitching of the facial muscles, blinking of the lids, sudden turning of the head, or a gesturelike movement of the hands. Such tics may represent dramatization of psychic experiences. Because of the suggestion of defense that they manifest, they may appear purposive. Care must be taken not to confuse hysterical tics with the more complex, coördinated tic-like movements observed after epidemic encephalitis and certain other organic diseases of the brain.

Sensory symptoms, like other physical disturbances, are usually those of functional incapacity. Among the more frequent ones are anesthesias, paresthesias, and disturbance of special sense organs, such as blindness or deafness. Hysterical anesthesia does not follow the distribution of a nerve but involves an extremity up to a sharply defined line above which sensation is normal. It follows what the patient believes to be the distribution of the nerve, which is represented in the patient's mind as a functional unit. One-half of the body may be anesthetic, in which case the special senses—hearing, smell, taste, and sight—may be lost on the same side. Hysterical anesthesia may be extended in area by the suggestive and repetitious procedure of the physician in examination. Anesthesia probably cannot be produced *de novo* by the physician's examination, although this was believed by Babinski. The area and degree of the anesthesia may vary from one examination to another. Hysterical disturbances of vision are of various forms, the most frequent ones being blindness and narrowing of the visual fields. Hysterical blindness usually has a sudden onset. The pupils continue to react to light, and usually, but not always, the patient avoids objects that would injure him if he came into collision with them. The onset is usually either closely related to some distressing visual experience or has a fairly obvious symbolic relation and significance.

Painful complaints are often hysterical in nature and may sometimes be hallucinatory. This conversion symptom is perhaps the commonest expression of the illness at the current time and is frequently misdiagnosed and mistreated. As with other hysterical symptoms, the patient presents a bizarre or unusual account of the symptoms that is not easily recognizable as a result of the usual physical illnesses, or he may exaggerate the pain of a relatively minor physical disturbance. In spite of his insistence on the severity and disabling nature of the symptom and his demands for medication and care, he may be observed frequently to appear indifferent and undisturbed by the symptom. Placebos may relieve the symptom. There is often an intermittent history of its occurrence, and exacerbations may be found related to incidents arousing emotional conflict. In taking the history, the examiner may induce many hysterical patients, apparently indifferent to the symptom, to complain at the point where the psychiatrist touches upon the emotionally disturbing relationship or incidents in his life. If the psychiatrist is easily dissuaded from the task of history taking in an effort to provide immediate relief of a sudden complaint of pain offered by the patient during the interview, a valuable opportunity and a significant clue pertaining to the emotional connotation of the symptoms are missed. Reintroduction of the anxiety-ridden topics or associated themes often gives rise again to painful complaining. The arousal of painful complaining may be regarded as perhaps hallucinatory. It may occur in the course of psychoanalysis when the patient associates pertinent information symbolizing the conflicting needs that underlie the symptom.

The determination of painful complaints appears to rest on any one of the following parent-child interactions.

Oversolicitude by the mother following minor painful experiences may establish the predisposition to obtain gratification, in the face of conflict, by means of painful complaining in later life. Envious observation of the attention given to another sibling or home member sometimes arouses fantasies of suffering that are repressed until the later conflictful period and are then aroused as a substitute means of allaying anxiety. Of greatest importance are the childhood experiences of pain that lead to *masochistic* suffering in order to obtain gratifying affectional responses. In some instances, parents suffer guilt on punishing the child for misdeeds and then lavish affection following punishment as a means of assuaging their own anxiety. If this is the means by which the patient as a child repetitively obtained emotional satisfaction, a pattern for later masochistic pain and suffering is established. Another method, described by Freud, has to do with the guilt suffered by a child after secretly enjoying the punishment offered an envied brother or sister. To assuage this guilt, he must then suffer some distress. In all these instances, the basic issue is the wish for the affection and acceptance by the parent or parental substitute. With the masochistic expression, pain or distress must be expressed in order to obtain the wished-for affection and acceptance denied in reality.

Organic Factors and Conversion Reactions

The existence of organic symptoms does not exclude the presence of conversion ones also. Symptoms of organic disease that still exist may be exaggerated, or symptoms may persist after the organic basis for them no longer continues. In such cases, the symptoms produced by the disease were found to serve some psychological purpose, to be of value in themselves. Because of their usefulness in providing protection, escape, or advantage, they are unconsciously exaggerated or prolonged. Hysterical symptoms of this nature occur particularly in industrial, insurance, and traumatic neuroses, but they are by no means confined to them, since there are many situations in which physical symptoms may serve some useful function. At times the organic disease may impose sufficient additional stress so that emotional problems can no longer be dealt with in a realistic manner. Exhaustion, whether a result of fatigue or of anxiety resulting from prolonged indecision or from emotional conflict, may predispose to a hysterical retreat from a situation that would otherwise have been met with ease. The person already having some organic disease will often, if his situation does not demand some other special symptom, select one related to the organic disorder with which he is already familiar. The organic symptoms may merge imperceptibly into the hysterical one.

Psychodynamics

It is not surprising that theories formulated to account for the etiology and nature of a personality disturbance that may manifest itself in symptoms apparently purely physical in nature should be various. As would be expected, these theories have been influenced by the concepts that have prevailed during different periods relative to natural phenomena in general, and human behavior in particular. Among these theories are the teaching of Hippocrates that hysteria is caused by the wandering of the uterus through the body in search of humidity, the belief of the 17th century that its striking manifestations seen in that period were a result of witchcraft or demoniacal possession, and the conviction now generally accepted that it is an adjustmental technique to which the personality may resort.

Among those who have contributed most to our understanding of conversion and of dissociative reactions are Charcot, Janet, Bernheim, Babinski, Morton Prince, and Freud. Although his point of view was entirely neurological, Charcot was the first to demonstrate that the dramatic manifestations of hysteria could be produced and allayed by hypnotic suggestion. He thus demonstrated that psychological influences could affect bodily mechanisms, although, with his lack of aptitude for psychological investigation, he assumed that a hereditary degeneration was an essential prerequisite for hypnotic or hysterical phenomena. His discovery did, however, lay the foundation for investigative work by others.

Bernheim expressed the opinion that all hysterical symptoms are the result of suggestion. Babinski added the opinion that not only could all hysterical phenomena be produced by suggestion but they could be removed by persuasion.

It is now universally agreed that conversion hysteria and dissociative reactions are of psychogenic origin. The greatest influence in creating this point of view is to be found in the contributions of Freud. Most psychogenic theories as to the nature of conversion hysteria go back to the concepts of conflict and of repression. According to Freud, the wish or other repressed material, although not permitted frank expression, obtains release in disguised form through the mechanism of conversion, by which the psychic conflict is transformed into a physical or mental symptom. Freud explained the hysterical symptoms as caused by a conflict between the superego and some wish that, because of its consciously objectionable nature, is repressed by the superego. This repression is not, however, entirely successful, and the wish therefore obtains disguised expression by its "conversion" or transformation into the symptom. The nature and localization of the symptom thus produced are such that it symbolizes or provides disguised expression of the repressed wish and at the same time provides some degree of its fulfillment or of relief from the emotional conflict. Many psychiatrists who accept the role of repression in the production of the hysterical symptom hesitate to accept Freud's belief that a repressed Oedipus complex is an essential condition for the development of hysteria.

At the present time, the most widely accepted explanation of the mechanism known as conversion is that impulses and unadjusted, repressed elements in the personality, highly charged with emotion, are productive of anxiety. The anxiety is then mitigated or dispelled by being "converted" into functional symptoms manifested in the voluntary musculature or in special sense-organ systems. The exact process involved in this "conversion" is uncertain.

In conversion hysteria, we find an excellent illustration of both *primary* or neurotic gain and of *secondary gain*. The conversion mechanism yields a primary or neurotic gain through its anxiety-defense function. It also yields a secondary gain by producing something to the advantage of the patient. A hysterical paralysis, for example, may enable one to evade some situation that he feels incapable of mastering.

The manner in which conversion, or the transformation of an anxiety-producing emotional conflict into a specific symptom, can alleviate the anxiety caused by the patient's conflicting desires, and at the same time yield a secondary gain that enables the patient to escape from an extremely unpleasant situation, is illustrated by the following case.

M., a young man who had been a dancer and an acrobat in a circus, enlisted in the army during peace time. Here he found the discipline rigid, his duties irksome, and his experiences monotonous. He longed for travel, excitement, attention, and the opportunity for exhibition enjoyed in his former life. The situation became quite intolerable, but to leave meant that he would be treated as a deserter. A hysterical conversion reaction, induced by two conflicting motives, the one to conform to the requirements of military life, the other to secure escape from a hated situation, provided a solution that permitted him to gain his own end, i.e., to obtain immunity from unpleasant experiences and tasks, and at the same time alleviated his anxiety and enabled him to maintain his self-respect. On arrival at the mental hospital to which he was transferred, he could neither walk nor stand, and his legs were anesthetic to even vigorous prickings by a pin. At the same time, he displayed a significant attitude of unconcern (*la belle indifférence*) as to his disabilities, although, as far as he was consciously aware, they were complete and incurable. His absence of concern is to be explained by the fact that the penalty was less than the gain, although one must not conclude that this weighing of advantages and disadvantages was at all a matter of conscious reflection. A few months later, the man was discharged from the army on a surgeon's certificate of disability. Soon the suspended motor and sensory functions began to return. Persistent efforts to walk met gradually with success, and in another three months he left the hospital practically well.

In the case of this soldier, it can be seen how a psychological mechanism "converted" the anxiety stemming from his repressed hostile drives against those in authority and his wish for release from military service into an overt and incapacitating symptom that, however, yielded a definite secondary gain.

The hysterical conversion reaction may provide the patient with a defense against anxiety, enable him to maintain his self-respect, and at the same time accomplish some purpose, the achievement of which respect for self would otherwise have been forbidden. It may make possible an escape from an intolerable situation; it may afford an exoneration for oneself, an excuse for one's failures, serve as an attention-getting device, or enable one to evade some duty, shun a responsibility, express some spite, or realize some purpose that would not bear the scrutiny of consciousness.

Hysteria has its analog in many acts of everyday life, when many psychological processes considered normal take place without full consciousness of their methods and motives, particularly if there is some reason for hiding the truth from oneself. The hysteric is always desirous never to disclose to himself the real nature of his illness, an effort that is successful, since the conscious personality has no access to the cause of the illness. Universal, too, is the tendency to project one's difficulties upon something tangible. Similarly, any physical basis for an explanation of the symptom is welcomed and assigned an important place.

In connection with conversion reactions such as the one cited, it should be kept in mind that several factors usually play a role in determining the specific nature of the neurotic reaction. This concurrence and integration of adaptive functions unconsciously served by the symptoms are known as *overdetermination*. Through this process, a single symptom or neurotic reaction may be a complex compromise

formation, to the production of which several needs have simultaneously and unconsciously contributed. If an overdeterminative process is analyzed, it will be found that in many neuroses there are anxiety-relieving values that have been produced by the symptom, together with further advantages that the patient secondarily derives from his illness once it is established. Two or more birds are killed with one stone, so to speak.

As already indicated, these two sets of values derived from the neurosis are the primary and the secondary ones. The *primary gain* is the defense against anxiety supplied by the symptom. The *secondary gain* is a material advantage that is contributed by the symptom. In the case of the soldier just mentioned, the conversion symptom (hysterical paralysis) relieved him from the anxiety incident to his ambivalent wishes. It also afforded what was to him a very important secondary gain: it rendered him unable to perform military services and therefore made his discharge necessary. Conversion reactions usually meet some immediate need of the patient and are therefore associated with more less obvious "secondary gain." The secondary gain is not always material but may be emotional or social, e.g., the extraction of love, sympathy, or consideration from other people. Usually the element of "secondary gain" secured from the disturbing conversion symptoms seen daily in the general practice of medicine is less apparent than in the case of the soldier. Frequently, in fact, when symptoms of anxiety are also present, the element of secondary gain may be slight.

In the case of the soldier, comment was made concerning the attitude of unconcern manifested toward his disability. This satisfied indifference and pathological tranquility, characterized by Janet as *la belle indifférence,* is of diagnostic significance in a conversion reaction, representing as it does the characteristic use of denial as a means of defense. The conflict having been solved and anxiety having been relieved through conversion of the repressed impulses and wishes into a functional symptom, an outward calm follows, even though the symptom produced is so disabling that it would presumably be a source of great concern.

Accident or Compensation Neurosis

Industrial accidents, in which a question of indemnification for a real or presumed disability may arise, are frequently followed by a definite psychoneurotic reaction. So, too, with the vast increase in automobile traffic accidents, they appear often following such occurrences. The presenting features of these reactions may be those of anxiety, hypochondriasis, conversion, or mixed types. Frequently the conversion symptoms are sufficiently prominent so that compensation neuroses are often classified among the hysterias. It was formerly considered that a desire for what the patient considered adequate compensation was the principal, if not exclusive, factor in the production of neuroses following industrial accidents. In recent years, closer studies of the patient's personality have shown that other factors also are usually dynamically important.

Persons of a paranoid tendency, those who are insecure, and those who crave sympathy and attention are predisposed to compensation neurosis. The same is true of the individual who finds himself in an employment situation that is becoming progressively more unbearable. The necessity, because of financial obligations, for continuing work beyond mental or physical capacity, or the failure to derive satisfaction from one's work may predispose to a traumatic or compensation neurosis. Some incidental gain resulting from an injury, such as escape from dreary or wearisome conditions of employment, may be an important contributing factor.

Oversolicitude on part of the patient's family or an injudicious remark by the physician in the first days or weeks after an injury concerning its severity may create fear in the mind of the patient and predispose to the development of a neurosis. Experience connected with bodily helplessness, disturbance of business resulting from the accident, or worry about cure may conduce to its development. Not only a desire for financial gain but the conviction on the part of the patient that he has the right to expect indemnification may be motivating factors. Social custom and public opinion tend to encourage the development of accident neuroses by their attitude toward the question of responsibility.

The probability of developing a compensation neurosis following a relatively slight injury is greater than if the injury is so disabling as to be obviously compensative. Mild traumatic residuals may become heavily overlaid with hysterical elaborations. The traumatic or accident neuroses rarely occur when the victim of the injury must bear the brunt of the financial responsibility for the accident, as in the case of injuries sustained in sports. There is usually an incubation period between the injury and the appearance of the mentally determined symptoms. This interval before the development of the chronic disabilities is of value in excluding an organic source. It is usually occupied with vague ruminations that tend to be of an imaginative, affective, resentful, wish-determined, and suggestive nature.

SYMPTOMS. The symptoms of the accident neuroses are various, but these neuroses differ in no essential feature from others except in the matter of compensation. Frequently the symptoms include irritability, stubbornness, argumentativeness, crying spells, anxiety, depression, sleeplessness, headache, and dizziness. The patient is garrulous in describing his feelings and may complain of poor memory and inability to concentrate. If the foreman, "company doctor," or insurance adjuster questions the genuineness of his symptoms or the validity of his claim that the injury was sustained while at work, the patient frequently reacts with an indignation and resentment that aggravates and prolongs his symptoms. The fact that a hysterical reaction may be superimposed on an organic injury that has escaped attention should not be forgotten. Sometimes the neurotic symptoms do not become seriously troublesome until after the patient has returned to his employment when they become so aggravated that he gives up work.

Tremors, paralyses, and other motor and sensory conversion symptoms occur. At times the necessary form of treatment for the original injury may be instrumental in suggesting a disability to a person of a hysterical type. Immobilization by splints of an injured extremity, for example, may be followed by its paralysis. As in other psychoneuroses, symptoms may be firmly fixed by overexamination or by overtreatment based on wrong premises. The development of symptoms through suggestion is, of course, in no way limited to accident neuroses involving the matter of compensation. A repetition of physical examinations may aggravate symptoms when organic disease exists and produce them when no disease exists. The fact that the physician's words and acts may have a suggestive effect upon the patient imposes a special responsibility upon him. In those cases in which indemnification is a participating motive, the patient remains unaware of such an influence and denies that he desires compensation, declaring that he would gladly forego any financial satisfaction could he be restored to health. He complains of his symptoms, but he rarely asks how he may get rid of them. Underlying feelings of guilt may be overcompensated and experienced as self-pity.

Workmen's compensation acts and industrial accident insurance have greatly increased the incidence of compensation neuroses. The effect on the worker of the general practice of awarding compensation for injury is to create a receptive mental state so that, when injury occurs, there follows an unconscious wishing for compensation. This does not at all mean that a worker who, following an industrial accident, complains of symptoms without organic basis is a malingerer or that

compensation is not merited. The disability, it is true, would not have occurred had the results of the injury not possessed potential benefits in some form. The misfortune is that the injury in the "damage-suit" hysteria occurred in a person who was psychologically predisposed to a neurotic reaction. The existence of litigation tends to maintain the patient's focus on his injury, particularly if legal processes are prolonged. Contrary, however, to a frequent belief, the end of litigation does not always terminate the symptoms promptly. A termination does usually, however, have a salutary effect on the symptoms by removing one factor that has tended to keep the patient's attention focused on himself.

Mention should be made of the *occupation neuroses,* a large proportion of which, particularly those characterized by spasms, are to be looked upon as hysterical. In these neuroses, the patient, on attempting to execute some specialized movement in an occupation requiring the coördination of groups of muscles, suffers from a spasm of the muscles involved in this act. Their function remains unimpaired when an attempt is made to employ the same muscles for the performance of some other act.

Diagnosis of Conversion Reactions

In addition to differentiation from the other neurotic reactions, features of which it often shares, hysteria is to be differentiated from organic disorders, malingering, schizophrenia, and the psychophysiological reactions. A conversion reaction may simulate an astonishing variety of organic symptoms, in making a differentiation from which certain principles should be held in mind. One should, of course, ascertain if sensory and motor disturbances are consistent with known anatomical and physiological facts regarding the distribution and function of the central and peripheral nervous system. Conversion symptoms often change from time to time and with suggestion. Reflex and trophic disturbances do not accompany hysterical disturbances aside from the changes that may come from chronic disuse following a paralysis. Before deciding that a physical sign or somatically expressed symptom is of psychogenic origin, one should carefully attempt to ascertain if a setting of affective dissatisfaction existed before the appearance of the sign or symptom.

The patient's attitude of satisfied indifference toward his disability and the circumstances under which the disorder arose are often significant. The coincidence or immediate sequence of an acute emotional state and the appearance of physical phenomena are suggestive, especially if the connection between the psychological event and the sign is unrecognized by the patient. In actual physical disease, the patient readily accepts or even suggests the statement that his disability is of mental origin. On the other hand, the patient whose disability is psychogenic eagerly seeks for a physical basis. Both patients, of course, are really attempting to avoid the truth. It is always well for the physician to ask himself if the signs and symptoms serve a purpose in the life of the patient (secondary gain) and not let the apparent loss or suffering exclude hysteria from consideration. In making the diagnosis of conversion hysteria, too, one should not rely solely on the presence of conversion symptoms but should also consider whether the patient is an emotionally immature type of person. It must be remembered, too, that organic disability and a conversion reaction are not mutually exclusive. Organic neurological disabilities are not rarely complicated by superimposed conversion phenomena.

The confusion of a conversion reaction with malingering is most apt to be made by persons who consider all hysterics as malingerers and mistakenly believe that the hysteric could control his symptom if he wanted to. Discrepancies, contradictions, and exaggerations of symptoms are more frequent in malingering; also, the malingerer usually expresses much concern about his symptoms. The use of appropriate psychological tests, such as the Minnesota Multiphasic, may suggest the tendency to lying and deception. In the classic form of major conversion hysteria, the patient manifests little concern about symptoms. Because, however, of the considerable component of anxiety often accompanying a recently established conversion reaction, the patient may show signs of concern. Surprise examinations or observation of which the patient is unaware may reveal the deception in malingering. Conversion reactions and malingering have much in common. The difference is largely one of the relative degree to which consciousness participates in the reaction. In malingering there is a subtle interweaving of conscious and unconscious factors.

Since there may be reactions in schizophrenia strongly resembling hysteria, the diagnosis is not always easy. The native temperament of the patient may be somewhat indicative, that of the hysteric person having been characterized by more easily shifting emotions. In hysteria a dominant affect usually exists, there are no inconsistencies in symptoms and no disturbance of associations, there is a greater response to any emotional reaction on the part of nurse or relative, and there is no deterioration in habits of dress or cleanliness. In hysteria there is an apparent desire to be the center of attention, and it will usually be found that either parent or mate has been accustomed to exhibit a sympathetic and exaggerated emotional reaction to any illness on the part of the patient. Here the aid of the clinical psychologist may be most helpful, particularly as the usual diagnostic interviewing with the hysterical patient is distorted through his unwitting use of denial and the force of repression.

Attention is called in Chapter 25 to the fact that conversion reactions should be distinguished from psychophysiological reactions, in which tension and anxiety arising from psychological conflicts and emotional stresses are allayed, not by channelizing them through voluntary muscular and special sense systems (conversion), but through the vegetative nervous system into visceral organ symptoms and complaints. Yet many patients show combinations of both varieties of reaction.

Prognosis

The degree to which conversion mechanisms can be eliminated depends to a considerable degree on the extent to which evasions become habitual in early life and on the maturity and independence of the personality pattern. The prognosis depends, too, upon the strength or weakness of the patient's personality resources in relation to the environmental demands and to the other stresses that he will be called upon to face. If the patient's capacity for social adaptation has been limited, if it has been his habit to deal with minor difficulties by evasive methods, or if he has led an aimless existence without drive or ambition, it is probable that further conversion defenses will be employed. Symptomatology alone is a poor guide to the future. If the patient was formerly well adjusted and the conversion reaction was brought on by unusual stress, the prognosis is favorable, provided return to the precipitating situation is not required.

The patient who has consciously thought how his difficulties would be solved by the chance appearance of disabling illness may easily and unconsciously permit the thought to become a reality. The presence of felt anxiety, with its indication that the conversion reaction is not providing an adequate defense, makes the prognosis less favorable. The childish egocentric patient who becomes increasingly dependent on his conversion symptoms has a poor prognosis. His conversion reaction becomes a more or less permanent mode of life, and he grows increasingly dependent on his symptoms.

The conversion reaction, in many instances, is engrafted upon a basically schizoid personality structure. With such persons, the psychotic reaction eventually becomes apparent. This is particularly so in groups of patients diagnosed as hysterical and followed for years after their initial admission to a mental hospital. On the other hand, similar follow-up studies over a period of a decade on patients who presented in a general hospital or out-patient clinic a monosymptomatic conversion make it clear that, even with treatment by measures designed only to modify the symptoms without restructuring the personality, the majority remained well and made excellent social adjustments. The outlook is best in the monosymptomatic hysteria that occurs in adult life rather than adolescence. Presumably here the response takes place in the face of a severe stress.

Treatment

In the treatment of a conversion reaction, the psychiatrist attempts to ascertain the purpose of the symptom and to discover the factors causing anxiety so great that it could be handled only through the mechanism of conversion with functional physical symptoms. Since the patient's disorder arose through mental causes and through the operation of mental mechanisms, the treatment should basically be that of psychotherapy.

The nature and energy of the dynamic factors that have led to the patient's symptoms are concealed from his recognition, and any explanation of the underlying mechanism is often received with resistance and protest. The patient's conversion reaction may, too, appear so remote from his emotional problem that only a searching analysis can uncover the relationship between the two.

Before beginning psychotherapy, the physician should first make a thorough physical examination. If no evidence is found that there is physical disease, no more physical examinations should be made, even though new symptoms occur. Continued examinations and long hospitalization may cause new symptoms to appear and old ones to become fixed.

The psychiatrist should remember that he must deal with two distinct although related problems: one, the removal of the symptom, the other, that of enabling the patient to apprehend the source of his anxiety and the significance of his symptom in order that he may form a more constructive method of action for the future. It is much easier to dispel a conversion than to help the patient to achieve further emotional growth.

It is important to make a correct estimate of the patient's personality stability and maturity and of his intellectual resources. If the personality limitations are relatively minimal, the treatment may be psychotherapeutic and based on analytical principles, with an investigation of the dynamic factors of repression. In the person of low intelligence and in the unstable individual who develops a conversion reaction in a relatively uncomplicated situation, the principal therapy will probably have to be limited to suggestion, hypnosis, and reëducation. In no case must the patient be accused of dishonesty or of a lack of desire to get well.

When the conversion symptom presents as a major disability incompatible with return to social and vocational activities, consideration must be given to its rapid reduction by the methods just described. In making this clinical judgment, the psychiatrist keeps in mind the defensive nature of the symptom and should evolve a concept of what the symptom defends against. With its rapid removal, he is aware that there will occur either overt anxiety or substitution by another symptom with equivalent symbolic significance. Either of these alternatives may be more suitable than major paralytic symptoms, blindness, choreiform states, or astasia-abasia. However, in those instances in which rapid symptom removal is likely to induce a serious disruption of self-esteem with anxiety, shame, and guilt, associated with regressive phenomena, this judgment is avoided. Serious regressions of this type are likely in those in whom the personality is essentially schizoid or there exist other symptoms indicative of an underlying schizophrenic reaction.

Narcosynthesis, persuasion, or hypnosis, as described in Chapter 31, are the therapeutic measures of choice for rapid removal of symptoms. Once the acute symptomatic disability is modified, the psychiatrist will then determine the potential for character change through the use of a dynamic psychotherapy. If this potential is considered to exist, psychoanalytic psychotherapy is recommended as a means of avoiding further symptomatic recurrences. These methods of treatment are described also in Chapter 31.

Evidence for the presence of a schizophrenic disturbance may be gained by careful assessment of the developmental history. Family history of psychotic disturbance or preëxisting information of a dependent, withdrawn, and isolated life with resort to fantasy or other disordered behavioral traits should arouse suspicion. Often, because of denial by the hysteric in presenting his life history initially, valid information is not obtained. Many consider that the aid of psychological tests, particularly the projective methods, should always be sought in such instances before treatment goals are determined and therapy is initiated. Such tests may provide clues as to the potentiality of severe regressions that will require hospital treatment if sudden removal of symptoms appears to be the method of choice. The author has been impressed with the frequency of such regressions in patients who present numerous pure color reactions in their Rorschach responses.

In the treatment of *accident neuroses* there are certain factors that require special attention. In case of injury any suggestion that it is serious should be carefully avoided. If possible, the injured person should be kept at work, and, if his condition does not permit this, he should return as promptly as possible. Care should be exercised that the treatment of any physical complication is not prolonged. The attitude of the physician toward a patient suffering from a traumatic neurosis should never be one of suspicion or antagonism. If he approaches the patient with a biased, skeptical attitude, disregards his complaint, and makes but a superficial examination, he destroys the possibility of any therapeutic rapport and may even contribute to further psychological elaboration.

A hope for indemnification on the part of the injured employee makes it impossible for him to disregard unpleasant sensations or unpleasant subjective experiences or to adjust himself to them. In contrast to an athlete similarly injured, the workman, doubtless unwittingly, is prompted to magnify rather than ignore the discomforts resulting from his injury. The harshness and disregard of complaints by representatives of insurance companies, a ready assumption of intent to swindle, and the delays and technicalities of court procedure tend to stimulate unwholesome patterns of reaction. Such attitudes engender resentment and discouragement and may force the injured person to resort to a primitive (conversion) mode of response. Whether a compensation award granted to the workman suffering from a traumatic neurosis is paid in a single sum or extended through a number of installments makes little difference so far as the neurosis is concerned. It is important, however, that a settlement be made promptly and that any litigation be terminated.

OBSESSIVE-COMPULSIVE REACTION

In the obsessive-compulsive reaction, the patient's anxiety is automatically controlled by associating it with persistently repetitive thoughts and acts. The patient recognizes that his unwanted thoughts and ritualistic acts are unreasonable, but he is unable to control them. The obsessive-compulsive reaction may be expressed in three clinical forms: (1) the persistent recurrence of an unwelcome and often distressing thought; (2) a morbid and often irresistible urge to perform a certain repetitive, stereotyped act; and (3) an obsessively recurring thought accompanied by a compulsion to perform a repetitive act.

Obsessive ideation may be concerned with various topics. Frequently the patient must fight against thoughts that are repugnant to his conscious moral and esthetic feelings, such as thoughts of a blasphemous nature or fantasies of killing a beloved member of his family. Although horrified that he should entertain such thoughts the patient is unable to rid himself of them. The intruding and constantly recurring thought may be pointless and absurd, such as the case described by Ireland, whose well-educated patient persistently wondered why a chair had four legs instead of one leg, or a ruminative preoccupation and speculation on such topics as creation, infinity, or other philosophical or religious questions. The condition of being obsessively preoccupied with an apparently indifferent topic, with marked exclusion of other interests, is sometimes known as an obsessive-ruminative state. The greater the effort to dispel obsessive thoughts, the more stubbornly they return. Ritualistic activities may be performed in an effort to dispel or counteract the thoughts. Practically never do such patients carry out any recurring thoughts suggesting an immoral or violent act, although they may become very apprehensive lest they do so. The inability of the patient to free himself from the distressing thought may occasionally lead him to suicide.

Types of Obsessive-Compulsion

FOLIE DU DOUTE. Some obsessive thinking assumes the form of *folie du doute* characterized by persistent doubting, vacillation, and indecision, usually with compulsive ruminations that lead to repetitive acts aimed to dispel the irrational doubts. Because of them, the patient must check and recheck even the simplest acts. He may, for example, lock the front door at night, but no sooner has he reached his bed than he is in doubt about the security of the door. He must therefore return and try the lock. Even then his doubts may recur after he is again in bed and require further visits to verify that the door is locked. Obsessive doubts and indecisions not rarely arise in case of conflict between desire and counterdesire.

Insistent, obsessive thoughts are defensive in purpose. The persistent idea is not to be taken at face value, so to speak. It is a substitute for another idea and thereby serves an anxiety-preventing function. Other affects are concealed behind the apparent content. The real sources may be any impulse, tendency, or wish that would be consciously intolerable to the patient. A hidden feeling of guilt is not an uncommon source. The manifest and recurring idea is the result of an effort to keep something else out of the mind and is formed by the mechanisms of displacement, symbolization, and condensation. The process is much the same as that occurring in a dream, where the latent or true content is concealed by these mechanisms so that the idea, wish, or impulse appears in the conscious dream in distorted and symbolized form.

COMPULSIVE ACTS. A second clinical type of obsessive-compulsive reaction is that of compulsive acts. In this there is the obligatory repetition of a certain act. The forces that produce the compulsive act are, of course, unconscious. Since the symbolic act cannot adequately satisfy the forces that produced it, the act is stereotyped and repetitive. When the patient is asked the reason for his behavior, he may either offer some explanation that he knows he has no rational basis or he may admit that it is absurd and purposeless. Usually the patient consciously experiences some rejection and resistance to the carrying out of his defensive, compulsive act, but tension and anxiety mount until the urge to repeat becomes irresistible. If the patient is prevented from carrying out his compulsive ritual, overt anxiety appears. One of the most frequent forms of obsessive-compulsive rituals is that of handwashing, which has for its purpose the warding off of anxiety.

Most obsessive-compulsive acts consist merely of such simple useless acts as touching or counting, or excessive ones, such as repeated handwashing. Some, however, become elaborate rituals or ceremonials. They superficially appear as meaningless formalities and are only recognized as neurotic ceremonials when a necessity for renouncing them is accompanied by discomfort and anxiety.

The ritualistic ceremonial described by Freud in one of his earliest papers (1896), entitled "The Defense Neuropsychoses," is often quoted and is an excellent illustration of the complexity that may be assumed by these compulsive devices designed to protect against anxiety:

"An 11-year-old boy had instituted the following obsessive ceremonial before going to bed. He did not sleep until he had told his mother in the minutest detail all the events of the day; there must be no scraps of paper or other rubbish on the carpet of the bedroom; the bed must be pushed right to the wall; three chairs must stand by it and the pillows must lie in a particular way. In order to get to sleep he must first kick out a certain number of times with both legs and then lie on his side."

The function of compulsive acts also is to allay or bind anxiety. The compulsive act that the patient performs has, it will be found, a symbolic significance. This symbolic act serves as a sort of magic ritual by which he undoes or annuls the possible effect of his unrecognized impulses and achieves a distorted satisfaction, self-punishment, and atonement. It temporarily dispels the dangerous situation; as long as it can be carried out, the intensity of the anxiety is reduced. If the performance of the ritualistic substitutive act is resisted or impossible, the effectiveness of the protective obsessive-compulsive defense is eliminated, and the forbidden wishes and impulses arouse anxiety. The need for ritualized behavior increases, since the unconscious striving threatens to erupt into consciousness; more and more symptoms must be constructed to provide defenses against the forbidden tendencies. In many respects, the defensive patterns of the compulsions resemble penances, atonements, and punishments, or serve as precautions, prohibitions, and restrictions. In many ways, they are closely allied psychologically to the ceremonies and taboos that primitive people devise as protections against demonological and other supernatural forces.

Compulsive acts are not uncommon in children and adolescents, in whom they originate as expiatory ceremonials or as means whereby, through attributing a certain magic-like power to an act, a particularly desired wish may be attained. The acts then become established through habit, but they normally disappear as repressed tensions subside and more adequate social adjustments are established.

PHOBIA WITH COMPULSION. The third type of reaction is that in which a phobia or obsessively recurring idea is associated with a compulsion to perform a repetitive act. This association occurs when there exists an overpowering fear of intolerable impulses. Usually considerable anxiety is observable. One of the commonest examples of this type of reaction is a repetitive handwashing, the result of an obsessive fear of dirt or uncleanliness. Whatever object the patient touches has, he is confident, left his hands contaminated. Since he can scarcely avoid touching objects, he must repeatedly wash his hands. As every object is a possible source of contamination, the patient may resort to complicated and troublesome means of avoiding the touching of objects. He may open doors with his elbows or handle articles with gloves or other coverings. One patient washed each Saturday the church pew she expected to occupy the following day. Because of this tension, preoccupation, and irresistible handwashing, the capacity for gainful employment may be destroyed.

Here, too, are found the same mechanisms of displacement and undoing. The real fear is, of course, not of dirt but of intolerable impulses or guilt-laden strivings that have been displaced and symbolized by constant preoccupation with fear of dirt. The anxiety to which they have given rise is temporarily alleviated by the compulsive washing, with its symbolic cleansing significance.

The following case illustrates many of the features of a mixed phobic and compulsive reaction.

S. K. was admitted to a mental hospital at the age of 29. The family history revealed no significant history. During the second and third grades of school "he was a problem to the nuns because of his stuttering. They would ask him to read a paragraph over two or three times." For a considerable period at this age "he felt he had to bless himself a certain number of times in the evening." When in the fourth grade and after an illness "he was afraid to go to sleep at night for fear he might die. He would call his mother two or three times before going to sleep. He would not go to sleep unless she reasssured him that he would not die. This lasted for two or three months." He bit his nails until he was 16 years of age.

At the time of his admission, the patient's mother and wife were requested to describe his adult personality characteristics. He was, they reported, a quiet, serious, honest, thrifty, saving, stubborn, and somewhat worrisome person. "He was ambitious. He wanted to go through college and be more than an ordinary working man. In college he studied very, very hard, and was an honor student." When 18 years of age the patient drank excessively for a period of several months. He then suddenly stopped and became so opposed to liquor that, to quote his wife, "He wouldn't touch a drop, and I remember once when we were both young he walked out of a home where liquor was being served because he was so opposed to it."

He enlisted in the Marine Corps. When, after his admission to the hospital, he was asked what prompted him to volunteer, he replied, "Well, I felt uneasy a little bit with my scrupulosity. I wasn't too uneasy, but I thought somehow the service would take it away." Asked what he meant by 'scrupulosity,' he said "I was doubtful about my confessions." Asked if he was doubtful that he didn't confess enough, his answer was, "That's right; I didn't have enough sorrow for my sins." When the admitting physician asked the patient about his duties in the military service, he replied, "I had a job cleaning urinals. I probably was very good. I tried to do a thorough job. I saw cigarettes, but I always kept on cleaning all the time. It could have been done in 2 or 3 hours, but I worked 8 or 9 hours. I volunteered for the job." Two years later he wrote his fiancée that he wished to break his engagement as he was going to study for the priesthood after discharge from service. Six months later he wrote again, saying he had decided not to became a priest and asked that their engagement be renewed. Twenty-four months later he was married but had no sexual relations with his wife until 17 months later.

After his discharge from military service two years later, the patient entered college, from which he was graduated, although several months before graduation his neurotic reaction had become so disabling that he was unable to continue his studies for the final two months of his senior year.

Soon after the patient's admission to the hospital, his wife was asked to give a history of the

patient's illness. She reported that he had exhibited a compulsive handwashing for several
months but that it became more serious. "He used
to wash his hands and keep the water running for
15 minutes at a time. After he had washed them,
he would turn off the spigot with his elbow. He
had to count and wash and rinse his hands a certain number of times. If he had touched the door
or door knob, he would go back and wash his
hands again. One time he began to wash his hands
at 1 o'clock in the morning. After we moved into
our own house, he refused to use the front door or
to turn the knob on the door for fear there might
be germs. He used to go to the back window and
call me to go to the front door and open it for
him. He reached the point where he would climb
in and out of windows so that he wouldn't have
to enter the doors at all." The wife described also
the following compulsion: "He also had the idea
that when he walked there was something under
his shoe. He would stop and look on the sole of
his shoe, but there would be nothing there. He
also worried as to whether or not his shoe laces
were tied. He would pick up his foot and look to
make sure. He had to do that a certain number
of times before he was absolutely sure they were
tied. When he walked down a street, if he kicked
a stone he felt that he should put it back in the
same place. If he walked on a line, then he would
have to walk on all the cracks in the sidewalk."

On arrival at the hospital, the patient stated to
the admitting physician, "I like to wash my hands
many times a day in order to get them good and
clean." While talking to the physician, he stood
with his arms folded in order to avoid touching
anything. He readily acknowledged that he was
worried about touching objects lest he give others
disease. As he seemed somewhat depressed, he was
asked about suicidal thoughts. He replied that he
felt he would be better off dead than to be thinking of the things he did but added that he would
"not really" commit suicide. He then added,
"When I say things, they have to be said a certain
way. If I don't say them properly, I must apologize. I do this all the time. This irritated my wife
and was another reason why she couldn't live with
me. I would leave my books to apologize to her.
It was the apologizing that was bothering her—
not being at peace. I thought if I rubbed my hands
88 times, shut the water off, and then went back
again, it would be all right. Then I thought maybe
it hadn't been 88 times."

A month after the patient's admission, his ward
physician entered the following note in the clinical
record: "This patient has become extremely disturbed over his obsessive-compulsive ideation during recent days. He stops his physician at every
opportunity and repeatedly asks the same questions, which include the following: "Should I wash
my hands after I go to the bathroom and just do
number one? Should I wash my hands when I go
to the bathroom and have a bowel movement? My
penis touches the toilet seat. Do you think I should
wash it off with soap and water so there won't be
a spread of disease? I wouldn't want anyone to get
this disease. There's a rash there. Do you want to
look at it? I think it is some sort of disease. I'm
afraid everybody will get it. I don't know, doctor,
I'm afraid something is going to happen. I have a
feeling that I might go crazy or something. Someone asked me if I thought these things were silly
and I said, 'Yes,' but now that I think of it, they
don't seem silly. I just can't quite explain them.
They must not really seem silly to me or I wouldn't
have to do them like I do." The patient manifested
an interesting inability to make any definite statement or to take any decisive action. When discussing a point he would say such things as the following: "Well, doctor, it's just like this. Well, no,
it isn't exactly like that. I should say rather that's
a little on the order of—well, that isn't quite right
either. Perhaps I should put it this way. It's more
of—uh—well, no, that isn't it."

Under therapy, the patient gradually improved.
Two years after his admission he left the hospital
for employment in a brick plant. A report received a year later stated that, although not entirely well, he was successfully employed.

Psychodynamics

Psychogenetically, the origin of obsessive-compulsive behavior is believed to
rest in the early struggle of the growing
child between his drives for omnipotent
self-assertion and the necessity to conform
to the demands of his parents in order to
maintain their love and respect. The early
period of toilet training initiates the conflict. Often the later obsessive-compulsive
individual is one brought up by a rigid
compulsive mother, who insistently demands compliance and threatens both
loss of love and various forms of punishment for failure to behave properly. The
growing child is then exposed to repeated
arousal of rage through the insistent requirements for cleanliness and compliance
but must repress them in order to retain
his relationship with the parent. Very
early he learns to regard his underlying
thoughts of hostile reprisal to be taboo,
and therefore subject to punishment and
requiring penance. He may learn, by
observing the parents, that his defiant
behavior provides gratification in the attentions of the parent, yet at the same time
he must then atone both by carrying out
the parental desire as well as an associated

expiatory act. This train of behavioral responses, derived from the long-continued relationship with such parental figures, becomes internalized and unconscious so that each thought reflecting rage or hostility sets in action the psychodynamic train of ambivalently balanced action and counter-action symbolizing rage, gratification, compliance, and expiation.

In the following brief summary are the free associations of a compulsively neat and fussy young woman lawyer given during psychoanalysis and following an observation by the therapist that she seemed to wish to be messy in the office judging by the way she dropped cigarette ashes on the furniture there.

"It is hard to believe that I do something like being messy or neat to annoy somebody. Being messy was a way to annoy mother. It seemed to me that mother's cleaning up and criticizing me for not being neat was a way to annoy me and father, I felt I had no way to get back at her. I never felt more angry toward anyone than mother. Being messy was a way I learned of getting back at her, of rebelling. She once told me how upset she was when I broke something that was valuable. . . . I became like my mother in camp when I was with Ruth. She was so neat, shiny. Everyone liked her and admired her. She inflicted her standards on everyone. Recently I met her and thought she was a snob."

Prognosis

When the obsessive-compulsive state has onset in childhood or early adulthood, the course is usually chronic but variable, with many patients suffering episodic periods of severity although able to adapt socially. This reaction does not increase the risk of suicide, homicide, or drug abuse of any kind, or of prolonged hospitalization. The patient's compulsive needs frequently interfere seriously with his comfort and efficiency. In extreme cases his constant preoccupation with his protective rituals renders him socially impossible. Some psychiatrists characterize the obsessive neuroses as intermediate between neuroses and psychoses. The obsessive-compulsive states of children usually disappear with time if not taken seriously in the presence of the child. Such compul-

sions grow out of childhood anxiety, often a single one. The prognosis is much more serious if the onset is during adolescence or early adult life.

Diagnosis

A diagnosis between early schizophrenia and the obsessive-compulsive neuroses is at times exceedingly difficult. The obsessive thinking of the psychoneurotic may not be unlike the subjective rumination of the schizophrenic, and the compulsive ritual of the former may suggest the mannerisms of the latter. The symbolisms seen in the compulsive acts of the neurotic individual, as well as the substitutive nature of the phobias, are close both in resemblance and in relationship to the symbols seen in schizophrenia. It not infrequently happens that what is first thought to be the ruminative and obsessive tension state of a neurotic subsequently becomes an obvious schizophrenic reaction, usually of the paranoid type. In general, it may be said that the greater the rumination and the less the tension, the nearer does the reaction approach that of the schizophrenic. A failure on the part of the patient to regard his phobias and compulsions as absurd and particularly to refer them to external influences indicates a malignant schizophrenic origin. The compulsive neurotic never loses the capacity for discrimination between subjective experiences and reality, as is the case in schizophrenia. Finally, as Bleuler points out, the compulsive neurotic struggles *against* his obsession, whereas the delusional patient struggles *with* his idea.

At times the genuine depressions of manic-depressive psychosis may be accompanied by obsessive ideas. In differentiating such cases from compulsive states, one will inquire which appeared first, the depression or the obsessive idea.

Treatment

Fully developed obsessional and compulsive reactions are even more refractory to treatment than the milder psychoses. It is therefore important that treatment be early. The obsessive-compulsive neuroses usually develop in individuals who have been characterized by compulsive personality traits. The neurosis is in many ways an exaggeration and caricature of that pattern. Effort is made, therefore, to discover the factors that, through their dynamic action, led first to the personality make-up and then to the neurosis. Treatment, then, should be psychotherapeutic and either consists of a formal psychoanalysis or is based on analytical principles. Guided by the therapist, the patient's unconscious is explored and his apparently irrational fears and compulsions take on new meaning when understood in terms of chronologically earlier experiences and early life dynamics. In all cases, but particularly in rigid personalities and in those of limited intellectual development, reëducational measures should be employed. The patient should be encouraged to evaluate the relative importance of matters and to learn that indecision and perfectionism should be curbed, even at the cost of errors and mediocrity. Such attitudes as excessive guilt and overconscientiousness should be discussed. Cultivation of latent interests may help to reduce the ruminative thinking to which these patients are often addicted. Self-preoccupation and self-analysis are to be discouraged.

Prefrontal leukotomy has at times been followed by improvement. It should, however, be confined to cases so severe that the patient is practically confined to his home and incapacitated for any useful activity because of his compulsions. Results are better when there is evidence of persistence and drive and when the obsessional symptoms are accompanied by considerable anxiety.

HYPOCHONDRIA

The term *hypochondria,* or hypochondriacal reaction, is one that has been long applied to a group of psychoneurotic symptoms. The reaction is characterized by an obsessive preoccupation and concern of the individual about the state of his health or the condition of his organs. Often he expresses a multiplicity of complaints about different organs or body systems, which, the patient reiterates, must be incurably diseased. The hypochondriac is not only aware of various sensations that most persons disregard, but he also magnifies the intensity of normal sensations of fatigue, et cetera. In many cases, the hypochondriasis seems to be a displacement of anxiety onto the body, with the resulting somatic complaints. Some hypochondriacal reactions may become excessively and persistently obsessional, and associated compulsions may develop.

DEPRESSIVE REACTIONS

In the psychoneurotic depressions, anxiety becomes masked by self-depreciating behavior and depressive affect. Such reactions include the many instances of pathological grief, the prolonged mourning that takes place following the death of a close family member. In most instances the onset of the reactive depression follows shortly after a significant and evident loss through death or separation or takes place subsequent to a defeat in the social, economic, or personal life. These crises, then, may be the breaking of an engagement; a jilting; a divorce; the death of a spouse, lover, or parent; or the sudden loss of a fortune, a prized possession, or a valued function. Less commonly the depression follows the achievement of a wanted position—the so-called *success depression.*

In every instance the loss induces the affective state of sadness and also anxiety and frequently guilt or shame. The general response differs in no way from that described earlier for the affective psychotic reaction. With the neurotic depressions, however, the symptoms of profound somatic regression such as anorexia, weight loss, constipation, sexual impotency, extreme retardation, and agitation are not seen. On the other hand, other reactive character changes may take place as well as the resorting to oral gratifications. Crying appears to be more frequent in the neurotic than psychotic depressions.

The reactively depressed usually are drawn from those with one of the neurotic character structures. Thus there are the excessively timid and self-depreciating, the overbearing or arrogant, and the compulsively self-righteous. When such persons are faced with a loss, there is the expected sadness with mourning and self-depreciation, and in addition, there is often usually guilty anxiety due to surging up of unacceptable rage and aggression toward the lost object relation. Sometimes the depressed attempt to overcome the guilty anxiety and tension by taking alcohol or drugs. Others seek dependent support through hypochondriacal complaining. The reactively depressed are common in general medical clinics with their symptoms of aching pains and backaches and preoccupation with various organ functions. A few others attempt to solve their rage and anxiety by impulsive acting out in various antisocial ways, such as promiscuity or indulgence in varieties of sexual excesses. The majority, however, complain of fatigue, lassitude, and difficulty in sleeping and in working. They deprecate their past, are pessimistic and self-pitying, but manage a precarious continuance of their general activities. In the instance of the loss of an ambivalently loved partner the virtues of the wife or husband are extolled, the rituals of mourning are prolonged, pictures and memories are displayed and conspicuously commented upon, while all recollections of disharmony are denied.

Depression that emerges after a presumed post of responsibility has been achieved accomplishes the aim of preserving the person with success phobia from the anxiety associated with assumption of a position of authority and acclaim wherein the need for firmness and the acceptance of reward expose the sufferer to the fears of retaliatory rage and envy, attitudes which he himself has held toward authority in the past.

Psychotherapy is the therapeutic method that most frequently provides the needed emotional support, and when coupled with psychodynamic understanding will bring about resolution of pathological guilt and shame. The anti-depressant drugs, preferably commencing with imipramine or one of its analogs as described in Chapter 32, should be tried in all cases, although their administration has proved much less effective than in treatment of the affective psychoses. Hypnotics generally are needed for the insomnia.

GROSS STRESS REACTIONS

Following severe threat to life, whether as the consequence of stress in civilian life in the form of catastrophes such as accidents, floods, tornadoes, or volcanic eruptions, or as the stress of warfare, combat, or the horrors of concentration camp existence, a well-defined personality disorder frequently results. This condition, known much earlier in the German literature as fright (*schreck*) neurosis and in the English as a traumatic neurosis, may occur as an isolated disturbance or may complicate preëxisting personality disorders. In the United States, it probably occurs most commonly, and is most frequently unrecognized, after automobile accidents. Adler differentiates two types of post-traumatic states: those with immediate, and those with delayed, onset.

Stressful situations with threats or induction of fantasies of annihilation are not necessarily conducive to the ego-disorganizing neurotic stress syndromes. Under certain conditions stress-inducing situations lead to personality growth and increased ego potential for emotional control. In a series of studies of the immediate reactions to acute stress of differing kinds, Janis described obsessional staring initially as a response to disaster. Such staring is also observed in those who converge on the disaster scene. Both victims and observers are preoccupied by thoughts and fantasies as to what might have happened to them during the disaster, or of what might happen in the future. When suffering or threats of death or annihilation extend over months, as with prolonged illness or in sadistic prison camp experiences, the process of working through is prolonged and profound attitudinal changes may be noted. As Janis reviews the evidence, working through, that is, the "work of worrying," seems to be a means of increasing the level of tolerance for subsequent threat or signals of danger. In a series of experiments he found that the more thorough the preliminary and anticipatory fear, apprehension, and worrying have been, the more reality-tested the individual's self-reassurances are likely to be and the more emotional control he is likely to exhibit under actual stress of life threat or deprivation. When the stressful event is so sudden as to eliminate the potential for worrying, when adequate prior warning of disaster or stress is not obtained, when the individual is given false reassurance, or when he is given to suppression of anticipating anxiety by means of the defense of denial through overoptimism or avoidance of warnings, the subsequent stress-induced reaction will be much more profound than in those prepared through anticipatory fear.

Perhaps the most closely related experimental model of the acute stress reactions or traumatic neuroses is the conditioned emotional response induced in animals and studied at length by Hunt and Brady. In this condition the emotional response is greater to the conditioned stimulus than to the unconditioned; that is, to put it in terms of human thinking, any perceptive thought or other associations to the traumatic event both continue and magnify the response disruptive to ego functions. The reader is referred to Hunt's review of the studies upon the continued emotional response as noted in Chapter 3 and particularly his assay of the varying effects of psychopharmaceuticals and electro-shock in its control.

In the current nomenclature, this syndrome is not listed under the neuroses but under the Transient Situational Personality Disturbances as "gross stress reaction." This classification is unsatisfactory, as the accumulation of evidence from studies of both war veterans with combat neurosis and the survivors of concentration camps has exposed the long-continuing persistence of disruption of personality functions. Kardiner and Spiegel defined the enduring disruption of ego functions in American veterans of World War I which they referred to as a *physioneurosis* in the belief that severe stress effected a disorganization of the physiological processes responsible for ego-integrative function. But the investigation of the survivors of concentration camp experiences, where on a mass scale men and women in the millions were exposed over years to the imminent threat of death, repeated brutalities, separation and loss of emotional support from family and friends, and physical deprivations of the most extreme kinds, has established the existence of a chronic stress state. Eitinger's study of the *concentration camp syndrome* provides today the most extensive study of these enduring fragmentations of personality functioning through exposure to overwhelming stress.

Since the clinical picture in both acute and chronic forms of stress reaction simulate most often the anxiety neurosis, these conditions are described here. As the response to combat in war has been the most thoroughly examined of the acute stress reactions, it is provided extended discussion as the prototype of the acute stress reaction. The concentration camp syndrome similarly is described as that of the chronic syndrome.

Combat Neuroses

Presumably combat neuroses have long been associated with warfare, although their real nature and psychopathology were not recognized until relatively recently. During the Civil War, DaCosta described the "Irritable Heart of Soldiers." This was undoubtedly a neurosis induced by the stress and anxiety of combat and closely resembled the "Disordered Action of the Heart," 80,000 cases of which, it is said, occurred among British soldiers during World War I. It is of interest that this high incidence was not reported in World War II, presumably because its nature had become recognized so much more fully and it was designated as a neurosis.

In World War I, artillery fire reached a new intensity, with a fear-producing potential probably never before attained by weapons of warfare. It was noticed that with this terrifying shellfire, often combined with fear-inspiring air attacks, soldiers developed a striking variety of symptoms, including paralysis, gross tremors, mutism, blindness, confusion, or intense anxiety. In apparent absence of other etiological factors, it was at first concluded that the brain must in some undetermined manner sustain damage by a blast concussion attending the nearby explosion of a shell. The term "shell shock" was therefore applied to these psychiatric casualties and prolonged hospitalization was prescribed for their treatment. Gradually it was recognized that "shell shock" was primarily a psychological problem. Late in the war it became apparent, too, that prolonged hospitalization merely fostered and fixated the mental symptoms, which, because they prevented return to combat and even brought a compensation pension, provided a considerable secondary gain.

Before the end of World War II, it became apparent that functional disability was much less likely if the patient with an acute, battle-induced neurosis was treated near the front lines and returned to duty as soon as possible. It was also noted that the percentage of recoveries was greater if the attitude of the psychiatrist indicated that no organic damage had been sustained and if the name by which the neurosis was known to the soldier implied that the disability was temporary and recoverable.

Extreme and repeated battle fear, with a constant threat of death plus intense fatigue, are the precipitating factors in the production of combat neurosis. Physical exhaustion alone is not sufficient to produce the neurosis, but it does serve to lessen resistance so that psychodynamic forces are more easily released. The greater, however, the element of decreased physical efficiency resulting from fatigue, lack of food and sleep, or intercurrent illness, the more easily does emotional breakdown occur and the greater is the possibility of the soldier's not returning to active duty.

Personality factors, too, predispose to the combat neuroses. It is not easy to select the man who will maintain emotional equilibrium in combat and eliminate the one who will prove inadequate for the stress. It is not always the unstable and neurotic man who, as might be supposed, lacks resistance to the terror that accompanies long and intense combat. In general, it is the timid and passive person who cannot mobilize and externalize his anger and react aggressively toward the enemy and thus discharge his tension who is prone to develop a combat neurosis.

Most men, although wishing to meet the demands of their country, are inducted into the armed forces without strong, conscious desire for military life or for combat experience. Many at the time of induction are still emotionally dependent on their families, perhaps overprotected by their mothers and intimidated by cruel fathers. It has been found, too, that an unduly large number of combat neuroses occurred in individuals from broken or distorted homes unfavorable for the development of a well-integrated and mature personality. Induction into military service is accompanied by the abrupt loss of emotional support provided by family and friends, the deprivation of female companionship, and the loss of individuality and privacy. Frequently, too, the unseasoned soldier has a feeling that he is not appreciated and nurses resentment resulting from the change from the relatively flexible and permissive civilian pattern of living to one of subjection to strict discipline, regimentation, and subordination.

The stresses and conflicts to which the soldier is exposed during his training period are relatively mild and are handled by most trainees without the development of protest symptoms in the form of neurotic or psychotic syndromes. Even though the period of training is not accompanied by the hazards of combat, normal gratifications are renounced and destructive goals are substituted for the constructive ones of previous civil life. New relationships that would meet the soldier's emotional needs in the strange and abnormal state of affairs have to be established. Under these circumstances, the most constructive relationship is the soldier's identification of himself as an integral part of his unit, and his unit as a part of himself. He should have confidence in his unit and in the character, capability, and bravery of his leader. With the formation of deep emotional relationship with his leader and his buddies, the soldier's feelings of security and power are increased and his morale, or those attitudes, feelings, and beliefs that promote participation in a united effort, is promoted.

Fear, it will be remembered, is an emotion experienced in response to a stimulus having actual reality, one that either constitutes a present threat to the individual or portends real danger. Anxiety, on the other hand, is an expectation of danger, an emotional state of apprehensiveness, uncertainty, and insecurity, that may be produced either from situations symbolic of external danger or from internal conflicts and tensions present in the unconscious. Frequently it springs from the threats of repressed hostility, aggression, or resentment. Although this distinction between fear and anxiety can be made, in war situations they operate jointly. Their feeling-tones and their accompanying physiological expressions are the same. Although anxiety really arises from internal threats, it is attributed to (projected upon) some real external source. In the war neuroses, this projection is upon a dangerous external situation that is also provocative of fear. Both fear and the feeling of apprehension and insecurity characteristic of anxiety may therefore seem to have a common source. In the

battle situation, fear and other powerful external and emotional forces play upon the internal tensions and threats, upon the unconscious sources of anxiety. Of these sources of emotional stress in combat, fear is the most potent, its somatic and physiological effects being a source of great strain. Under combat circumstances, the various external and internal stresses conspire to produce a conflict that may become intolerable. The psychological defenses of the ego, hitherto effective, collapse, with a consequent rise of anxiety and the emergence of infantile patterns of behavior which constitute the neurotic picture. Anxiety and its management constitute, therefore, one of the basic problems in war neuroses.

FACTORS CONTRIBUTING TO WAR NEUROSES. As already indicated, fear and an impairment of the ability to repress fear reactions are highly provocative of anxiety. A breakdown of group morale or an attitude of defeatism within the combat unit greatly increases the psychological strain. Such a loss of morale is particularly prone to exist in case of lack of faith in commanding officers, in the absence of identification with one's unit, or during a retreat. The quality of leadership is one of the most important factors in the incidence of neurotic breakdown in any given unit. Prolonged periods of enforced inactivity during which men are exposed to danger predispose to an anxiety reaction. So does the loneliness of foxhole fighting with the usual inability to communicate with comrades. Repeated narrow escapes, high combat losses, and repeated exposure to the mutilation and death of close friends increase apprehension and stimulate guilt and anxiety. Fear of being a coward or of losing one's self-control, a realization of the responsibility for the lives of others, and an insufficient understanding of war or a lack of conviction of the need to fight, all predispose to war neuroses. A sense of guilt over expression of hostility is at times a psychogenetic factor. The regimentation and frustration of service life, separation from home, and the existence of domestic difficulties are often of much greater significance than more dramatic events.

The necessity that the man "sweat it out" in a continuously hostile environment results almost inevitably in at least some degree of anxiety; there are also certain internal as well as external factors that tend to increase anxiety. One of these internal problems is the soldier's handling of his hostilities. During his civilian life he was called upon to inhibit any hostile or aggressive drives. Whereas he formerly had the value of human life constantly impressed upon him, the soldier is expected to kill as many men as possible. His hostility, which through long inhibition had become well repressed, is now to be released to kill men like himself. This release of hostile and aggressive drives in their most destructive expression evokes anxiety. The problem of control of aggressive impulses is probably one of the soldier's heaviest psychological burdens. The combat situation demands release of aggression. Whatever their origin, any anxieties and tensions that add to the burden of the ego weaken its defensive functions and increase the possibility of a neurosis. Frustrations, such as unfair treatment in regard to promotions, citations, or leaves of absence, also bring to the fore resentment, hostility, and anxiety.

Feelings of guilt provoke anxiety as well. Such feelings may arise from the soldier's thought that he has been responsible for the death of someone else, perhaps of civilians as well as an enemy. Again, the death of a comrade toward whom the patient entertained ambivalent feelings or whom he had identified with a sibling rival may create feelings of guilt with anxiety or depression. An unconscious hostility may lead to a conviction on the part of the patient that he has actually caused the death of a comrade. At times, following the death of a buddy, a man develops a feeling of guilt through a belief that he failed to take care of his friend. Frequently the loss of a buddy or of a respected officer, by creating the feeling that one is being left alone, helpless, and deserted, deprives the soldier of emotional support and leads to an unendurable anxiety.

One important factor, then, in the production of combat neurosis is the excessive mobilization of emotions that have always been important in the personality but have not previously strained or overwhelmed the forces of control. Neurotic anxiety in battle may be rooted in passivity, hostility, or aggressiveness, and in the character of the personality defenses constructed against them in early life.

NEUROSIS-PREVENTING FACTORS. One of the most important mechanisms in strengthening the ego against factors productive of anxiety and other neurotic reactions is the soldier's identification with his unit. By this mechanism, he transfers a considerable share of his personal self-love to affection and pride in his outfit. His feelings of obligation and loyalty, having their source in this mechanism, overrule selfish, personal interests and provide one of the strongest motivations for combat and most effective protections against any expression of his conflicts.

The group relationship and its emotional bonds are among the most constructive and integrative forces for the individual. Similarly, an intense loyalty to each other on the part of the fighting men and their immediate leaders promotes morale and raises the threshold against anxiety. A resolute personal motivation, good morale, sustained by pride in one's organization, good leadership, respect for officers and fellow soldiers, confidence in equipment, the feeling of being properly trained, and high quality of food together with adequate recreational outlets are of great importance in preventing war neuroses. Other factors that aid in warding off anxiety are the desire to avoid loss of the esteem of the group by any failure in courage or in other demands of military tradition and also the habit of obedience and of disciplined behavior established by military training.

An additional factor that doubtless assists as an aid in the prevention of war neuroses is education through a series of lectures concerning the nature of fear. He is told that fear is a normal emotion of battle and to experience it should not be considered as occasion for censure or self-depreciation. The soldier is given simple information concerning its physiological manifestations and the nature of the nervous reactions it produces. His recognition of fear and his effort to deal with it on a conscious level tend to minimize its anxiety-stimulating influence.

NORMAL BATTLE REACTION. To protect itself from an overwhelming threat to its existence, the organism becomes completely and continuously alert. This leads to severe and continuous emotional tension. In spite of the various factors that aid in the prevention of combat neuroses, such stresses as exhaustion, excitement, and mortal terror inevitably produce reactions that would be considered abnormal in a civilian setting, yet are not so incapacitating as to demand removal from combat. Unless extreme, such reactions must under the circumstances be considered within the range of normal. Many of the reactions represent psychosomatic responses to stress and fear. Among them are sensations of pulling or pressure over the back of the head and neck, muscular tension, shaking and tremor. In some cases, the soldier may be transitorily immobilized. Excessive perspiration is common, and some soldiers experience anorexia, nausea, vague abdominal distress, mild diarrhea, and urinary frequency. Tachycardia, palpitation, breathlessness, and a sense of thoracic oppression and of faintness together with generalized muscular weakness and lassitude often exist. Many soldiers experience difficulty in sleeping and have repetitive nightmares of battle and "startle" reactions to theatening noises. Irritability is normal in the soldier subjected to long-continued battle, and resentment is common among those who have lost friends and withstood privations and dangers.

An 18-year-old Navy radioman was admitted to a hospital with symptoms of anxiety and depression. The patient was the youngest son in a happy family of four children. He was the favored child and throughout his early life gave no indications of instability. At school he was an average student and later was president of his high school class and an outstanding football player. At the outbreak of the war, he enlisted in the naval service with the consent of his parents, and immediately after completing his recuit training was detailed aboard a destroyer, where the morale was high. He made many close friends, and with the personal assistance of the communications officer, who helped him with the radio work, made a rapid advancement in rate.

The destroyer was part of the screen of an aircraft carrier engaged in the Coral Sea Battle, the raid on the Gilbert and Marshall Islands, and later the Battle of Midway. At the onset of each engagement, the patient felt apprehensive, but once firing commenced, he became entirely composed and attentive to his duties. While the destroyer was lying alongside a stricken aircraft carrier following a bombing attack during the Battle of Midway, the patient saw "torpedo wakes" approaching the ship; he resumed his post, until suddenly he was thrown out of his seat when the torpedo exploded beneath him. He plunged overboard, reached a nearby raft, and was later taken aboard another destroyer. He was then cognizant that his best friend, his immediate chief, and the communications officer had all been killed. On being taken aboard the ship, he collapsed. Following his return to the naval base, it was learned that he had suffered blast injury to the chest and abdomen that eventually necessitated intestinal resection. During convalescence from this operation, he first had terrifying nightmares in which various scenes related to the sinking of the destroyer were continually repeated, and during which he awoke in a state of anxiety. Sudden noises also produced unusual apprehension.

There was no evidence of physical disease, but insomnia, anorexia, constipation, and fatigue were observed and psychiatric study was requested. The patient was listless, dejected, and emotionally labile. Discussion of his battle experiences was distressing to him, and he described in detail his sensitivity to sounds and various combat scenes in motion pictures. The latter stimulus invariably led to anxiety. After one month of treatment on the psychiatric service, he became more energetic and content, slept well, commenced to eat, gained some weight, and again desired to return to duty. Nightmares were infrequent and sounds were less disturbing to him.

NEUROTIC REACTION. As indicated, such symptoms as those described should, if of moderate degree, be considered as a gross stress reaction and as the base line from which pathological reactions should be evaluated. The combat neurosis consists therefore of pathological degrees of the reactions mentioned.

The most frequent form of combat neurosis is the *anxiety state*. This constitutes over 75 per cent of acute war neuroses. In moderate or mild anxiety states, the patient shows tension, tremor, apprehension, weeping, depression, feelings of guilt, dizziness, tinnitus, urinary frequency, insomnia, and repetitive nightmares and dreams of battle trauma. Less frequently than in World War I, and usually in men of poor integration, the neurosis may consist of a *conversion reaction* with paralyses, sensory losses, aphonia, deafness, partial or total blindness, speech defects, astasia-abasia, a fixed stooping posture known as camptocormia, and occasionally a persistent amnesia. Such patients exhibit little visible anxiety and may manifest *"la belle indifférence."* In the most severe reactions, the onset is acute and sudden. A coarse tremor is not uncommon. It may be difficult or impossible to establish contact with the patient. Even though no longer under fire, he may believe himself still in battle and behave accordingly. He may, with expressions of terror, call to his friends to look out for the shells. Some show highly dramatic reactions and excessive startle patterns in response to slight stimuli. In extreme cases, the soldier's behavior is one of panic reaction, in which there is apparently a complete disruption of personality organization. His uncontrolled, catastrophic reaction may vary from wild, impulsive flights to "freezing," or primitive protective withdrawal, with stupor, catatonia, or mutism.

Some cases of combat neurosis assume the form of *depression*, usually preceded by anxiety. The depression may not be particularly obvious until after the effort to control anxiety has failed. The depression is frequently precipitated by the death of a comrade to whose loss the soldier was unable to reconcile himself. The conscious mental content is dominated by ideas of failure, guilt, and self-condemnation. The patient is convinced that he has let his buddies down or that in some way he has been responsible for their deaths. Frequently such depressions arise in cases in which the patient has had ambivalent feelings directed toward a comrade. Upon the death of his buddy, the unconscious hostility that existed in these feelings stimulates the conviction that he actually caused the death of his comrade. This evokes guilt, depression, and self-punishment. The clinical symptoms are characterized by a rigid, masklike face, by paucity of movement, and by ideas of self-accusation and self-depreciation.

A 17-year-old seaman had seven months' active duty prior to admission to the hospital with a tentative diagnosis of intracranial injury.

He was the third of four boys in a family of six. His father was a "shell-shocked" veteran of World War I, now alcoholic and a chronic complainer. The mother was migrainous. The home was kept discordant by parental quarrels; nevertheless, the patient, though of retiring and quiet nature, adjusted well at school, was accepted by his classmates, and was not considered temperamentally unstable.

Following his enlistment in the naval service, he received three weeks of basic training and was detailed aboard a transport for drill in amphibious operations. The patient had hoped for duty aboard a combat ship of the line. Three weeks prior to the departure of the convoys for the North African engagement, he was transferred to another ship. There he was barely acquainted with his new shipmates when the engagement opened. His immediate chief was regarded by him with little respect as an "old man." The seaman was extremely apprehensive as his landing boat approached the beach during the opening operations, but he quickly regained composure when not exposed to fire. The following day he was frightened to the point of believing his legs were paralyzed when an enemy plane strafed the ship and he threw himself on the deck. The fourth day the ship was suddenly torpedoed. He was blown against the bulkhead and struck his head but was not injured and quickly climbed down a net into a tank lighter below. While throwing out lines to men struggling in the water, he was fascinated by their cries and amazed to see some cast aside their life jackets. After helping one man aboard, the patient felt so weak that he lay upon the deck and later had to be assisted ashore. The following day a plane killed a French woman in town, and he morbidly examined her body and the leg wounds of a sailor wounded in the same raid.

He then realized how tense and anxious he felt, and in the following weeks had difficulty in sleeping, being repeatedly awakened by dreams in which his ship was torpedoed or he was shot in the leg. While aboard the transport returning home, he and the men in his division were quartered in a forward compartment. During a prolonged storm, the group repeatedly rushed to the boat deck in panic when a loose hatch cover slammed above them. He was given a 30-day leave after arriving in this country, but the change in his personality was so conspicuous to his family that his mother shortly sought medical advice concerning his symptoms.

On return to duty, the patient complained of headaches and dizziness and was transferred to the hospital for study. As there was no evidence of organic disease, psychiatric examination was requested. His extreme restlessness, amounting to agitation, and his inattentiveness and irritation were immediately apparent. He was unable to concentrate, expressed death fears, and presented the history of nightmares and sensitivity to sounds reminiscent of combat. His sleep was broken almost nightly by terrifying dreams. With sedation and psychotherapy there was some diminution in the restlessness, the insomnia, and his response to startle. He put on weight but continued to complain and insisted upon his inability to return to duty. It was evident that he would not again adjust in the service and, accordingly, he was recommended for discharge.

This youthful seaman, who was reared in a discordant home by a neurotic, alcoholic father and a high-strung mother, presented no evidence of emotional instability prior to his traumatic combat experience. He then developed nightmares, a startle reaction, and a personality change marked by agitation, anxiety and preoccupation, with the complaints of headaches and dizziness. The case study illustrates the importance in determining the neurotic reaction of a disturbed home life with the possibility of neurotic identification, and the contributing factors of inadequate training, indifference to leadership, and low morale. The repeated panics during the voyage home probably further served to deepen the patient's anxiety by the process of conditioning.

PSYCHOPHYSIOLOGIC SYMPTOMS. Physical symptoms often associated with anxiety constitute a frequent form of psychiatric disability in military service. Such symptoms may be referred to any part of the body and may appear in the soldier's training period or may be precipitated or aggravated by battle stress. Sometimes they are seen in areas of the body previously the loci of disease, wounds, or injuries. The soldier then suffers pain or other discomfort out of all proportion to physical signs. In other cases, the emotionally upset soldier reports "sick" with types of disability—rheumatic, asthenic, gastrointestinal—that are acceptable to his group as having originated through no fault of his own but providing, nevertheless, a relatively nonpunishing escape from a psychologically intolerable situation. The somatic manifestations discussed in this paragraph should be regarded as physical expressions of anxiety rather than as conversion phenomena. If such cases are subjected to prolonged study and treatment, the symptoms may become fixed, and the patient may become a permanent military loss.

PSEUDOPSYCHOTIC STATES. In some cases the soldier, in his anxiety and panic reaction to combat stress, is so out of contact with reality and so confused and dissociated and his behavior so bizarre that he appears psychotic. The onset is usually sudden, and the clinical picture suggests schizophrenia. Many patients are disoriented and fail to reply to simple questions. Some cases resemble catatonic stupor; others suggest a catatonic excitement. These psychotic-like pictures occur in individuals who have not been psychotic in their previous reactions or in their basic personality structures. Such short-lived "three-day" psychoses usually disappear when the patients are removed from the traumatic situations. Sometimes sedation or electroconvulsive treatment is advisable.

PROGNOSIS AND TREATMENT. In dealing with these neuroses in the armed forces, emphasis is placed on preservation of medical discipline, early and vigorous treatment, the shortening of the period of hospitalization, the avoidance of unnecessary hospital atmosphere, and the promotion in the patient of the expectation of return to full duty. In his treatment, care is exercised to preserve the patient's identification with the combat group, to minimize the secondary gain of neurotic illness, and to avoid any suggestion of illness and disability. It is a basic principle in the attainment of these objectives that treatment should be as far forward as possible. So far as practicable, soldiers who show symptoms of becoming psychiatric casualties on the battlefield receive what may be called psychiatric first aid from members of their own combat units. Here company officers promote morale by counsel, reassurance, exhortation, and leadership. Soldiers with relatively minor complaints may frequently be prevented from entering medical channels where the dissolution of group ties and the factors of secondary gain and suggestion tend to fix their symptoms.

If his motivation has been reasonably good, the combat exhaustion patient responds rather well to proper therapeutic handling. If formal medical treatment is required, the patient is evacuated to the battalion aid station. Here most patients are those suffering from mild to moderate anxiety states complicated by physical exhaustion and the effects of exposure. They are usually wet, cold, dirty, and physically worn out. If the anxiety state is no more than moderate, the patient is kept at the aid station for 24 hours, where he is cleaned up, dried, adequately fed, and given sedation in the form of 7½ to 10 grains of sodium amytal orally. By his manner and remarks, the battalion surgeon indicates that he expects an early return to duty of the soldier after he is rested. Many of the patients evacuated to the battalion aid station are simply suffering from normal fear reactions, with the somatic and psychological manifestations of that state. The patient has usually become alarmed by these symptoms that he has interpreted as those of cardiac, gastrointestinal, or other physical disorder. A careful physical examination is made. If no organ involvement is found, the cause of the symptoms is carefully explained to the soldier, who is assured that there will be no lasting effects or disability. After 24 hours of rest and psychotherapy consisting of reassurance, support, and exhortation, many patients are so greatly improved that they may be returned directly to duty.

Those with the more severe and the pseudopsychotic reactions are unsuited for management in the battalion aid station and are therefore transferred to the division clearing station. These patients exhibit marked anxiety states, extreme agitation and tension, acute panic, hysterical manifestations, or symptoms of acute psychosis. Upon arrival at the division clearing station, active psychiatric treatment begins. Sedation is given at once to those who have not already received it, and they are placed in adequately heated tent wards, are provided with cots for sleeping, and are given an abundance of hot food.

The psychiatrist combines an attitude of respect and sympathy for the patient, yet he is also firm, decisive, and realistic. He permits no doubt to arise in the patient's mind that he will return to full combat duty after a brief rest. If the patient is allowed to ventilate his fears, hopes, and resentments, prompt symptomatic relief often follows. Since loyalty and sense of duty to his comrades are among the most important supports of the soldier in combat, an effort is made to strengthen these forces. Motivations for rejoining his outfit and active duty are strengthened. An attempt is made to avoid any suggestion of illness in the organization and atmosphere of treatment stations and in the attitude and action of the psychiatrist. As much care is used to avoid suggestion of serious psychiatric illness as of physical disease.

Both at the battalion aid station and at the division clearing station, in order to emphasize the precipitating role of physical exhaustion, to imply a rapid recovery after a brief rest, and to avoid giving the impression of incurable mental illness, the term *exhaustion* is used for psychiatric casualties.

At one period in World War II, intravenous barbiturate narcosis was extensively used in severe anxiety states and in hysterical conversion reactions. During the narcosis, strong suggestion was used, with resulting emotional release, during which the patient relived his battle experiences. Few patients treated by this method recover to a degree that permits return to combat duty. It is now used in selected cases only.

The earliest possible return to duty prevents progress of the neurotic symptoms, minimizes secondary gain from their existence, and has a desirable therapeutic value in lessening guilt over separation from the group.

Inasmuch as psychiatric patients in the combat area are easily convinced that they are seriously ill, either physically or psychiatrically, it is important that, after proper physical examination, they be assured that they have no serious physical illnesses, that the psychiatric disability is temporary, that it is a reaction to the situation in which the soldier has been placed, that it has no relationship to "insanity," and that there should be no permanent after-effects. It is explained to the soldier that his psychological and somatic symptoms are but a frequent and essentially normal result of battle fear.

Since a neurotic illness occurring in battle places the patient in a safe situation with possible permanent removal from combat, it is important that the element of secondary gain be avoided so far as possible. If it is determined that a patient will not be returned to combat duty, he is informed of this decision and given reason to believe that it is final. The tension and pressure accompanying the anticipation of possible return to combat are thus eliminated, together with a further unconscious striving for the secondary gains of the illness. Such a soldier should, however, be returned to some type of duty as soon as possible lest prolonged rest and inactivity in comfortable hospital surroundings provide opportunity for brooding, tend to fixate the neurosis, and lead to demoralization and invalidism. Such measures should help to prevent permanent neuroses, so many of which followed the combat neuroses occurring in World War I. It should be remembered that the burden of guilt that a soldier may assume if he is evacuated from combat for less than excellent reasons may in some arouse intolerable and persisting guilt, by which the personality may be influenced morbidly or from which neurosis results.

Chronic Stress Reactions

Those survivors of the concentration camp experiences of World War II are today the largest group of sufferers of the chronic stress reactions. Others are veterans of combat, or civilian groups who have been exposed to catastrophes either collectively or individually. As the *concentration camp syndrome* is the most widely recognized clinical example, it is taken for description here.

Those millions confined to concentration camps consisted of groups exposed to differing kinds of intensities of stress. The threat of imminent death or permanent incarceration was suffered by all. The intensity of the threats was variable. Those exposed to the open brutalities and killings and executions of other prisoners and who were required to participate in prison camp persecutions and burials while surviving separation from family members and friends suffered differently from others incarcerated and deprived physically owing to severe shortages of food, clothing, housing, activity, and opportunities for needed human contact, emotional support, and stimulation. The vast majority of those survivors who now have symptoms impairing their personality functioning experienced the full range of terrifying and despair-creating stresses: personal assaults of all kinds, perceptions of brutality and killings of others, desecration of bodies, separations from families and friends, and physical illness and deprivations. Many became "living corpses" in the concentration camp.

Those who have survived did so through the mobilization of a variety of psychological defenses and adaptations—as well as through being among the group fortuitously saved by circumstances. The mobilized adaptations and defenses are considered to have been called into play while the established ego and superego attitudes were eroded under a continuing barrage of exhausting challenges. These stresses broke down successively the ego integrative processes evolved over the many years of personality development, and particularly those successful for emergency control of emotions in ordinary civil life.

The sufferers of the concentration camp syndrome complain of increased fatigability, impairment of memory, difficulty in concentration, emotional lability, bitterness, depression, lack of pleasure in any effort, apathy and indifference to others, persisting disturbances of sleep, recurrent nightmares and daytime preoccupations and fantasies of these past experiences, irritability, restlessness, and headaches.

Restlessness, tension, and chronic anxiety with inability to forget or put aside memories of the concentration camp persecutions often lead the sufferer to isolate himself socially from his environment as a means of cutting off associations that intensify these symptoms. The numerous physical symptoms represent the psychosomatic expressions of anxiety. There is some indication now that concentration camp survivors are more subject to those conditions associated with specific tissue damage such as peptic ulcer.

Others who have lost their families, homes, and vocations are apathetic, indifferent, depressed, and guilty. Enduring and burdening guilt responses follow as the sufferer realizes that he is the sole surviving member of a family or group or even a single relationship. The guilt often is in response to a sense of implication in the death of others. Those with a predisposition to psychoses or with previous psychoses express their symptomology in the defenses characteristic for their personality make-up. Some evolve paranoid persecutory attitudes. Those who were exposed to the concentration camp early in life often express their personality restrictions in antisocial behaviors. Yet the psychiatrist will note the surmounting symptoms expressive of the chronic stress reactions. These emerge in the perpetual preoccupation with the past, the terrors of the experience, the recapitulating nightmares and either restlessness, irritability, and irascibility or apathy, hopelessness, and indifference.

Psychodynamically these symptom expressions have been interpreted as an erosion of ego and superego functions. With the threat to self and the loss of relations with others, the sense of personal identity is impaired and depersonalization occurs. This is followed by eruption of intense anxiety and terror which evoke in turn the primitive psychological adaptations and defenses such as passivity, sadomasochistic traits, and identification with the aggressor. These infantile modes of adaptation and defense remain even after removal from the camp. The capacity to redevelop defenses and adaptive processes seems impaired or permanently damaged. There is a loss of more mature volitional, cognitive, and affective processes.

There is reason to believe that this form of personality disruption is irreversible in many, particularly those who have suffered head injuries and other cerebral or general physical disability as the result of deprivations.

Prolonged psychotherapy has had only limited success in such patients.

Those who have attempted psychotherapy with the sufferers of the concentration camp syndrome have pointed up their frequent reluctance to enter treatment. This stems in some from their unwillingness to subject themselves to the emotional vicissitudes of reviewing the persecutory events. In others, treatment threatens their uniqueness—their sense of omnipotence in survival which seems to serve as a defense against terrifying anxieties of loss and abandonment and/or death.

In those who enter treatment it is necessary to work through the anxieties associated with abandonment and death. At first such patients may express their disappointment with their present situation and accuse their physician of a lack of understanding and warmth. Such patients will not be concerned with their losses and the associated guilt until late in treatment. Some are concerned early with the working through of grief and guilt, others with projections to the therapist of destructiveness.

The major therapeutic problem for all is the fear of a new close human relationship. Avoidance of therapy represents this anxiety, as does the frequent aggression toward the therapist used as a defense against involvement and the anxious helplessness of potential abandonment.

For psychotherapy to be successful many believe the patient must be offered or have available opportunities to express realistically his aggressive strivings. This is in keeping with Ostwald and Bittner's finding that presumed successful life adaptation of survivors of Nazi concentration camps often has been based upon aggressive single-minded drives toward outward attainment. In many of these untreated persons the outwardly successful aggressive drive state obscures the underlying anxiety, depression, and hostile defenses against others.

Treatment for many then will remain directed at amelioration of symptoms through emotionally supportive management and use of appropriate drugs.

BIBLIOGRAPHY

Alexander, V. K.: A case study of a multiple personality. J. Abnorm. & Social Psychol., 52:272–276, 1956.

Berrington, W. P., Liddell, D. W., and Foulds, G. A.: A reevaluation of the fugue. J. Ment. Sci., 102:280–286, 1956.

Breuer, J., and Freud, S.: Studies in Hysteria. Translated by Brill, A. A. Washington, D.C., Nervous and Mental Disease Publishing Company, 1937.

Davis, D., Lambert, J., and Ajan, Z. A.: Crying in depression. Brit. J. Psychiat., 115:597–598, 1969.

Eitinger, L.: Concentration Camp Survivors in Norway and Israel. London, Allen and Unwin, 1965.

Errera, P., and Coleman, J. V.: A long term follow-up study of neurotic phobic patients in a psychiatric clinic. J. Nerv. & Ment. Dis., 136:267–271, 1963.

Fenichel, O.: The Psychoanalytic Theory of Neurosis. New York, W. W. Norton & Company, Inc., 1945.

Freud, S.: Collected Papers (5 Vols.). London, Hogarth Press, 1924–1925.

Freud, S.: The Ego and the Id. London, Hogarth Press, 1927.

Freud, S.: The Basic Writings of Sigmund Freud. New York, Modern Library, 1938.

Freud, S.: The Problem of Anxiety. New York, W. W. Norton & Company, Inc., 1936.

Fry, W. F.: The marital context of an anxiety syndrome. Family Process, 1:245–242, 1952.

Goodwin, D. W., Guze, S. B., and Robins, E.: Follow-up studies in obsessional neuroses. Arch. Gen. Psychiat., 20:182–187, 1969.

Haefner, H.: Psychosocial changes following racial and political persecution, in social psychiatry. Res. Publ. Assn. Res. Nerv. & Ment. Dis., 47:101–117, 1969.

Janet, P.: The Major Symptoms of Hysteria. 2nd ed. New York, The Macmillan Company, 1920.

Janis, L.: Psychodynamic Aspects of Stress Tolerance in the Quest for Self Control, pp. 215–246. New York, Free Press, 1965.

Janis, L.: Some implications of recent research on the dynamics of fear and stress tolerance in social psychiatry. Res. Publ. Assn. Res. Nerv. & Men. Dis., 47:86–100, 1969.

Kelly, D., Guirgnis, W., Mitchell-Heggs, N., and Sargant, W.: Treatment of phobic states with antidepressants. Brit. J. Psychiat., 116:387–398, 1970.

Kennedy, A., and Neville, J.: Sudden loss of memory. Brit. Med. J., 2:428–433, 1957.

Krystal, H. (ed.): Massive Psychic Trauma. New York, Int. Univ. Press, 1968.

Kubie, L. S.: The relation of psychotic disorganizations to the neurotic process. J. Amer. Psychoanal. Assn., 15:626–639, 1967.

Laughlin, H. P.: The Neuroses in Clinical Practice. Philadelphia, W. B. Saunders Company, 1956.

Ljungberg, L.: Hysteria: A clinical prognostic and genetic study. Acta Psychiat. Neurol. Scand. Suppl., 112:1–162, 1957.

Marks, I. M.: The classification of phobic disorders. Brit. J. Psychiat., 116:377–386, 1970.

Ossipov, V. P.: Malingering: A simulation of psychosis. Bull. Menninger Clin., 8:39–42, 1944.

Ostwald, P.: Life adjustment after severe persecution. Amer. J. Psychiat., 124:1393–1400, 1968.

Ovesey, L.: The phobic reaction: A psychodynamic basis for classification and treatment. In Goldman, G. J. and Shapiro, S. (eds.): Developments in Psychoanalysis. New York, Hafner Publishing Company, 1966, pp. 41–68.

Raskin, M., Talbott, J. A., and Meyerson, A. T.: Diagnosis of conversion reactions. J.A.M.A., 197:530–534, 1966.

Richman, J., and White, M.: A family view of hysterical psychosis. Amer. J. Psychiat., 127:280–285, 1970.

Seitz, P. F. D.: Experiments in the substitution of symptoms by hypnosis. Psychosom. Med., 15:405–424, 1953.

Tan, E., Marks, I. M., and Marset, P.: Bimedial leucotomy in obsessive-compulsive neurosis: A controlled serial enquiry. Brit. J. Psychiat., 118:155–164, 1971.

Taylor, S. J. L., and Chave, S.: Mental Health and the Environment. Boston, Little, Brown & Company, 1964.

Thigpen, C. H., and Cleckley, H. M.: The Three

Faces of Eve. New York, McGraw-Hill Book Company, 1957.

Whitlock, F. A.: The Ganser Syndrome. Brit. J. Psychiat., *113:*19–29, 1967.

Woodruff, R. A., Clayton, P. J., and Guze, S. B.: Hysteria: Studies of diagnosis, outcome and prevalence. J.A.M.A., *215:*425–428, 1971.

Ziegler, F. J., Imboden, J. B., and Meyer, E.: Contemporary conversion reactions: A clinical study. Amer. J. Psychiat., *116:*901–910, 1960.

Chapter 25

"The sorrow which has no vent in tears may make other organs weep."

Henry Maudsley

Psychophysiological Autonomic and Visceral Disorders

The reactions included under the caption of psychophysiological autonomic and visceral disorders comprise those that are more frequently referred to as "psychosomatic disorders." To put it in the language of general systems theory, these disorders relate particularly to the malfunctioning of those two critical subsystems found in all living states: the organs functioning to process matter to energy and those directed to the same purpose but also to process generational biological information. Malfunctioning takes place, however, owing to failure on the part of a third subsystem, the informational system of the brain, to effectively process the incoming symbols from all sources and integrate the operations of all three systems.

To put it in more human terms, the affects of anxiety and/or fear or their derivatives in guilt and shame are aroused and maintained to levels of intensity that break through the usual psychological defenses. Anxiety leads to disturbances that are expressed predominantly through physiological processes rather than symbolically. The expression of affect being through viscera, its feeling or subjective part is repressed and therefore largely prevented from becoming conscious. Neither is its expression under full voluntary control or perception. The long-continued and exaggerated physiological expression of anxiety may eventually lead to structural change in the organ or viscus

through which it is expressed. The physiological and the organic are secondary to vascular disturbance, smooth muscle dysfunction, and hypersecretion or hyposecretion of glands, innervated largely by the sympathetic and parasympathetic divisions of the autonomic nervous system.

The tendency, however, to delineate only such psychosomatic disturbances as those that are expressed through the pathological mediation of the autonomic nervous system is not in keeping with the structural or functional organization of the organism. Furthermore, it tends to provide too narrow an interpretation of psychosomatic interrelations and their disturbances. The broader concept used here is to classify as psychosomatic all those disturbances involving the organs of internal economy, of instinctual function, and of the body image as a whole. It is evident that the internal organ systems located within the body cavities are largely controlled through the connections of the central nervous system and various metabolic and hormonal feedbacks. The organ systems that have direct contact with the external environment are used for the intake and elimination of needed bodily substances and for procreative activity (respiratory, gastrointestinal, and genital apparatus) and are controlled in part at their orifices by the voluntary nervous system and also by the autonomic through the integrative activity of the central nervous pathways. Here is seen initiation of the functions by utilization of the voluntary nervous system followed by increasing degrees of automatization through the sympathetic and parasympathetic innervations.

In the instances of the body image disturbances, the total organism is involved, and not a single organ or series of organs. Excluded, then, from the area of the psychosomatic disorders are dysfunctions of the central nervous system subserving the external relations of the individual, his perceptual and conative activities, communicative systems, orientations in space and time, and his capacity to organize and integrate the information provided him from the outside world. It is clear that the borderline between the disorders subsumed under the body image and those of the integrative functions of the nervous system in contact with the external world may not be sharply delimited and subtly merge with personality growth.

Emotional Components of Physical Illness

Within this chapter, consideration is given as well to the emotional factors and problems incident to physical illness. Their importance in medical practice is so great that an awareness of personality-illness relationship should be constantly in the physician's mind.

The manifestations of a physical illness are frequently much colored by the patient's personality. Many persons who already have a well-defined disease of chronic nature experience exacerbations or complications of it in relation to severe life stress. The course and outcome of the organic process may be greatly influenced by the mental attitude of the patient. Illness, therefore, of a clearly established physical nature is often attended by important psychological concomitants that, because of their importance in both prognosis and treatment, should be recognized by the physician. A patient suffering from serious and progressive physical disorder is very prone to develop some psychological responses to it. Among such psychological responses may be repression, denial, or perhaps exaggeration of symptoms through a desire for pity and attention. At times the damage suffered by the emotional life and mental health of the patient through somatic illness or disability may be more serious and permanent than are the physical results of the organic lesion. It is therefore not only illness or disability in itself that is of psychiatric importance, but also what a particular ailment means to a particular individual. The meaning of the illness or its symptoms often assumes paramount importance to the individual.

Many fears and exaggerations of the importance of disease arise from feelings of guilt, particularly from a sense of guilt concerning early sex activities or indiscretions. A slight indisposition may be attributed to a regretted lapse and may be magnified into disabling or fatal illness and regarded as a just desert.

ATTITUDE TOWARD ILLNESS. The attitude that the patient manifests toward his disability should be taken into consideration. The patient must adapt himself not only to his disability, but also to the idea of his disability. Faced with physical disease, the patient may readily accept or even suggest that his disability is of mental origin. He may neglect his symptoms or deceive himself as to their seriousness. On the other hand, the patient whose disability is of psychic origin seeks for a physical basis. Instances in which the patient consciously desires cure from a physical disability but unconsciously wishes that the symptom may continue are not uncommon. The patient sincerely believes that he desires to be cured but unconsciously clings to his disability with a tenacity that may defeat the physician's therapeutic efforts.

The motives that *delay recovery* may be various—self-punishment, self-importance, revenge, or protest. For various psychological motives, too, certain patients may welcome or request surgical operations. With some patients, surgery may be an attention-gaining device, with others a means of punishing themselves for feelings of guilt or of escaping responsibility or irksome drudgery. If psychic or emotional components accompany definite physical disease, a failure to treat them also will often tend to prolong convalescence or encourage a reaction of chronic invalidism. If the physician concentrates his attention on symptoms without an adequate attempt to ascertain or remove their causes, he may aggravate or permanently fix them.

SOCIAL ENVIRONMENT. Factors arising from the patient's social environment or from interactions between the patient and his social setting may be important in the causation of illness and require consideration in its diagnosis and treatment. It is not always easy to determine if his symptoms are to be attributed entirely to his disease or in part or even largely to his personality disturbance or to his environment. A study of an unselected series of patients who consulted the out-patient clinic of a large general hospital showed that in 65 per cent of these patients there were adverse social conditions related to their illnesses. In 35 per cent of these cases there were emotional reactions that were largely responsible for their illnesses. The physician should remember that in the general hospital, conditions and situations may constantly arise that tend to produce various stresses and tensions and thereby promote unhealthy mental reactions or physical complaints, perhaps with visceral disturbance. Among them may be protracted convalescence, awareness of incurable or crippling disease, fear of death, conflicting medical statements or advice, or the misinformation and misguided advice of other patients.

PSYCHOLOGICAL NEEDS. Every specialty is accompanied by procedures or situations heavily weighted with elements potentially disturbing to emotional life or personality. In ophthalmology, for example, the bandaging of both eyes during a prolonged convalescence in a darkened room may precipitate a panic reaction of a delirioid nature. In gynecology, there may be problems connected with contraceptive practices, illegitimate pregnancy, or the occurrence of cystoscopy addiction. In urology, psychiatric problems connected with impotence, frigidity, dyspareunia, or premature ejaculations are common. In surgical disorders, a fear of mutilation or disfigurement or of loss of vital structure or capacity may threaten the patient's sense of security. Today, with the increasing resort to organ transplantation or reliance upon such synthetic organ substitutes as the artificial kidney, there has arisen a host of new stresses for the patient, his family, and his associates, as well as for those in the health professions attending him. These stresses, too, have been cause for precipitation of anxiety and/or other affects with arousal of pathological behaviors, psychological defenses, and further organ malfunctions.

Convalescence from a serious physical illness often constitutes a psychiatric problem. The patient may be reluctant to give up the luxuries of the sick room and the unconscious secondary gains of illness. He may be resentful as the warmth of feeling and interest previously manifested by his family seem to lessen. More frequently, the family may insist on continuing to be protective and the patient on being babied, with the result that regressive personality characteristics persist. He may even create new symptoms as they are needed. The longer the patient defers his return to his responsibilities, the harder it is to come back, and the more firmly are fixed any unwholesome personality reactions that have been established. His convalescence and rehabilitation may be largely dependent on his adjustment to an existing emotional problem.

PERSONALITY PATTERNS. Frequently the manifestations of the patient's illness are determined more by his personality characteristics than by the nature of the etiological agent producing the disease; he experiences his illness in accordance with his personality make-up and established types of reaction to stress. These patterns are brought particularly into the foreground in the case of chronic disabling illness. Some patients accept their handicap in a spirit of apathy and refuse to make any active effort to overcome their handicap. They may regress to a dependency pattern. In some instances, the reaction may be one of depression and anxiety; again, there may be a greater feeling of optimism and well-being than may rightly be expected. The patient may attempt to maintain a feeling of health by means of psychological mechanism. If the patient feels that there is an implication of inferiority, abnormality, or incurability associated with his disease, he may, through brooding and resentment, develop various compensatory and defensive reactions, perhaps of an aggressive nature.

Among the psychological concomitants of chronic illness, the physician should remember the unwholesome effects that may result from the continued presence in the family of a member suffering from prolonged disability, particularly if the patient reacts to his disease with irritability or aggressiveness or in some other unpleasant way, or if the responsibility for his care means the frustration of deeply cherished desires on the part of some other member. At times, too, chronic invalids suffer more from diseased family relationships that have grown out of the disability than from the disease itself.

Whatever the individual's physical disability may be, a certain amount of anxiety is added to the burden imposed by the disease or injury itself. The clinical picture may therefore be directly influenced by this anxiety and the particular reactions of the patient to it.

Diagnosis

Because chronic emotional states frequently associated with physiological malfunctions are often closely related to the everyday problems of living, the physician or psychiatrist takes a careful and extended look into the whole development and experience of the patient. Home life and its jealousies and frustrations, as well as working conditions—which frequently involve the boredom of constant repetition or a perpetual striving for security or achievement, with the attendant drives for prestige or comradeship in relation to those in authority or to other persons—are common stressful problems, yet ones that may lead to a variety of symptoms that are unrelated to detectable pathological changes in organs or cell structure. Cumulative problems of interpersonal relationships produce a large share of the tensions and anxieties that beset the human being and upset his physiology. Lack of emotional satisfaction in one's life may act likewise. Anxiety reactions to situational difficulties and crises seem particularly prone to be expressed in psychosomatic symptoms. The psychiatrist inquires, therefore, for personal situations that may give rise to anxiety, hostility, aggression, guilt, bottled-up resentment, smoldering discontent, and other disturbing emotions and unwholesome attitudes that may act as the cause or as an aggravating factor in the production of much ill health manifested at the somatic level.

Sometimes a temporal relationship can be established between the onset of the apparently physical symptom and some emotionally disturbing event. Again, it may be possible to identify experiences of early life that seem highly relevant to adult attitudes and diseases. Ruesch makes the observation that the psychosomatic disorders as organ reflections of psychological tension are most common in the middle class, with its greater burden of self-required striving, conforming, and repressing. There seems, also, to be a greater tendency for emotionally introverted persons to show somatic complaints than for those who are extroverted.

Physical symptoms are the presenting ones and so dominate the clinical picture that their mental source is not superficially recognizable. The patient rarely complains of his anxiety, depression, resentment, or sexual tension, but rather of his disorder of bodily functions, such as anorexia, vomiting, backache, headache, or palpitation.

Psychosomatic medicine deals with several groups of patients: (1) In the first group are those who suffer from various physical symptoms but who do not have a bodily disease that may serve as a cause for the symptoms. As the result of the failure to recognize that such illnesses are of emotional origin, they have often been called "functional." (2) In another group of psychosomatic disorders, a physical disease exists, but the original, causative factors were of an emotional nature. The pathological condition resulting from the action of the emotional causes reaches a point where it is no longer reversible. (3) In a third group of psychosomatic disorders, the patient does have actual organic disease, but certain of his symptoms arise not from this disease but from mental factors, perhaps from anxiety arising from some situation in relation to other persons. In disorders of this type, the disability is often out of proportion to the physical disease.

Psychological Stress and Physiological Functioning

Early in the century the physiological studies of Cannon demonstrated that various changes in secretions, muscle tensions, and circulation might be produced by arousal of emotions in animals. The research of Pavlov went further, as it showed that in animals such emotional arousal with induction or inhibition of organ functions might be learned, a symbol acting as a conditioned stimulus, substituting for the original situational ("unconditioned") stimulus that produced emotion. The influence of emotional factors on physiological functions was well demonstrated by Wolf and Wolff in their patient with a gastrostomy with herniated gastric mucosa. It was found that pleasurable emotions of appetite led to some increase in secretion and vascularity of the mucosa, with increased motility of the stomach wall. Sadness, discouragement, and self-reproach led to prolonged pallor of the mucosa and hyposecretion. Anxiety produced hyperemia, hypersecretion, and

hypermotility. Aggressive feelings, including resentment and hostility, led to a great increase in secretion and vascularity and to some increase in motility.

The same investigators showed also, in the case of portions of exposed colons in persons with fistulas, that situations productive of conflict, resentment and hostility were associated with hypermotility and hypersecretion of the enzyme lysozyme and of mucus. In some patients with sustained hyperfunction during anger and resentment the appearance of petechial hemorrhages was noted. Dejection and fear were associated with hypofunction of most of the large intestine.

Learning by association to respond to specific cues in the environment such as the presence of another person who may symbolize release of tension or its arousal takes place very early in life. The differentiation of gut responses to such social stimuli, so apparent in the Wolf and Wolff experiments, also was found by Engel and Reichsmann in their studies of an infant girl with a gastric fistula. After a time her stomach responded physiologically as though it were receiving and processing food whenever her physician was present. It is on the basis of these experiments and a variety of clinical observations that Engel has hypothesized that the precipitation of psychosomatic disorders is largely on the basis of unresolved feelings of separation or loss of a significant human relationship, associated with profound feelings of helplessness. However, psychological stress, even in the animal world, is more complexly determined than by the threat or actuality of loss of a dependency relationship. Thus in the experimental situation described by Brady an "executive monkey" placed in a training situation where he could learn to work to avoid electric shocks developed gastric ulcers; his companion monkey who was not allowed to control the shock schedule remained without a somatic lesion.

These experiments and others suggest that inflexibly continuing activation or inhibition of organ systems in a manner that is often inappropriate to the immediate environmental situation is the culmination of a specific genetic makeup, the patterning by the nervous system, through a long-continued experiencing of responses which in themselves contain poorly understood and critical variables that lead to their impress. Thus experiences arousing emotions of high intensity, owing either to their suddenness or unexpectedness or to their variable or sometimes prolonged recurrence, all have potentials for establishing disruptive patterns of physiological functioning, as both clinical and laboratory observations now show.

The complex interrelationship that is set up over time between the functions of component parts of the brain—the hypothalamus, limbic system, and cortex (described in Chapter 3, Brain and Behavior)—forms the neural pathways determinative of psychophysiologic expression of symptoms. The fact that emotions may influence physiological functions and dysfunctions is now well established by both clinical and experimental observation. That a patient suffering from physical disorder, especially if it is of a serious and progressive nature, is very prone to develop some psychological response to it is equally well established.

Psychodynamics

The psychophysiological responses may be interpreted as the inappropriate perpetuations of organ reactions adaptive to, or protective against, some stress in human life experience. They are *not*, as some psychoanalysts once considered, direct symbolic expressions of neurotic conflicts in the same way as are the conversion symptoms in hysteria. Thus, no longer would one lay credence to the interpretation of heavy breathing as a disguised wish for coitus or necessarily of vomiting as a rejection of oral sexual desires. The symptom expression is recognized primarily as an activation or deactivation of the organ or system on the basis of arousal of an affect. To be sure, secondarily, the act may have attached to it symbolic meanings, but the crucial clinical question is the primary affective state and the sequence of events which led to its precipitation.

As has been shown in previous chapters, stress reactions include not only those caused by assault by other organisms and physical agents, but also those consequent to man's capacity to interpret symbols as indicative of danger derived from his past experiences, including the threats resulting from necessary conformity to family and cultural mores that in themselves lead to deprivation of certain innately desired satisfactions. In response to the stress imposed by various threats and conflicts, organ reactions, in conjunction with various feelings and attitudes, occur to assist in adaptation or to prepare for emergencies to protect the individual. The perpetuation of the organ reactions beyond the period of stress leads to sustained responses that are inappropriate and may end in tissue damage.

The psychosomatic symptom represents the physiological concomitant of an emotional state. In the acute emotional state of rage, for example, it is a normal vegetative process for the blood pressure to be raised. This rise in blood pressure will subside if the angry man releases his emotional tension by physical or verbal attack on the object of his anger. If, however, a persistent, inhibited aggression (chronic rage) continues, the patient's emotional tension does not subside, his blood pressure does not become less, and he suffers from "essential" hypertension. In other words, a chronic emotional tension has activated bodily changes resulting in vascular hypertension. The physical symptoms of some cases of hypertension are therefore of psychosomatic origin. If a chronic emotional tension acting through the vegetative nervous system stimulates muscular or secretory activity of the gastrointestinal tract, then the psychosomatic symptom will be referable to that system. The physiological expressions of anxiety may then be interpreted by the patient as "stomach trouble." Through introspection, these self-diagnosed conditions may be exaggerated.

Psychoanalysts have postulated that the symptoms represent physiological regressions in much the same way as psychological symptoms often express recurrence of infantile behaviors as an attempt at solution of conflict. In these views the physiologic expression is due to the failure of the ordinary psychologic defenses to maintain homeostasis. The symptoms are seen as analogous to the undifferentiated organ responses characteristic of the infant when his needs are frustrated.

The regression hypothesis does not provide any clues as to the organ system selected for disturbance in the individual patient. Adler's early suggestion of organ inferiority as a means for determination of specific symptoms led later to other efforts. Most psychiatrists now agree that the conception of Dunbar of a personality constellation specific to each psychosomatic disorder has no sound foundation. Alexander and others stress rather a *specific emotional conflict* as determining the disordered function in a specific organ. Thus, hyperthyroidism, the specific emotional conflict thought to precipitate this organ disturbance, centers around the arousal of death wishes toward one to whom the sufferer holds an exaggerated and gratifying dependency relationship. Among the objections to this hypothesis are the fact that similar conflicts may be discovered in patients who have other psychophysiologic disturbances, and that many patients have symptoms referable to disordered function in several or multiple organs.

Groen particularly has emphasized the phenomenon of *syndrome shift,* the sequential replacement of one illness syndrome for another, as for example the occurrence of bronchial asthma in babies or young children as their infantile seborrheic eczema disappears. Such shifts may take place after apparently successful therapy of the initial symptom complex. They have occurred following the use of pharmacologic and surgical measures, psychotherapy, and electroconvulsive treatment. Groen suggests that syndrome shift is a manifestation of the nervous system's ability to substitute one form of illness used adaptively for another. The phenomenon frequently involves a shift in the gross personality reaction, such as the neuroses and the psychophysiologic reactions or vice versa. Such shifts may be seen as a means of maintaining a precarious homeostatic adaptation through illness where the personality of the individual and the preëxisting stress which induced the reactive syndrome remain unchanged, while the reactive syndrome has been modified by an environmental modification—a therapeutic intervention which has left uninfluenced the basic personality structure and the impinging and stressful threat.

Although many such shifts have been reported (agitated depressions to rheumatoid arthritis, compulsive and hysterical neurosis to duodenal ulcer, ulcerative colitis to schizoid and depressive psychosis, asthma to psychosis), the evidence for them is uncertain. It seems true, for instance, that the rate of rheumatoid arthritis is much less in hospitalized psychotic patients than in the general population. Yet O'Connor, in a recent paper, discovered only one instance of symptom alternation during treatment of over three hundred patients classified as having psychosomatic disorders. In the overwhelming number of cases reviewed by him, exacerbation of physical disease was associated with onset of psychotic and neurotic processes. On the basis of his findings, he warns against using the concept of symptom alternation in determining appropriate medical management.

Another view is that the organ system affected by the emotionally acting influences is determined not by psychological factors but by an inherited tendency to respond somatically to stress and conflict in a fashion consistent for each person. This view, presented by Wolff, differs from the earlier ideas of inherited or acquired systemic or organic weaknesses. That some constitutional determinants exist for specific psychophysiologic disturbance is supported by Mirsky, who has recorded the pepsinogen and uropepsin levels in patients with peptic ulcers as significantly higher than in the population at large. Such levels are higher, commencing at an early age in some persons who he believes are prone under particular psychosocial stresses to develop symptoms and signs of ulcer.

The psychosomatic symptom alone, however, does not fully account for the patient's distress. More influential is the underlying anxiety that gave rise to the symptom and threatens to break through failing defenses. In a way, therefore, the psychosomatic "functional" symptom may be considered an emergency measure to prevent the patient from being overwhelmed by anxiety. He may consciously want relief from his neurotic, defensive symptom. The psychosomatic patient, like the neurotic, has an unconscious resistance to the relinquishing of measures that are largely or in part defensive. In his endeavor to stress a purely somatic origin of his symptoms and to deny even the possibility of psychological causes, the patient may seem to protest too much. His conscious negation of such an origin amounts to an unconscious acknowledgment. One objective in therapy is to help the patient to understand the relation of his symptoms to the particular personality difficulties and maladjustments that are a source of anxiety.

If the physician fails or refuses to recognize the importance of emotional factors in illness, or by a useless repetition of previously negative examinations he continues to search for an organic pathological condition, the patient becomes even more convinced that his trouble is organic. The doctor's attitudes may, too, be important factors in perpetuating or provoking illness. By his tone of voice, gestures, et cetera, his own anxiety may readily be transferred to the patient. If some incidental pathological condition is found, the patient's anxiety becomes fixed on the system in which the pathologic condition, often unimportant, is found. In emotional disorders misidentified and mistreated as organic diseases, the patient's troublesome symptoms, instead of improving, tend to become chronic.

The identification of some recent event, such as the loss of a significant relationship or conflict-inducing emotional arousal, provides inferences as to the precipitating stress. From such inferences and a study of the predispositions found in the personality of the patient, one may formulate a rational approach to therapeutic management. Emotional support, environmental separation or continued contact, the utilization or avoidance of medical or surgical therapies, or various psychiatric treatments become appropriately determined when the *total history* of the afflicted patient is obtained.

Postoperative Reactions

The most frequent type of postoperative syndrome is delirium, with its confusion, disorientation, hallucinations, paranoid delusions, fear, apprehension, and restlessness. Similar disturbances may follow amputations of limbs and other external appendages. In these instances, the clinical picture is complicated by the patient's reaction to the "phantom phenomenon." A not uncommon postoperative mental syndrome is that which occasionally follows the removal of a cataract. The patient becomes suspicious and confused and manifests fear and panic-like excitement, particularly at night. The loss of familiar landmarks adds to the sense of insecurity. It is now thought that those psychotic reactions which occur due to the covering of the eyes after cataract removal are induced by deprivation of visual perception.

Manic states, depressions, and schizophrenic reactions determined by long-standing personality factors may be released by emotional, toxic, or other agents incident to the operation.

Surgery may be accompanied by trauma not only to the body but also to the personality. Psychological factors such as those mentioned may also act in the production of anxiety and occasionally of hysterical syndromes. In addition to these factors, ill-considered remarks by the surgeon or his assistants, technical bedside discussions, or the demonstration of charts or roentgenograms that create apprehension on the part of the patient may produce alarm in the insecure personality. Hysterectomy or oöphorectomy in the woman highly desirous of bearing children may prove so frustrating that a permanent neurosis results. Although scarcely pertinent to the present topic, it should be borne in mind that many a failure of surgery to relieve a disabling symptom occurs because an attempt has been made to remove surgically the somatic expression of an emotional illness. All too often such attempts merely lead to their repetition.

Metabolic changes may in some instances act as contributory agents to many postoperative mental disturbances. These should be included among acute brain syndromes resulting from metabolic and endocrine disorders. It is probable, however, that other factors, both somatic and psychogenic, are of equal or greater importance. Postoperative anxiety and other neurotic states are, too, more frequent than postoperative psychoses. Their source is to be sought in emotional factors.

Physical agents, other than metabolic changes, causing disturbances may include the anesthetic and sedative drugs. Other factors may be toxic and infectious complications and also nutritional disturbances with associated dehydration, ketosis, or avitaminosis. Among psychological factors are fear and apprehension preceding the operation. The fear of mutilation, of loss of part of one's body, and of possible death is important. The strangeness of the setting, the sights and sounds in the operating room, and all the other preoperative procedures, including anesthesia with the fear of losing consciousness, contribute to the tension and apprehension. The importance to the patient of the particular organ operated upon affects the possibility of a postoperative psychosis and will influence the character and content of any psychotic ideas. There is usually a postoperative interval of three to ten days before the onset of the psychosis.

Prevalence

Good figures do not exist for the prevalence of the various physiologic reactions. The wide differences which exist between the several available reports are due apparently to the survey techniques employed. As Pasamanick has discussed, the household survey carried out by questionnaire has many weaknesses and must be validated by proper medical study before one may accept the high rates found using this method of investigation. The Baltimore study conducted by the Commission on Chronic Disease provided prevalence figures from a sample of 1200 persons of whom approximately two-thirds underwent thorough clinical and laboratory study. Per 1000 white persons the age-adjusted rates were as follows: diabetes 23; asthma 12; hypertension 57; hay fever 20; heart conditions 92; and arthritis 74. While it has been proposed that rates differ between those of differing socioeconomic classes, at this time such variations remain dubious.

TYPES OF PSYCHOPHYSIO-LOGICAL REACTIONS

It has been pointed out that emotional conflicts produce anxiety that through prolonged action on the vegetative nervous system may seriously disrupt the autonomic regulation of the body, with resulting manifestations of symptoms referable to various visceral vegetative organs. These symptoms tend to be manifested in disturbances of certain systems, particularly the cardiovascular system, the gastrointestinal tract, the endocrine system, the respiratory tract, the skin, and the genitourinary system.

Because the resulting symptomatology is so definitely referred to viscera, many of these disorders were known as "organ neuroses." If the emotionally generated autonomic impulse produced physiological disturbance of heart action, the disorder was known as a "cardiac neurosis." If the disturbance was of the stomach, it was known as "gastric neurosis." Clinical experience shows that at times an individual may successively or simultaneously have disorders affecting several organ systems. For the purposes of classification, the dysfunctions are separated into those of various systems.

CARDIOVASCULAR SYSTEM

For various reasons, perhaps largely because the heart is generally regarded as the most important bodily organ and because the idea of sudden death is often associated with it, anxiety, under conditions creating prolonged tension, may readily become attached to the heart. It has been demonstrated that stress inducing anxiety tends to increase the heart rate, cardiac output, and blood pressure, as well as to cause changes in the rhythm and the electrocardiogram. Dejection and despair are associated with diminution in the cardiac rate and output and lowering of the blood pressure. With anxiety and resentment, exercise tolerance is impaired. Such functional derangements may become the neurotic focus, particularly if associated with injudicious comment or procedure by the examining physician, or if some suggestive but not significant symptom adds a contributive influence.

Without Structural Disease

The clinical picture known as *neurocirculatory asthenia,* or effort syndrome, and characterized by breathlessness, easy fatigability, palpitation or heart consciousness, trembling, fainting, giddiness, headache, and fear of effort, is not of organic but of psychosomatic origin. The term "effort syndrome" is a misnomer, since the symptoms of the syndrome are not confined to effort. The term "effort intolerance" has been suggested as more appropriate. To a varying degree, the symptoms of anxiety coexist and assume the form of bad dreams, apprehensiveness, sweating, depression, trembling, and a tense restlessness. The symptoms described in many instances represent the physiological expression of the hyperventilation syndrome that is precipitated by situations that arouse acute anxiety or fear in the individual. This condition, although not always the physiological source of the "effort syndrome," is readily recognizable and is described later in this chapter under the heading of Respiratory System.

Most sufferers of this syndrome have been described as overly dependent and immature. First described clearly by Da Costa during the American Civil War, the "effort syndrome" has attracted much attention during each succeeding war effort when large numbers of men are inducted into military service. Yet it is not confined in its expression to males.

While no evident physiological deficit has been detected in those so diagnosed, the question remains unanswered whether there is a predisposing potential to express symptoms of emotional arousal through the cardiorespiratory systems. Thus in his recent studies Lacey has defined a group of cardiac "labiles" and "stabiles." The former exhibit much sinus arrhythmia and generally are sensitive to environmental cues. They are, therefore, more easily aroused. The cardiac stabiles exhibit little sinus arrhythmia and tend to ignore the environmental stimuli.

With Structural Disease

It is assumed generally from clinical data that stress inducing emotional change contributes to the development of *coronary artery disease, angina pectoris,* and *myocardial infarction* and their expression in various forms of heart failure. These conditions are determined by multiple factors, including genetic and constitutional, which are reflected in biochemical predispositions (lipid metabolism), the latter probably modifiable through external stress. It should be recognized, however, that good validating support from carefully controlled studies is weak. Yet in a recent study by Rosenman and Friedman a group of middle-aged men was selected for their behavior patterns of great drive, ambitiousness, competitiveness, and a sense of urgency of time, which derived from their commitment to executive positions in which they were involved persistently in multiple vocational and avocational activities; these men had a higher level of blood lipids as well as predisposition to coronary heart diseases. In these respects they differed significantly from another group of men of similar age who were not under similarly urgent competitive stresses.

The recent Liljefors and Rahe study of coronary heart disease in identical twins demonstrated that those more severely ill devoted more time to work, were less able to use leisure time, and had a greater number of conflictive home interactions. These authors suggest that the most significant variable was the manner in which the individual perceives his work and other aspects of his life. Those who experience satisfaction and enjoyment from their work and their home life, in spite of work and conflict, may not be as vulnerable to coronary heart disease.

Fear and anxiety are common to all patients with angina pectoris and coronary heart and are complicated as well by pain in those with acute coronary occlusion. Fear and pain may subside with recovery from acute attacks of occlusion. In those with personality defects adaptation to the illness is difficult and various neurotic defenses are mobilized. Sometimes excessive dependency needs or needs to control the environment may prolong an invalidism for secondary gain. As in the case of other disabling illnesses, the patient may use his invalidism to escape from some emotionally troublesome situation and may be reluctant to relinquish this defense as he improves physically. Again, the threat of his illness may be so intolerable to the patient as to lead to an irrational and rebellious denial of its existence.

Cumulative evidence seems to support the contention that emotional stress precipitates attacks of congestive heart failure. Also, proper psychiatric attention to the anxiety-producing situations incurred by those admitted to coronary care units or returned home from such units seems to reduce mortality among those so attended and facilitates maximal adaptation on discharge.

With arousal of stress, it is postulated that the release of adrenergic catecholamine and glucocorticoids enhances the myocardial need for oxygen. In the normal heart the need is met by augmenting the coronary blood flow, but with coronary artery sclerosis or myocardial insufficiency the augmentation fails to occur, thus leading to myocardial hypoxia, depletion of cardiac magnesium and potassium, and increase in sodium, owing to the contributing action of the adrenal glucocorticoids. Cardiac hypoxia is again aggravated, establishing the vicious circle precipitating the congestive failure.

Cardiac Surgery

With the increase in the use of surgical procedures for correction of both congenital and valvular defects in the heart, numerous early and late postoperative failures in personality functioning have been reported. Thus after open-heart surgery and following a lucid interval of approximately 48 hours, a very high percentage of adults develop an acute brain syndrome (delirium) which subsides several days after transfer of the patient from the recovery room. Symptomatically the patients suffer anxiety, illusional and hallucinatory experiences, disorientation, and paranoid ideation. This acute postoperative disturbance appears related to the duration of the operation and of cardiac bypass. The combination of the induced cerebral insufficiency, of environmental factors in the recovery room which prevent sleep and lead to a deprivational state, and of the intense anxiety associated with the threat imposed by operation on the organ, impairs ego functions.

Postcardiotomy delirium has declined in recent years, so that now up to two thirds of the operated patients no longer so suffer. This has come about through correction of the contributing factors, such as prolonged time on the cardio-pulmonary bypass pump, changes in the frightening and disturbing aspects of the recovery room, and reassurance through preoperative interviews by psychiatrists.

Beyond the recovery period from cardiac surgery, evidence of psychological maladaptation takes place often when potential for increased physical activity exists with less need for support from others. Those patients who have become dependent through long invalidism or have utilized the illness to avoid anxiety-provoking situations are most prone to respond to the surgical procedure in this manner.

Overdetermined reactions of anxiety often are found to be related to path-ologic identification with a relative or important love object who has suffered presumably similar symptoms or illness. Distorted perceptions of the illness derived from childhood experiences or parental admonitions, or suppressed and repressed acts and thoughts related to pro-hibited rage or sexuality and conceived as shameful or sinful and therefore causative, often will be discovered to be readily accessible and to contribute directly to the emotional disturbance. Frequently their verbal discharge rapidly allays the pathological affect.

In the instances of chronic invalidism and persistent inability to readapt even though cardiac functioning is restored, more often long-standing patterns of passivity and dependency are discoverable which require continuing support and authoritative encouragement to effect improved social and physical functions.

Treatment

When cardiac function is greatly disturbed by a serious somatic lesion, a load of anxiety added from the psychic side may be sufficient to throw the balance in the direction of decompensation. If a patient is found to have frequent breaks in compensation when there is but relatively slight damage of heart muscle, a search should be made for complicating psychic factors the elimination of which may determine the course of the illness. Frequently the patient is deeply threatened by his symptoms and by the implications, often irrational, conveyed by the diagnosis. The physician should utilize his knowledge of psychopathology in dealing with the lowering of personality defenses that may occur in the face of fear of possible impending death. A strong, dependable, and constructive doctor-patient relationship should help the patient in handling both intrinsic and extrinsic tensions and the emotionally disturbing life situations that frequently exist.

In heart disease, particularly in coronary thrombosis, the physician should seek to dissipate the patient's fear of the disorder as an incapacitating or fatal ailment. Unwarranted fear is too often fostered by the gloomy predictions of the physician.

Hypertension

Vascular hypertension is not, of course, a specific disease but rather a systemic reaction that may be induced by a variety of causes. The cases of primary interest to the psychiatrist are those in which a major factor is emotional tension operating through the vegetative nervous system to cause vasoconstriction. Some are of the opinion that the unrealized inner tension that often accompanies hypertension is to be attributed to the mobilization of excessive rage in the face of a threat to the dependent relationship of the hypertensive patient. This emotion is seen as partly repressed and suppressed and inadequately discharged through verbal or motor activities. The personality of many hypertensive patients is one of outward serenity and affability, but it covers conflicting attitudes of readiness for aggressive hostility with needs to conform in order to maintain often strong dependent attachments, particularly to those in positions of authority. However, hostility is not peculiar to hypertension. Many hypertensives are neurotic, with strong perfectionistic and compulsive tendencies. It must not, of course, be assumed that psychodynamic factors are the only ones that contribute to essential hypertension.

Some patients with early hypertension suffer also from gastrointestinal symptoms, head discomforts, and fatigue. Such symptoms cannot usually be accounted for on the basis of the hypertension itself but are presumably a result of the same emotional factors that contributed to, but did not cause, the hypertension. With the patient's discovery of the hypertension, the "blood pressure phobia" may dominate the clinical picture.

No final statement can yet be made concerning the influence of psychological factors in the production of essential hypertension. There is much reason to believe, however, that many of the symptoms attributed to hypertension are of emotional origin. Investigation of the life situation and psychotherapy will often make the patient a more contented and effective person, even though the hypertensive disease itself is not significantly influenced by psychotherapy.

Migraine

Although the conspicuous feature of migraine is the episodic and usually unilateral headache, the syndrome consists of a widespread neurovascular dysfunction and other somatic symptoms accompanied as well by disturbance of mood in individuals of a driving perfectionistic personality.

SYMPTOMS. Before the onset of headache, there exists for some hours or days evidence of mood change, associated with increased variability in the contractile state of the blood vessels, particularly of the head. Irritability or moodiness at this time is often associated with flushing or pallor of the face due to contraction or dilatation of the extracranial blood vessels. Visual phenomena, including scintillating scotomata and unilateral or homonymous hemianopia, occur in about 15 per cent of the patients in the hour or two preceding the headache, owing to vasoconstriction of the retinal vessels. As these symptoms disappear, the typical throbbing unilateral headache ensues, usually located opposite to the side of the perceived visual disturbance. The headache is due to vasodilatation of the common carotid and external carotid arteries and may be relieved by pressure upon them by the actions of vasoconstricting pharmaceuticals. With the persistence of vasodilatation for several hours, there occurs edema or tenderness in the vessels, which become incompressible and less amenable to the actions of vasoconstricting drugs. Also at this time, redness or tearing of the eye and swelling of the nasal mucosa, and, in some patients, painful contraction of the neck musculature follow. With some patients, nausea, vomiting, fluid retention, and other variant phenomena are associated or may represent minor variants of the migraine attack.

Recently, Lance and his colleagues have found that total plasma serotonin falls sharply at the onset of the migraine attack to about 40 per cent of its former level. It remains depressed throughout the attack. Before the headache, plasma serotonin rises. Serotonin injected into the common carotid artery produces extracranial vasoconstriction. Administration of reserpine will induce a headache and a drop of serotonin in plasma in those susceptible to migraine. Intravenous injections of heparin (150 to 175 mg.) will abort a migrainous attack shortly after onset.

ETIOLOGY. The migraine sufferers tend to come from ambitious, highly conventional families that attach great significance to attainment and in which children are required to conform to strict behavior patterns that limit the direct expression of aggression by either physical or verbal activity. Failure to conform threatens the family attachment. Thus hostile feelings toward parents or other respected or loved persons are repressed. Consequently, the arousal of rage or hostile wishes leads to conflict and anxiety, and this condition acts as precipitant for the pathophysiologic neurovascular response. Migrainous patients often disclose in psychotherapy hostile fantasies toward siblings and other family members. Frequently they have fantasied smashing the head of the person toward whom they have felt hateful. The arousal of sexual drives, which in turn are rejected by their overly strict superego, may lead again to the secondary emergence of rage and consequent precipitation of headache. The personality of the majority of those with migraine is one expressive of consideration to others, control, and outward calm, and the individual is often thought of as an effective driving and perfectionistic person. Just prior to the migraine attack, some personality traits and moodiness more directly expressive of the concealed rage may become evident. There is frequently a family history of migraine, and women are affected more often than men.

TREATMENT. Treatment for the acute migrainous attack is directed to symptomatic relief by providing a vasoconstricting agent. The administration by mouth of 1 mg. of ergotamine tartrate and 100 mg. of caffeine sodium benzoate (available in tablet form as Cafergot) repeated at 30-minute intervals up to six doses usually effectively relieves or aborts the headache. If the patient is nauseated or vomiting, a subcutaneous injection of 0.25 or 0.5 mg. of ergotamine tartrate may be given.

As a preventive for migraine, methysergide maleate (1-methyl-D-lysergic acid butanolamide bimaleate), a serotonin antagonist, given in tablet form, 2 mg. three times daily, has been effective. It has no value in aborting the acute attack. Its adverse side-effects in order of frequency are nausea, dizziness, epigastric pain, restlessness, drowsiness, and leg cramps. The drug is contraindicated with pregnancy or with presence of any vascular disease. Retroperitoneal fibrosis has developed in some patients administered this drug over prolonged periods. It has been recommended that a urogram be obtained at the start of methysergide therapy and be repeated at six-month intervals to detect any evidence of silent ureteral obstruction owing to such a growth.

Psychotherapy is recommended when the migrainous episodes are so frequent or so disturbing as to affect the general life adaptation of the sufferer. Treatment should be directed to allowing more direct and constructive expression of the rage and aggressive drives and to reducing the exaggerated superego demands.

Tension Headaches

Tension headaches are precipitated in other individuals of essentially the same personality make-up by similar emotional conflicts, or they may complicate the migrainous state. The tension headache typically produces diffuse and sustained aching pain in the forehead, back of the head, shoulders, and neck. It is frequently encountered as the somatic component of a chronic anxiety state or in those whose personality characteristics and development are described in Chapter 24. Hence the pain is due to prolonged and sustained contracture of the cervical musculature.

Symptomatic relief from these headaches may be obtained with the use of drugs relieving anxiety and by muscular relaxants. Meprobamate, 400 mg., may be prescribed with barbiturate medications, such as sodium amytal, repeated at three-hour intervals. Again, the frequent or prolonged occurrence of such headaches indicates the prescription of dynamic psychotherapy to allow recognition of conflict and modification of the underlying pathological structure of the personality.

Both types of headaches are to be discriminated from those due to other physical illness, as well as those symbolic complaints of head pain or peculiar head sensations seen occasionally in the schizophrenic that represent in some way derogatory inferences to intellectual functioning or doubts as to social or emotional capacities. Patients with such a concept frequently speak of their complaints in a vague and bizarre manner, in contrast to the usual stereotyped descriptions of headache provided by those with an organ illness or neurovascular or neuromuscular dysfunction involving the head and neck.

ALIMENTARY SYSTEM

It is hardly surprising that the gastrointestinal function provides the most frequent focus of psychosomatic syndromes. In life experience, the first contact of the infant with another person comes in relation to the nursing process. The infant here experiences his first relief from physical discomfort and tension through the intake of milk. The satisfaction of relief from hunger through this experience becomes strongly associated with feelings of wellbeing in maturity. On the other hand, deprivation of food or its irregular presentation is associated with feelings of tension and rage. Compounded with the somatic disturbance and the attending emotions are the gradually developing perceptual processes in relation to contacts with the mother and mother surrogates.

Hunger, as a percept to which the individual responds, depends, too, on the learning reinforcement which comes in the transactions between child and mother. Central percepts of need or satiety in feeding as well as sensations of gastric motility seem to form the basis of this important percept. Hunger and satiety as percepts serve as a guide for the need to consume or to fast. The successful development of these percepts is a requisite for maintenance of food intake and the establishment of an internal homeostasis which regulates the healthy establishment of bodily reserves expressed in acceptable weight.

In addition to the growing awareness of the dependence on the mother with satisfactions and frustrations coming as they do through feeding, there is also the similar interpersonal conditioning that takes place through the eliminative activities of the lower end of the gastrointestinal tract. Here again the infant is brought to eliminate and retain fecal matter in terms of relating to the mother.

Thus it is seen that the satisfactions gained through the early sucking process are associated with the emotion of being loved and the development of feelings of security and satisfaction. On the other hand, the bowel training process again provides opportunity for the feelings of approval through cleanliness or of stubbornness through retention and constipation. Frustration of the pleasures of feeding mobilizes aggressive activity in the form of biting, taking, greed, and envy. Again the process of eating is surrounded both in the family and in the culture with many opportunities for pleasure and conflict in interpersonal reactions. This is less apparent in respect to eliminative processes, which are usually solitary.

Symptoms of disturbance of the alimentary system are widespread, as they extend from those focused in the oral cavity and most frequently encountered by the dentist to the multitude of expressions of disordered function of the stomach, large and small intestines, and the related major secretory organs. The most common are anorexia, nausea, "nervous indigestion," vomiting, belching, distress from gas, pain, diarrhea, and constipation. Less common are burning sensations in the mouth, pain and clenching of the jaws, difficulty in fitting dentures, and canal tenesmus with pain. Frequently the abdominal pains and discomforts are attributed to "chronic appendicitis," and the patient is subjected to surgery. This is soon followed by a recurrence of symptoms. In other cases the gallbladder is removed. Spastic or mucous colitis with diarrhea and constipation represent another phenomenon of this disturbance of the gastrointestinal tract. In addition, obesity and anorexia nervosa may be considered psychosomatic expressions of this system.

Peptic Ulcer

Not only the clinician but also the lay person is aware that functional gastric symptoms commonly follow worry, business reverses, family quarrels, and other emotionally disturbing experiences. Similarly, for many years physicians have considered that psychogenic factors are of importance in the etiology of peptic ulcer. The evidence to support this clinical impression is impressive. It includes the early observations of the effects of emotional arousal on gastric functions as observed by William Beaumont through the fistulous opening into the stomach of Alexis St. Martin, the more precise but similar studies of Wolff and Wolf on their patient Tom, and most recently those of Engel and his colleagues upon the infant Monica. Anxiety and aggressive strivings increase motility, vascularity, secretion, and even the electrical activity of the stomach; sadness, depression, and discouragement equally depress these functions.

Yet we do not have a precise explanation of ulcer formation. The ulcer patient and his parents probably are genetically predisposed. Mirsky has demonstrated that the ulcer patient habitually has higher levels of uropepsin in his bloodstream and urine. From a population of persons with this idiosyncrasy one may predict a later population of ulcer sufferers. Also, the ulcer patient when anxious is said to secrete more hydrochloric acid than those without ulcers.

For many years it has been known that lesions placed in the hypothalamus in animals often lead to gastric ulcer or hemorrhage. Most likely the induction of ulcers experimentally in this manner is due to a profound disruption in the delicate balances established between autonomic systems concerned with vascularity, regulation of neurohormones, and secretion in the gastrointestinal tract.

Thus it would seem that the ulcer sufferer is predisposed as a persistent gastric hypersecretor and becomes symptomatic only when exposed to certain psychodynamically important stress situations.

At any rate, the ulcer syndrome is now among the most frequently encountered of psychosomatic conditions. It is of interest that the incidence of peptic ulcer has significantly changed within the past half century in western European societies. At one time it was extremely prevalent in women, but now it occurs chiefly in men. The change in the sex ratio is unexplained. Recent pediatric studies have shown that such ulcers occur as well in children. Peptic ulcer is much more frequently seen in those subject to depressions and alcoholism and is uncommon in the schizophrenic.

Peptic ulcer may occur under a number of circumstances. It may be seen as an acute transient reaction in the face of unusual stress. Such stresses may be the serious threats of military life, or, on the other hand, internal inhibition may lead to frustration, mounting tension, and consequent psychosomatic expression through the gastrointestinal tract. In addition, there is a group of individuals in whom dependency longings are so exaggerated that they may not be satisfied or are bound to remain ungratified because of the ordinary demands of living. These are individuals with essentially infantile personalities.

Alexander has defined the specific emotional conflict determining the peptic ulcer psychophysiologic reaction. From psychoanalytic studies peptic ulcer patients were found to have a persisting strong infantile wish to be loved and cared for, conflicting with the adult drive for independence. Thus the conflict, heightened often by adverse external circumstances, induces shameful anxiety. The drive to be cared for is equated by Alexander with that to be fed and hence associated with gastric hyperactivity. This basic striving is held to be common to all peptic ulcer patients no matter what the personality characteristics—that is, whether they are overtly aggressive, ambitious, and driving or dependent, irresponsible, and inactive. In the former case the overt behavior is considered a reaction to the infantile wish.

Mahl and others, however, have suggested that any conflict inducing anxiety will lead to gastric hyperactivity and thereby ulceration. Studies of women with peptic ulcer have recently shown that the onset is often related to surgical procedures or other events that have threatened in reality or in fantasy their sexual functioning. Since threat to the sexual functioning may also simultaneously be seen as a threat to the dependency relationship of the patient, the production of ulcer symptoms may well be related to the conflict situation described by Alexander.

From the therapeutic point of view, the psychiatrist may seldom function successfully as the therapist for these patients. There are on record some excellent therapeutic results from prolonged psychoanalysis, but whether these outcomes exceed the frequency in patient groups treated by medical measures alone has not been demonstrated. It may be recommended that the repressed dependency needs of the patient be gratified directly or indirectly without inducing shame, guilt, or resistance. This can be done by environmental manipulation, including vacation, enlisting the support of key figures in the patient's environment, or strengthening the patient-physician contact through regularity and frequency of visits. In those individuals with an infantile personality, facing the conflict during psychiatric treatment may well lead to serious depression and a more disturbing personality reaction than that accompanying the primary ulcer symptomatology.

Mucous Colitis

In this disease we meet with a group of symptoms into which anxiety-producing problems are not infrequently translated. Among these symptoms are constipation and the discharge of mucus-containing stools. Shreds of membrane are discharged in masses or mixed with soft or liquid fecal matter. The patient complains of indigestion. The appetite is poor and capricious, and the patient resorts to an increasing restriction of diet in an attempt to find one that will not cause discomfort. Distention of the stomach, belching, flatulence, heaviness or pain after eating, nausea, and other gastric symptoms are common. Many patients are asthenic and show diminished output of energy. In many cases this physiological disturbance appears to be in response to anxiety, guilt, sensitivity, overconscientiousness, and resentment. It is common for the symptoms to be attributed to various alleged causes varying from chronic prostatitis to gallbladder disease. All too frequently the patient is advised to have colon irrigations or an operation. It is stated that mucous colitis is responsible for the removal of more undiseased appendices than any other cause.

Ulcerative Colitis

A relationship between periods of emotional stress and the onset of exacerbation of symptoms has been recognized in those with ulcerative colitis. Quite frequently the attacks commence three or four weeks after a sudden, unforeseen threat to the patient's security, commonly in the form of bereavement through death, separation, rejection, disillusionment, loss of a part of the body, or changes in psychological status, such as graduation, failures at school or at work, and other causes of diminished self-esteem. Although those patients who have been studied psychiatrically often appear to be highly intelligent, their emotional lives suggest impaired capacity for appropriate affective experiences. Yet they seem keenly perceptive and sensitive to the emotional responsiveness of others. With ambivalent human contacts, they respond to loss with depression and rage, accompanied by disorganization of bowel function. Many patients whose primary affective need was the protective care of a maternal figure were disturbed through their early conditioning in relationship to dominating, hostile, or rejecting mothers, so that they expected humiliating rejection. Again, in the family setting physical symptoms often had signified preferential care. With emerging hostility or rage toward the wanted person, such patients frequently responded with guilty fear of retaliation. It has been noticed that both men and women with ulcerative colitis, when referred for psychiatric treatment, have shown considerable evidence of disturbance of psychosexual development.

Treatment of the patient with ulcerative colitis must generally be carried out by the physician or internist. The psychiatrist's contribution initially is that of assisting in or advising the establishment of a solid dependency relationship that will again provide the patient with a feeling of mastery over himself and his environment. Dramatic interruption of attacks of colitis has been obtained by some psychiatrists through assuming a simple supportive and protective role for the patient and demanding little. Margolin goes so far as to establish what is termed anaclitic therapy, in which the patient is regarded as a helpless infant and is encouraged to regressive behavior. Here the therapy is somatically directed. It is generally recognized that intensive psychotherapy or analytic therapy is not possible during the acute phases of the illness. Others have criticized anaclitic therapy even in later stages of the illness as implying too extensive a commitment of the therapist to the patient's emotional and psychological demands. Some patients are unable to accept extreme solicitude and sympathetic behavior because of their own personality make-up and their expectation of further rejection. On the other hand, the effort suggested by Lindemann to restore the patient's former equilibrium in a dependency relationship through attempting to replace the lost supportive figure may fail if the patient's expectations in such a role are not fulfilled.

There is evidence from carefully controlled follow-up studies by O'Connor and Daniels and their colleagues that those patients who receive intensive dynamic psychotherapy over time more effectively manage their symptoms and present other evidences of improved social, sexual, and emotional functioning compared to patients who receive little psychotherapy. Such treatment leads to improvement in physiologic functioning of the bowel but does not modify significantly the lesions in the colon as visualized by the proctoscope. In this series of patients, a high proportion was schizophrenic, and the severity of the illness and ultimate prognosis for those with this personality disorder was much less hopeful than for those with other types of personality organization.

Obesity

Obesity has been understood largely from the standpoint of an increased drive to eat. Both physiological and psychological studies have been directed toward the unraveling of this source of pathological drive. It now appears, from the physiological demonstration of two hypothalamic areas subserving separately the act of feeding and the accomplishment of satiation, that overeating must be recognized as a much more complex problem than a simple increase in a drive to provide satisfactions of a need. In the laboratory, diminution in the capacity for satiation through specific brain lesions causes hyperphagia without increase in hunger.

But other regulatory processes than those concerned with determination of hunger and its satiation determine lipogenesis. Thus Cohen has shown that the storage of lipid increases when food is forced through intermittent heavy feedings in contrast to unregulated and free patterns of ingestion. Much more attention has been directed to the processes that favor excessive eating, and too little to those which bear upon the patterning of eating habits.

As our knowledge of the physiological processes underlying feeding behavior and satiation have enlarged, so also has that pertaining to the parental influences on personality growth that affect the development of eating behavior. It is necessary that the growing infant and child stabilize within his personality a hunger awareness as well as one of satiety if his impulses for eating are to be controlled. Bruch contends that at birth a discriminating awareness of hunger does not exist. That discrimination comes about through the reciprocal transactional feedback patterns established in the relationship with the mothering person responsive to the infant and child's demands. The same inference may be adduced as regards satiety. For the majority of patients, these latter factors are probably the major determinants in the obesity syndrome. Without their recognition and consideration, the treatment of the overweight patient often fails and on some occasions leads to serious disruptions of personality functioning.

What constitutes obesity or overweight is not well defined. As Bruch has made clear, the changes and fluctuations in weight measured over a period of time provide a better index of weight disturbance than the percentage of weight excess computed from the standard height-weight tables. Stability in weight, then, is recognized when the individual maintains a relatively constant poundage without concern over dieting. Some individuals maintain weight curves close to the average but only through a perspective on life that is fixed on maintenance of weight through dieting, a measure that for them is abnormal. The study of the extended temporal weight curve provides important clues for the treatment of the obese person who is seeking help.

Among the obese, then, there may be defined three groups: (1) those whose weight is stable or who have arrived at a stationary stage of obesity; (2) those who show dramatic fluctuations in weight; and (3) the hyperobese, with weights exceeding 660 kg. (300 pounds) and much more.

With evidence of many fluctuations up and down, with or without medical supervision, inference may be made that additional attempts at weight reduction will be unsuccessful, since the previous failures and successes have not been comprehended in their fullest meaning. Here a study of the weight changes in relation to the total personality functioning, which includes an estimate of the sense of well-being and adequacy of performance in the individual's spheres of life action, becomes as important as the weight changes. Stability in weight is a reliable guide to estimate whether the obese person is adapting well to his life experiences. This is particularly so during childhood and adolescence. A degree of overweight in these periods, if stable, becomes disturbing only when the growing person is involved in a ceaseless struggle owing to family and cultural pressure, enhanced in Western society in these times by the insistence on slimness as a desirable bodily trait. Thus the relationship between obesity and social class has been found in New York City to be strikingly different between women of high and low status. Obesity is six times as common among those in the latter groups. Furthermore, obesity was less likely to be found in families upwardly mobile in socioeconomic status and was less frequent the longer a family had lived in the United States. In some families and cultures obesity is accepted and even encouraged. The psychiatric and psychoanalytic studies of the obese have been made for the most part on middle class individuals who were aware of some personality problems in connection with their somatic disturbance.

In recent years the statistical evidence that overweight contributes significantly to increased death rates resulting from circulatory disturbance has been strongly challenged by new information and analysis. Yet the health emphasis on weight reduction continues. It is accepted in many medical circles that a weight 20 per cent above the standard for a particular age and sex constitutes pathological overweight. The concept, although useful in the clinic in detecting individuals at the extremes of the weight curves and providing clues pertaining to pathological disturbances and their changes, fails to do justification to the genetic and constitutional differences in individuals. It is perhaps wiser to think of a "preferred weight" for the individual as Bruch does.

The development of obesity often occurs in a family setting in which the parents compensate for their own life frustrations and disappointments through their attachment to the child. In most instances the mother is the dominant family member and holds the obese child or children by anxious overprotection, including a pushing of food. The mother frequently has high expectations for achievement for the child, achievement to compensate for the failures of the parents and those of their children. The child is not cared for as an individual with particular problems that require emotional support, and, as the aims of the parents are predominant, the child fails to develop personal independence or self-esteem. Often the mother's attitudes reflect her own early sufferings and hardships coupled with resentments toward her family's and her own childhood experiences. Toward herself she appears self-pitying, yet intent on saving her children from similar experiences. In many instances the obese child is not a wanted child. He is often one who has passively accepted the indulged role without rebellion because of his own demanding attitude, which cannot be met outside the home. On the surface, the obese individual, as a child and as an adult, is most frequently seen as submissive and unaggressive. Yet this is not really the case. His demands are met in the family setting by the balance provided through the food expression of love and satisfaction.

The overweight adult often is unable either to notice the existence of hunger contractions or to estimate as well as others the amount of his food consumption. Bruch has suggested that there occurs through the family feeding processes a distortion of the perception of the growing child's bodily sensations that prevents him from properly identifying and responding to hunger and satiation appropriately. This takes place by the parental figure telling the child how he feels and forcing food as a means of alleviating the parent's anxiety but not in relation to the bodily demands of the child. This perceptive distortion is considered by Bruch as crucial for the understanding of developmental obesity. Also contributing to the

condition is the greatly limited physical activity of the obese person. Research by Bruch, Stunkard, and their colleagues has demonstrated that such a perceptual distortion exists in the obese who fail to perceive changes in gastric motility associated with food limitaton or intake as do others.

When exposed to social frustrations with their consequent arousal of hostility, the overweight person seeks his satisfaction in overeating and by this means symbolically obtains an expression of his aggression, as if the food represents to the patient evidence that he is the best loved. Oftentimes the overeating is done at night time in association with insomnia and is then accompanied by morning anorexia. There is some indication that the uptake of glucose by the tissues in the obese is accelerated in periods of anxiety. If this is the case, satiation might well not occur physiologically.

In time, the obese body image also comes to have high emotional significance, as it often represents the desire to be strong and powerful and actually, in life, provides satisfactions. The child is conspicuous and may receive attention through this source, even though denied it by other socially more acceptable means. Loss of weight becomes difficult not only because of inability to face the physical discomfort of hunger, but also because of the symbolic loss of love and revenge that eating had provided, and later because of fear of loss of the power symbolically represented by the obese frame.

During a 15-week period of hospital weight reduction produced by limiting diet to 600 calories daily, quantitative observations by Glucksman and his colleagues on the behavioral changes of severely obese nonpsychotic persons revealed the following affective, perceptual, sexual, and feeding changes. Anxious and depressive symptoms occurred during and following weight loss, with appearance of hostile aggressive actions only while undergoing caloric deprivation. Perceptual alterations in the period of weight loss were shown in concern over change in bodily size and "permeability of ego boundaries." Figure drawings then showed expanded waist diameters, and total body areas. Subjectively the patients reported feelings of obesity following weight loss. Also in this period there occurred augmentation of sexual psychopathology, dreams and fantasies of food and eating, as well as acting out in diet breaking, and increase in interpersonal transactions.

With the concept of specialness and power that the obese child develops from the maternal association and later attaches to his size, the psychological life becomes filled with grandiose daydreams, particularly in those persons who daily suffer defeat in their major aspirations. These fantasies are usually conscious and not deeply repressed as in many with psychoneuroses. The fantasies differ from those of the psychotic because the obese person has awareness of their unreasonableness. Obesity at a later stage then becomes, in itself, the rationalization for failure. In some, the overweight is used as a means of escaping the anxieties requisite for the pursuit of a creative social existence. The overweight person's attitude toward himself is further complicated by his felt rejection by family and friends because of his obesity, particularly since he has a deep need to be accepted as he is.

Sexual maturation is complicated for both the overweight boy and girl. In many fat men, there is marked lack of interest in women and failure to establish heterosexual relations. Yet homosexuality seems rare. The clear concept of the man as a masculine personality is often lacking. Overweight women are usually outgoing with men and succeed in establishing marriage relationships.

The term "reactive obesity" has been used by Bruch to separate out those problems of overweight that occur suddenly after a psychologically traumatic incident in persons who have not previously been evidently stout. Yet indications from the study of such persons show they have previously reacted to stress with overeating, and the family patterns and personality development are very similar to those with "developmental obesity." Most frequently the incident leading to reactive overeating has been either the death, or the anxiety associated with the possible loss, of a close and significant person. Among those who may be considered as reactively obese are individuals who have for periods been deprived by starvation. Obesity has been frequently observed in those who have spent long periods in prison camps, deprived of love, happiness, and recognition and have substituted eating for satisfaction.

The satisfactions of overeating appear protective in some with incipient psychoses. Not infrequently such a person develops a full-blown psychotic state when undertaking to lose weight by dieting. This is particularly so in the schizophrenic, while in the depressive individual we most frequently encounter anorexia with weight loss. A number of patients overeat and become overweight, sometimes with reversal of depressive mood to manic behavior.

The psychology of the obese person, as discussed, explains the usual failure of medical therapies to effect continuing change in the overweight state. Since simple loss of weight in those with developmental obesity threatens their psychological defenses, symbolized by the satisfactions of eating and the personal concept of strength in size, the failure to obtain gratifications either through fantasy or through becoming slender results in relapse. Before yielding to the wish of the overweight patient or of his parents for treatment, it is necessary to determine whether the desired change is likely to threaten the physical and psychological balance of the individual. The threat to physical health in terms of later cardiovascular disease appears to be over-emphasized, and the physician and psychiatrist should take into account possible serious psychological and emotional disturbances that may result from efforts at weight reduction.

Successful treatment of the obese person requires a knowledge of his total personality, also that the goal of treatment be directed beyond the mere reduction of weight. With young people, these aims are not likely to be obtained unless the parent in the parent-child symbiosis that led to the overeating is also willing to participate in the treatment, even in some instances to the point of undertaking simultaneous psychotherapy. When psychotherapy is utilized, it is unwise to attempt weight reduction initially and then discontinue therapy at the point the patient has attained an ideal weight. The timing of the dieting, in association with psychotherapy, needs careful consideration. The nature of the diet and its palatability are important. There is again a growing appreciation that exercise, coupled with diet, is important in reducing weight and maintaining a slender figure. Since inactivity, like over-eating, is often an essential facet of the personality of many obese individuals, a simple medical authoritarian approach is unlikely to increase the exercise of the sick patient. In individuals in whom eating provides the major satisfaction in life and other gratifications are not available, psychotherapy is often not successful.

Many of the obese who will accept the group therapeutic approaches with their social rewards and punishments as contained in the programs of such organizations as "Weight Watchers" and "TOPS" do very well in effecting and maintaining weight reduction.

For some of the hyperobese, unresponsive to all the previous therapeutic measures, surgical bypassing of the small bowel by use of jejuno-transverse colostomy has given good results in weight reduction, although fatty hepatitis has been reported as an occasional complication. Weight reduction by this means has led some of the hyperobese to recognize their essential character weaknesses and to request and work in psychotherapy following the operation.

Anorexia Nervosa

A somewhat uncommon psychophysiologic gastrointestinal reaction is that known as *anorexia nervosa*. The disorder was first described in 1868 by Sir William Gull and given the name anorexia nervosa in 1874. In a classic paper, he called attention to its neurotic peculiarities. The reaction occurs largely in young, single women. Most patients are intellectually superior and in personality characteristics are introverted, stubborn, selfish, perfectionistic, and overly sensitive, and manifest compulsive and self-punitive behavior.

While disgust for food or lack of appetite has been described as the cardinal symptom, the essential symptom appears to be a compulsive drive for *thinness* often coupled with an attitude to being fat. Bruch has suggested from her studies of a sizable patient group that the majority are relentlessly driven to maintain thinness and, while they often exhibit bizarre eating habits, the primary concern is not phobic avoidance of food per se. Many in this group indulge in episodic gorging with food, coupled later with guilt and sometimes induction of vomiting. In a second but smaller group the primary drive is phobic avoidance of food and eating per se, and the act of taking in has symbolic representation in terms of disgust or various sexual meanings.

In addition to the loss of appetite, there is an extreme emaciation with a remarkable preservation of bodily vigor that, as Gull pointed out, cannot be reconciled with inanition caused by constitutional disease. Other symptoms are amenorrhea, constipation, low metabolic rate, dehydration, dryness of skin, falling of hair, and restless activity. Roentgenographical gastrointestinal studies are negative, and no evidence of pituitary disease is demonstrable by roentgen ray examination.

Dally has suggested that patients diagnosed as suffering from anorexia nervosa may be separated into three differing groups, when one examines their symptoms as regards hunger, appetite, attitudes to eating, food, treatment, the presence of overeating, vomiting, their activity, concern over physical health, sex and amenorrhea, prevalent mood, and compulsion to mirror gazing.

In the primary form hunger persists,

as does appetite. The patient consciously fears eating because of possible weight gain and consciously restricts this activity. She may insist on eating alone. Paradoxically she often has an intense preoccupation over cooking, and reads or may collect cook books. Her attitude toward treatment is usually devious or negative, and she will employ subterfuges to avoid eating, although sometimes "surrendering." Overeating may alternate with periods of refusal to eat. Vomiting, sometimes voluntarily produced, often occurs after the excessive indulgence. In spite of the restriction of food, she is noted for her excessive activity and energy but often complains of exhaustion as a consequence. Fearful of sex, she is not concerned greatly after her amenorrhea nor about her health in general. Depression with shame are the prominent moods. Mirror gazing is common. The general character structure is obsessive.

To Dally, the second group tends toward a hysterical makeup. Here hunger and appetite are denied from the beginning, and eating is feared because of intestinal discomfort. Her eating experiences are social, but there is no interest in cooking. This group does not overeat and vomits only occasionally. Overactivity is less obvious. Sex is abhorrent or avoided, and concern over amenorrhea is denied. Affective changes are denied, and there is little concern over body image as shown through mirror image gazing. These patients often remain amenorrheic after gaining weight.

The third group comprises those with anxiety and conversion reactions, including the schizophrenic. Aside from those with anxiety, the prognosis is poor even if weight gain occurs. This group differs in that energy seems lacking and overactivity does not occur. The effect is depressive.

Onset of anorexia nervosa is generally noted between 10 and 15 years of age at a risk of 5 to 75 per 100,000. The mortality rate is high (5 to 15 per cent). A variable morbidity rate of from 34 to 65 per cent is reported as concerns psychopathology and sexual functioning.

Anorexia nervosa does occur in males, although rarely.

The patient, a married woman, was referred for consultation to determine whether lobotomy should be performed to relieve her serious condition of anorexia nervosa. Thirty-seven years old, she stated that she became nervous and excitable following her first pregnancy ten years ago. Her symptoms worsened during her second pregnancy five years later. Prior to her last pregnancy she began to lose weight. Following the termination of that pregnancy, she commenced to take laxatives. She could not recall if she vomited or induced vomiting, but that vomiting occurred there was no doubt. In her conversation she advised that she weighed only 65 lb., a weight level of which she was afraid to inform her husband.

The patient declared that her husband was very angry about the third pregnancy and stated that he was in no position to support more children. It was her impression that she resented the child at birth.

Before the last pregnancy, she commenced to see a psychiatrist regularly, one hour per week. He gave her tranquilizers, and she was entered in group therapy. She considered herself very amusing to others in the group; yet the experience did not help her condition. Following the pregnancy she became so weak that she was unable to stand. Multiple sclerosis was suspected. She then entered a psychiatric hospital for a period of six weeks, where it was discovered that she had a potassium deficiency. In her treatment there she gained 5 pounds. The treatment consisted of psychotherapy two or three times a week, multivitamins, and necessary ions. One year later she was admitted to a general hospital, where 14 electroshock treatments were given but without improvement.

The patient stated that both her parents were living. Her mother, some 5 feet tall, had always been heavy, and now weighed approximately 150 lb. Her father was a big eater and a hard worker, and her mother was a "fantastic cook." The mother always bragged that she had enormous meals for her children and told her friends that when they were at school she arranged that they eat well by having the dinner at noontime. She urged her son and daughter to eat. Her famous expression at meals was: "Finish it." The children's threat toward their mother when defiant was to say, "I won't eat."

The patient declared that she was always overweight, but that this was fluctuant. At age 19 her poundage was 135. Her early development seemed to be normal. She was a good student and entered a university. Her marriage took place 12 years before the consultation. There was some loss of weight following the birth of her first child when she commenced to take laxatives during pregnancy. This was done to prevent gaining weight. There were two sons, aged 11 and 5, and the daughter, aged 2. The marriage had never been satisfactory so far as sexual relations were concerned. She stated that she had never enjoyed such relations. Since the end of the last pregnancy she and her husband failed to have intercourse together.

Discussion of her eating habits disclosed that she would eat if her mother cooked for her. But at such times she forced all the food at one big sitting. Then she spent the rest of the day, following the taking of a cathartic, in the bathroom attempting to get rid of the food. In recent months she advised her mother to discontinue giving her "goodies." Since then she did not remain up at night forcing food into herself or taking laxatives. She declared that mother always disliked her being overweight, and that her mother is domineering and aggressive. She hated her mother's way of managing money and spoke of it as "Jewish."

The patient declared that she was the one in the family who loved to go to restaurants and have fine food. Also, she collected cookbooks. She liked the taste, the smell, and the difference in consistency of food most of the time, but sometimes rejected all. An account of the eating schedule in her home indicated that she prepared a regular dinner for her husband and children but that all other meals were irregular. She no longer prepared breakfast for her children. When she had no taste for food, she ate eggs or Chinese food, as they went down easily. One time, food seemed to get stuck as she swallowed it.

Also, she had great concern over constipation. Her mother always said that she could not leave the home until her bowels had moved. Her mother forced prune juice upon her, and gave her enemas and suppositories.

At times she attempted to discontinue the taking of cathartics. After stopping a day or two she would eat an enormous amount of food. If she had no laxative, she nibbled and got very hungry.

Her husband stated that she was a failure as a housekeeper and a mother. She did not perform her housework, did not take care of the baby, and gave no time to other members of the family.

A niece entered a psychiatric hospital over a year ago and was treated successfully for anorexia nervosa.

The patient died within 60 days of consultation when further hospital treatment had been suggested. Her husband indicated that she had discontinued eating at home.

There is often a preceding history of obesity and over-eating, with a feeling of shame at being fat. Usually there are unhappy home relations, often taking the form of hostility between mother and daughter. The pursuit of thinness is used sometimes as an act of hostile and defiant compliance by the patient against the mother who has insisted on dieting to avoid obesity. Thus the illness often comes on suddenly in adolescence. Psychodynamically it has been suggested that the syndrome arises from impairment of psychosexual development, arising from the early mother-daughter relationship. The adolescent girl, faced with the feminine individualization of adolescence and threatened by the loss of her family dependency, responds to the conflict by an aggressive regression to an infantile-maternal relationship with craving for the feeding experience denied in her bulimia.

The ambivalent relationship between the patient and the mother sometimes is strikingly demonstrated in the hospital where the mother refuses to part from her child. The latter in turn may reject all food or accept some only to be found inducing vomiting shortly thereafter. With removal of the parent, the patient commences to eat once again. There may also be sibling rivalry and jealousy. In a striking number of cases there is a history of frustration in heterosexual adjustment. In some cases, a pregnancy fantasy seems to have prompted the patient to begin to diet.

Probably, however, the neurosis can have many varied conscious and unconscious psychological roots. Some psychiatrists point out that the patient seems to achieve both primary and secondary neurotic gains through the reaction. They suggest that, through working out her hostilities and by provoking the environment to acts of punishment that alleviate a sense of guilt, a primary or internal gain is obtained. The illness brings, too, a secondary, but unconscious, gain in the form of desired attention, affection, and sympathy from the family. In some instances it seems to lead to a diversion of family notice from a supposedly more popular sibling.

Care must be taken not to confuse anorexia nervosa with Simmonds' disease, which results from insufficiency of the anterior lobe of the pituitary, or Sheehan's acute pituitary necrosis, which occurs secondary to pregnancy and parturition. While excretion of pituitary gonadotropins and other hormones is much reduced in anorexia nervosa, there is no indication of panhypopituitarism with failure of hormone production. Furthermore, feeding leads to an increase in hormone production. Likewise the alkalosis and hypopotassemia seen in those patients who have starved themselves severely disappears with ingestion of an adequate diet.

Treatment will depend upon the condition of the patient when first seen. If she is seriously starved, with evidence of vitamin deficiency and electrolyte imbalance, infusions and spoon and tube feeding may be necessary to preserve life. In this condition efforts other than the establishment of a supportive, encouraging therapeutic relationship are unwise. The patient should be brought by suggestion to initiate intake of portions of food perceived by her as less than her capacity, slowly increasing these portions over days. When much transactional conflict is evident she should be protected from intrusion of family members. Dally and Sargant have reported on the potential of rapidly increasing weight in such patients by combining chlorpromazine and insulin therapy. In a few hospitalized patients, Blinder et al. have found that behavior therapy in the form of operant reinforcement, wherein the reward for eating was the privilege of physical activity, produced rapid weight gain.

Later on, in those with psychoneurotic personality makeup, insight therapy may be undertaken. In many over long periods of time the outlook for social adaptation and even freedom from symptoms is good. Some with schizophrenic makeup may die or become permanently incapacitated.

Oral and Dental Conditions

Since the mouth is involved in the complex relationship between the dependent infant and the mother from the earliest period of life, and since the satisfactions and frustrations of both ingestion and denial of food are centered there, it is not surprising that it is the focus of many emotionally determined symptoms. The mouth and its teeth have significance through both use and symbolic representation as an orifice concerned with aggressive and sexual behaviors.

It is the dental practitioner who is confronted most frequently with complaints or actions symptomatic of emotional disturbance fixated in the mouth. Sometimes these expressions are in terms of either compulsive sucking or chewing movement or avoidance of these actions. Lack of chewing, in turn, may contribute secondarily to the development of such conditions as *malocclusion* or *periodontitis*. Again, some avoid dental care or neglect needed assistance because they fear pain or loss of control and possible sexual attack under anesthesia, while others deny the presence of a defect by totally or repeatedly rejecting a prosthesis that is indicated for the correction of some dental abnormality.

Some patients have abnormal habits of chewing, of which the condition *bruxism* is the best known. Its persistence produces pain and may lead to damage of oral structures. Pain from abnormal habits of sucking and chewing may develop in the temporomandibular joints, as well. Also, dental and oral procedures occasionally are the precipitating external event for the development of the syndrome of atypical facial pain. Then there are the subjective symptoms of burning pain referred to the tongue and oral mucosa designated as *glossodynia* and discovered often in those with hysterical or obsessive personalities. *Xerostomia,* excessive dryness of the mouth, often is a source of neurotic complaint. This condition is to be differentiated from the dryness of the mouth secondary to administration of phenothiazine and antidepressant drugs.

Moulton found that the majority of patients seen by her with glossodynia in a dental clinic were chronically anxious and complaining. Cancerphobia was a major problem in many. Of the women, many had empty lives and were sexually dissatisfied, rigid, tight mouthed, and often openly hostile.

Bruxism, the persistent grinding of teeth in adults even during sleep, associated with pain and trismus of the jaw, has been found in overly dependent individuals, expressing much hostility. It seems to occur as a tic-like preoccupation in obsessive individuals as well; it is detected often in those with a rigidly controlled facial expression owing to a tight-set mouth. Such conditions may relate to the habitual finger sucking of children. The psychiatrist called in to consult should recommend treatment based on analysis of the personality structure and situational factors confronting the patient. Moulton and Lefer both give case examples. Drug therapy has been used with success in certain patients when the symptoms have been expressive of a related involutional psychosis.

MUSCULOSKELETAL SYSTEM

Rheumatoid Arthritis

Psychiatric interest in rheumatoid arthritis stems from the repeated observation that the onset or exacerbation of the illness has been related to a period of emotional stress. The patient with rheumatoid arthritis often has been described as an individual who is composed emotionally, seldom expresses his feelings overtly, and appears to derive gratification from being of service to others. He is usually active physically and intellectually and is inclined to outdoor and competitive sports. His dependence on others is masked. The majority of such persons were brought up in families in which the mother was the domineering parent, while the father was gentle and compliant. This led to a strong dependency, with fear of the maternal figure and, in girls, a competitive relationship toward the father and brothers. Control of the intense hostility is accomplished through neuromuscular activity, domineering position, ability to control the environment, and overvaluation of physical functions.

The precipitating events leading to the arthritis have ranged from the death of the mother and threat of the father to remarry, separation or rejection from the husband or other important figures, to birth of a child, miscarriage, or disappointments in the personal relations of the patient. It is believed that the common factor in these various events has been an unconscious increase in the feelings of resentment, rebellion, and hostility associated with guilt that had been previously handled through self-sacrificing activity and service to others. In a number of patients exacerbations of rheumatoid arthritis have occurred following the suppression of feelings of grief on the loss of an important family member. Sometimes such exacerbations are seen as anniversary reactions to the loss associated with feelings of depression.

There is a frequent association of rheumatoid arthritis with duodenal ulcer. Although it has been stated that individuals with psychoses seldom suffer from rheumatoid arthritis, yet in a study of a number of arthritic patients by psychoanalytical technique, covert psychotic defenses were noted, and in the course of treatment several became overtly disturbed.

At the time of onset of rheumatoid arthritis, or during emergencies, the therapy is essentially one of management of acute illness by the internist, with restoration of the patient's sense of security. The psychiatrist at this time is most effective as a consultant and advisor unless the patient has been in psychiatric treatment previously. Here active support without too rigid control of therapeutic needs is important. Patients with rheumatoid arthritis do poorly in classical psychoanalytical treatment. They respond best to activity on the part of the therapist and for a long time accept activity, rather than words, as security. Psychiatric therapy may be of assistance in those in whom tissue damage is extensive and the extent of disability exceeds the impairment of neuromuscular function. Many patients with this illness deny their need for help, yet with the establishment of a regular regimen of therapeutic interview arranged on the authority of a physician, they often do well over long periods of time on little more than supportive treatment. Only in occasional instances can the patient be freed from his often unrecognized hostile identifications with lost persons.

Colostomy

This surgical procedure, producing as it does a mutilation of the abdomen, an unsightly open orifice, difficulty in control of fecal discharge, and sometimes sexual malfunction, is often productive of post-operative emotional reactions. Some depression is almost universal, even though the surgical removal of a carcinoma or relief from the symptoms of ulcerative colitis ensue. Many colostomy victims are shamed to the point of arranging personal isolation through their doubts of controlling fecal discharge or flatus. Still others suffer failure of ejaculation or impotence or both owing to damage to the sympathetic or presacral nerves during surgery.

Careful preparation by the surgeon and the nursing staff, for both the patient and, if married, his spouse, is helpful in alleviating the personality reactions subsequent to this surgical procedure. Colostomy clubs, too, have done much to assist in adaptation. In the instance of serious personality reactions, psychiatric treatment is indicated.

RESPIRATORY SYSTEM

Emotional behavior involves the respiratory system both in its expression and in its action. Crying and laughter, screaming, or speech involve change in respiratory action; overbreathing and its obverse both typify responses in contrasting periods of action or relaxation. According to Dudley and his associates, one of the main factors in contemporary life which may determine the response to psychologic distress through either hypoventilation or hyper-

ventilation is orientation toward action. Thus arousal of anxiety or anger leads to hyperventilation, as does exercise. Conversely, apathy and depression, like sleep, bring about hypoventilation. Dudley suggests that neural factors make the major contribution to hyperventilation in response to action, and his studies show this response in the majority of persons in the face of sudden or short-lasting life stresses. The experienced clinician has been aware for years that the hyperventilation syndrome is the most frequently encountered of the psychophysiologic disturbances. It is also the symptom complex most recurrently unrecognized and mistreated.

Hyperventilation Syndrome

Subjective symptoms resulting from overbreathing are frequently not recognized by either the psychiatrist or the internist. Hyperventilation is the common physiological means by which the subjective disturbance noted in the usual acute anxiety attack takes place. It may be induced by any condition producing fear and not uncommonly occurs in the course of other personality disturbances when anxiety becomes manifest. Its recognition is of importance since in the medical clinic the afflicted patient is often considered to have heart disease, angina pectoris, asthma or other respiratory disease, or even painful lesions presumed to be a result of spinal cord disease. In the psychiatric clinic, many patients have been exposed to time-wasting therapy in which efforts were made to interpret the symbolic meaning of the subjective phenomena produced by overbreathing.

The sufferer usually does not recognize that he is overbreathing. The increase in the depth and rapidity of respiration may be so slight that they go unobserved. It is well known that an irregular respiratory rhythm occurs in anxious individuals and is accompanied by sighing and yawning. Furthermore, these respiratory disturbances, if sufficiently prolonged, lead to reduction in the alveolar air and the carbon dioxide tension of the arterial blood with a fall in the blood bicarbonate. Consequently many physiological systems are altered. The acid-base equilibrium is disturbed, the urine composition and volume are affected, circulatory changes take place, and neuromuscular and electro-encephalographic alterations ensue. It is not surprising that subjective disturbances take place.

The initial subjective feeling resulting from overbreathing is light-headedness or giddiness. If overbreathing continues, the individual has the sensation that he is about to faint; he may perspire profusely, and, if walking, his gait may seem unstable. There then follows a sensation of air hunger or shortness of breath and feelings of pressure in the thorax. Some patients speak of palpitation or of pain in the heart; others describe a bandlike feeling about the chest. With mounting anxiety over presumed lack of air, many consciously increase the depth and rate of breathing, thereby exacerbating the initial cause of the subjective symptoms. The more commonly recognized symptoms of hyperventilation consist of tingling paresthesias in the fingertips, perioral region, or toes, followed by tetanic contractions. If overbreathing persists over a sufficiently prolonged period, disturbance of awareness may result, associated with pallor, vasomotor collapse, rapid, irregular, and weak pulse, and ending, in many instances, in loss of consciousness or in convulsions.

In those instances in which the psychiatrist sees a patient who complains of attacks of breathlessness, palpitation, and dizziness or perspiration, consideration should be given to the symptomatology as representative of episodic attacks of hyperventilation precipitated by acute situational anxiety. Such patients frequently are able to define well the situations in which the attacks occur and provide excellent descriptions of disturbing interpersonal contacts, with arousal of unbearable feelings of hostility, resentment, or sexuality. Not infrequently the attack of hyperventilation takes place as the consequence of a disturbing dream or nightmare. The diagnosis of a hyperventilation syndrome as the source of the symptoms of the individual patient may be easily determined by requesting the patient to overbreathe for a period of two minutes in a sitting position.

In order to carry out this test effectively, it is frequently necessary to provide a brief demonstration of what is required, also strongly to encourage the patient to continue overbreathing, as many will attempt to desist after 30 seconds of hyperventilation. At the end of this test the patient may be asked to describe his subjective symptoms. If he is unable to elaborate them spontaneously, the psychiatrist should inquire as to the presence of giddiness, breathlessness, palpitation, shortness of breath, perspiration, and pins-and-needles sensation. The patient then may be asked if he identifies the subjective sensations of overbreathing as those that he has suffered in the episodic attacks of which he complains. Not infrequently the neurological symptoms that occur in the course of this disturbance are unilateral. In general, the carbon dioxide–combining power of the blood and the blood calcium are unchanged. However, in those instances in which chronic hyperventilation exists, venous alkalosis has in some instances been demonstrated. Occasionally with chronic, persistent hyperventilation, a compensatory acidosis, with reduction in blood carbon dioxide, has been reported.

Hyperventilation may result not only from sudden emotional stress and anxiety but also in the course of febrile illnesses, high-altitude anoxemia, high external temperatures over a prolonged period, and occasionally in the course of encephalitis.

In some sufferers, the reduplication of the characteristic symptom complex by means of requested hyperventilation provides immediate and continuing relief of symptoms. On the other hand, in those individuals who have clear-cut evidence of chronic anxiety usually associated with phobic symptoms or with depressive or schizophrenic personality disorders, the demonstration of the physiological source of the symptomatology is effective only in providing an intellectual interpretation of the acutely disturbing symptoms and not in providing them with continuing relief. In these instances, it is recommended that the patient receive psychotherapy. In the course of such treatment, a modification of the personality structure that predisposes to the eruption of anxiety precipitated repetitively in particular situations may be brought about. The following case report provides an example of the need for psychotherapy in patients who present the hyperventilation syndrome.

A 57-year-old woman who had been under medical care since her menopause at the age of 50 was referred for psychiatric treatment. At the onset of the menopause she had complained of headaches, nausea, tremulousness, and cold sweats. Her blood pressure was usually about 180 systolic, 90 diastolic. She made regular visits to her physician, who treated her with diet and Theominal. The patient did well for a period of five years until her treatment by this physician was abruptly terminated by her husband.

The patient was brought for psychiatric treatment two years later by her husband, who stated in her presence that he could no longer stand her "huffing and puffing." In the intervening two years he had taken her to several other physicians for her increasingly frequent and severe attacks of apparent shortness of breath. The patient described these as occurring only in the morning upon awaking. She would then seem short of breath and soon become dizzy and weak. She next suffered from palpitation, followed by tingling and numbness about the mouth and tips of the extremities. The attacks had increased in frequency to one daily. Each morning they prevented her husband and daughter from going to work and kept her from prepairing the breakfast and doing the housework. The patient had been advised to "snap out of it," and had been given sedatives and ammonium chloride without avail.

The only abnormality observed on physical examination was a slight elevation of blood pressure. She was requested to hyperventilate and it was demonstrated to her that her symptoms could be reproduced by this procedure. The patient was considered to have essential hypertension complicated by attacks of hyperventilation resulting from chronic anxiety.

From spontaneous remarks made by the patient at this time, it was learned that during the period of overbreathing she was concerned about dying— not the possibility of her own death, but the death of her husband. She spoke of the recent death of her brother from heart disease and cancer, she went on to state that her children had now grown up and no longer needed her and she commented that the family had threatened to place her in a hospital for mental disorders. Her past history indicated that the patient was a driving, energetic woman who had been completely immersed in her family. It was inferred from her remarks about death that she harbored repressed resentment toward her husband, who showed little sympathy with her during the initial interview. It soon seemed apparent that situations arousing repressed hostility toward her husband and family, feelings that were unacceptable to her as a conscientious person, and threats of separation from her family induced the acute anxiety attacks manifested by overbreathing.

It was learned that the patient had married her husband suddenly after having been jilted. At that time, too, she had given up an excellent job. Her own daughter had been jilted some six months prior to the consultation. The patient described her husband as self-centered, buried in his work, disinterested in social life, and disparaging in his attitude toward her church and recreational activities. He was seen and advised to spend more time with his wife.

In four subsequent visits she was encouraged to ventilate her unacceptable feelings concerning her family and husband. She commented on the fact that she wished to resume typing and playing the piano. She was frank in speaking of her anger toward her husband for his years of indifference, obstinacy, and ridicule, culminating when he forbade her to continue to attend the doctor who had helped her so well throughout the menopause. The patient was encouraged to plan activities outside the home that might help to make her less dependent on the family. She responded quickly. Within six weeks she was free of overbreathing attacks, did not require medication, and had returned to her house work. She then decided that further treatment was unnecessary, since her immediate symptoms had been relieved.

This case illustrates several important factors in the management of the hyperventilation syndrome. First, the patient was made aware of the physiological mechanism underlying the attacks by intentionally hyperventilating. This test also made her realize that her symptoms were regarded as significant in themselves. Second, a series of simple psychotherapeutic discussions allowed the patient to express herself freely concerning her emotions and attitude toward her family. This discussion of her feelings, interspersed only with a few directional questions related to possible anger and resentment, relieved her of her symptoms. Third, this patient was an excellent choice for brief psychotherapy as she gave a history of previous satisfactory adjustment at home, at work, and in marriage.

Asthma

That a relationship exists between emotional arousal and the precipitation of an asthmatic attack has been a matter of comment since the time of Hippocrates. Despite the fact that it is generally conceded that the asthma occurs in individuals with a constitutional predisposition, there are now on record many cases in which the attacks were initiated by events other than the presence of a specific antigen. The well-known instance of "rose asthma" is representative of this type of induction, in which the patient regularly had an attack when she was brought into contact with roses but also had asthma when she was shown a papier-mâché rose. Other similar precipitating instances are recorded in which patients have their asthmatic attack at a regular hour each day, when they hear a particular song or type of story, or react on hearing comments about a parent, or visit the parent's grave. Under such circumstances, the asthmatic attack is regarded by some as the conditioned response to the situational cue—that is, as a conditioned reflex to a conditional stimulation. It has been shown experimentally that one may establish in animals a conditioned asthmatic reflex by associations of a cue to presentation of an allergen used as the unconditioned stimulus. Undoubtedly the process of precipitation is more complex. Hyperventilation leads to bronchial spasm; its precipitation through induction of anxiety also may be causative in initiation of the asthmatic episode. Freeman and his associates have reviewed recently and critically the considerable literature on this subject. In some surveys of allergic patients as many as 75 per cent were found to have an emotional component influencing their attacks.

The asthmatic personality often is one of irritability and quickness to respond, coupled with lack of confidence, submissiveness, and anxiety. Most clinical observers have noticed that there is an unusually strong maternal dependency that arouses conflict when aggressive or sexual drives threaten the relationship. The exaggerated dependency drive has arisen either through the relationship of the child to a rejecting mother or through too early urging by the parents that the child assume independence, a pseudo-independent façade thus being forced. The attack has been thought to represent symbolically both a protest against separation from the mother and also the wish to reëstablish this relationship through crying; thus it is considered equivalent to a repressed cry. Others have stressed the relationship of the asthmatic attack to arousal of repressed conflicts relating to bodily odors, particularly concerned with excretions and secretions and thereby presumably involved in early childhood rearing relative to cleanliness, dirtiness, or sexuality. There is evidence that asthmatics show significantly greater blocking of associations on exposure to various odors than do other groups.

In addition to medical care to prevent and also treat the acute seizure, many asthmatics may profit by psychotherapy particularly directed to resolution of the dependency problem, which is often associated with repressed hostility. It has been found that children with asthma frequently respond promptly on separation from their parents. Permanent improvement for such children requires, as well, effective counseling and psychotherapy for the involved parents.

ENDOCRINE SYSTEM

Diabetes Mellitus

Among the more striking examples of the influence of emotional disturbances on somatic functioning is that observed in certain patients suffering from diabetes mellitus. Personality factors and the consequent emotional responses to the treatment regimen of this condition relate to almost all the issues pertaining to the therapy of diabetes. The psychiatrist may make a major contribution in the treatment and management of those difficult patients with "brittle diabetes." Psychosomatic investigations in recent years have clearly elucidated the disturbances in glucose metabolism and variations in ketonemia resulting from changes in the emotional state of the individual.

It has been suggested that the onset of diabetes is often related to periods of severe emotional distress after such experiences as disruption of the home, or frustration associated with long periods of grinding work. Although the inquiry into the personality structure of the diabetic has failed to demonstrate a uniform personality picture, many psychiatrists have emphasized the passivity and immaturity with which diabetic patients look for attention and affection. Psychoanalytical studies of a few patients suggest that certain diabetics are frustrated when their demands for love and attention cannot be met. Others have stated that the psychological trauma derives from reactivation of dependency needs by new exposure to rejection and deprivation through the loss of another person.

On the physiological side, it has been shown that urinary and blood glucose levels are elevated following periods of emotional stress and that the glucose tolerance curves may be modified at such times. In general, the glucose tolerance test has been found to indicate a higher degree of diabetes when the individual is feeling more hostile and depressed, and it approaches the healthy curve when the patient feels accepted and cared for. It has been shown that an increase in ketone bodies in the blood stream may occur in similar situations; also, that with increasing diuresis, the diabetic may lose sugar, ketones, and chlorides, with depletion of fixed base and a rapid fall of glycogen in the blood stream. Such physiological changes, associated with the metabolic defect, lead to acidosis and may precipitate coma, particularly when the anxious patient neglects his diabetic regimen, as frequently takes place.

Since the customary regulation of diabetes requires both control of the diet and the administration of insulin, the management of the disease is often complicated by the fact that the symbolic significance of the feeding process and its relationship to provision of emotional support through love may modify the therapeutic indications. It is particularly true that the giving of food and its deprivation become paramount in those homes where tension exists between parents and a diabetic child. The illness magnifies the difficulty between the child and the parents. Those parents with perfectionistic, aggressive attitudes may bring their children to good control of the diabetes but with the creation of a behavior difficulty. On the other hand, parents who pity themselves or blame the child and reject it may foster poor control of the diabetes.

The need to limit food often becomes a battleground between the child and parents and the child and physician. This is particularly so since the giving of candy or of food is often a token of approval in the family. The child has an excellent weapon that he can use against rigid punitive parents by refusing to eat when he is denied his wishes. Other children, under treatment for diabetes mellitus, finding themselves starved for food or affection, express their hostility through eating as they wish and then lying convincingly. Thus the rigid dietary management insisted upon by the physician and the family often leads to rather serious emotional disturbance in the child, with concomitant change or modification of the glucose metabolism and probable ketosis, or to psychological conflicts that deter the proper acceptance of the therapeutic needs of the illness. In such instances, the psychiatrist is needed as a means of working through the emotional conflict of the child with the parents, in assisting the parents to understand the child's problem and occasionally in providing advice to the internist in regard to the personality reactions of the child and the need to modify the dietary regimen and insulin requirements in conformity with the emotional problem that exists.

Because this 16-year-old lad had been hospitalized nine times in a general hospital for diabetic acidosis or coma during the preceding six months, he was referred for psychiatric consultation. There was a history of diabetes commencing three years previously, when his mother noticed he had lost weight and suffered abnormal thirst and frequency of urination.

Previous to the onset of the diabetes the boy had been able to engage in all activities with friends of his age. He withdrew from his contacts with other children following the commencement of his treatment due to their teasing of him as "diabetic kid" and "sugar blood kid." His physicians advised him that if he did not care for his diabetes by restriction of diet and proper use of insulin, he might lose a limb or his sight or be subjected to overwhelming infections if he were hurt. His diabetic treatment proceeded well during the first year under the care of a firm, insistent, older physician. However, difficulties arose when this physician retired and the patient transferred to another more permissive doctor. In view of the inability to control him under general medical care and as the result of the psychiatric consultation, it was decided to hospitalize him in a psychiatric nursing unit.

On admission the patient advised that his problem was simple. He stated he was a compulsive eater and that all he had to do was learn how not to eat. When his mother was consulted, she appeared anxious and expressed feelings of depression and hopelessness in regard to the patient. She described her deep feelings of guilt toward him but explained she was unable to cope with his rebelliousness. Her three other children were obedient. She stated that he seemed to awaken at all hours of the night and had taken to stealing food, frequently failed to give himself insulin injections, and strongly resisted the mother's attempts to administer them. He refused absolutely to perform the urinalysis, and he falsified reports to the clinic physician. He told his mother that he would rather have cancer and die than continue with the diabetes. He was openly aggressive toward her, and when angry he threatened to refuse to take insulin the next day. His relationship with his father was similar to that with the mother.

The mother admitted that she constantly argued with the patient to persist with his diet and to take insulin as prescribed. At the same time, she forbade mention of the diabetes at other periods. The father saw the patient's diabetes as a severe blow, as he had long hoped that the patient would be able to assume the financial support of the family. The father described his discontent in the marriage and accused the mother of forcing him into marriage. The patient was born as an illegitimate child. However, approximately 2 years later, the parents married following the mother's second pregnancy. The father spoke of his resentment toward his very active son because of his noisy play and admitted frequent beatings of the boy.

The developmental history revealed that the patient was a feeding problem from birth onward. He cried frequently at night and was awake for most of the day. Following an early circumcision, he developed projectile vomiting. Throughout his childhood he was a poor eater and required small feedings eight to ten times daily. His mother held and fed him until he was three years of age. With the birth of his sibling, there was evident rivalry and hostility. Since the father worked at night, this boy had slept in the mother's bedroom until the onset of the diabetes.

It was formulated that this young patient had suffered early affective deprivation that established an exaggerated need for a dependent emotional relationship. Also, the early feeding pattern had formed a demanding need for satisfactions that were not being met through the restricted and rigid diabetic dieting. In addition, it was considered that the boy was fearful of expressions of hostility due to the threatening relationship with the father and the threats provided him by the physicians in charge of his case. In reaction to his exaggerated dependency needs, he had developed an air of defiance. It was accordingly arranged that on admission to the hospital he would be allowed a permissive diet, with the privilege of controlling his own utilization of insulin, and that treatment should be conducted by a relatively firm male physician.

The patient was seen twice weekly in psychotherapy over a period of one year. Initially he was grandiose, defiant, and a braggart, both in relation to other patients on the ward and during treatment hours. Much anger was expressed toward his father, and he suffered mood swings. Some 10 weeks after admission, he burst into tears while describing an incident in childhood when his father had locked him in a room. At this point he verbalized the reasons for his hostile feelings toward his mother and also became defiant toward the nurses on the wards. Many fears were then expressed relative to mutilation and death that were traced to the father's early threats of bodily harm.

Following a home visit, when he had an argument with the father, he developed a stuporous condition simulating a diabetic coma on return to the hospital. This was recognized as a hysterical dissociation; it was treated conservatively and later studied in psychotherapy. In the course of a succeeding therapeutic hour, he acted out his rage toward the father in relation to the therapist. When no harm resulted, there were no further recurrences of the dissociated activity, diabetic coma, or acidosis. He was discharged home to his family, continuing on the permissive diet and personal control of insulin.

Control of diabetes with evident improved relationship and understanding between the patient, parents, and sibling were evident in follow-up visits extending two years after his discharge from psychiatric hospitalization. The diagnosis was character neurosis with diabetes mellitus, juvenile type.

Adult diabetics who repeatedly go into acidosis are usually individuals who are seriously disturbed. Such individuals either give up all dietary control or cease taking insulin as a means of expressing their depressive and suicidal drives. Although this is the case in the majority of instances, other persons are precipitated into states of acidosis by serious transient emotional disturbances. Sexual difficulties are common in both men and women with diabetes. Diabetic women are concerned over child bearing, while diabetic men are frequently impotent. Childbirth itself may activate regressive cravings for care and affection in diabetics of either sex. The new child may be seen as a rival for the affection of the husband or wife. Thus the dependent cravings of the patient may be magnified, with resulting feelings of anxiety and depression that disturb the metabolic balance or lead to despair and diminished motivation for control of diet. Obese diabetics who are addicted to sweets or to over-eating are likely to overeat when anxious in spite of threats of physicians concerning their future health if they fail to adhere to the diabetic regimen. Here, again, the need for psychiatric aid becomes important.

Hyperthyroidism

The most important of the endocrine glands as related to psychosomatic medicine is the *thyroid*. Although as early as 1803 reference was made to the occurrence of sudden fright preceding hyperthyroidism, yet not until relatively recently has the possibility that emotional troubles may play an important part in the cause and course of the disease received adequate attention in the treatment of thyrotoxic states. This recent knowledge is detailed in Chapter 17 of this book.

SKIN

A recognition of the importance of psychological factors in many dermatoses is by no means recent. Sydenham (1624–1689), for example, writing of the "hysteric diseases," described angioneurotic edema affecting one leg. Since the skin is an organ subject to the direct influences of the autonomic nervous system and the indirect effect of endocrine activity, as well as subject on the body surface to compulsive contact or self-inflicted damage representing unconscious conflict, the means of expression of the psychological disturbance vary greatly from one type of lesion to another. In the past few years, with the increasing recognition of psychological factors in the genesis of somatic diseases, the dermatologists have emphasized a high degree of association between various skin diseases, such as pruritus, neurodermatoses, hyperhidrosis, and other reactions, and evidences of difficulties in adjustment of personality to stressful life situations. Some dermatology clinics have reported that psychiatric factors were found to be of significance in over 75 per cent of their patients.

There have now been carried out numerous experiments indicating that the skin inflammatory responses in the same individual are variable depending upon his mood and attitude and the situational stress. Depression is associated with low responsiveness. High responsiveness occurs in association with evidence of diminished adrenal cortical function.

In cases of the dry type of *neurodermatitis,* it has been considered that excoriation of the skin is more fundamental than the pruritus usually complained of by these patients. The itching often represents a voluptuous or tantalizing sensation. Events that produce the emotions of anger, with depression and feelings of guilt, generally precipitate the exacerbation of the cutaneous eruption. The family constellation is often that of a hostile dependent maternal relationship, in which itching and scratching symbolize anger at the mother figure handled masochistically due to guilt.

In the exudative type of neurodermatitis of children (atopic dermatitis), there has been found evidence of maternal rejection. Here the emotional disturbance is thought to be expressed primarily through a psychophysiological mechanism that induces vesiculation. In *urticaria* the psychodynamic explanation is very similar to that of asthma, with the lesions precipitated by situations that induce resentment and frustration resulting from a threat to an important dependency relationship. With *pruritus of the anogenital* area, repression of various sexual conflicts has been observed. *Dermatitis factitia* has been recognized for many years as psychologically determined. Sado-masochistic mechanisms associated with the need to maintain a gratifying passive dependency again underlie the self-infliction of the lesions in many such instances.

Various methods of treatment for the neurodermatoses have been devised. Frequently separation from the significant family members brings about clearing, with recurrence noted on return to the family. The following case report represents a trial with a brief psychotherapeutic method of the type recently described by Sietz.

The patient, a 46-year-old retired policeman, was seen with the chief complaint of a skin rash. The onset of his dermatitis occurred 25 years previously when, shortly after his marriage, he noted the gradual appearance of a diffuse scaling eruption of the scalp. Some time later he developed redness and scaling in the groin, and a more or less generalized eruption, especially around the sides of his neck and in the creases of the knees and elbows. The rash was intensely pruritic, and the patient frequently scratched until he bled. Two years prior to admission, the eruption became generalized. No relief was obtained from steroid therapy and a multitude of other medications. Because of a life-long history of emotional problems, he was referred for psychiatric consultation.

The patient was the second of six children. His father was described as a strict disciplinarian who beat the children regularly with a cat-o'-nine-tails. Until 17 years of age, the patient was not allowed to stay out in the evening without his father's permission, and if he arrived home late he was beaten.

The mother was described as a warm, understanding person who was affectionate with the children but showed little love toward her husband. The patient's older brother was a fireman, who had retired 10 years previously following an acute psychotic episode. The other four siblings appeared to be in good health. The patient explained their good fortune with the statement, "By the time they arrived, my father had mellowed."

The patient's early development was unremarkable and his progress at school was average. He remembered that he was never able to express anger and never disobeyed his father's detailed instructions.

As an adolescent the patient was a shy, sensitive boy who was self-conscious and avoided social relationships with girls. There were exaggerated guilt feelings over masturbation. When confronted with social situations that were threatening, he would turn to drinking. He stated, "I had a terrific inferiority complex and liquor helped me to overcome it."

Since a civil service position offered a secure position and pension, he joined the police force at the suggestion of his father. When 20 years of age, he married in the hope of getting away from home. From the first there was marital difficulty, and he began to drink a quart of liquor daily.

Fourteen years before psychiatric consultation, the patient, during a riot, was struck on the head and sustained a concussion necessitating a brief hospitalization. Following his discharge he became tremulous and complained of extreme nervousness. His alcoholic intake increased in an effort to alleviate the pruritus, his anxiety, and the constant fear that he was about to die. He was discharged from the police force with a pension and the diagnosis of post-traumatic psychoneurosis.

During the subsequent two years he separated from his wife and child, lost contact with his family, and lived with an alcoholic woman who was suffering from cirrhosis. There were several episodes of delirium tremens, and he was hospitalized for alcoholic neuropathy, hepatic cirrhosis, and hematemesis.

Eight years prior to this consultation and following the death of his female companion, he was warned by a physician that if he continued drinking he would probably not survive another year. He discontinued drinking, was reconciled with his wife, and his dermatitis cleared, leaving only a few eczematous patches. He returned to work as a law clerk, attended church regularly and, in his own words, "became a model citizen." He maintained a rigid routine involving difficult hours of work. He dressed meticulously and attempted to do a perfect job at the office.

During the past two years his rash again became generalized and intensely pruritic. His wife informed him that, while asleep, he scratched as if he were intent on killing himself. He was admitted to a hospital in the hope that separation from his family and job would help in the treatment of his skin condition.

When seen in psychiatric consultation, he appeared as a well-groomed, neatly attired, middle-aged man, alert and accurate, who spoke of his past experiences with obvious embarrassment. His memory was good, and he was well oriented, with an average intelligence and a normal fund of knowledge. He seemed anxious to please the interviewer and stated that he needed psychiatric help. During consultation he scratched freely. He volunteered that scratching usually brought him great relief and, at times, a satisfaction not unlike that of sexual pleasure. When psychotherapy was suggested, he quickly agreed. It was explained that he would be seen once a week for a period of 10 weeks by the psychiatrist in the outpatient department and that immediately preceding the interview he would be seen by the dermatologist for a brief examination.

During the first two interviews, an anamnesis was obtained, with particular emphasis on his current activity. He discussed the present fear of his father and the avoidance of situations that would bring him in contact with him. His wife frequently accused him of being a coward because of this, but he could not admit his fear to her. He described his wife as a stubborn, outspoken woman who was usually the disciplinarian with his 17-year-old-boy. When he attempted to punish his son, his wife became outraged and pointed out to him how good it had been of both of them to accept him back eight years ago. He nevertheless denied that there was friction in the household and stated that, in many ways, they were an ideal family. His son had recently been arrested on a minor charge, and it was suggested to the patient that perhaps he was failing as a father by not setting limits for the son.

During the third visit it was noted that the scratching had increased, and there was no improvement in the skin condition. He stated early in the interview, "I followed your advice and asserted myself with the boy but was careful not to become angry." His wife had been angry with him, but he pacified her by taking her out for a drive. He admitted that he dared not express anger toward her for fear she would leave him. Scratching was frequent, especially when his fear of expressing anger was discussed. His wife insisted upon knowing what was going on in therapy. He resented this but felt he could not refuse to tell her. He was told that it was not necessary to tell her, and he appeared to have considerable anxiety over this.

At work he was accused by a colleague of being a perfectionist; he admitted being angry at this criticism. When it was suggested that he deal more directly with the problems confronting him at work and at home, he scratched and talked of his extreme loneliness. When the patient attempted to discuss early experiences and relationships, he was referred back to current areas of conflict.

At the fourth interview, his skin condition was much worse, and he was unable to attend work. He had purchased two suits of clothing without consulting his wife, who usually accompanied him. He made some rather feeble attempts to tell his wife that he preferred shopping without her but felt that it was unsuccessful. He turned to the interviewer and asked, "Doc, tell me, what do you do when you become angry?" There was a fantasy of telling off a co-worker, and he remarked that recently he felt resentful and angry, wondering if his increased scratching was related to this.

At the time of the sixth interview, his skin remained unchanged. He expressed his fear of losing control of his anger and appeared more aware of his current problems. He talked of his helplessness and became angry with the interviewer for not being of more help to him.

With the seventh interview, his skin looked considerably better. He had informed his wife that he was the boss around the house and, following a minor altercation with his son, had told him that he was "not yet dry around the ears." He appeared surprised that his wife was "snapping to," and that his son was spending more time around the house.

In the ninth week, his skin improved remarkably. He related an incident with pride in which, when his wife refused to prepare breakfast for him, he had advised her that she had better behave herself, ordered her to the bedroom, and had intercourse with her. That evening he took her to the movies and noted that she was affectionate.

He remarked that during the previous week he had been able to tell his employer that too much of the work fell on him and that this should be changed.

Treatment was terminated after twelve visits. The patient was seen in dermatology clinic two months later. His skin had cleared completely except for a small area of dermatitis behind the knees. He was feeling well, had no difficulty sleeping, required no medication, and was much satisfied with the changes in his relations with his family and employers.

Schoenberg and Carr have found that patients who respond promptly with remission of neurodermatitis to this brief psychotherapy may be selected by their evident overt hostility during initial diagnostic interviews and by a high frequency of hostile content responses on the Rorschach test. The existence of overt psychotic symptoms did not preclude the active psychotherapeutic approach.

GENITOURINARY SYSTEM

As a consequence of the close anatomical relationship of the sexual and excretory organs and the prolonged exposure of the growing child to the conflicting biological drives and the attitudes of his family and society to excretory patterns and sexual behavior, it is no wonder that in no other system, except perhaps the gastrointestinal, are disturbances of function so common. During development, ideas pertaining to urination, defecation, and sexuality become associated with feelings of shame, disgust, guilt, fear, and hatred. On occasion the anatomical-physiological functions of these organs are not properly discriminated and the result is confusion of function and attitude. Although such attitudes are often caused by faulty and deficient education, in many instances they represent a symptomatic expression of a general personality disorder that requires for their solution skilled psychiatric treatment. Even though urologists and gynecologists have become increasingly aware that the majority of such disorders are the consequence of personality maldevelopment and educational defects, far too many men and women continue to be subjected to unnecessary surgical and physical procedures that usually only serve to fix a conviction of physical illness, thus impairing the potential effectiveness of the indicated forms of treatment.

In men, the common psychosomatic symptoms are impotence and premature ejaculation. Frigidity, dysmenorrhea, dyspareunia, premenstrual tension, and the drive for abortions and other castrating operations are common expressions of psychopathology in women.

Impotence and Premature Ejaculation

Various degrees of impotence may be recognized, extending from complete failure to obtain an erection with no interest in coitus, a partial or inadequate erection with limited interest, periodic failure of erection coupled with limited libido, ability to establish erection but lack of sexual gratification with ejaculation in coitus, to premature ejaculation.

For the successful completion of the sexual act, there is needed a certain sexual drive (libido), an attractive partner, a situation that provides freedom from distraction and anxiety, allowing in turn erection, penile insertion, and the muscular activity that provides penile friction and stimulation to mount to eventual ejaculation accompanied by a distinctive pleasure and climactic orgasm.

Impotence, then, may follow either when there is lack of attraction to the partner or when the coital environment is threatening or distracting. Much more commonly, however, are those often unconscious and conflictual loves, due either to persisting infantile attachments to the mother, sister, or some other important succoring woman in early life, or to instances of latent homosexual attachments. Again, anxiety may prevent potency owing to underlying hostilities toward women stemming from childhood experiences in which the opposite sex is perceived as critical, punitive, and capable of damaging the male genitals. Guilt, anxiety, or shame may lead to impotency in which the sufferer fears disapproval by parents or society, has unconscious wishes to damage the partner, or considers exposure of his body or his sexual performance as subject to ridicule. Also, fears of contracting venereal disease or of dying sometimes inhibit potent behavior. Impotency is a common accompaniment of the depressive reactions, in which it often is obscured by the symptom of backache, which serves to prevent efforts at coitus.

To establish the diagnosis of psychogenic impotency, a careful history must be taken that will determine the situations in which failure at intercourse has occurred. Particular attention should be paid to the attitude toward the partner, the environment of the coital acts, the frequency of sexual relations, attitudes toward and desires for various forms of precoital stimulation, and a study of the attitude of the partner. Note should be made of any fantasies that take place during intercourse. Some men undertake relations while thinking of another partner or are dissatisfied in the belief that their partner will not allow precoital stimulation of various kinds when they desire it; others find themselves impotent only with certain women. As an example, a man may be unable to have satisfying successful relations with his wife, yet may be potent with prostitutes or in extra-marital affairs. Those who use intercourse as a means of defense against unconscious homosexual fears are likely to fail. The attitude of the partner is most significant. If the woman is domineering or competitive with men, her persistent derogation of her husband or lover may not only induce but also perpetuate the impotence.

Impotency due to such illnesses as multiple sclerosis, syphilis, diabetes, or other disorders involving the sacral segments of the spinal cord, the lumbar parasympathetic outflow, or the lumbar sympathetic chain should be excluded by general medical and neurological examination. In psychiatric patients treated with phenothiazines, impotency may be a toxic effect of drug administration.

Aside from those occasional instances in which the symptoms may be rectified by simple advice relative to disturbing situational conditions, such as attempting intercourse in the parental home or bedroom or avoidance of an unwanted partner, the indicated treatment is psychotherapeutic and preferably with psychoanalytic orientation. In most cases of failure of erection, the patient should be advised initially to avoid intercourse and failure as a means of preventing further lowering of self-esteem. Such advice is probably unnecessary and unwise in the instances of premature ejaculation, in which more frequent attempts may reduce the anticipatory tension. When impotency is a symptom of depression, the patient may be advised that the symptoms will disappear with subordinance of the affective disorder, which should, of course, be treated appropriately in its own right. Relief of the symptom is less likely in the elderly or in those cases in which the sexual partner is consistently intimidating or threatening. In the majority of instances in which impotency occurs in marriage, the partner should be involved in the treatment.

Nonspecific Urethritis

This condition, frequent in young men, in some instances probably represents a psychosomatic response to continuing sexual fantasies, perhaps associated with excessive secretion from the urethral glands. It may be complicated by a secondary nongonococcal infectious process.

In a few young women the history and recurrent attacks of interstitial cystitis were considered by Cohen to be similar to a migraine-like syndrome. He reported that ergotamine prophylaxis and psychotherapy led to remission of such symptoms.

Hemodialysis and Kidney Transplantation

Psychiatrists in general hospitals are now called upon to assist in decision-making as regards the patients with renal failure most likely to successfully adapt to the stresses attached to prolonged treatment by the technique of renal dialysis, to treat those who developed neurotic reactions during therapy, and to assist in and aid the family, the donor, and others involved in that network when renal transplantation is planned.

Regarding renal dialysis, my colleague, M. Viederman, is of the opinion that for successful treatment by this method the candidate must have the capacity to adaptively regress to a state of dependence without conflict. Such regression allows acceptance of the machine, the varying personalities of the treating staff, an open willingness to follow dietary instructions, and acceptance of pain. To him the usual criteria for judging health and psychopathology do not serve as reliable indices of the individual's capacity to adapt to this treatment procedure.

Many patients selected for hemodialysis have demonstrated self-destructive drives, with an expression of suicidal behavior computed by Abram and his colleagues at a rate of 400 times that of the general population. The suicidal behavior has been expressed through withdrawal from the programs, failures to follow the prescribed regimen of treatment, direct suicidal efforts, and numerous extraneous accidents.

Hemodialysis as a therapeutic measure presents the patient with a constant reminder of the existential threat. There are few indeed, needing such treatment, who sooner or later do not suffer some evidence of psychopathology. Each patient suffers constantly from the anxieties attending the enduring perception of his eventual mortality, but also from the pain that may not be escaped owing to his continuing physical illness. Although the dialysis improves the subjective sense of well-being, it by no means restores the sense of health.

Just as the dialysis procedure affects the individual patient, his experience and the change in his behavior usually bring about changes in the family homeostasis which may or may not be conducive to the maintenance of his precarious existence. Here, too, the psychiatrist is often the member of the hemodialysis team who must intercede to assist in maintaining the necessary family stability.

In the case of renal transplantation there may be a need initially for the psychiatrist to investigate the unconscious fantasies of the donors—their expiatory, reparative, or rescue dreams—and their motivations as related to the recipient. Whether rejection of a transplant may in any way be related to a specific unconscious conflict selected psychosomatically is unknown and has not been researched.

Menstrual Disorders

With the regular fluctuation in hormonal control that maintains the menstrual cycle throughout the child-bearing period, there occurs parallel shifting in emotional state. At the onset of the cycle and coincident with the gradually rising production of estrogen, there occurs an active drive to heterosexual contact with the biological aims of copulation. This phase is commonly one of emotional

well-being and may be recognized in the behavior, conscious activities, and desires of healthy women. If the drives of the phase remain ungratified, tension with irritability and restlessness betray the frustration. On the other hand, in the inhibited or immature woman the activated heterosexual drive of this period may be defended against by hostility toward men. With ovulation, there occurs readiness for conception, and the behavioral tendencies just commented upon reach their height.

Relief of tension takes place after ovulation, when both estrogen and progesterone are secreted simultaneously. At this time, according to Benedek's description, there occurs a shift from the heterosexual to a receptive-retentive phase, which, in neurotic young women, may bring out infantile wishes to be cared for as a child. This may be expressed through increasing need for attention or dissatisfactions due to lack of care.

Coincident with the fall in hormonal production in the premenstrual period, there generally follows a depressive mood, with inclination to bodily complaints, preoccupations, and emotional regression with less control. At the onset of menstruation, and associated with the sudden decrease in hormonal production, tension and excitability again decrease. Overdetermined responses to this recurring cycle of psychophysiologic preparation for sexuality and conception constitute the basis for many of the menstrual disorders.

PREMENSTRUAL TENSION. The symptoms of the premenopausal syndrome consist of one or several of the following: irritability, depression, tension, headaches, energy loss, and sensations of swelling. It seems to occur in several forms. In one it is first noticed with menarche and persists throughout the menstrual period; in the second, it commences initially several years after the menarche. In the former, sexuality and menstruation have been presented to the developing girl in a derogatory way by her mother. The feminine role is derogated by her, sexual activity is presented as immoral or disgusting, and the menses are spoken of as illness. The menarche is experienced by girls identifying with these mothers as a messy, unwanted event that they complain about as sickness and for which they often demand excessive care. Such young women live in a hostile, dependent relationship with their mother, who herself is living in marital discord. With the delayed form of premenstrual tension, there is more likely to be found guilt over sexual temptations or transgressions in recent life experiences. However, there is a greater initial acceptance and pride in the female experience of menarche. Oral contraceptives have been observed to reduce premenstrual irritability and tension in most women; edema and headaches have not been much improved. There have been some recent efforts to modify the edema with lithium therapy.

DYSMENORRHEA.   Severe dysmenorrhea and the less recognized condition of *pelvic pain,* which may be related to vascular congestion, seem to occur also in women ambivalent concerning their sexual and feminine role in life owing to early anxieties, doubts, or lack of healthy identification and training for feminine sexual, maternal, and home-making roles.

AMENORRHEA.   Although amenorrhea may be the consequence of delayed sexual maturation owing to hypogonadism, it may also occur as a defense against sexuality. It is seen as well in depressions in women and, similar to the impotence of depressed men, disappears when recovery takes place. It is a common symptom of anorexia nervosa. Menses cease also with *pseudocyesis* when, influenced both by the wish for and fear of pregnancy, certain immature women present themselves for examination with many of the signs of the condition, including distended abdomen, changes in the breast, and increase in weight. The majority of women with pseudocyesis are dependent hysterical personalities who seek to preserve a marriage in which they perceive themselves as unwanted unless they bear children. On some occasions, sexual relations have not occurred.

Amenorrhea then must be recognized as a multidetermined symptom. It seems evident that the hypothalamic regulatory system which influences the activity of pituitary, ovarian, and adrenal glands through the autonomic nervous system and direct hormonal action is itself subject to influence by the cerebral cortex, wherein are laid down the perceptions of childbearing and sexuality.

MENOPAUSE.   Menopausal symptoms again represent a complex of physiological and psychological responses to which the mature woman usually adapts more effectively than those who have neurotic or psychotic personalities or in those whose sexual and maternal functions have been frustrated. With the diminution of hormonal secretions, neurovascular control becomes labile, and there result episodic periods of perspiration, flushings, tension, or moodiness. Associated may be increasing anxiety and agitation, with exaggerations of all personality defenses. The prescription of synthetic hormones will alleviate the physiologically determined symptoms but not those aroused as the consequence of growing awareness of fading opportunities to fulfill the primary biological functions of womanhood or those secondary to loss of parental responsibility, when grown children are separated from the home and deprive the mother of satisfaction in their immediate care.

Frigidity, Dyspareunia, and Infertility

In considering the response to sexual intercourse, it must be kept in mind that the climax of coitus in women is not analogous to orgasm in the male. Even the anatomical structure of the feminine genital tract differs from that of the male. Sensory cells similar to those found in the glans penis are confined largely to the clitoris, with some located in the labia minora and lower vaginal muscles. The vagina is homologous with the penile shaft and therefore cannot respond to sexual stimulation in the same way as the phallus. The widely held notion or expectation of many women of rapid and climactic orgasm similar to that of men is probably incorrect. For satisfactory sexual relations, women must find themselves with a desirable partner, be devoid of anxiety and guilt, and must then be provided with appropriate stimulation in order to achieve a slower but more enduring gratification. Many women believe they are frigid due to misconceptions about feminine arousal. Much has been learned of sexual arousal in women through the work of Masters and Johnson; this knowledge is imperative to all psychiatrists concerned with evaluation of symptoms indicative of sexual dysfunction.

Frigidity often is related to fear of injury in intercourse or of pregnancy and may spring from envy of and hostility to men. Unfulfilled expectations of their response arouse in some women feelings of shameful inadequacy or rage at their partner. Less anxious women and those who accept a more giving and passive role are often gratified even without full clitoral stimulation and orgasm. Dyspareunia and vaginismus are the consequence of the same anxieties and fears that impair sexual satisfaction in women. It appears likely that infertility also has its origins in suppression by central mechanisms of ovulation through persisting anxieties and doubts of pregnancy and childbearing.

When it is evident that emotional factors are the primary factor determining the existence of these conditions, analytic psychotherapy is the indicated treatment. It is more likely to prove beneficial in those whose inhibitions are due to unconscious feelings of guilt, disgust, or repressed hostility than in women with a strong maternal fixation and infantile personality make-up.

Reactions to Abortion, Sterilization, and Contraception

Those medical and surgical procedures that prevent or deprive women and men of their reproductive function are bound to produce psychological conflict and emotional disturbance. Since the ideal concept of healthy human growth includes in the attainment of adult status sexual maturity, including the capacity to conceive and bear children, measures that prevent the realization of these aspirations are likely to arouse feelings of sadness, shame, inadequacy, envy, and hostility toward the more fortunate, including those who are seen as responsible for the frustration. Furthermore, anxiety and depression are mobilized, with their attendant defenses. Such emotional responses may be expected and do occur more frequently in those who have not attained the satisfaction of marriage and the bearing and rearing of children. It is not surprising that women are more frequently disturbed than men following surgical operations on the genitalia, since marriage and the maternal function play a significantly greater role in the realization of a satisfying self-concept than the attainment of fatherhood.

The physician and psychiatrist today are ever more frequently called upon to make judgments pertaining to therapeutic abortions, sterilization procedures in both men and women, hysterectomies, and the use of contraceptives.

With the now ready availability of controlling conception by a multitude of available techniques and with the concern over the need to control population, there are underway worldwide changes in human values regarding sexual activity and freedom. A recent survey of a college population in the United States by Eisner et al. revealed that 84 per cent agreed on the desirability of limiting family size; yet a majority (65 per cent) desired three children or more, only 30 per cent favored two, and only 5 per cent one or less. As regards contraception 53 per cent favored the contraceptive jells over all other methods. Other contraceptive devices such as condoms, diaphragms, and intrauterine devices were preferred first by 13 per cent. Only 6 per cent indicated a willingness for vasectomy after family size had been achieved; the number favoring ligation of oviducts was 2 per cent. A majority of both sexes indicated that they would *never* accept sterilization. Many did not understand the implications as to sterilization in either sex; biology students were as lacking in such information as those in the humanities and other sciences. The survey has implications for those recommending contraceptive aid in providing current knowledge of those techniques likely to receive cultural support or to be rejected. Also, it makes apparent the continuing ignorance of the effects of the various methods on sexual functioning.

Medical and surgical skills have decreased the frequency of indication for therapeutic abortion for such illnesses as heart disease, tuberculosis, and diabetes. At the same time, the number of abortions performed on the recommendation of psychiatrists has increased rapidly in the past two decades, both abroad and in the United States. Although there is little difference in the recognized indications for therapeutic abortion on the grounds of physical disease, the range of indications on social-psychological grounds varies tremendously from country to country throughout the world. In some states and countries, therapeutic abortion may only be recommended legally when the life of the mother is threatened by the pregnancy's coming to term. In other countries, notably the Scandinavian, therapeutic abortion may be recommended for economic, social, and psychological reasons. In these countries, there has been brought to light much information from the careful studies of the emotional responses of women who have been recommended for and denied abortions that they requested. The insistent biological urge to conception shines through clearly. In Ekblad's series, over a third of the women who were not sterilized at the time of abortion became pregnant again. A number do so consciously, and soon after the abortion. As many as a fifth of the women allowed therapeutic abortions later expressed regret for accepting the procedure, although in a tenth these personal reproaches were of short duration. Al-

though it seems that these unfavorable psychological sequelae are seldom severe, when one considers the advisability of allowing therapeutic abortions literally to all women, there remains a substantial group of women who react with continuing psychopathology. The majority in this group will be found to have had preëxisting personality disorders and unsatisfactory family relations during childhood and adolescence, to be unmarried, and to have undergone previous abortions. Even in instances in which therapeutic abortion is performed, the risk of a postabortion psychiatric disability is greatest among those women previously ill psychiatrically or predisposed to such illness. However, clinical experience has shown too that if the request for abortion is denied to this same group of women they are again most prone to unfavorable personality disturbance.

Solution of the clinical problem confronting the psychiatrist called upon to determine whether abortion or any sterilizing procedure should be performed demands not only a full knowledge of the life experiences, expectancies, and personality weaknesses of his patient, but also awareness of the legal status of therapeutic abortion and sterilizaion in his community. From the study of many psychiatrically ill patients, the conclusion is inescapable that those women who do not wish to bring a particular conception to birth seldom make a satisfactory mother for that child. The experienced clinician, however, will not easily accept the initial verbal declaration of patients that they do not want to bear; in some instances these declarations are made to gain or regain love and attention or may be compliant demands made at the request or insistence of a consort who does not wish to bear his responsibility for the child.

Experience does not show that pregnancy and birth of the child influence adversely the course of the schizophrenias, manic-depressive illnesses, or the majority of the psychoneuroses, but they may be the precipitating factor for a period of serious ego decompensation. Even women who have a postpartum psychotic reaction often go through later pregnancies without ego disorganization. Suicidal threats are used frequently to force recommendation for abortions. Here again, experience has shown that execution of the threat is uncommon when the mother is allowed to go to term. If suicidal attempts have been made previously, if a psychotic disorder is known to exist, or if previous postpartum personality disorders have occurred, there exist grounds for psychiatric considerations for therapeutic abortion. The eventual psychiatric recommendation must rest not only upon the personality of the patient and the past sexual and maternal satisfactions, but on her needs for future stability. Allowing the birth of a child, even in the face of a physical illness, is indicated for the future preservation of mental health for certain women. In such instances, however, all arrangements must be made to assume the needed medical and psychiatric care both through term and beyond parturition.

Sterilization procedures for men, such as *vasectomy,* too often are requested by those with preëxisting defects in personality functioning. In the series of men followed by Johnson after vasectomy, over 10 per cent were hospitalized for psychiatric illness within a year, and almost 25 per cent had been or were in the process of divorcing their wives. Multiple marriages were common in both members of the marital couple that decided on vasectomy. The operative procedure was followed usually by feelings of inadequacy, shame, or guilt. In only a few marriages did a better sexual relationship follow surgery. Too frequently the vasectomized male wished a reconstruction. Thus it is clear that the psychiatrist will undertake careful assessment of the personality and motivation of those men who either seek his advice or are brought to consultation before vasectomy.

Although the use of *contraceptive devices* is increasingly accepted, for many, sexual conflicts are complicated by this very fact. In assessing the sexual complaints of individual patients, both the wishes and attitudes of each partner toward the use of contraceptives should be explored. In some instances, the type of contraceptive device may impair sexual gratification, as for example, in the limitation of frictional stimulation experienced by some men with the use of condoms or in the feeling of disgust or lack of spontaneity induced by the use of a diaphragm in certain women. Again, family or religious training may contradict the use of such devices, and yet fear of pregnancy may induce their trial and so lead to guilty anxiety. No less difficult are those interpersonal conflicts in which the responsibility for the use of the contraceptive is foisted upon an unwilling partner as a means of expressing hostility or neurotic dependent demands and intimidating the partner by denying sexual relations when he or she complains or fails to accept this responsibility.

Both physician and psychiatrist should be fully acquainted with the various types of contraceptive measures that may be prescribed as well as the commonly accepted views of various religious groups toward their application. With the recent development of effective oral contraceptives it has been possible to offer a safe method of preventing conception that has proved widely acceptable. These agents have physiologic actions similar to the natural estrogens and progesterone which inhibit secretion of pituitary gonadotropins and thus prevent ovarian follicular maturation and ovulation. It is reported by Kane et al. that they also influence the metabolism of the biogenic amines. In the United States there are available at least ten different synthetic steroids. There are excellent reviews on their structure, biologic properties, mechanism of action, and side-effects. The latter have consisted largely of headache, nervousness, abdominal pain, dizziness, nausea, and vomiting. At this time there have not been recorded any serious personality disturbances from their administration.

There have been several cases reported of psychotic reactions developing after withdrawal of an oral contraceptive. In these instances the patients have suffered previously from postpartum psychosis or a similar disturbance while taking other contraceptives.

NERVOUS SYSTEM

Disturbances of the Image of the Body

Although our modern conceptions of the body image derive from the studies of Schilder, the knowledge of phantom phenomena, which demonstrate so strikingly the validity of this concept, extend well back into medical antiquity. They were known to Ambroise Paré and surgeons before his time. They were the subject of study by Weir Mitchell over a century ago. It is now recognized that, with growth, the individual develops a total perception of his own body as well as certain attitudes toward his physical self that many consider the core structure in the development of the ego. The body percept slowly evolves through the multiple sensory experiences of the infant in the discovery of his body parts. The various sensory impressions conveyed by means of kinesthetic, visual, and tactile apparatus to the cortex lead to an expanding and growing perception of body awareness, presumably organized and integrated in the parietotemporal cortex of the brain.

In addition to this physiological substratum acquired over the years by postural, tactile, and visual percepts, each individual attaches to this appreciation of body surface and its various parts attitudes with emotional overtones that derive from his early experiences in the family and as a result of the parental evaluations of his physique. The attitudes are ingrained through verbal remarks, nonverbal indications, and the expressions of valuation pertaining to desirable physical traits and attainment. The comparison of his own physique with that of his parents and peers and the emphasis on the differences play a large role in the body image of the growing child. The parents imply that the child's body and its parts are good or bad, pleasing or repulsive, clean or dirty, loved or disliked. Thus, in some families in which physical strength and physical accomplishment are emphasized, a boy's attitude toward his body is determined to a large extent by the parents' feelings and attitudes toward development of his limbs and muscles. In a similar manner, the parents or the culture may overemphasize physical beauty or particular physical attributes in girls. The American cultural overemphases are evident in our advertising and writing.

It may be mentioned that certain families and ethnical groups tend to derogate various body parts that have sexual significance. This, in turn, reflects in part on both conscious and unconscious conceptions of body parts in certain individuals. The loss of a hand, for example, may have a very different meaning to a violinist than to a professor of history, and a resulting disturbance or disorganization of the personality would therefore be much more apt to result in the former. Lesions in parts of the body that psychologically represent organs of marked value for the personality—such as eyes, breasts, sexual organs—may be highly disturbing, even though the disease, objectively considered, is not serious. Disturbances of the personality rarely follow operations upon the appendix or other organs not invested with deep emotional value. On the other hand, psychiatric complications following operations upon highly valued ones, such as the reproductive organs, are not uncommon.

Disabling physical handicaps, such as crippling, blindness, and deafness, which put the patient at a disadvantage with his fellows, may have profound effect upon emotional health. The sensitive, even paranoid, reactions of the deaf, at times more disturbing to the individual's social adjustment than the deafness itself, are familiar observations. In girls, particularly, a serious physical handicap may produce mental problems that completely overshadow the defect.

Because of the high evaluations placed upon their biological functions and because any conditions that adversely affect these functions may seriously jeopardize their personal, economic, and social security and happiness, women are particularly subject to fears and emotional conflicts when such functions are disturbed. Lack of attractiveness, or physical defects that preclude offers of marriage, an inability to bear children, the loss of physical charm through age or disease, the presence of conditions that make discontinuance of marital relations necessary, or the approach of the involutional period may constitute problems to which emotional adjustment is difficult or impossible within the limits of mental health.

For the clinical psychiatrist, disturbances of the body image will be observed in association with many of the major psychoneurotic and psychotic disorders. However, there are certain expressions of primary body image disturbance of particular interest that may be recognized as separate entities. Among these are the various phantom phenomena and the efforts on the part of the individual to adapt to these phenomena, as well as such conditions as neurasthenia and hypochondriasis.

Phantom Phenomena

Phantom phenomena are considered the expression of the enduring concept of the individual's body image persisting after loss of a body part. It is significant that phantoms have not been noted in those with absence of a limb resulting from a congenital defect or from infantile amputations. The phantom is not explainable, then, on the basis of wish fulfillment or "gestalt" psychology. The observation of a phantom limb after amputation occurs in some 98 per cent of amputees. Such phantoms are initially perceived as consisting of the whole extremity. Usually the distal portion of the phantom, such as the hand or foot, is most conspicuous. As time passes, the phantom appendage tends to shrink and may eventually disappear into the stump. Movements of the amputation stump may induce the impression of movement of the phantom extremity provided kinesthetic sensation remains in the stump.

Three kinds of sensory phenomena may be noted in the phantom limb. In all patients with a phantom, there occurs a mild tingling, the basic phantom phenomenon, which may be regarded as dependent upon the function of the sensory-motor cerebral cortex. A stronger momentary pins-and-needles sensation may be provoked in the phantom by touching neuromas in the stump; this sensation is dependent upon functional activity of lower spinal centers. Also included under the second type of sensory phenomena are sensations referred into the phantom in the presence of disease of other organs, such as referred pain of cardiac origin. Referred sensations into the phantom may be elicited by deep pressure on the amputation stump, less often with algesic skin stimulation, and least by tactile stimulation.

The third type of painful sensory disturbance in the phantom is the common cause of the amputee's referral for psychiatric or neurologic consultation. Questioning usually reveals that the patient is concerned about sensations that he describes variously as "twisting," "burning," "pulling," or "itching." In most instances, the symptom is intermittent. It is more often annoying than agonizing. The introspective, observant amputee notes its aggravation by stimulation of the stump, sometimes by micturition in those who have lost a leg, by changes in weather, and in many instances by emotionally disturbing incidents.

Limb phantoms are common; mammary, penile, rectal, and nasal phantoms are rare. But Simmel's recent study has shown that mammary phantoms, after mastectomy, are much more frequently present than was heretofore thought. About 50 per cent of women will report no change in their body sensation following surgery; if subjected to a body sway test, the phantom breast sensation is more frequently and vividly noted. However, the phantom breast is less vividly presented as a hallucinated phenomenon than the phantom limb. Phantoms of the bladder and rectum have rarely been observed in paraplegic patients, while those of the flaccid penis and erect penis are more frequent. The existence of phantom images of other internal organs is not generally accepted as occurring, although it has been suggested that the occurrence of phantom pain in the abdomen may explain the recurrence of peptic ulcer pain in the patients who initially report the disappearance of such pain after vagotomy.

The admission by an amputee of a limb phantom should be regarded as a healthy psychological response. Subsequent to an amputation, the healthy individual slowly reorganizes his body image by means of the new sensory experiences related to the changed body form. The persistence of a physical defect irritating the afferent nerves from the amputated part will delay this reorganization and may cause pain.

The healthy amputee accepts his defect, resumes his family position, returns to his occupation, and, with an adequate stump, makes use of an appropriate prosthesis. On the other hand, those who complain of persistent or intermittent pain in a phantom incapacitating them for a return to life in society, in whom the painful symptom does not conform to the recognized descriptions of the sensations resulting from irritation of known structures, with referral into recognized areas of nervous distribution, and in whom there is resistance to the acceptance of a prosthesis or poor family, marital, or occupational adaptation, are usually suffering a serious personality disturbance. Such disturbances, though rare, occur as amputation leads to an upsurge of anxiety owing to the distortion of the patient's

concept of his body and therefore of himself and his relations with others. This distortion requires readaptation in relation to others and to society. Also, hostile feelings may emerge in the amputee toward those people with whom he identifies, on whom he is dependent, and whose rejection he now apprehends. The painful symptom thus may symbolize the need for, and apprehension relative to, a possible loss of dependency.

Kolb found that in many instances the amputee with the painful phantom has identified in a hostile way with another amputee significantly related to him in his early life. In those amputees with a hysterical personality make-up and identification with another amputee, the fantasy life often discloses superstitious rationalization to explain the existence of the phantom phenomenon. The rationalizations are concerned with the loss and the fantasied disposal of the amputated part. In association with these fantasies, the amputee attempts to master his grief and mourning over the loss of the amputated part. He desires to have the part disposed of tenderly and respectfully as if the whole body were to be buried.

The neurotically over-determined painful symptom has been relieved by a variety of psychiatric therapies, including suggestion, hypnosis, narcotherapy, electroshock, lobotomy, and more recently by the tranquilizing drugs. The therapeutic procedure of choice must be determined on the basis of the over-all personality disturbance observed in the individual patient. The following report lllustrates an acute emotional disturbance associated with the phantom phenomenon.

A 14-year-old boy came to clinic complaining of a "knot in his leg." He said he had bumped the lower part of his right leg against a step one month previously.

On examination a hard, fixed, tender mass was noted in the middle third of the injured part of the leg. Roentgenograms showed a primary malignant tumor involving the anterolateral cortex of the right tibia. Three days later, amputation of the right leg was performed through the lower third of the femur. The pathologist reported an osteogenic sarcoma of the tibia. The patient complained of pain in the phantom right leg shortly after recovery from the anesthesia. Within two days after operation, large doses of narcotic agents were being employed in an attempt to relieve him of pain. By the ninth postoperative day, the patient was complaining bitterly of a burning pain, was over-active, thrashed about in bed, and spoke of jumping out of a window. Special nurses were required at this time, and psychiatric consultation was requested. The patient was found to be fearful, disoriented, and confused. Administration of all drugs except morphine was discontinued in order to alleviate the mild toxic delirious state.

The next day the patient was rolling about in his bed, with his eyes closed, apparently oblivious to those about him. He cried out repetitiously, "Help me, help me. Do something for the pain." It was believed that frightening rationalizations as to the origin of the phantom contributed in part to the state of painful panic. The boy was therefore asked if he was aware of the feeling of a phantom limb after operation. Surprisingly, the boy immediately became silent, opened his eyes, and responded affirmatively. Under questioning he stated that a year previously one of his school teachers had casually discussed amputations with his class. The teacher told the class a story of a man who had undergone an amputation, after which a severe stinging pain developed in his phantom limb. The story went that the limb was disinterred and that ants were discovered burrowing into and stinging the amputated part.

When inquiry was made as to what disposition the boy believed had been made of his own amputated extremity, he stated that he thought it was being burned. He was reassured and informed otherwise. The complaint of pain and his wild overactivity subsided to a large extent immediately after this interview. It was possible to discontinue the use of all morphine within 24 hours and to discharge the patient's special nurse shortly thereafter.

Complete relief of his pain, however, required four additional hours of psychotherapy. It was learned that the boy had been severely upset by his mother's death from cancer of the breast five years previously. The boy never spoke of his mother after her death but was morbidly inquisitive whenever anyone became ill and would inquire of his father if the person were about to die. The mother had undergone amputation of the breast. The latter hours of treatment brought to awareness the boy's repressed hostility toward his mother, with whom he identified as an amputee, and his ambivalent feelings toward his father.

When he was dismissed from the clinic 25 days after operation, the boy had no pain, did not require medication, was active on crutches, and was eager to have a prosthesis fitted. A year later his stepmother wrote that he was without pain and was wearing a prosthesis. He had returned to school, was doing well in his studies, and had been elected to a class office.

Athlete's Neurosis

Men and women whose senses of personal esteem rest largely upon their athletic abilities are high risk subjects for neurotic reactions. These reactions often are long enduring and difficult to manage. They are not unlike the middle-aged neurotic reactions of women whose ego strength has resided largely in the adulation given them for their earlier but now fading beauty. The usual precipitating causes are direct threat to physical well-being, injuries and illnesses. In contrast to other neurotic reactions, the response must be seen as one of deprivation or loss of the overvalued body concept of physical prowess. There is, then, a strong reactive depressive element in the neurotic reaction often obscured by the extroverted and sociable personality evolved by many successful athletes. Hypochondriasis and anxiety attacks are frequent symptoms, but any neurotic or psychotic constellation may develop in these athletes, who are vulnerable through their obsessive preoccupation in the satisfaction of their sport.

Neurasthenia

The concept of neurasthenia has undergone many manifestations, and one might say abuses, since the term was first introduced by Beard in 1867 to describe a condition caused, he believed, by an exhaustion of the nerve cells through depletion of their stored nutriment. Today most of the symptom complexes formerly classified as neurasthenia fall under the category of psychophysiological asthenic reactions.

General fatigue, with its feeling of overwhelming exhaustion and of diffuse "nervousness," is the predominating complaint in the reaction that should be regarded as a response to emotional conflicts and their attendant anxiety. The causes therefore are psychological. It is no longer believed that "neurasthenia" is caused by a generally impaired or exhausted physical state, as a result of which the nervous system is drained of its energy in the manner of a partially discharged battery of low voltage. Some complaints seem to be disappointment reactions, while others appear to be the expression of sexual dissatisfaction or conflicts. Sometimes repressed hostility or other anxiety-exciting factors produce the reaction. In other instances, the asthenic reaction seems to arise from constant failure, frustration, and disappointment. Boredom, monotony, and absence of goals may serve as contributory causes. It will be found that many patients have had a difficult childhood, with little interest or affection from their parents. The existence of family or social problems should always be considered.

SYMPTOMS. The premorbid personality of the patient with psychophysiological asthenic reaction has usually been characterized by dissatisfaction and by a sense of being thwarted and rejected. The premorbid characteristics often merge so insidiously into the symptoms of the reaction that no definite time of its onset can be stated. As already indicated, the asthenic reaction patient has a long-continued subjective sensation of overwhelming exhaustion. Any exertion, either mental or physical, seems too great. An exaggerated degree of attention is paid to the bodily organs and their functions. The patient may complain of dizziness, of a feeling of pressure on the head, and perhaps of pain at the nape of the neck. There is an intolerance of noise, bright lights, and cold, and complaints about muscae volitantes are common. Associated gastrointestinal discomfort is frequent. Indigestion, constipation, and diarrhea may occur.

Palpitation, extrasystoles, and tachycardia, symptoms of an associated anxiety state, increase the alarm of the patient. Vasomotor instability is frequent so that the skin is at times flushed and again sweating or cold. Patients with this vasomotor instability wrap themselves in mufflers and are in constant fear of catching cold. Complaints of "fallen stomach" or "loose kidney" are common. The sexual functions of the male are disturbed; impaired potency, nocturnal emissions, and failures at intercourse are common. The significance of these symptoms is magnified, and the patient is greatly distressed. Women with asthenic reaction often suffer from dysmenorrhea. Paresthesias and hypesthesias are common.

The patient may suffer from broken sleep and disturbing dreams. In the morning he awakes with a feeling of exhaustion. As the day progresses, the patient feels better, and in the evening he may be comparatively free from his sense of exhaustion. He complains of poor memory, but this defect is a result only of preoccupation and lack of concentration. Many patients are shy, awkward, and irritable, lack confidence, and exhibit irresolution, indecision, and irascibility. They are pessimistic and lack initiative and ambition. Asthenic patients are often critical, whining, dissatisfied, envious, and resentful. A tendency to projection is not uncommon. Some patients develop a complaining attitude and may appear to take pleasure in finding fault with and annoying others. Moderate depression is the rule. Varying degrees of anxiety are present.

The neurasthenic is characteristically preoccupied with his bodily weakness and a multitude of minor subjective physical perceptions that are overlooked or disregarded by the active and healthy person. He comes to rationalize his failures and dissatisfactions, which are accompanied by underlying emotions of rage, guilt, and anxiety as to these subjective perceptions, and, in turn, they allow much in terms of secondary gain through attention and consideration by others not available through socially constructive adaptations. The persisting underlying anxieties feed back into the various systems mediating psychophysiologic responses and continually maintain the opportunity for bodily preoccupation, with the psychological defenses of weakness, lack of strength and persistence, and helplessness. Many patients with predominant neurasthenic defenses have been reared in families in which somatic symptoms or illness were used in a similar manner by parents or siblings. Thus the symptom choice rests often on the process of identification.

DIAGNOSIS. One of the most important differentiations to be made is to distinguish the asthenic reaction from the depressive form of manic-depressive psychosis. Many mild cases of this psychosis do not come to the attention of the psychiatrist, and the patients are considered by the general practitioner to be suffering from neurasthenia. Manic-depressive psychosis occurs in more definite episodes, with intervals free from symptoms of mental disorder, while the asthenic reaction is a more continuous, or at least prolonged, process, and the patient, even when comparatively well, is solicitous as to his health. The chief complaint of the neurasthenic is of weakness and shifting physical ailments, which he is eager to discuss on every occasion, whereas that of the manic-depressive is depression. Although the neurasthenic is apparently depressed, his emotional manifestations and responses are well marked and even excessive, whereas the depression of the affective psychosis remains unchanged by experience or environment. Sometimes it is difficult to distinguish early schizophrenia from the asthenic reaction. The schizophrenic does not usually have so great a variety of physical complaints, and sooner or later they become obviously delusional. The neurasthenic lacks the listless apathy and the indifference to external circumstances usually manifested by the schizophrenic. The neurasthenic, unlike the schizophrenic, is not given to daydreaming.

Neurasthenia-like symptoms first manifested at middle age should arouse the suspicion of neurosyphilis. Experience suggests that some cases of chronic brucellosis have been diagnosed as neurasthenia. Thiamine deficiency may produce an asthenic reaction syndrome characterized by generalized feelings of weakness, fatigability, poor appetite, poor sleep, various somatic complaints, and subjective difficulties in concentration and memory.

TREATMENT. The treatment of the asthenic reaction is psychotherapeutic. Usually encouraging results are limited to relatively early cases.

BIBLIOGRAPHY

General and Theoretical

Alexander, F.: French, T. M., and Pollack, G. H.: Psychosomatic Specificity. Experimental Study and Results. Chicago, University of Chicago Press, 1968.

Cannon, W. B.: Bodily Changes in Pain, Hunger, Fear and Rage. 2nd ed. New York, D. Appleton Century Co., 1929.

Hofling, C. K.: Textbook of Psychiatry for Medical Practice. 2nd ed. Philadelphia, J. B. Lippincott Company, 1968.

Kubie, L. S.: The central representation of the symbolic process in psychosomatic disorders. Psychosom. Med., 15:1–7, 1953.

Lief, H. I., Lief, V. F., and Lief, N. R.: The Psychological Basis of Medical Practice. Hoeber Medical Division, Harper & Row, New York, 1963.

Lipowski, Z. J.: Psychosocial aspects of disease. Ann. Int. Med., 71:1197–1206, 1969.

O'Connor, J. F.: Symptom alternation. Arch. Gen. Psychiat., 16:432–436, 1967.

Pasamanick, B.: Prevalence and distribution of psychosomatic conditions in an urban population according to class. Psychosom. Med., 24: 352–356, 1962.

Pavlov, I. P.: Experimental Psychology. New York, Philosophical Library, 1957.

Ruesch, J., et al.: Chronic Disease and Psychological Invalidism. Berkeley and Los Angeles, University of California Press, 1951.

Titchener, J. L., and Levine, M.: Surgery as a Human Experience. New York, Oxford University Press, 1960.

Wolff, H. G.: A concept of disease in man. Psychosom. Med., 24:25–30, 1962.

Cardiovascular Reactions

Editorial: Emotional stress and heart disease. J.A.M.A., 218:89–90, 1971.

Elkind, A. H., Friedman, A. P., Bachman, H., Siegelman, S. S., and Sacks, O. W.: Silent retroperitoneal fibrosis associated with methysergide therapy. J.A.M.A., 206:1041–1044, 1968.

Heller, S. S., Frank, K. A., Malm, J. R., Bowman, F. O., Harris, P. D., Charlton, M. H., and Korn-feld, D. S.: Psychiatric complications of open heart surgery. New England J. Med., *283*:1015–1020, 1970.

Kolb, L. C.: Psychiatric and psychogenic factors in headache. In Friedman, A. D., and Merritt, H. H. (eds.): Headache: Diagnosis and Treatment. Philadelphia, F. A. Davis, 1959.

Lance, J. W., Anthony, M., and Hinterberger, H.: Control of cranial arteries by humoral mechanisms and its relation to the migraine syndrome. Headache, 7:93–102, 1967.

Layne, O. L., and Yudofsky, S. C.: Postoperative psychosis in cardiotomy patients. New England J. Med., *284*:518–520, 1971.

Liljefors, I., and Rahe, R. H.: An identical twin study of psychosocial factors in coronary heart disease in Sweden. Psychosom. Med., *32*:523–542, 1970.

Reiser, M. F., and Bakst, H.: Psychology of cardiovascular disorders. In Arieti (ed.): American Handbook of Psychiatry. Vol. I. New York, Basic Books, Inc., 1959, pp. 659–677.

Rosenman, R. H., and Friedman, M.: Behavior patterns, blood lipids, and coronary heart disease. J.A.M.A., *184*:934–938, 1963.

Timberline Conference on Psychophysiologic Aspects of Cardiovascular Disease. Psychosom. Med., *26*:405–538, 1964.

Alimentary Reactions

Bell, E. T., Harkness, R. A., Loraine, J. A., and Russell, G. E. M.: Hormone assay studies in patients with anorexia nervosa. Acta Endocrinologica, *51*:140–148, 1966.

Blinder, B. J., Freeman, D. M. A., and Stunkard, A. J.: Behavior therapy of anorexia nervosa: Effectiveness of activity as a reinforcer of weight gain. Amer. J. Psychiat., *126*:1093–1098, 1970.

Brady, J. V.: Ulcers in "executive monkeys." Sci. Amer., *199*:95, 1958.

Bruch, H.: Anorexia nervosa in the male. Psychosom. Med., *33*:31–47, 1971.

Cohn, C.: Neuroendocrine aspects of feeding behavior and obesity. In Endocrines and the Central Nervous System. Res. Publ. Assn. Nerv. Ment. Dis., 63, Baltimore, Williams & Wilkins Co., 1966.

Dally, P.: Anorexia Nervosa. New York, Grune and Stratton, 1969.

Dally, P., and Sargant, W.: Treatment and outcome of anorexia nervosa. Brit. Med. J., *2*:793–795, 1966.

Drenick, E., Simmons, F., and Murphy, J. F.: Effect on hepatic morphology of treatment of obesity by fasting, reducing diets and small bowel bypass. New England J. Med., *282*:829–834, 1970.

Druss, R. G., O'Connor, J. F., Prudden, J. F., and Stern, L. P.: Psychologic response to colectomy. Arch. Gen. Psychiat., *18*:53–59, 1968; *20*:419–427, 1969.

Engel, G. L., and Reichsmann, F.: Spontaneous and experimentally induced depressions in an infant with gastric fistula. J. Amer. Psychoanal. Assn., *4*:428–452, 1956.

Glucksman, M. L., Hirsh, J., McCully, R. S., Baum, B. A., and Knittle, J. L.: The response of obese patients to weight reduction. Psychosom. Med., *30*:359–373, 1968.

Goldblatt, P. G., Moore, M. E., and Stunkard, A. J.: Social factors in obesity. J.A.M.A., *192*:1039–1044, 1965.

Goldman, M. C.: Gastric secretions during a medical interview. Psychosom. Med., *25*:351–356, 1963.

Karush, A., and Daniels, G. E., O'Connor, J. F., and Slone, L. C.: The response to psychotherapy in chronic ulcerative colitis. Psychosom Med., *30*:255–276, 1968; *31*:201–226, 1969.

Kaufman, M. R., and Herman, M. (eds.): Evolution of Psychosomatic Concepts. Anorexia Nervosa: a Paradigm. New York, International Universities Press, Inc., 1964.

Long, D. M.: Hypothalamus and gastric ulceration or hemorrhage. Arch. Neurol., *7*:167–175; 176–183, 1962.

Mayer, J., and Thomas, D. W.: Regulation of food intake and obesity. Science, *156*:328–337, 1967.

Mendelson, M.: Psychological aspects of obesity. Int. J. Psychiat., *2*:599–616, 1966.

Mirsky, I. A., Futterman, P., and Kaplan, S.: Physiologic, psychologic and social determinants in the etiology of duodenal ulcer. Amer. J. Digestive Dis., *3*:285–314, 1958.

Rowland, C. V. (ed.): Anorexia and Obesity. International Psychiatry Clinics. 7. Boston, Little, Brown & Company, 1970.

Schoenberg, B., Carr, A. C., Kutscher, A. H., and Zegarelli, E. V.: Chronic idiopathic orolingual pain. N.Y. St. J. Med. *71*:1832–1837, 1971.

Ziegler, R., and Sours, J. A.: A naturalistic study of patients with anorexia nervosa admitted to a university medical center. Comp. Psych., *9*:644–651, 1968.

Respiratory Reactions

Brown, E. B., Jr.: Physiological effects of hyperventilation. Physiol. Rev., *33*:445–471, 1953.

Dudley, D. C., Martin, C. J., and Holmes, T. H.: Psychophysiological studies of pulmonary ventilation. Psychosom. Med., *26*:645–660, 1964.

Freeman, E. H., Feingold, B. F., Schlesinger, K., and Gorman, F. J.: Psychological variables in allergic disorders. A review. Psychosom. Med., *26*:543–575, 1964.

Kalogerakis, M. G.: Role of olfaction in sexual development. Psychosom. Med., *25*:420–431, 1963.

Purcell, K., Brady, K., Chai, H., Maser, J., Molk, L., Gordon, N., and Means, J.: The effect of asthma in children of experimental separation from the family. Psychosom. Med., *31*:144–164, 1969.

Wheeler, E. O., While, P. D., Reed, E. W., and Cohen, M. E.: Neurocirculatory asthenia. J.A.M.A., *142:*878–889, 1950.

Endocrine Reactions

Geist, H.: The Psychological Aspects of Diabetes. Springfield, Ill., Charles C Thomas, 1964.
Levine, M. (ed.): Endocrines and the central nervous system. Proc. Assn. Res. Nerv. Ment. Dis. 63. Baltimore, Williams & Wilkins Company, 1966.

Skin Reactions

Ely, N. F., Veehey, J. W., and Holmes, T. H.: Experimental studies of skin inflammation. Psychosom. Med., 25:264–284, 1963.
Schoenberg, B., and Carr, A. C.: An investigation of criteria for brief psychotherapy of neurodermatitis. Psychosom. Med., 25:253–263, 1963.

Genitourinary Reactions

Benedek, T. F.: Sexual functions in women and their disturbances. *In* Arieti, S. (ed.): American Handbook of Psychiatry. Vol. I. New York, Basic Books, Inc., 1959, pp. 727–748.
Brown, E., and Barglow, P.: Pseudocyesis. Arch. Gen. Psychiat., 24:221–229, 1971.
Calderone, M. S. (ed.): Abortion in the United States. New York, Hoeber-Harper, 1958.
Cohen, R. L.: The treatment of "interstitial cystitis" as a migraine equivalent: Report of four cases. Comp. Psych., 4:58–61, 1963.
Daly, R. J., Kane, F. J., and Ewing, J. A.: Psychoses associated with use of sequential oral contraceptive. Lancet, 2:444–445, 1967.
Ekblad, M.: Induced abortion on psychiatric grounds. A follow-up study of 479 women. Acta Psychiat. Neurol. Scandinav. suppl., 99:1–238, 1955.
Engels, W. D., Palter, C. J., and Wittkouer, E. D.: Emotional settings of functional amenorrhea. Psychosom. Med., 26:682–700, 1964.

Gutheil, E.: Sexual dysfunction in men. *In* Arieti, S. (ed.): American Handbook of Psychiatry. Vol. I. New York, Basic Books, Inc., 1959, pp. 708–726.
Hamilton, J. A.: Postpartum Psychiatric Problems. St. Louis, Mo., C. V. Mosby Company, 1962.
Hastings, D. W.: Impotence and Frigidity. Boston, Little, Brown & Company, 1963.
Herzberg, B., and Coppen, A.: Changes in psychological symptoms in women taking oral contraceptives. Brit. J. Psychiat., 116:161–164, 1970.
Jansson, B.: Mental disorder after abortion. Acta Psychiat. Scand., 41:87–110, 1965.
Kane, F. J., Lipton, M. A., Krall, A. R., and Obrist, P. A.: Psychoendocrine study of oral contraceptives. Amer. J. Psychiat., 127:443–450, 1970.
Masters, W. H., and Johnson, V. E.: Human Sexual Response. Boston, Little, Brown & Company, 1966.
Peel, J., and Potts, M.: Textbook of Contraceptive Practice. New York, Cambridge University Press, 1969.
Psychiatric Aspects of Renal Failure. Amer. J. Psychiat., 127:1185–1204, 1971.
Ziegler, F. J., Rodgers, D. A., and Prentiss, R. J.: Psychosocial response to vasectomy. Arch. Gen. Psychiat., 21:46–54, 1969.-

Nervous System Reactions

Druss, R. G., Symonds, F. C., and Criklair, G. F.: The problem of somatic delusions in patients seeking cosmetic surgery. Plastic & Reconst. Surg., 48:246–249, 1971.
Kolb, L. C.: Disturbances of the Body-Image. *In* Arieti, S. (ed.): American Handbook of Psychiatry. Vol. I. New York, Basic Books, Inc., 1959, pp. 749–769.
Little, J. C.: The athlete's neurosis—a deprivation crisis. Acta Psychiat. Scand., 45:187–197, 1969.
Schonfeld, W. A.: Gynecomastia in adolescence. Personality effects. A.M.A. Arch. Gen. Psychiat., 5:46–54, 1961.
Simmel, M. L.: A study of phantoms after amputation of the breast. Neuropsychologia, 4:331–350, 1966.

*". . . and a sick soul is always astray and cannot either attain
or endure, never does it cease to desire."*

Cicero

Personality Disorders

The group of personality disorders includes a wide range of cases in which malfunctioning is expressed in inflexible and limited patterns of behavior. At times these personality patterns and traits are compatible with social success and satisfaction in cases in which the particular features of the individual makeup are both accepted and rewarded by the culture and the special vocational opportunities that are available. In such instances the inflexibility of the personality or its special vulnerability to particular stresses remains unnoticed except perhaps in the form of some peculiarity or eccentricity until that individual is required to adapt to another environment or is exposed to some personal or environmental pressure that he has previously avoided or escaped. In other forms, difficulties in social and sexual adaptation are evident and occur repetitively throughout life, in spite of adequate intellectual capacity.

The personality disorders differ then in that the psychopathologic manifestations do not present themselves in the grossly regressive disturbances of the behavior, affect, or thought of the psychoses or in the exaggerated and fixed psychological defenses that characterize the psychoneurotic. Nor does the disorder present itself in the form of somatic symptoms due to an expression of anxiety or other affect through disruption of psychophysiologic functions.

Those personality disorders listed as the paranoid, cyclothymic, and schizoid are recognized as forms of personality organization that contain many features similar to those found in patients with the various types of affective and schizophrenic reactions, but in the individuals in whom these disorders are present ego functioning and reality testing remain intact and allow an effective social adaptation. Presumably those with the paranoid, cyclothymic, schizoid, obsessive-compulsive, and hysterical cyclothymic, or melancholic make-up form a reservoir of persons vulnerable to manic-depressive or involutional reactions when exposed to a sufficiently severe and appropriate loss or frustration, with concomitant stress and emotional arousal. Similarly, from the reservoir of schizoid personalities derive those reactive schizophrenic and paranoid disorganizations that occur in the face of affective arousal beyond the capacity of containment by the ego adaptive and defensive development.

The trait disturbances, as presently described, contain the *compulsive* and *hysterical* personalities. Also grouped here are the large number of individuals characterized by inability to delay or control their drives and associated emotions or to establish a personal autonomy and independence. This ill-defined aggregation of cases is classified as *passive-aggressive, emotionally unstable, explosive,* or *inadequate personalities.* For the most part, this latter group of disordered personalities and those classified in the antisocial group come to medical or psychiatric attention through contact in or referral from social institutions such as the courts, prisons, military organizations, and special schools. They now constitute problems in civilian life for large organizations such as the various labor unions. Together they were formerly considered as "psychopaths."

It was formerly believed that the unmodifiable behavior patterns of such persons were matters of inborn disposition and were constitutionally influenced or directed. Not only has the assumption of a constitutional basis failed to yield any understanding of the behavior of such persons, but it is only logical that such behavior disturbances should be susceptible of explanation by theories that are analogous to those that have been so fruitful in rendering other reaction types intelligible.

Thus the pathologic behavior of the psychopath presumably has a psychogenetic origin. The major defect in the personality rests in failure to establish an identity with constructive and socially useful adaptations or to evolve those controls that allow the delay and repression of impulses to action often generated by anger. Loss or absence of parents and parental substitutes and limited contacts with other adults and peers often deprive the growing child who later presents psychopathic features of the experiences necessary to establish an ego identity through the process of identification. In some instances his behavior may be the result of frustration in his efforts to achieve a satisfaction of such fundamental needs as love, security, recognition, respect, and success. The child who was rejected may react by becoming resentful, rebellious, and antisocial, and thus establish a "negative identity," which brings him some ego satisfactions.

The origins of these personality disorders can best be regarded as the expression of an arrested or deviated development of personality. Whether this behavior represents the consequence of a development fault—an experiential lack in the process of emotional maturation through deficiency of interpersonal contact or a character neurosis—it denotes the continuing activity of psychopathological forces set in motion very early in life. The persisting drive to or reaction to aggressiveness, passivity, frustration, or deviated sexuality gives a compulsive chronicity to the psychopathic behavior.

As the result of studies of children deprived of early parental care through loss, or placement in foundling or foster homes, as well as by the developmental studies of animals exposed to maternal or peer deprivations at certain critical periods in early development, there is reason to consider today that such experiential deprivation often leads to persisting defects in social and sexual behavior. Whether such behavioral pathology may be modified by substitutive experiences later in life remains uncertain. For the growing child, neither the critical periods for social experiencing nor their duration or intensity are established or fully defined. It has been suggested from studies of "acting out" in children, adolescents, and adults in psychoanalytic therapy that the critical experiences which initiate impulse control take place during the second year of life. At this time the growing child undergoes those series of transactions with the mother or her substitute designed to establish control of activity and the somatic functions of bladder and bowel so that he may become socialized. At this same time he commences to evolve the highly complex motor activity concerned with speech. Impairment in development of language has been pointed to as a common finding in children and adolescents who display delinquent and antisocial behavior. Inconsistent or deficient mothering at this stage is thought to lead to limitations of those ego and superego functions which characterize later behavior of the adult with a personality disorder. Here, future research promises to provide a more precise understanding of the deficits in family transactional processes which underlie later intrapsychic inadequacies.

Since all but the antisocial disturbances have been described in Chapter 6, Psychopathology, the remainder of this chapter is directed to consideration of the antisocial and the sexual deviations.

THE ANTISOCIAL
PERSONALITY

Formerly the majority of patients now classified as antisocial personality were designated "constitutional psychopathic state" or "psychopathic personality." The present term provides a more restrictive application and is referred to those chronically antisocial individuals without the capacity to form significant attachments or loyalties to others, to groups, or to codes of living. Thus they are callous and given to immediate pleasures, appear devoid of a sense of responsibility, and, in spite of repeated humiliations and punishments, fail to learn to modify their behavior. They lack in social judgment, yet frequently are capable of verbal rationalizations that often convince them their actions are reasonable and warranted.

The essential defect in the character structure rests in the failure to develop a socialized superego and ego ideals. If they exist, they are directed to personal self-aggrandizement, acquisition of money and material goods, and the control of others for immediate pleasures and satisfactions.

Etiology

The future antisocial personality is often that of a child born to parents who did not want him, and not infrequently he is of an illegitimate birth. The mother's own early life and development have been unhappy, and her departure from her parents has been motivated by a wish to escape from them. She has little resources to offer others and thus comes to term feeling herself deprived. Any suffering with the birth or failures to realize her fantasies in the child serve only to increase her negative attitude toward the infant. Even when the parents have married, their relationship usually terminates in desertion or divorce. Thus the child may have been passed frequently between others or institutionalized. If he remains

with the parents, he has been exposed to violent tempers, abuse, and a variety of brutalities and sexual observations that occur in parents frequently addicted to alcohol and to promiscuity. In this type of family, authority goals for the child are not clearly established and never are based on a foundation of mutual affection, tenderness, and trust. The attempt by school and other authorities to establish some control for the acts of the child are treated indifferently, openly defied, and fought off by the parents. The child is deprived again of other sources for establishing healthy identifications with those accepting the social values of the community. Further, both the attitude of the parents to outside authority and the child's own resentments are often deepened and embedded.

Even in childhood, the future pathological personality usually shows signs of emotional maladjustment and unwholesome personality traits. Typically, he is characterized by an emotional immaturity reflected by his impulsive and instant response to his feelings. His personality seems to be dominated by primitive drives to the exclusion of rational behavior. Certain lines of conduct, particularly of a socialized nature, are never learned. Some of these children are sensitive, stubborn, and given to tantrums or to outbursts of rage; frequently these preadolescent psychopaths steal, run away, suffer from enuresis, are destructive, quarrelsome, sulky, deceitful, obstinate, defiant, boastful, shameless, and erratic. Antagonism or open rebellion against a dominating parent may be shown. The adolescent resists the ideals and mores of his family and tends to socialize at a lower level. With approaching maturity and the weakening of the restraining forces of the home and with the increase of responsibilities and of environmental contacts and demands, the earlier tendencies become outspoken manifestations. These are elaborated in some as they obtain gratifications through cupidity, deceit, or sadistic acts as the only few means learned in such family environments to respond to their own needs and desires.

Many psychopaths, although not intellectually deficient, seem emotionally so. They therefore lack keenness and delicacy of sentiment. The psychopath is typically affectionless, selfish, ungrateful, narcissistic, and exhibitionistic. He is egocentric, demanding much and giving little. His excess of demand is, in fact, one of the outstanding characteristics. He has no critical awareness of his motives and is unable to judge his own behavior from another's standpoint. In spite of the fact that his conduct is so inadequate or so hostile from a social standpoint, the psychopath is satisfied with it. He shows few feelings of anxiety, guilt, or remorse. He lacks definiteness of objective, and his usual state of restlessness may result from a search for the unattainable. Occupational application and efficiency are usually faulty; routine is intolerably irksome. He demands immediate and instant gratification of his desires, with no concern as to the feelings and interests of others, with whom he forms few emotional relationships or stable affectional ties. He does not, either, build up a sense of social values as normally should occur through the process of identification. As a result, such a sense is frequently distorted.

He is often plausible and talkative but absolutely unreliable. Frequently the only environment to which he can adjust is the one that he can dominate. Surprising irregularities of ability and inconsistencies of behavior are constantly demonstrated. A certain number escape from a difficult situation by way of a psychotic episode, while others at the slightest stress resort to alcohol or drugs. Many psychopaths bear alcohol poorly and under its influence become noisy, quarrelsome, and destructive. The sociopathic personality projects his own insecurity by blaming others. His behavior prevents proper psychosocial adjustment and ranges from "queerness" to criminality, with a large intermediate group made up of cranks, extremists, eccentrics, habitual delinquents, and other social misfits.

Sometimes one sibling in a family may manifest the behavior and personality characteristic usually associated with the sociopathic personality, while other siblings may present mature and well-adjusted personalities. Presumably this difference in personality characteristics is because of the fact that the effect of a particular emotional experience or social influence in the family was highly specific to the individual. This type of psychopathic behavior probably develops more often in upper or middle class families than that previously described. The superego defect or lacuna, as it has been termed, may be limited to a single form of behavior—such as stealing, running away, or promiscuity.

In this respect, concurrent studies of children exhibiting antisocial activity and of their parents provide new insights into both the form of deviant behavior adopted by the child and its impulsion for gratification. Johnson and Szurek have found that the more important parent, usually the mother, has unconsciously encouraged the amoral or antisocial behavior in the child. Although the parent verbally protests such behavior both to the child and to others, yet it is accepted, either unconsciously or with a guilty permissiveness, by the parent. The permissiveness has appeared to gratify vicariously neurotic needs of the parent that derive from her own lack of current satisfactions or unmet needs of childhood, or both. Since the parent's permissiveness is uncertain and incomplete, the child, and later the adult, is inconsistent and confused. Healthy discipline is not administered by such a parent—discipline combining firm prohibition with reward for socially acceptable behavior. Through his own overt acts, inconsistencies, innuendoes in speech, or various nonverbal means of communication, the child has been found to recognize the partial permissiveness. But since the child is both partially gratified and encouraged in his action and partially frustrated by the parent, there are associated with the act feelings of hostility toward the parent and perhaps of guilt. In instances in which this variety of family interaction exists, the antisocial behavior is fixed unless the several participating persons can be brought to understand and modify their behavior or they are completely separated.

Psychopathology

These sociopathic individuals show a moral and ethical blunting, a lack of sympathy for their fellow men, and a behavior destructive to the welfare of the social order. As children they are often self-willed, play truant, commit petty thefts, are cruel and untruthful, and as they grow older they may be inaccessible, boorish, and without a sense of responsibility. Their emotional life is superficial and affectively cold. They seem incapable of mature emotional relationships. They cannot organize an acceptable, constructive expression of their aggressions. They appear to lack ambition, application, seriousness of purpose, and foresight. They are irritable, arrogant, unyielding, characterized by a brutal egoism, and rarely feel remorse for their most serious offenses against person or property. Frequently they show a rebellious attitude toward authority and society. Changes in mood are sudden and often without apparent cause. They are cynical, devoid of a sense of honor or of shame, and are lacking in sympathy, affection, gratitude, and other social and esthetic sentiments. When frustrated, they may be dangerous to others. Their offenses may constitute the whole register of crime—theft, embezzlement, forgery, robbery, brutal sex attacks, and other acts of violence. Many take pleasure in their struggle with the law and feel pride in their accomplishments. They are unable to identify themselves with society and its laws. Punishments are considered as expressions of injustice and have no deterrent effect.

Merely to indicate the wide variety of behavior patterns that the antisocial personality may manifest, a description is given of a group formerly characterized as pathological liars and swindlers. In this group are egocentric individuals whose social maladaptation consists of extravagant, often apparently purposeless, lying, frequently combined with swindling. They exhibit a marked excitability of imagination combined with an instability of purpose. They are usually good-natured, of agreeable manners, optimistic, of a light-hearted geniality, and make social contacts easily. A glibness of tongue, and unusual aptitude for the use of language, a self-confident manner, a frequently assumed dignity, and a misleading appearance of knowledge readily enable them to convince the credulous as to their statements. They acquire a smattering of art, literature, or technical parlance, which they employ to their own profit and to the expense and humiliation of their victims. They spin remarkable tales concerning past experiences and paint their future with a careless disregard for reality.

Some are guilty of sex offenses and others obtain large sums of money under promise of marriage. When discovered in their delinquencies, they profess amnesia, and if charged with offense, they often stage an emotionally affected exhibition designed to impress observers and arouse sympathy. They are restless and unstable and are incapable of exertion or responsibility. They never learn to meet the struggle for existence with industry and perseverance but live in a world of imagination and seek to acquire the necessities of life by deceit and fraud. They are unable to accept the limitations of reality. Their theatrical imitation, their tendency to daydream, to boast, to avoid realities, and to surround themselves with an imaginary world suggest a childish immaturity of personality, while their wish-fulfilling fabrications have much in common with the fantasies of childhood. Many times their flagrant lying is defensive in purpose. On a less conscious level is the extravagant and often apparently purposeless romancing known as *pseudologia phantastica*. This egregious disregard of the truth seems to result from a pressing need to indulge in extravagant castle-building in order to make up for a reality that appears to be too onerous or prosaic. Inasmuch as the content of the fantasy is generated by unconscious forces, the patient is not entirely aware that his statement is a fabrication. His unusually rich imagination, stirred into active expression by acute emotional needs, enables the patient to live in a dream world. Psychometric tests usually disclose a normal or superior intellectual capacity, but as with other psychopaths, intelligence has little regulating influence on behavior. At times it would appear that such personality characteristics grow out of a feeling of inferiority, envy, or jealousy.

DIFFERENTIAL DIAGNOSIS. Not all delinquents and criminals, even though guilty of repeated offenses, are to be considered as antisocial personalities or psychopaths. In previous chapters mention has been made of criminal behavior as an incidental manifestation of the neuroses, the affective and schizophrenic reactions, and the mental deficiencies. However, the personality structure and its precursors in the constitutional and psychogenetic history differ from that of the psychopath.

But, in addition, it must be kept in mind that cultural, economic, and social forces also may determine antisocial behavior and in some instances release it, as, for example, in times of war, when the ordinary standards of social interaction are overturned or reversed even for those with well-established social values. There exist in many societies subcultures that live through their adeptness in defying the usual social codes, the members of which constitute a separate criminal class. Persons in these groups differ from the psychopath or antisocial personality in their personality structure. As an example, in a recent study of a group of thieves, Medlicott concluded that stealing may be a symptom of a depressive illness. Among fifty thieves he found 14, all women, with depressions resulting from recent bereavement, many in the menopausal or postmenopausal period, who acted out their rage at frustration through presumably senseless thefts. In contrast to the antisocial personalities, individuals of this group are capable of warm and strong loyalties to others and to their group. To Jenkins and others they represent a criminal occupational group motivated as other citizens to gain, but through illegal means; as such, they learn, plan, and adapt as others without significant personality disorder. The major differences rest in their group loyalties and the nature of the early development, which has fostered the capacities for interpersonal contact and trust but through continuing life in a delinquent or criminal subculture that has limited its expression to behavior acceptable to those groups. Certain of the antisocial adolescent gang activity, now widely reported but known for centuries, represents culturally determined antisocial behavior.

Particularly to be distinguished from the sociopathic group are the *neurotic characters*. Here the neurotic conflict is resolved through asocial or antisocial behavior rather than through a symptom neurosis; the psychopathology is expressed in antisocial behavior rather than in neurotic symptoms. In the antisocial neurotic character, his compulsive "acting out" relieves anxiety that would otherwise be distressing. Oftentimes the "acting out" is motivated by a pathological sense of guilt due to an abnormal superego. The "acting out" is performed for the purposes of relieving the guilt through apprehension and punishment. Intellectually such patients are aware of the potentialities for punishment and humiliation but are unconsciously impelled to the repetitive antisocial act in order to assuage the unconscious guilty anxiety and need for punishment. The neurotic character then differs from the antisocial personality in that he, like the dyssocial personality, has evolved an ego structure that allows for trust and attachment to others and has internalized social codes.

Thus he has available superego structure, but this is distorted and creates a persisting unconscious irrational sense of guilt, shame, or unworthiness.

A characteristic of all antisocial psychopathological behavior is the fact that the drive or motivation behind it is intense and forceful. The immediate urges are stronger than any rational considerations. The pathological personality who repeatedly commits some antisocial act appreciates intellectually that he will doubtless be caught, and if so, will face severe punishment. His need for his customary anxiety-relieving means impels, nevertheless, the compulsive continuance of his behavior. He may make a genuine effort to "go straight" and yet find his efforts futile in the face of strong unconscious forces. At times this may be the result of a vicious circle. His dynamically motivated aggressiveness, for example, may generate anxiety, and his anxiety, in turn, may generate antisocial aggressiveness. Although from a psychopathological standpoint the sociopathic personality may be looked upon as not responsible for his conduct, from a legal point of view he is regarded in most American courts as accountable for any violations of the legal code. The projective psychological techniques may yield significant information concerning personality structure and underlying psychopathology as well as reveal the areas around which the patient's major problems revolve. The Minnesota Multiphasic scales also are most revealing in assisting in this diagnosis.

Prognosis

There has been an impression that over time those with antisocial personality disorders slowly mature and become less involved in criminal and other disruptive behavior as they age. Maddocks' recent report of a five-year follow-up of social adaptation of a group of untreated psychopaths belies the full validity of this impression. Although he discovered that conviction rates fall with increasing age, some three out of five psychopaths do not establish a satisfactory social adjustment in later life. Maddocks suggests that although they leave the circuit of detention in prisons as they age, many then enter the medical care system as an expression of their continuing maladjustment.

In another follow-up study Tölle addressed himself to the differing courses the antisocial personality takes in his attempt at "mastery of life." Some were found to do so by increasing social withdrawal and abnormality; others improved slightly in their capacity to utilize the opportunities for social improvement offered them; whereas another group succeeded partially by limiting their range of activity. The mastery of others was highly successful in spite of considerable stress. About one-third pursued the first two lines of adaptation; another one-third the second; and the remainder the last mode.

Treatment

One must not oversimplify the factors that have determined the behavior of the sociopathic personality. Pernicious social and cultural influences may contribute to the creation of the sociopathic personality, although they do not serve as the basic genetic agents. Often there is an interplay between psychological and social factors. If environmental influences are contributory, either their modification or the patient's removal from them is desirable.

The rational treatment of the antisocial and dyssocial must differ from that of those neurotics who perform delinquent or criminal acts. Essential to any effective therapy is the placing of the individual in an accepting and warm human environment where he may find it possible to develop a therapeutic relationship with some member of the treatment group whom he perceives as having his interests at heart and to whom he can give some trust. In dealing with delinquency of late childhood and adolescence, it is often found that one of the most effective corrective measures is a warm, authoritative father figure with whom boys can identify.

With the older psychopaths, this initial step becomes increasingly difficult and often is impossible owing to the inherent ego defect of basic distrust. Psychiatrists and others treating such patients must be highly motivated and endowed with a mature patience to effect the development of the therapeutic relationship.

When the treatment relationship is established, through either individual or group identification, pressure through personal and verbal behavior must be initiated toward certain goals and standards of social relationship. Usually such efforts must be made continuously and slowly, and infractions should be treated by withdrawal of privileges and their reinstitution on improved behavior. The treatment relationship, whether established through the medium of a single psychiatrist or a group, makes clear certain standards of behavior, and their abuse is managed by frustrating loss of satisfaction in other areas. A sense of authority is consistently and firmly maintained. This treatment regimen cannot be attained frequently without some type of institutional care. It clearly differs from the continually permissive attitude necessary for the treatment of the neurotic child or adult. If such permissiveness is adopted for treatment of the psychopath, no focus will be established for superego growth, and, if anything, the permissiveness may aggravate the antisocial behavior.

In this respect the use of group process through exposure to the "therapeutic community" has been on trial for many years. Whiteley has reported that of over 122 patients so treated and released for two years, during that period 40 per cent remained without conviction or psychiatric hospitalization. In examining the factors indicative of good social outcome from this therapeutic exposure, those adapting socially had previously achieved some success in school, at work, and in interpersonal relations, as well as exhibiting a capacity for emotional responsivity and involvement with others. He suggests that for the more immature, persistently acting-out psychopath the therapeutic community is both unbeneficial and sometimes harmful. For the egocentric, impulsive, thought-disordered, and aggressive psychopath, little benefit may be achieved by this treatment.

When the antisocial behavior of a child or adolescent has its origins in the family interactions described by Johnson and Szurek, in order for treatment to succeed, in most instances the parent of the patient must be treated as well or, in the case of a child or young adult, separated during the course of psychotherapy. Such separations are resisted by parents, whose major gratification comes from their dependent relations with the "scapegoat" child. In some instances, separation of the patient from the parent or change in the behavior of the patient during treatment has led to serious behavior disturbance in the symbiotic parent.

Treatment for those with a neurotic character of the antisocial type that has led to repetitive antisocial behavior should conform to the psychoanalytic model as described in a subsequent chapter. Here the hope of the therapist is to relate past conflicts that have led to the erection of a pathological sense of guilt and its expressive force in masochistic "acting out." Since the patient has already established a set of values, it is unnecessary to intervene by providing an environmental setting that prevents actions and denies or punishes for failure to comply.

Sometimes the patterned response to pathogenetic factors is so fixed that it is not modifiable. Again, the patient seems to lack capacity to experience anxiety with its resulting desire for relief. The hostility, too, often shown by the psychopath may generate hostility in others and hamper treatment. Sometimes a secondary gain from his neurotic-like symptom neutralizes any wish for a change in his behavior.

A prison environment is a handicap to therapy. If the sociopsychopath's behavior brings him before court, the judge may be aware that ideally the treatment of the prisoner's behavior is by one of the several forms of psychotherapy. Like the psychiatrist, he may realize that punishment without recognition of the prisoner's emotional problems may intensify his social maladjustment. On the other hand, a person cannot be sentenced to therapy.

Frequently the psychiatrist is confronted in the case of the sociopsychopath with the question of criminal responsibility. As a scientific psychiatrist, he should seek to ascertain if the criminal behavior is susceptible of psychopathological interpretation, but he should also remember that it is not easy to prove or disprove such interpretations, that society cannot yet evaluate them, and that it cannot yet, and perhaps should not, establish them as criteria of responsibility. The matter of judgment of responsibility rests solely with the law. The psychiatrist's only function is to provide his opinion as to the motivating forces for the criminal act and their origins as determined from the personality study.

SITUATION PSYCHOSES

If, according to the view expressed, the maladaptation of the antisocial personality is fundamentally an attempted solution of the individual's problems rather than the result of unwholesome social influences, we should expect a higher incidence of psychotic reactions among these poorly integrated individuals than among well-adjusted persons. This assumption is found to be true. The great majority of such reactions are schizophrenic, affective, or paranoid but some, occurring under circumstances involving great emotional distress, represent attempts, through disorders of belief or of sensorium, to escape from the hard and uncompromising reality of some specific, difficult situation and are therefore called "situation psychoses." Frequently situation psychoses are in the nature of confused states, paranoid episodes, or periods of irritability, excitement, or depression.

Prison Psychoses

Since the most difficult situation into which the behavior of the antisocial usually leads him is confinement, which he bears poorly, the most important of the situation reactions are the prison psychoses. It must not be concluded that all psychoses developing among prisoners belong to this group; in fact, but a minority of them belong to the true prison psychoses, in which delusional ideas tend to be ideas of persecution, innocence, or pardon. The majority of the psychotic reactions observed among prisoners are of the usual clinical types, especially schizophrenia and paranoid states, the stress of imprisonment acting merely as the releasing agent.

Prison psychoses that begin after the prisoner has received sentence are most likely to occur among long-term prisoners and comparatively early during the period for which they are sentenced. The forms assumed by the psychotic reactions are various. Occasional forms are sudden excitements manifested by intense emotion, violent rage, cursing, and destructive attacks on the environment. Such attacks, usually brief, may, psychologically, represent a protest against an intolerable situation. Episodes characterized by delusions of persecution, ideas of strange influences, olfactory hallucinations of gas, or anxiety, irritability, and uneasiness are not common. Manic-depressive reactions rarely develop among persons held under indictment or sentence, and some psychiatrists of extensive experience report that they have never seen this form of psychosis in the case of life prisoners.

There are two forms especially typical of prison psychoses. One, expressing a deep-seated dissatisfaction, is characterized by querulousness. Patients suffering from this form have numerous delusions of ill treatment. They constantly grumble and maintain that all sorts of obstacles are placed in their way and that attempts are being made to annoy them. Frequently their complaints sound plausible.

One of the most frequent forms of prison psychoses found among long-term prisoners is that characterized by delusions of innocence or of pardon. The patient may experience auditory hallucinations wherein he is told that he has been exonerated from his alleged crime and is now to be liberated. Other, but similar, wish-fulfilling ideas are heard. As the patient believes himself an innocent and unjustly persecuted individual, he becomes bitter toward those who fail to set him at liberty.

Most of those with the acute prison psychoses recover after transfer from the prison to the hospital, where the general attitude is treatment rather than the maintenance of fixed and rigid discipline. Many life prisoners thus transferred fail to recover but gradually deteriorate mentally. One of the most important elements in the treatment of the prison psychoses is to render the patient's points of contact as little irritating as possible. Occupation, games, amusements, and a friendly, although necessarily firm, attitude are helpful.

Ganser Syndrome

An interesting type of mental disorder sometimes occurring in the case of prisoners under detention and awaiting trial was described by Ganser. It develops after commission of a crime and, therefore, tells nothing about the patient's mental state when he committed the offense. This syndrome is described in Chapter 24.

SEXUAL DEVIATION

Persons whose biological sex urges are directed toward a normal heterosexual goal but who, because they are segregated from those of the opposite sex, casually seek sexual satisfaction through various perversions are scarcely to be considered as sexual deviates.* In the true deviate, the offending sexual act is the surface symptom of a more profound personality disturbance.

In the opinion of many psychiatrists, the term sexual psychopath, or deviate, should be limited to the individual whose sexual impulse, through defects in the step-by-step development of personality, either has remained immature or has undergone deviation in the course of its maturation. The arrest or deviation in development is not, of course, in the anatomy or physiology of sex organs but in the psychosexual, i.e., the emotional, dispositional aspect of sexual expression. Psychosexual maturation may lag behind biological maturation or be so blocked that mature heterosexual impulses are not established. The emotional and instinctive aspects of sex are not harmoniously integrated into the total personality. Satisfaction of the sex impulse is therefore sought through such expressions as voyeurism, exhibitionism, homosexuality, rape, pedophilia, masochism, sadism, and other means.

If the family and social environment are not favorable to a healthy, mature psychosexual development, the drive toward mature heterosexuality will be blocked or deviated. Thus a boy held closely by his mother through his growing years and deprived of close association with a father, through the latter's absence, indifference, or hostility, is likely to have homosexual relations as his preferred form of sexual gratification in adulthood. There is much evidence from both the clinic and the laboratory that effective

---

* "It is said that only a small proportion of males convicted of sex offenses have been involved in behavior which is materially different than that of most males in the population. This small group, which numbers in the neighborhood of 5 to 10 per cent, is that which engages our attention as psychiatrists. They are hereinafter designated as psychiatrically deviated sex offenders." Group for the Advancement of Psychiatry, Report No. 9: Psychiatrically Deviated Sex Offenders.

heterosexual development in man and animals depends upon continuing contacts with members of both sexes throughout growth.

Homosexuality

From the Kinsey studies, it is clear that there is a wide range of homosexual behavior in both men and women. Whereas some live an exclusively homosexual life and receive all adult sexual gratification from a partner of the same sex, others are predominantly but not exclusively satisfied in this way. With a large number of adolescents and adults, the major sexual expression is heterosexual, yet occasionally or incidentally these individuals have homosexual contacts. Such incidental contacts may take place when the person is deprived of heterosexual contacts, after alcohol debauches or head injuries, or in situations of homosexual license.

The term homosexuality is often used in ways other than to indicate a personality disorder wherein the predominant mode of sexual expression is with a member of the same sex. "Latent homosexuality" refers to the existence of a personality make-up similar to that of the overt homosexual, and associated even in some cases with fantasy formation of homosexual activity, but without overt homosexual activity. Unfortunately, homosexuality is now used frequently as a derogatory designation, and some neurotic patients designate themselves as homosexual due to their feelings of failure and inability to express and utilize successfully their aggressive drives to mastery.

Among the groups of men charged with homosexual behavior in courts, one finds the female impersonator, as well as the isolated and dull person who has not had a loving relationship in the past, the resentful antisocial, those generally compensated individuals who are apprehended after an overt act while drinking in later life, and those whose homosexual behavior is a single component in a more serious psychotic disorder, most frequently schizophrenic or mentally defective. There is a group of homosexuals whose personality development and ego functioning otherwise appear intact and who conduct themselves both effectively and constructively in society. Yet all these individuals exhibiting homosexual behavior do show certain common features in the personality. They have difficulty in reconciling dependent and assertive drives, an ambivalent maternal relationship, and a high frequency of rearing in a broken home.

Homosexual behavior is determined on the basis of defect in psychosexual maturation. While Kallmann found a large number of identical twins concordant to homosexuality, more recently a study of a number of identical twin pairs showed one to be heterosexual and the other homosexual. In such twin pairs the opportunity is optimum to examine the differing psychogenetic forces that relate to the several forms of sexual behavior, and the findings of these studies gives a strong support to earlier psychodynamic formulations.

For a healthy psychosexual development, the child should form an identification with the parent or a member of his own sex. The future homosexual male has an inordinate attachment to his mother, fostered by her and leading to identification with her. This attachment flowers in the absence or indifference of a father or when the child fears or hates this parent or derogates him as the mother often does. The homosexual who has identified with the mother as the dominant person seeks out males as sexual companions, motivated either through fear of incest or loss of the maternal relationship that is threatened in his contacts with women. Then there are underlying castration fears and resentments toward women derived from the repressed hostilities toward the mother. The homosexual relationship may express as well his hostility to men. In a few instances, male homosexuality arises when the child has been separated from women and reared by men throughout life. Here he is deprived of the experience of heterosexual contact and also fears women.

Pedophilia

Pedophilia, or a pathological sexual interest in children, is regarded as a variant of homosexuality in which homosexual strivings are directed toward children. It occurs largely in weak and impotent persons. The pedophil acts toward the child as he unconsciously wished his mother to behave toward himself. Another, and perhaps more logical, explanation of the pedophil's behavior is that he functions on an immature psychosexual level because of his fearfulness and doubt concerning himself. As a result of these feelings, he expects rejection and failure in adult, heterosexual advances. His sexual expression is therefore released toward children.

Fetishism

Fetishism is a perversion peculiar to men. The fetishist is unable to love a real person but becomes attached to some material object having a feminine association, such as a lock of hair or an undergarment. This object attains a highly exaggerated value and becomes a special source of erotic gratification, a reliever of both psychic and sexual tension, as contact with it leads to orgasm. The fetish always has a genital meaning; it serves the purpose of denying the anatomical difference between the two sexes, a discovery of which caused an overwhelming genital fear.

Fetishism has usually been considered as a substitutive genital drive necessary as the consequence of fears of castration. Some psychoanalysts consider the fetishistic attachment an effort to gain an ego identification through contact with a substitutive satisfying object and point to the fetishistic attachment of little children to blankets, toys, or other objects as a means of satisfaction in the absence of the mother. Thus, the act may be seen as one satisfying a pregenital wish.

Transvestism

Another deviation is that of transvestism, the impulse to dress in the clothing of the opposite sex. Formulations of the psychopathology of fetishism and of transvestism are still largely speculative. Transvestism occurs more frequently in the male than in the female. Usually the patient's mother wanted a girl and literally reared her son to be one.

Transvestism is not to be confused with homosexuality. It consists in the desire to wear clothes of the opposite sex and thereby attain sexual gratification. Most transvestites are oriented to heterosexual relations as well as to social relations with the opposite sex. They often marry.

Transvestism usually commences between the ages of five and 14 in the association of articles of feminine clothing with sexual gratification through masturbation. The behavior is reinforced if the growing youngster's potential for heterosexual development is impeded through passivity or opposing family or social forces which he cannot overcome. According to Buckner the transvestite then elaborates his masturbation fantasies to develop a feminine self through the process of identification and fantasy. By so doing he is able to act out the heterosexual patterns without the anxiety-provoking presence of a person of the opposite sex. By the late teens the transvestite pattern becomes fixed.

The term transvestite has been used often to refer to others who derive satisfaction from cross-dressing. Thus there are other heterosexual and homosexual persons who find gratification in this act, although they do not have the developmental history or the psychodynamics of the transvestite as just described. It has been used as well to label transitory cross-dressing in children who later may or may not become homosexuals. So, too, have been designated erroneously males who adopt a ritualistic fetish of wearing special articles of female clothing openly or concealed beneath male clothing and also male homosexual "drag queens" who periodically cross-dress.

Trans-sexualism is not to be confused with transvestism. The term has come into use since the introduction of gender transmutation by surgical or endocrinological means. A trans-sexual is presumed to be a biologically normal person with an unalterable conviction that he is a member of the opposite sex. He argues that throughout life he has so regarded himself. Such persons often attempt now to join the desired sex through requests to reshape their genital organs by surgical or endocrinological means. By so doing it is their hope to achieve their enduring fantasy in reality. Kubie and Mackie have discussed in depth the many serious issues which have arisen as the consequence of the numerous recent surgical operations done to effect gender transmutation.

Exhibitionism

In exhibitionism, one of the commonest sexual deviations, one usually finds that the offender is a son of a dominant, aggressive mother who resents her feminine role and tries to live her life through her children, especially the sons. The father is frequently a weak and ineffective person who has exerted but little influence in shaping the son's emotional development. Because of the mother's spoiling and showering the boy with unusual affection, he comes to identify himself with her and incestuous wishes develop as well. With a strong taboo against such insistent but consciously forbidden wishes, the boy must build compulsive but unconscious defenses. The symptom of exhibitionism with genital exposure to others functions to reassure him against castration.

Pathogenesis of Perversions

A characteristic common to all forms of sexual perversions is their repetitive, compulsive, patterned nature. Such behavior represents the expression of an uncontrollable urge, committed without logic or rationale and apparently for the purpose of securing relief from an unbearable tension. The satisfaction derived from the commission of the sexually deviated and compulsive act is symbolic and substitutive; it is therefore temporary and requires repetition. These characteristics constitute the criteria of the neuroses. There is, in fact, an increasing tendency to regard the true sexual perversions as basically psychoneurotic in their psychopathology and therefore as a kind of mental illness. As in the case of compulsive handwashing, the apparent motive is not the real, or at least not the only, motivating factor. The real motive is to satisfy aggressive or various other immature and deviated aspects of the psychosexual component of the personality.

A majority of serious sex offenders are unable to comprehend the reasons, the inner compulsion, for their actions. The sexual psychopath's behavior is not a substitute for normal heterosexual relations. It is a form of sexual activity that satisfies some very specific need ungratified by normal sexual activity. The added fact that the offender is usually unable to comprehend the reason for his actions, that their motivations are to a large extent unconscious, gives the psychopath's behavior a neurotic characteristic. In general, sexual psychopaths are people with deep-seated personality disorders of which sex deviation is but one manifestation.

Recent studies in the pathogenesis of the sexual deviations make it appear that overt antisocial misbehavior may be caused by parental, often unwitting, seduction. In infancy, nudity, fondling, and virtual absence of privacy are appropriate and even necessary. If, however, such evidences of kindly parental affection persist until childhood or adolescence, they become pathological. Under the guise of "motherly" or "fatherly" affection, boys and girls may be bathed by parents, often of the opposite sex, until adolescence. Sleeping with children of the opposite sex may be prolonged into the teen-age period. Undressing may habitually occur in the presence of children. Sometimes legitimate parental embraces of affection extend into the sphere of frank bodily petting of adolescent children. Stimulated by parental behavior, the boy finds no outlet for his aroused sexual impulses. Eventually, mounting frustration and anger force him to follow one of two courses. One is regression to the safety of more infantile attitudes of sexual behavior. The other is sexual aggression toward women. Neither course resolves the rage or dissipates the overstimulated unconscious sexual drives. The result may therefore later be a direct, sexual, destructive acting-out of the conflict.

In contrast to the direct, hostile acting-out stemming from the repeated seduction and frustration incident to the child's intimate association with the parent of the opposite sex, such sexual aberrations as exhibitionism, voyeurism, and transvestism may be traceable to the unconscious tendencies of the parent. In such cases, the instinctual sexual development of the child seems to represent or constitute an acting-out of the unconscious wishes of the parent.

Treatment

Before considering therapy, a word should perhaps be said concerning the prevention of sex deviation. This requires a knowledge of its origin, also a recognition and emotional acceptance by the public of the fact that true deviation, in contrast to methods of sexual gratification adopted in absence of opportunity for the satisfaction of a biologically normal heterosexual impulse, is a manifestation of a development fault in the mental life that had its beginning in the early forma-

tive years of childhood. Any progress in reducing sexually psychopathic behavior must remain exceeding slow. The most hopeful approach is doubtless through more and proper sex education in childhood, the establishment of identifications consonant with the child's sex, and assistance in a constructive sublimation of sexual and aggressive impulses that may be misdirected by the vicissitudes of childhood.

Psychotherapy utilizing psychoanalytical principles is the rational treatment for the sex deviate. Some sexual psychopaths have no conscious desire to be cured of their behavior. Ideal conditions for therapy exist when the deviate has not been guilty of offense against the person, has therefore not committed a serious social offense, and has voluntarily sought therapy. If his offense has been so serious that the community must be protected, the deviate must be confined. The prison environment and routine are not, however, conducive to successful therapy. The personality factors and emotional conflicts that led to the crime will not, of course, be worked through by simply spending a certain amount of time in prison. If the offender has not been guilty of violence, it is usually desirable that he be confined in a hospital atmosphere in which the therapist may supervise the surroundings in accordance with the needs of the patient as the therapy progresses. Through therapy and subsequent parole, some such offenders, if their desire for improvement is strong, may be enabled to channel their impulses into constructive activites.

The Committee on Forensic Psychiatry of the Group for the Advancement of Psychiatry, to whose report reference has been made, gave thoughtful consideration both to the psychiatric aspects of sex deviation and to legislation to be recommended for dealing with sex offenders. It suggested that a psychiatric examination be made of any persons convicted of sexual offense and that if the psychiatrists report the offender suffers from a fundamental personality disorder, the judge, if he deems it wise, should, in lieu of sentence, commit him for an indefinite period to an institution equipped to give psychotherapy. Such a law would satisfy the aims of both community protection from the potentially dangerous offender and treatment under conditions favorable to restoration. "If the offender is curable he can be eventually released to society; if not, he should never be released. . . . The Committee is unreserved in its opinion that the committed sex offender should be actively treated in a non-penal institution. . . . The stigma of sex offenses officially attached to the sex offender committed to a penal institution creates a formidable obstacle to treatment. At best consistency demands that if we diagnose the sex offender as mentally disordered he should be treated as a mental case in a facility for that purpose."

Not all persons concerned with the disposition of sex offenders recommend treatment in state hospitals for mental diseases. They contend that such institutions lack facilities in both housing and personnel, that sex offenders do not mix well with others, that treatment is unsystematized and difficult, and that there are no criteria of recovery.

BIBLIOGRAPHY

Aichhorn, A.: Wayward Youth. New York, Viking Press, 1935.
Alexander, F.: The neurotic character. Internat. J. Psycho-Analysis, *11*:292–311, 1930.
Bieber, I., et al.: Homosexuality. New York, Basic Books, Inc., 1962.
Buckner, H. T.: The transvestic career path. Psychiatry, *33*:381–389, 1970.
Cleckley, H. M.: The Mask of Sanity. St. Louis, C. V. Mosby Co., 1941.
Eissler, K. (ed.): Searchlights on Delinquency. New York, International Universities Press, Inc., 1949.
Ford, C. S., and Beach, F. A.: Patterns of Sexual Behavior. New York, Paul B. Hoeber, 1951.

Glueck, E. T.: Identifying juvenile delinquents and neurotics. Ment. Hyg., *40*:24–43, 1956.
Green, R., and Money, J.: Transsexualism and Its Management. Baltimore, Johns Hopkins Press, 1969.
Guttmacher, M. S.: Sex Offenses: The Problem, Causes and Prevention. New York, W. W. Norton & Co., Inc., 1951.
Hooker, E.: A preliminary analysis of group behavior of homosexuals. J. Psychol., *42*:217–225, 1956.
Jenkins, R. L.: The psychopathic or antisocial personality. J. Nerv. & Ment. Dis., *131*:318–334, 1960.
Johnson, A. M., and Robinson, D. B.: The sexual deviant (sexual psychopath)—causes, treatment and prevention. J.A.M.A., *164*:1559–1565, 1957.
Johnson, A. M., and Szurek, S. A.: Etiology of antisocial behavior in delinquents and psychopaths. J.A.M.A., *154*:814–817, 1954.
Kennedy, A.: Psychopathic personality and social responsibility. J. Ment. Sci., *100*:873–881, 1954.
Kolb, L. C., and Johnson, A. M.: Etiology and therapy of overt homosexuality. Psychoanalyt. Quart., *24*:506–515, 1955.
Kubie, L. S., and Mackie, J. B.: Critical issues raised by operations for gender transmutation. J. Nerv. Ment. Dis., *147*:431–443, 1968.
Lorand, S., and Balint, M. (ed.): Perversions: Psychodynamics and Therapy. New York, Random House, 1956.
Maddocks, P. D.: A five year follow-up of untreated psychopaths. Brit. J. Psychiat., *116*:511–515, 1970.
Marks, I., Gilder, M., and Bancroft, J.: Sexual deviants two years after electric aversion. Brit. J. Psychiat., *117*:173–185, 1970.
Medlicott, R. W.: Fifty thieves. New Zeal. Med. J. *67*:183–188, 1968.
Rainer, J. D., Mesnikoff, A., Kolb, L. C., and Carr, A.: Homosexuality and heterosexuality in identical twins. Psychosom. Med., *22*:251–259, 1960.
Redlich, F. C., et al.: Narcoanalysis and truth. Amer. J. Psychiat., *107*:586–593, 1951.
Rexford, E. N.: A developmental concept of the problems of acting out. J. Amer. Acad. Child Psychiat., *2*:6–21, 1963.
Swanson, D. W., Bohnert, P. J., and Smith, J. H.: The Paranoid. Boston, Little, Brown & Company, 1970.
Tölle, R.: The mastery of life by psychopathic personalities. Psychiatrica Clinica, *1*:1–14, 1968.
Whiteley, J. S.: The response of psychopaths to a therapeutic community. Brit. J. Psychiat., *116*:517–529, 1970.
Yalom, I. D.: Aggression and forbiddenness in voyeurism. Arch. Gen. Psychiat., *3*:305–319, 1960.

"... his sense of happiness—was now. Nothing more than a thin cover beneath which anguish and the obsession of death were awakening."

André Malraux

Drug Dependence

During the last decade, drug-seeking behavior, drug dependency, and addiction have increased markedly, particularly among the adolescent and young adult populations of the world. Many factors have influenced this trend. Thus the number of new drugs produced synthetically has gone up enormously. Some of these, notably the hallucinogens, have been advertised to the public as "mind-expanding" agents that are presumed to give the taker unexpected personal powers. Widespread communication of information regarding drugs between countries through radio, television, and other media, along with wide advertising of the use of pharmaceuticals in general as means of relieving pain, distress, or discomfort or enhancing well being has established an international cultural milieu of acceptance of drug taking. The vastly improved and rapid means of transportation, as well as those of supply and improved individual purchasing power, have provided an availability of drugs to populations never before exposed. In contrast to the economic rewards of drug production, distribution, and sale which have facilitated usage, legal control measures throughout the world directed against abuse have proved incapable of effective application.

In countries where certain drugs known and advertised as capable of producing physical harm, such as alcohol and tobacco, remain socially acceptable among older age groups, esoteric drug taking has become a means of defiant behavior by adolescents, of expressing dissent as to the hypocrisy they detest in their society. Also, in certain sections of this age group, peer acceptance provides the motivating force both for experimentation with drug taking and even maintenance to habituation. Above all, the biological driving force of curiosity as expressed in experimentation continues.

What has changed are the drugs abused and the styles in which that abuse is expressed between generations and cultures.

To comprehend the drug abuse problem today, the perspective must be one which includes all drug taking. Among those drugs used for euphoriant or anxiety-reducing effects which lead to habituation, addiction, or other physical disabilities, one must include in perspective those legally accepted by societies in which production and distribution are sometimes supported by the state, distributed, and even taxed by the society, as well as those in which the various states prohibit any aspect of production or distribution. In the United States alcohol represents a drug which is legally and socially accepted, in contrast to the narcotics whose distribution is legally prohibited except under government regulation.

In this chapter consideration is given to the psychiatric consequences of dependence on opium, its alkaloids, and derivatives; the synthetic analgesics with morphine-like effects; the barbiturates; other hypnotics, and sedatives; cocaine; *Cannabis sativa* (hashish and marihuana);

509

and other psychostimulants such as amphetamine and the hallucinogens. In general the majority of those who become habituated and addicted to these agents suffer from personality disorders. Others are neurotic and psychotic.

Definitions

The following definitions are those given by the World Health Organization in 1969. *Drug abuse* is persistent or sporadic excessive drug use inconsistent with or unrelated to acceptable medical practice. *Drug dependence* is a state, psychic and sometimes also physical, resulting from the interaction between a living organism and a drug, characterized by behavioral and other responses that always include a compulsion to take the drug on a continuous or periodic basis in order to experience its psychic effects and sometimes to avoid the discomfort of its absence. Tolerance may or may not be present. A person may be dependent on more than one drug.

Perhaps there should be further explanation of some of the terms contained in this definition as well as certain others relating to addiction. By *habituation*, or habit-formation, is meant a psychological dependence on the use of a drug because of the relief from tension and emotional discomfort that it affords. By *tolerance* is meant a declining effect of the same dose of a drug when it is administered repeatedly over a period of time. As a result, it is necessary to increase the dose in order to obtain the original degree of effect. *Physical dependence* refers to an altered physiological state brought about by repeated ingestion or administration of a drug in order to prevent the appearance of a characteristic illness called an *abstinence syndrome*.

Dependence on analgesic drugs is characterized, on their withdrawal, by autonomic dysfunction, such as yawning, lacrimation, rhinorrhea, gooseflesh, and symptoms reflecting general irritability of the central nervous system, such as twitching of muscles, insomnia, hypertension, and fever. Dependence on hypnotics and alcohol is manifested chiefly by the development of convulsions and delirium following withdrawal. Physical dependence is a self-limited process. The symptoms appear in a definite time sequence following withdrawal of the drug, reach maximum intensity at a definite time, and decline at a definite rate. The symptoms that follow withdrawal of drugs with relatively short lengths of action, such as heroin and Dilaudid, appear quickly, become intense in a short time, and decline rapidly. Symptoms that follow withdrawal of a drug with a long length of action, such as methadone, appear slowly, are never intense, and decline more slowly.

Another new definition is that of *physical dependence capacity* (PDC). This refers to the "ability of a drug to act as a substitute for another upon which an organism has been made physically dependent, that is, to suppress abstinence phenomena that would otherwise develop after abrupt withdrawal of the original dependence-producing drug."

Extent and Prevalence of Drug Abuse

A compilation of 38 studies made of the extent of drug usage among university, college, high school, and selected graduate students, hippie groups, and adults reported by Berg in 1969 documents the widespread experimentation in drug usage now taking place in the United States. *Extent* refers solely to the individual ever having used an illicit drug; thus it includes all persons ever having used such a drug (not necessarily current users), as well as regular users of one or more drugs. It contrasts with *prevalence*, defined as current regular users of illicit drugs. That the rates of usage vary widely is apparent. Rates from high schools were surprisingly like those among the college students. Marihuana rates of extent of use varied from 5.6 to 34.9 per cent, amphetamines from 9.5 to 21.5 per cent, barbiturates and LSD from 1.7 to 15.7 per cent, and opiates from 1.0 to 4.7 per cent.

As regards high school users, the rates were collected from institutions where a drug problem was known to exist. Also, in this group were many who tried a drug experimentally only once. Finally the schools surveyed were located in metropolitan areas; available statistical reports on rural schools show generally low rates of usage of illicit drugs. As to narcotics, juvenile users are usually those living in the urban ghettos; the increase is greatest among black and Spanish-speaking ghetto families.

At the site of entry into psychiatric services where serious disability, including addiction, habituation, and personality disturbance coincide, the pattern of drug abuse is well described by Hekemian and Gershon. From over 100 patient admissions to a city receiving hospital of those improperly using drugs, the majority of the heroin users fall into the group of antisocial personalities. Emotionally disturbed but younger groups tended to use marihuana, amphetamines, and the hallucinogens. One-half of this group were considered schizophrenic before taking drugs, and 40 per cent required prolonged hospitalization. The desire for euphoria, thought to be due to a wish to escape underlying depression, was the most frequently given reason for drug taking. Secondly blamed were the influences of friends or the need to escape the living environment. Almost all had taken more than one agent.

Opium and Its Alkaloids

ETIOLOGY. Addiction to drugs and the extent of its occurrence result from a complex interaction of cultural and familial forces that determine the availability of the pharmacologic agent, the opportunities for initiation to its usage, and the individual predisposition to con-

tinue its usage. In China and other Asian countries where opiates have been readily available in the past, addiction was common. Where the drug traffic offers opportunity for large profits and its usage is pushed, as in those areas of the United States offering sites of entry and distribution, prevalence of narcotic addiction is higher. Here, again, the initiation to its use takes a daring and defiant attitude that appeals to the adolescent and the immature. In those Western European countries, such as England, where narcotic addiction is managed as a medical problem, drug traffic is less profitable, and the culture does not place prestige on its use by overemphasizing its significance, the number of narcotic addicts is much smaller.

Those who become addicted are for the most part antisocial personalities, but the neurotic and psychotic also are predisposed in view of their affective problems. Those seeking the use of an addicting drug are motivated by the wish to induce and perpetuate the most satisfying state of personal existence even at the risk of impairing other values. Some who become addicts appear to try narcotics first as a means of seeking thrills, of facilitating self-esteem and self-assertion, or of expanding perceptual senses and hopefully gaining new insights and creativity so as to gain later appreciation from others. Another group achieves addiction because the narcotic agent is capable of reducing inhibitions, anxiety, and tensions, or else they seek separation from distressing affects through a life of partial stupor. No matter the initial motivation, whether to facilitate self-esteem or to relieve tensions, addiction reveals an imbalance in personality development and functioning.

Thus the large group of addicts is composed of individuals with personality disorders who became addicted to drugs through contact and association with persons already addicted. The addict often seeks to recruit new addicts, hoping to secure funds to supply his own needs by selling to others. Most members of this group are emotionally immature, hostile, aggressive persons who take drugs in order to secure relief from inner tension. They have few healthy resources or interests and are motivated by immature drives for immediate goals. The addict-to-be finds in the drug a release from tension, felt as a restless need for pleasurable or exotic sensations and the satisfaction of a longing for artificial elation or peace. Conscious discomfort is eliminated, repressed drives may be released, and responsibility is evaded. Another group consists of frankly neurotic persons with anxiety and obsessive-compulsive or psychophysiologic symptoms that are relieved by drugs. A third group consists of persons who, in the course of physical illness, have received drugs over an extended period and after the termination of the ailment have continued their use. However, probably all persons who acquire addiction in this manner have some fundamental emotional problem that caused them to continue the use of drugs beyond the period of medical need. Many addicts were intemperate in the use of alcohol before they became addicted to drugs. In practically all addicts, the previous adjustment to life was marginal or unsatisfactory.

PSYCHODYNAMICS. The majority of the narcotics addicts are those with arrests in the ego and superego development and, for the most part, fixed to an ambivalent maternal figure. The latter is both possessive and rejecting—on the one hand encouraging the addicted child to give up the habit, and on the other often offering or smuggling the addicting agent to him.

As in other families where psychopaths are reared, there has been an absence of a strong and consistent father figure. The addict fails to develop internal controls, hopes for immediate gratifications of his needs, and yet is continually frustrated due to his exaggerated demands, his psychosexual immaturity, and his lack of ego capacity that might bring satisfaction by delay and insistent efforts toward his goals. Whereas the psychopath is de-

prived of pleasure and pained by his frequent failures socially, the neurotic and psychotic suffer from either anxiety or depression, or both. Narcotics particularly, and other drugs as well, offer to such individuals both immediate reduction in the painful affects and the provision of a sense of pleasure or euphoria that provides a striking contrast to the usual state of those with personality disorders. The drug gives pleasure, satisfaction, and a sense of power as well as immediate relief from the tensions of disturbing affects.

The narcotic agents particularly reduce hunger, pain, and the frustration of threatening yet unrelieved sexual urge. Thus they alleviate the anxieties and tensions attendant on continuing frustrations or oral and sexual drive states. The drug then substitutes for satisfaction of the basic biologic drives. As the drug effect wears away, anxiety, depression or the customary feelings of loneliness or hopelessness recur, compounded with neurotic or psychotic sense of guilt. The drive to be relieved again becomes insurmountable, and additional doses are taken. The euphoric effects of the narcotics tend to subside with their increasing use. Here, again, in an attempt to regain the longed-for pleasure and relief from distress, the dosage is gradually increased.

PHYSIOLOGICAL THEORIES. Although there is no proved explanation for the phenomena of tolerance and of physical dependence, there are now two proffered theories. According to one theory, morphine has diphasic actions—excitation and depression. The excitant effects persist longer than do the depressant effects. For this reason, as doses of morphine are repeated, excitant effects are accumulated, larger and larger doses being required in order to obtain a sufficient degree of depression to mask the excitant effects. This is the suggested explanation for tolerance. Following withdrawal of the drug its excitant effects are released, thus accounting for physical dependence.

A second theory advanced to explain

the development of tolerance and physical dependence is that known as the theory of cellular adaptation. According to this hypothesis, the administration of opiates stimulates compensatory homeostatic mechanisms that oppose the depressant effects of the drug. These homeostatic responses become strengthened upon repeated administration of the substance. More and more drug is therefore required to induce the original degree of effect, and when the drug is withdrawn, the enhanced homeostatic mechanisms are released from the brake imposed upon them by the continued presence of morphine within the body, thus giving rise to physical dependence. This theory is based largely on the observation that manifestations of abstinence are always opposite in nature to those of the direct effects of opiates. Thus in the nontolerant, nonaddicted person, morphine constricts the pupils, lowers body temperature, reduces blood pressure, and causes sedation. Following withdrawal of morphine from the addict, there are noted dilation of the pupils, fever, a rise in blood pressure, and insomnia. Although the exact nature of the changes responsible for tolerance and physical dependence are not precisely known, they must be due to biochemical changes within the cells of the body. It may be that the narcotic agents given over time stimulate the drug metabolizing enzymes of the liver or brain microsomal system to excessive production, as Rubin and Lieber have shown for alcohol and barbiturates, thus producing increasing tolerance. If true, this explanation does not fully explain the abstinence phenomena.

Social conditioning, too, appears to play a major role in narcotic abuse and addiction. In Preble and Casey's study of the life of the "heroin user" in the modern urban American ghettos among blacks and Puerto Ricans, there are many social rewards for successful "hustling." In these deprived communities, where to sustain a mild habit requires the daily output of twenty or thirty dollars, the user aggressively expends his day in a career devoted to finding the monies to give him his fleeting moments of euphoria or surcease from distress and anxiety. The life of thievery to achieve his goals is active and may be seen as adventurous and challenging. The business demands liveliness and resourcefulness to hustle (rob or steal), seek victims, avoid police, find the dealers, purchase the heroin, adulterate it, and then cheat others. The competitiveness for monies is now so great that these users seldom associate other than in pairs. Then they steal and prey on each other, as well as their family members and those living in the neighboring communities. The successful hustler thus comes to be treated with respect by those in the "biz." The successive process of adulteration of heroin in the course of its passage through the lengthy chain of supply now has reduced the daily average to the bulk of heroin users to about 3 mg.—the estimated contents of one "bag." As Preble and Casey put it, "If they can be said to be addicted, it is not so much to heroin, as to the entire career of heroin user."

Still another process takes place as the narcotics user receives his drug from a peddler, injects it ("mainlining"), and responds with euphoria and relief of tensions. There is now good evidence, as in the research of Olds (who demonstrated that animals with implanted electrodes in areas of the midbrain and certain midbrain nuclei repeatedly stimulate themselves electrically as though receiving pleasure or a reward), of the drive of the nervous system to reinforce activities that provide satisfactions. It may be assumed that a conditioning process now takes place as well. Such a process, with the possibility of establishing as unconditioned stimuli the presence of another narcotics user, the offer of a drug, or a syringe, may well explain the propensity to relapse even long after a formerly addicted person has recovered from a state of physical dependence and perhaps has even been relieved of the painful affect that originally led to the pleasure in the drug.

Extent of Drug Addiction

When the Harrison Narcotic Act was passed in 1914, there were 175,000 narcotic addicts, mostly women, in the United States, which then had a population of 92,000,000. The rate equaled 1.9/1000.

In 1969 the Bureau of Narcotics and Dangerous Drugs reported 68,088 narcotic addicts (95 per cent heroin) in the United States, a number double that of 1968. However, using the dubious approach of computing the number of addicts from the number of heroin-related deaths, which in some states equal 1 per cent, the national total of addicts could have been above 200,000. This extrapolation fails to take into consideration the change in the pattern of heroin use with the greater frequency of "mainlining" (intravenous injection). The rapid increase in deaths from heroin usage is attributed in large part to this practice, as well as to drug-related infections such as septicemia. In 1970, in New York City, there were 1154 deaths as the result of narcotic addiction. Approximately 50 per cent of these deaths occurred in the young (aged less than 23), and the same percentage was due to overdosage. These high rates reflect the new patterns of narcotic use as well as the highly variable dosages available in supplies provided through the illicit market.

If the total of narcotic addicts equals 200,000 today, this is equivalent to one per 1000, far below the rates of the 1920's. So, too, as described earlier, although the extent of heroin use may be rising, the degree of addicted users in this country is, for the most part, less. It has been noticed that the abstinence syndrome of many of the heroin users arrested for trading in this country has become much less marked in intensity on withdrawal. Also, those who have observed addiction in opium-producing countries such as Laos are impressed with the much greater severity of the individual addiction there than in the United States.

Opiate Addiction

DeQuincey states in his "Confessions of an Opium Eater" that at one period in the history of his drug addiction he took 500 ml. of laudanum, or approximately 4.6 gm. (72 grains) of morphine, daily. Today, most addicts in the United States subsist on a much lower daily dosage, as mentioned earlier. Many addicts tolerate, without unfavorable symptoms, several times the dose they are accustomed to receive. This tolerance is destroyed following disappearance of the withdrawal symptoms. Addicts usually do not realize how rapidly they lose their tolerance for opiates. Sometimes during the "cure" addicts have obtained access to an opiate and have taken, with fatal results, what was the usual dose before withdrawal was instituted.

After recourse to his drug, the addict feels a sense of relief and perhaps of exhilaration, together with an increase in efficiency. The alleviation and sense of well-being obtained by the addict through a dose of the drug is so great that, as its pleasant effect diminishes, the desire for the satisfaction that the drug affords can scarcely be resisted. Although the continued administration of small amounts of the drug will prevent the distressing withdrawal symptoms to be described, increasing amounts are necessary to obtain the desired exhilaration and sense of increased capacity. As a result, the quantity taken is gradually increased until enormous amounts are required.

The eventual effect of the habit is impairment of a higher ethical sense, that is, the ego ideals. This moral and social deterioration is not a result of the direct effects of narcotics, but rather, of social consequences of the life of addiction. When the narcotic is taken in large doses, ambition and physical energy are lessened, lethargy is produced, and the pleasurable feeling that all is well makes the addict contented. As a result, he pays less attention to work and becomes an idler. Those who depend upon an illegitimate source for their supply of drugs are sometimes unable to work because of discomfort and weakness resulting from inability to secure the usual dose. When such patients, after a short period of deprivation, secure a supply, they often take more than is necessary to keep them comfortable. As a result, they alternate between physical and mental instability and physical and mental lethargy.

DIAGNOSIS. Frequently the individual admits that he is addicted to and needs drugs. If he denies the habit, the diagnosis can at times be made on the basis of needle marks, indurations, and the scars of abscesses. Miosis is suggestive but not definite evidence. Periods of restlessness, irritability, and anxiety, followed rather suddenly by euphoria and apparent relief and contentment, should be suggestive of drug addiction.

At times the only method of diagnosis may be isolation of the patient from a source of drugs followed by observation for signs of abstinence. The addict may be exceedingly clever in concealing a supply of his drugs. He may enter a hospital for the purpose of being cured of his addiction, yet at the same time have a supply craftily concealed in personal articles or even in body cavities.

A diagnostic test of considerable sensitivity has been developed that depends upon precipitating the abstinence syndrome by the parenteral injection of N-allylnormorphine (Nalline), a morphine antagonist. Before conducting such a test, it is advisable to obtain written permission of the patient or his guardian. This test is performed by injecting subcutaneously 3 mg. of N-allylnormorphine. In less than 20 minutes after injection, clear-cut signs of the abstinence syndrome will be noted in addicts using 60 mg. or more of morphine daily or equivalent amounts of heroin, dihydromorphinone, methadone, or Levo-Dromoran. Symptoms of the abstinence syndrome are described in the next section of this chapter. If the response to the first injection is negative or doubtful, a second dose of 5 mg. should be given 30 minutes after the first, and again a third 30 minutes after the second.

At this time, if abstinence symptoms have not become apparent and if the signs of the direct effects of the injected drug have appeared, the test may be read as negative. N-Allylnormorphine directly produces dizziness, pseudoptoses, mioses, and reduction in the respiratory rate, with a drunken experience. The absence of response to this test may occur in addicts who have been withdrawn from narcotics for as short as a week's period, or in addicts taking scattered doses. It is unreliable for meperidine (Demerol) addiction and contraindicated in the presence of serious organic disease.

WITHDRAWAL SYMPTOMS. Whenever opium or its habit-forming derivatives are abruptly withdrawn, a definite train of symptoms known as _abstinence_ or _withdrawal symptoms_ appears. If, within 12 to 14 hours after the administration of morphine, the dose is not repeated, the so-called withdrawal signs and symptoms begin to appear. Among the first are yawning, lacrimation, rhinorrhea, sneezing, and perspiration. These symptoms become more marked, and anorexia, dilated pupils, tremor, and gooseflesh are added. About 36 hours after the last dose, uncontrollable twitching of the muscles appears and cramps develop in the legs, abdomen, and back. The patient becomes intensely restless, is unable to sleep, and both pulse and blood pressure rise. Vomiting and diarrhea are frequent. These acute signs and symptoms reach their height about 48 hours after the last dose of morphine and remain at this height for 72 hours. They then gradually subside during the next five to ten days. As the withdrawal symptoms develop, the patient becomes restless, pessimistic, surly, fault-finding, and irritable and exhibits an unpleasant, increased psychomotor activity. He has a marked subjective feeling of weakness, and considerable prostration may occur. He may curse, cry, be impulsively destructive, and make suicidal gestures. To quite an extent, the intensity of withdrawal symptoms depends on the amount of drug the patient has been receiving. To some degree, the extent of the symptoms can be controlled by the patient himself. Any patient who appears comfortable during the period of withdrawal should be suspected of illicit possession of the drug.

PROGNOSIS. It should be remembered that narcotic addiction nearly always results from emotional problems, compounded frequently with a complex system of habit patterns that add to the difficulty of treatment. In general, these emotional problems are the same anxieties, conflicts, and neuroses as those with which other emotionally unstable persons are confronted.

More addicts than is commonly realized are permanently cured. The United States Public Health Service Hospital, Lexington, Kentucky, an institution for the treatment of addicts, found that only two-tenths of 1 per cent of the patients who left the hospital in less than 30 days remained off the drug, whereas 24 per cent of those who remained for the recommended period were believed to have remained free from addiction.

Some habitués, pretending that they no longer have any desire for the drug, eagerly look forward to an opportunity to return to their habit and devise every imaginable pretext to hasten their release from the hospital. Even those who believe they wish to be cured return to the drug on the slightest pretext, the alleged occasion being actually but a rationalization of their emotional defects and their psychological need for obliterating reality and its problems. They feel lost without the narcotic and the sense of physical comfort it imparts. Many, too, feel that they are not understood, are in a constant state of mild dissatisfaction, and long to return to the accustomed companionship of other addicts, by whom they feel they are understood and with whom they feel a sense of security and comradeship.

Often other addicts, sometimes for the sake of self-justification, sometimes because, as vendors of morphine, they see in their unhappy companion a potential customer, urge the recently "cured" pa-

tient to share the alleviating agent. The profits from this "cured" patient will replenish their own diminishing supply of the drug, of course.

It is often the pattern for the narcotics addict to waver between periods of voluntary or involuntary withdrawal for a decade or more. Recent long-term studies have found that by the age of 40 approximately three-quarters of persons addicted in early adulthood have withdrawn from drug usage. Stable abstinence takes place in about 40 per cent, and frequent relapse does not preclude recovery. In the group of former addicts who achieve abstinence the outlook for social stability is high; thus as many as three-quarters obtain full-time employment, support themselves and their families, and eschew abuse of other drugs and alcohol as well as criminality. Nor, according to Vaillant, do they succumb to depressive or psychosomatic complaints.

TREATMENT. On a rational basis, the preferable mode of treatment of the drug addict should be directed at relief of the distressing affective state that originally predisposed him to respond positively to the use of drugs. Such treatment would be directed to correction of the personality disorder or the psychoneurotic or psychotic state by the therapeutic process most applicable for the particular patient. Withdrawal of the drug then would not be undertaken until there had occurred the development of a firm dependent therapeutic relationship with a physician or other member of the therapeutic team. This relationship might sustain the patient through the period of abstinence and provide positive support to sustain withdrawal.

Unfortunately, therapeutic efforts today are directed largely to simple withdrawal of the drug, which must be undertaken in an institution where the activities of the patient and the sources of the drug can be controlled. The patient must remain long enough to be relieved of any physical ailments, to have opportunity to develop habits of living and working without drugs, and to be helped in discovering the source of his emotional difficulty.

WITHDRAWAL. It is not humane and it may be even dangerous to withdraw a narcotic abruptly. It may be withdrawn rapidly over a period of 10 days, in which case 30 mg. may be given every six hours for two days, with continued reduction thereafter until withdrawal is complete by the end of 10 days. It is probably more desirable to begin with the withdrawal of the narcotic, then shift to methadone, which suppresses the withdrawal symptoms in persons addicted. In this method, one should first ascertain the least amount of drug that will prevent the appearance of withdrawal symptoms. This is termed the stabilization dosage and can usually be determined in two or three days. Once the stabilization dosage is known, 1 mg. of methadone may be substituted for every 3 mg. dose of morphine or 1 mg. of heroin.

As methadone is a cumulative, slow-acting drug, the patient should be given one-half of his accustomed dose of morphine and one-half of his calculated dose of methadone during the first day of substitution. During the second day, only methadone is given. After substitution of methadone has been effected, the calculated dosage should be maintained for two or three days. The total dosage can be adjusted upward or downward, depending on the patient's response. Thereafter, methadone should be withdrawn over the course of 7 to 10 days, depending on the patient's response. Although withdrawal symptoms should be expected near the end of treatment, severe manifestations of abstinence are never seen when this method of withdrawal is used. Chlorpromazine is also useful in the tension states occurring in the withdrawal of opium and other narcotics. Great caution should be exercised in withdrawal of drugs from patients with evidence of myocardial insufficiency.

Sometimes the patient, without knowledge of the physician, has also been taking barbiturates before his admission. In that case the patient may develop an abstinence syndrome resulting from barbiturate withdrawal, as well. This will usually be in the form of a severe convulsion in which fractures may occur, or sometimes a delirious psychotic reaction. The prevention of this additional abstinence syndrome is the continued but gradually decreasing administration of a barbiturate.

An effort should be made to establish rapport and positive transference between the patient and physician during withdrawal. The patient usually has a resistance to gaining insight into the real causes of his addiction. Psychotherapy should, however, be directed toward his motivations, defenses, and adaptations. Many heroin users are now under treatment in various therapeutic groups. The outcome of such treatment remains to be evaluted. The usual recognition of drug addiction as a crime rather than as a disease reacts unfavorably on success of therapy. The vocational and social discrimination experienced by the addict following his discharge tends to lead to relapse.

The discharged addict should be required to report regularly for a period of five years to a center staffed with internists, psychiatrists, and social workers who are specifically trained to help him meet his problems. If left to solve his problems unaided, he usually returns to the use of drugs. It is frequently helpful if he joins the organization known as Narcotics Anonymous.

NARCOTIC ANTAGONISTS. *Cyclazocine Treatment.* Cyclazocine, a long-acting orally effective narcotic antagonist of the benzomorphan series is now under study as a therapeutic agent in the treatment of addiction. Like nalorphine, when given to an addicted person this drug will precipitate an acute abstinence state. In the previously addicted, the administration of this drug reduces or prevents the development of physical dependence on morphine-like drugs. Presumably it does so by preventing morphine from fixating to the usual receptor sites in the bodily tissues, including the central nervous system.

From 48 to 72 hours after completion of withdrawal from the addicting drug with the help of methadone, patients may be given subcutaneously two successive doses of cyclazocine of 3 and 4 mg. separated by a 30-minute interval. If no signs of abstinence are noted, cyclazocine administration is commenced at 0.25 mg. twice daily. This dosage is elevated by 0.25 mg. daily if no side-effects occur until such time as the daily dosage reaches 1.75 or 2.0 mg. The patient may then be seen once or twice weekly outside the hospital. Once the dose reaches 1.0 to 1.5 mg. per day, a single dosage may be given.

Initially the drug produces in some a degree of motor incoördination and slowing of thought. They must be advised not to give the drug to their friends who are narcotics users, as a serious or fatal reaction may be induced. However, the patient will not have discomfort if he himself takes a morphine derivative. The drug, if taken regularly, allows the addict to return to his usual environment but deprives him of the capacity to receive gratification from the use of narcotic addicting substances. Presumably then the reinforcement of the habituating drive is voided. It is not yet known what group of addicts will continue the use of cyclazocine; its immediate acceptance as therapy by addicts apparently is less than for the methadone treatment.

Naloxone (N-allylnoroxymorphone), another narcotic antagonist, has been tried in treatment as well. Unfortunately, its effects are less enduring than those of cyclazocine, as administration is required more than once per day. Nor is it very effective administered orally.

At this time the narcotic antagonists seem useful only in the treatment of the casual user of heroin with high risk for addiction, in the rehabilitation of the addicted who do not desire methadone maintenance, or in those entering treatmen who reject attachment both to a therapeutic community and to a methadone maintenance program.

Methadone Treatment. Maintenance treatment with methadone is based on the hypothesis that to achieve a homeostatic state, physiologically and psychologically, the confirmed narcotic addict must be provided with a medication to levels of narcotic tolerance freely which simultaneously protects him from the drive to obtain heroin or other addicting substances. The addict is considered to need the drug in order to obtain a comfortable physiological state which will allow social functioning. This addicted condition is considered analogous to that of the diabetic, deficient in substances needed to metabolize glucose and therefore physiologically in need and incapable of homeostasis unless receiving substitutes such as insulin.

Dole and Nyswander have placed confirmed heroin addicts on oral methadone commencing with doses of 10 to 20 mg. dissolved in a fruit juice. The dosage is increased gradually over a four-week period to levels of 50 to 150 mg. daily in a single oral dose. Too rapid elevation of the dosage may lead to oversedation, urinary retention, or abdominal distention. Too little methadone leads to abstinence with symptoms of malaise, sweating, lacrimation, and restlessness. On the full stabilized dose formerly refractive addicts with prolonged records of job instability, marital discord, and criminal recidivism have become socially productive. As yet, the long-term outcome of this maintenance therapy remains to be determined. It may be that the drug may be withdrawn after a successful period of social rehabilitation.

A longer-acting suppressant of the narcotic abstinence syndrome, *l-methadyl acetate,* has undergone tests by Jaffe and his colleagues as an adjuvant in methadone maintenance. This agent's supressive actions appear to last up to three days. To date it has been used as a weekend substitute for patients on methadone maintenance. Undoubtedly it will be tested as a full substitute for methadone.

Other Opium Derivatives

Heroin, taken both hypodermically and by snuffing, has great addiction ability. Many consider it the most difficult of all addictions to cure. *Codeine* has a definite, though low-grade, addiction liability. Both *Dilaudid* (dihydromorphinone hydrochloride) and *metopon* (methyldihydromorphinone) have high physical dependence and habituation liabilities. *Demerol* (meperidine hydrochloride) is a synthetic analgesic that is not chemically related to morphine but is nevertheless addicting. It possesses considerable habituation liability, and after prolonged administration its addicts develop physical dependence. Any differences in the addiction liability of the new analgesic drugs from that of morphine are differences in degree, not in kind. The general features of the morphine abstinence syndrome are also characteristic of these drugs.

Barbiturates and Other Sedative Drugs

INCIDENCE, ETIOLOGY, SYMPTOMS. According to reports of the United States Public Health Service, there has been a great increase in recent years not only in acute barbiturate intoxication but also in barbiturate addiction. Acute intoxication with barbiturates accounts for about 25 per cent of all deaths from acute poisoning among admissions to general hospitals, and more deaths are caused by barbiturates, either accidentally ingested or taken with suicidal intent, than by any other poison.

As in alcoholism and in narcotic drug addiction, the important factor in barbiturate addiction is an underlying personality difficulty. Many psychoneurotics become addicted to barbiturates through their prescription for insomnia. Persons with character disorders ("psychopaths") begin the use of the drug in order to experience its intoxicating effect. Mor-

phine addicts often use the drug when they are unable to secure morphine or in order to reinforce the effect of that narcotic. Alcoholics may begin the use of barbiturates to relieve the tension following a debauch and continue their use to induce toxic effects. In contrast to the situation in other narcotic drug addictions, a large proportion of the cases of barbiturate addiction results from administration by physicians. Especial care should be exercised in prescribing them for emotionally unstable persons. Simple insomnia alone is rarely a valid indication for the use of barbiturates.

Not only do the barbiturates induce acute brain syndromes but also they cause chronic delirious reactions in those who use the drug in large amounts over periods of time. In the latter there may occur, on sudden withdrawal of the drugs, an *abstinence syndrome,* again characteristically delirioid but often with an associated convulsive state. It is necessary to differentiate the two conditions (that due to intoxication and that due to abstinence); they differ in their clinical manifestations and their treatment.

With the development of the "minor tranquilizers" approximately a decade ago, these agents quickly found widespread use, entered illicit markets, and have been used as intoxicants as have the barbiturates. Since their pharmacological actions are very similar, the psychiatrist now encounters acute states of intoxication as well as withdrawal symptoms in periods of abstinence in their users. The following are some of the more widely prescribed and abused of the 25 or more agents marketed in the United States: meprobamate (Equanil, Miltown), chlordiazepoxide (Librium), ethchlorvynol (Placidyl), glutethimide (Doriden), diazepam (Valium), and chloral hydrate (Sominos).

Acute barbiturate intoxication occurs frequently in those with suicidal intent and sometimes as an accidental occurrence in some who are using such agents for insomnia. In the latter instance, in partial confusional states from previous doses that have failed to provide hypnosis, the patient automatically takes excessive amounts. Again, accidental overdosage may be observed in persons suffering severe anxiety who self-administer overdoses when the prescribed amount has failed to bring relief. Barbiturate intoxication often occurs in alcoholics or narcotic addicts when this agent is substituted for, or used with, the preferred addicting substance.

DIAGNOSIS. With acute intoxication, there is impairment of cognitive functions as with any form of cerebral insufficiency, lack of emotional control shown in bursts of laughing or crying, garrulousness, and poor judgment, followed later by progressive drowsiness, stupor, and finally coma. While the condition often resembles acute alcoholism, there is no odor of alcohol on the breath. It is characteristically associated with certain cerebellar signs such as a gross dysarthria, a constant nystagmus, ataxia in both gait and stature, and adiadochokineses. With deepening intoxication, absence of the deep tendon reflexes, Babinski reflexes, and contraction of the pupils develop. Respiration is characteristically slow, and in severe intoxication is shallow or even periodic. Peripheral circulatory collapse may supervene.

In states of *mild intoxication,* the patient is confused or, if drowsy, is easily aroused, judgment is defective, and the nystagmus is transient, with at best reduction in the skin reflexes (abdominal). Neither respiration nor blood pressure is depressed. *Moderate intoxication* may be estimated in the presence of sleep or drowsiness, with arousal only on vigorous stimulation, constant nystagmus, and dysarthria. There is depression of tendon reflexes and respiration is slow. *Severe intoxication* is judged when the clinician observes unarousable coma, absence of all reflexes, including the corneal and pharyngeal, periodic respiration, and the symptoms of shock.

The diagnosis may be confirmed by the finding of barbiturates in the urine and blood. With mild and moderate states, the electroencephalogram shows a characteristic fast wave frequency.

In the examination of a suspected barbiturate user a meticulous search should be made of his belongings and his person. The chronic user often secretes drugs in his clothing or even in his person in the mouth, rectum, or vagina.

A *"barbiturate test dose"* is sometimes useful in estimating tolerance and physical dependency in the suspected barbiturate addict. In the nonaddicted, 200 mg. of pentobarbital given orally should produce signs of mild intoxication after one hour. If the patient fails to show such signs he is probably tolerant. The signs of acute intoxication are dysarthria, ataxia, pseudoptosis, and presence of Romberg's sign. Many nonaddicted individuals will be asleep one hour after receiving the test dose.

TREATMENT. Treatment of acute intoxication should be conservative for all patients with mild and moderate degrees of barbiturate intoxication, since only the severe grades of cerebral insufficiency threatens life. In the former groups, gastric lavage is indicated if the drug has been recently taken. The patient should be kept awake and not allowed to sleep by use of such measures as talking, walking, and the administration of caffeine sodium benzoate, 0.5 gm. intramuscularly, or 10 to 40 mg. of amphetamine sulfate by mouth or intramuscularly.

Comatose patients who may be aroused by manual stimulation may also be treated conservatively. If stupor deepens, adequate pulmonary ventilation must be maintained and circulatory collapse prevented by intravenous administration of a plasma expander. Oxygen is of doubtful value as it may further depress respiration with the use of an automatic positive-pressure apparatus or a Drinker external respirator should be started. In some instances an endotracheal tube or tracheotomy is required. Supportive treatment of this type alone has given a better overall prognosis than use of a diuretic or dialysis.

It must be recognized that in the recovery phase from coma there again supervenes a delirious state which will require protective nursing until the patient fully recovers.

Addiction to barbiturates may develop; yet such hypnotics may be taken in doses of 0.5 gm. or less daily for prolonged periods without harm. Those who consume 0.8 gm. daily suffer definite impairment of mental functioning and will develop addiction as judged by the appearance of an *abstinence syndrome* if the drug is suddenly withdrawn after six to eight weeks of continuous ingestion. Those consuming amounts between these levels of 0.2 to 0.8 gm. daily show variable degrees of deficit.

Chronic cerebral impairment due to barbiturates produces signs similar to those described earlier for the mild states of intoxication, shown in fluctuations in intensity of the degree of confusion and in impairment in thinking, judgment, and motor activity. There exist persistent nystagmus and various degrees of dysarthria, dysmetria, and ataxia, with loss of the superficial reflexes. Often the condition of chronic intoxication is confused with multiple sclerosis. Again, the blood and urine will show evidence of barbiturates, and the electroencephalogram presents a characteristic fast pattern.

Sudden withdrawal of the drug in the addicted will precipitate an abstinence syndrome resembling the delirium tremens of the alcoholic. Within the first eight hours after discontinuing the drug, the patient appears improved as his confusion subsides. Then he develops anxiety, tremulousness, and severe weakness. Within a day following withdrawal, muscular twitching and severe shaking of the extremities appear. Body temperature rises as does the pulse rate. When the patient moves from a supine to a standing position the rate may increase 15 to 30 beats per minute. Postural hypotension is evident and muscle tonus increases, as is evidenced in more brisk tendon reflexes. Blepharoclonus can be elicited by tapping the glabellar area. In 75 per cent of patients, one or several grand mal convulsions take place during the second day of abstinence; they may be noted as late as one week after the drug is discontinued. In about 60 per cent, anxiety increases and complete insomnia follows. Between the third and seventh day of withdrawal, there develops a frank delirious reaction associated with vivid delusions and hallucinations, usually auditory. Recovery ensues some three to five days later with a prolonged bout of sleeping.

Treatment of the *chronic barbiturate user* requires careful evaluation of the extent of his habituation or addiction, which is often most difficult to assay. Here the word habituation is used to indicate psychological dependence on the drug, and the word addiction, to indicate physiological dependence with propensity for development of the abstinence syndrome on withdrawal. In no instance should abrupt withdrawal of the barbiturate be attempted in the chronic user. Since such patients often distort the amount of drug they consume daily, they should initially receive the maximum amount admitted. Withdrawal should be commenced at the level of 0.1 gm. daily. When half the stabilization dose is reached, reduction should be discontinued for several days before a decrease in the drug is continued again. The appearance at any time of anxiety, tremor, insomnia or weakness or the development of slow-wave activity in the electroencephalogram heralds the onset of the abstinence syndrome. Such symptoms call for termination of withdrawal and support with additional barbiturates. If the abstinence syndrome appears, a dose of 0.2 to 0.3 gm. of pentobarbital orally usually is sufficient to prevent its full symptomatic expression. Following a convulsion, 0.3 to 0.5 gm. of pentobarbital or amobarbital should be given parenterally or orally, followed by the oral administration of these drugs to the level of mild intoxication.

Smith and Wesson recommend the substitution of phenobarbital, a long-acting barbiturate. When the patient is chronically addicted to the short-acting agents such as seconal or nembutal. For each 100 mg. of the short-acting barbiturate, one may substitute 30 mg. of phenobarbital. A two-day period should be allowed for the switch.

During withdrawal, patients require careful nursing and observation. With the withdrawal complete, it then is necessary to ascertain the motivating forces which led to dependence and arrange for appropriate treatment of the primary psychopathology of the individual.

Barbiturate Addiction

Any of the barbiturates, when given daily for periods of three to six months in amounts approximately eight or more times the usual effective dose, produce addiction. Upon withdrawal, all patients who have been ingesting as much as 0.8 gm. or more of pentobarbital daily suffer anxiety, weakness, and tremor. Many will develop a psychotic reaction resembling delirium tremens, and probably a larger number has one or more convulsions. The nature of the biochemical and physiological disturbances responsible for the withdrawal symptoms is not yet known.

TREATMENT. Even a gradual withdrawal of barbiturates carries a certain risk. Patients should therefore be under constant supervision and observation during withdrawal, which should be carried out in a hospital. As already indicated, the drug in barbiturate addiction must not be withdrawn abruptly. For the first two days the patient will receive just enough of the barbiturates to maintain a mild degree of intoxication. This will usually be from 0.2 to 0.4 gm. of pentobarbital or an equivalent amount of another barbiturate. Thereafter the drug will be very slowly reduced, the total withdrawal period being extended over two to three weeks. If excessive anxiety, insomnia, or tremor appears during withdrawal, reduction of the drug should be stopped and the amount held constant until these symptoms disappear.

It is important to remember that acute barbiturate intoxication is frequently superimposed on barbiturate addiction. After patients who have been acutely poisoned with barbiturates have recovered from coma, it should be ascertained whether they have been taking the drug chronically. In such cases, barbiturate intake should be restored and gradual reduction begun. After withdrawal has been completed, there should be a long period of psychotherapy.

Many believe that addiction to barbiturates is more serious than morphine addiction. Abstinence from morphine is less dangerous than abstinence from barbiturates, and morphine addiction causes less mental and emotional disturbance.

Cocainism

For many years cocaine addiction constituted one of the major drug problems, but, because of legislation, its use among addicts is much less prevalent than formerly. At the present time, nearly all its habitués have acquired the addiction through other addicts. Strictly speaking, cocaine is not a narcotic. It produces a marked stimulation, a sense of exhilaration, euphoria, and self-confidence, an increased flow of ideas, and a pressure of speech and of activity. During this period of stimulation and sense of competency, there may be an actual increase in capacity for work. As the stimulus of the drug wears off, the patient feels weak, depressed, restless, morose, and irritable. Other abstinence symptoms are digestive disturbances, tremors, palpitation, specks in front of the eyes, muscular weakness, slight confusion, and impotence.

Frankly psychotic symptoms are common among those who continue the use of large doses of cocaine over a prolonged period. Such addicts may experience terrifying visual hallucinations, become suspicious, and perhaps show much excitement. Delusions of jealousy and of persecution are common and may lead to violence. A rather characteristic phenomenon is the frequent existence of formicative paresthesias, associated with which there may be the delusion that there are actually insects beneath the skin, the presence of which the patient may attempt to demonstrate.

The moral deterioration in the cocaine addict is even greater than in the morphine habitué. The prospects of any permanent cure of the habit are even less favorable than in the case of the morphine addict. Withdrawal of the drug is not accompanied by the painful experiences and tendency to collapse occurring in the withdrawal of opium derivatives.

Marihuana and Hashish

The rapid and enormous recent popularity in use of the products of *Cannabis sativa* represents the greatest shift in patterns of drug use and abuse in western societies. The interest in marihuana, particularly among adolescents and young adults, has aroused great controversy as regards its potential deleterious effects on personality functioning and general health and stirred heated debate as to the need for legal control relating to its production and distribution.

Marihuana is a crude preparation of the whole plant, including flowers, leaves, seed, and stems, whereas hashish is prepared by scraping resin from the tops of the hemp plant. Marihuana is five to ten times less potent than hashish and is by far the most commonly used preparation of cannabis. Tetrahydrocannabinal (THC) is the active ingredient contained in these drugs.

Among regular users of marihuana, smoking generally induces an enjoyable experience, consisting of a sense of exhilaration or euphoria, relaxation, calm, increased sensitivity, a sharper perception of sound, a change in time perception as though slowing occurs, increased thirst, and dry mouth and throat. Some 6 per cent of those who indulge have unpleasant or aversive experiences, with symptoms of anxiety, memory impairment, or a sense of depersonalization. Others in sizable numbers report pleasant and noticeable changes in which they have floating sensations, become more talkative or laugh and giggle, have increased desire for sweets, or become sexually aroused. Conjunctival infection is noticed in about a third of regular smokers.

Among heavy hashish users, uvular edema is reported as a diagnostic sign. Hashish users seem to be subject to various respiratory disorders, including bronchitis, asthma, and oropharyngitis. Diarrhea, hepatoxicity, and acne also seem associated with its use.

Following inhalation, the individual may sleep for one to six hours and awaken without exhilaration or other "hangover." There is no evidence that its usage leads to serious abuse or addiction to the narcotics.

Amphetamines

Chronic intoxication with the sympathomimetic amines, amphetamine (Benzedrine) or methamphetamine (Desoxyephedrine or Desoxyn), may be brought about by the continuing use of these drugs. It has been suggested that they produce chronic central nervous stimulation through accumulation of the biogenic amines, norepinephrine and epinephrine, releasing the latter by occupying their binding sites in the brain. The amphetamines physiologically are known to specifically block "fast" or REM (rapid eye movement) sleep, and their symptoms of chronic intoxication may thereby be similar in development to those seen with prolonged sleep deprivation.

Since these drugs bring about a sense of well-being and exhilaration, with relief from fatigue, their abuse is frequent among thrill-seeking adolescents and among those needing a "lift" from depression or from the after effects of other sedative agents and alcohol. Their stimulatory effect is succeeded again by fatigue and depression, and, as pharmacologic tolerance also occurs, increasingly larger doses are necessary to produce the desired euphoria. Some addicts of amphetamine have taken individual doses as high as 250 mg. and a daily dose equivalent to 1 to 1.5 gm.

The symptomatology of chronic intoxication is very similar to that of cocainism. Although subjectively the users report a sense of increased assurance and decisiveness with greater energy, they also frequently recognize tension and irritability. Amphetamine abuse may be suspected when an appearance of restlessness and rapidity of speech are noted, associated with unusual cheerfulness or euphoria. In other instances, the clinical evidence rests with irritability, anxiety, ataxia, and teeth-grinding movements. Physically there occur dry mouth, tachycardia, brisk reflexes, dilated pupils, increased pulse pressure, and fine tremulousness of the limbs. Nystagmus, cardiac arrhythmias, and weight loss may be observed. With severe intoxication, shallow respiration or circulatory collapse may be noted. Subjectively the user may complain of sleeplessness, headaches, or nausea. Apprehension, tremulousness, and jerky muscular twitches ensue with time. Mounting insomnia and anorexia develop, and there is increasing motor activity with loquacity.

Amphetamine psychosis seems to be a distinctive entity with recurrent psychopathology unrelated to the personality makeup, aside from the reflection of it in the content of the hallucinatory and delusional material. It is characterized especially by vivid visual hallucinations, ideas of reference, and persecutory delusions, without the loosening of thought processes noted with schizophrenia or the impairment of sensorium diagnostic of the delirious syndrome (acute brain syndrome or acute cerebral insufficiency). Upon withdrawal of the drug this syndrome disappears within a period of ten days, but it may be seen recurrently in those who return to use of the drug. In those addicted individuals with a schizoid or schizophrenic premorbid personality, long-continued paranoid states have been precipitated which differ from the simple psychotic state in the occurrence of other types of hallucinatory experiences (particularly auditory) and the usual disorganization of thought. Whether long-continued addiction leads to permanent personality disorganization and brain dysfunction, except in those with schizophrenic predispositions, is unknown.

Treatment requires immediate withdrawal of the drug and use of phenothiazines or other sedatives. Psychotherapeutic measures are indicated following recovery to correct the motivational forces underlying the need for the drug.

Hallucinogenic Agents: LSD-25 and Mescaline

For centuries the plant-derived hallucinogens have been used by man in religious ceremonies, in the hope of divining a prophecy, in producing euphoria, or as aphrodisiacs. *Amanita muscaria,* the mushroom, is thought to have provided the substance inducing madness in the Norwegian berserkers and to have been the deified soma transported to India by the Aryans over three thousand years ago. It was used by the Koryak women of Siberia to stimulate their men. Mushroom cults existed in central America and the mescal cactus, peyote, was used in Aztec religious practices. *Cannabis sativa,* or hemp, thought to be the most widely distributed hallucinogenic plant in the world, was known to the ancient Chinese and Assyrians and has been used as hashish in Asia Minor and Africa for centuries. Bhang is its designation in India and marihuana in South America. The myristicene family includes nutmeg.

To commune with their gods, Aztec priests are thought to have eaten ololiuqui, the morning glory, which has psychotomimetic constituents similar to ergot, which in turn relates to LSD. Datura of the Solanaceae is so used by the Zuni and Jivaro Indians of North and South America. Other ancient peoples discovered the hallucinogenic potentials of snuff prepared from leguminous trees, the hormala-alkaloid containing plants, and certain mints, including catnip.

The Western world's current interest and concern over the use and abuse of such drugs represents no more than an expanded revival of practices existing throughout the ages. The revival of interest comes at a time when the hopes of personal security promised in the advances of science and technology seem delusional to many.

It is surmised from various studies that the hallucinogenic agents also affect the biogenic amines within the brain and thereby produce their now well-known modifications of perceptual and other physiological functions. Thus it is hypothesized that LSD-25 exerts its effects by release of norepinephrine with consequent activation of various neuroreceptors while binding serotonin and histamine.

As a consequence of the ill-advised dissemination of public information on the hallucinatory properties of these drugs and the unsupported and extravagant claims made that they expand psychic activity and thereby enhance creative processes, they have been eagerly sought by the same types of individuals who have attempted to find release from their personality disturbances through the use of amphetamines, barbiturates, alcohol, or narcotics. The more widely disseminated and known of these agents are the synthetic drugs d-lysergic acid diethylamide-25 (LSD), an alkaloid of the ergonovine type, and mescaline, the best known of the various active compounds of the naturally occurring cactus *peyotl*. It has become known that morning glory seeds, which contain LSD, have hallucinatory properties, and the hallucinatory agent psilocybin has also been abused.

Under experimental conditions these agents produce vivid alteration of perceptions without clouding of consciousness, as well as certain symptoms caused by autonomic dysfunction, sympathomimetic in nature. The subjects report an impressive intensification of perceptions with kaleidoscopic visual hallucinations, hyperacusis, tactile paresthesias, and distortions of the body percept. The thoughts appear novel and illusory, are portentous, and are often interpreted in mystical terms. Feelings of estrangement and variations in mood take place. Psychodynamically it has been suggested that a release of primary processes occurs or that primitive percepts emerge as the result of toxic impairment of ordinary ego operations. For the latter reasons, certain psychiatrists have employed these agents to assist in therapeusis with, however, no well-established evidence of their effectiveness.

Abused by those predisposed through personality defect, LSD-25 has been implicated in the precipitation of frank schizophrenic reactions. Others have been admitted to hospital in panic states, and those taking the drug over prolonged periods have had intermittent episodes of panic even in periods of abstinence. Those in panic report terrifying experiences, with the emergence of haunting experiences of loneliness, depression, depersonalization, and visual hallucinations. Both homicide and suicide have been acted out in states of LSD intoxication.

A 21-year-old woman was admitted to the hospital along with her lover. He had had a number of LSD experiences and convinced her to take LSD to make her less constrained sexually. About half an hour after ingestion of approximately 200 μg., she noticed that the bricks in the wall began to go in and out and that light affected her strangely. She became frightened when she realized that she was unable to distinguish her body from the chair she was sitting on or from her lover's body. Her fear became more marked after she thought she would not get back into herself. At the time of admission she was hyperactive and laughed inappropriately. Stream of talk was illogical and affect labile. Two days later, this reaction had ceased. However, she was still afraid of the drug and convinced tnat she would not take it again because of her frightening experience.

"Sniffing" by children and adolescents of gasoline fumes and a variety of volatile substances containing aromatic hydrocarbons as a means of producing euphoria, erotic fantasies, and a general sense of intoxication has been reported in recent years. Knowledge of the biological actions of the volatile euphoriants and hallucinatory stimulants is incomplete.

The sufferers of the "bad trips," the frightening, strange, or panic-inducing crises precipitated in some after taking LSD or other hallucinogens, have increasingly come to treatment in recent years. Such crises, created in the user when he is overwhelmed by anxiety through threat of loss of control because of experiences of depersonalization, must be recognized today as caused often by the taking not only of LSD but simultaneously of other drugs, as well as unknown and sometimes toxic adulterants and contaminants. It is important to recognize "the bad trip" sufferer who has taken, in addition to LSD, anticholinergic drugs, particularly the belladonna alkaloids.

The recommended treatment of an LSD-induced crisis is administration of a phenothiazine. When adulteration with anticholinergics has occurred, the use of phenothiazines will enhance their action and may induce coma or cardiorespiratory failure. The differentiation should be made by attempting to obtain a history from the ill person or his friends of the drugs taken and their effects on others. Physically LSD and mescaline generally induce pupillary dilation and reflex hyperactivity, with a slight increase in pulse rate and blood pressure, sweating of palms, and tremor. The anticholinergic agents produce similar signs, but there is dryness of the mouth and absence of sweating.

Treatment of the "bad trip" is best carried out in the majority of cases by verbal reassurance wherein reality is repetitively defined by indicating that the frightening experience and the perceptual distortions are caused by the drug. Also, it has been helpful to maintain the patient's orientation by advising him of his identity, those who are with him, and his location. Moreover, assisting him to identify and examine concrete objects is sometimes helpful.

If medication is indicated owing to the severity of the patient's anxiety or the inability to control his behavior, 50 mg. of chlorpromazine may be given intramuscularly. Pulse and blood pressure should be followed. This dosage may be repeated in 45 to 60 minutes if no symptom improvement has occurred, and again at similar intervals providing that the circulatory system is maintained.

McGlothlin's follow-up study of 247 persons who had taken LSD either in experimental situations or during psychotherapy did not reveal any permanent personality defects. However, these individuals were not among the group of compulsive users.

Bromides

INCIDENCE, ETIOLOGY, SYMPTOMS. If administered in toxic amounts, several salts of bromide may produce acute brain syndromes. A decade or more ago, with the development of methods of determining the bromide content of blood, it was found that mental disturbances resulting from bromides were more frequent than had been realized. In some psychiatric clinics, 4 per cent of all those admitted were found to be suffering from bromide psychoses. The condition is now seen less frequently. About 50 per cent of the cases arise through the prescribing of bromides by physicians, the prescription being repeatedly refilled. All too frequently, additional amounts of the drug are given in an effort to rid the patient of symptoms already caused by the bromides. Many toxic states arise through self-medication, principally by the use of proprietary preparations containing bromides.

Symptoms of intoxication may be expected if the bromide content exceeds 150 mg. per 100 ml. of blood serum, although there is a wide variation in susceptibility to the drug. The mechanism of bromide poisoning is through the replacement of the chloride with bromide. Elderly or arteriosclerotic patients have a poor tolerance and may develop toxic symptoms even though the blood content be relatively low. Bromides are excreted slowly, and a mental disturbance may develop within two or three weeks after one begins to use amounts as small as 45 to 60 grains a day. Malnutrition, dehydration, and arteriosclerosis render the patient more susceptible to the effects of bromides. Their use is at times associated with alcoholism.

DIAGNOSIS. In mild intoxication there may be a feeling of tiredness or weakness, irritability, broken sleep, slowness of mental grasp, inability to concentrate, faulty memory, drowsiness, impaired attention, and perhaps even confusion. Physically one notes a dry skin, coated tongue, digestive disorders, impotence or menstrual disturbances, ataxic gait, tremors of tongue and fingers, and hyperactive, sluggish, or absent deep reflexes. Dehydration is common. Protein elevation in the spinal fluid is frequent. Acne, considered an ordinary sign of bromidism, is often absent. In more severe intoxication, the clinical picture is one of delirium with fever, confusion, clouding of consciousness, varying degrees of drowsiness or stupor, disorientation, difficulty in grasp, misidentification, motor restlessness even to the point of extreme excitement, fear, and memory loss accompanied by confabulations. Speech is thick, muttering, hesitant, and slurred, and the face is mask-like and expressionless. The mood is often one of fear or depression. In bromide as in other toxic psychoses, there may be a loss of the usual forces of repression, with a resulting appearance of hallucinations. The ideational content of the delirium may be colored by individual psychogenic factors. Paranoid ideas are common. Occasionally a schizophrenic-like syndrome is observed. Bromide delirium may continue for ten days to two months. Remissions and exacerbations with sudden changes in the mental state are not uncommon.

TREATMENT. The treatment consists of stopping the drug, the forcing of liquids, and the administration of 2 to 4 gm. of sodium chloride every four hours unless gastric irritation forbids such large doses. Most patients can take a total of 4 to 6 gm. a day in divided doses if it is given in enteric-coated tablets. Recent investigations seem to show that bromides are excreted more rapidly following the administration of ammonium chloride than after the use of sodium chloride. Ammonium chloride not only furnishes a chloride for displacing bromide but acts also as a diuretic. In some instances intermittent peritoneal lavage or the use of the artificial kidney might be considered to increase bromide excretion. Cathartics are usually necessary for the obstinate constipation that often exists. Paraldehyde may be advisable at night.

CLINICAL REPORT. The following clinical report of an acute reversible brain syndrome associated with bromidism illustrates not only the type of mental disorder associated with toxic states but also the sensorial and other disturbances often seen in delirium:

C. M., aged 38, was transferred to a mental hospital on October 22 from a hospital to which he had been admitted five days previously. His history prior to the present illness was without particular significance, although apparently he was of a somewhat immature, unstable personality. His wife commented, "He could not sit for five minutes. He had to have the last word in everything. He felt that he was never to blame for any difficulty. He lost his temper easily." For several years he had drunk moderately but was never intoxicated.

In September the patient became tense and greatly concerned because, after a brief and stormy marriage, his daughter had left her husband. About October 1 he began to drink more alcohol. Between October 9 and October 13 he consumed four "large bottles" of a proprietary drug product containing a large quantity of bromides. So far as was known, he took no alcohol during that period. On October 13 he appeared confused and showed a slurring of speech and an unsteadiness of gait. Soon, in addition to these symptoms, he stated that he would shoot his son-in-law, also other members of his family.

On October 17 he was admitted to the general hospital. There he was seen by a consulting psychiatrist who suggested that the patient's blood bromide content be determined. This was found to be 600 mg. per 100 ml. The patient was confused, refused to stay in bed, showed poor motor coördination, and one night locked himself in a closet. He thought he had a gun in bed with him. He made such irrelevant remarks as, "I know who shot him. I was behind the curtain." He told his wife that the patient in an adjoining bed had "killed the little girl on B Street," located near his home. No such incident had occurred.

On October 21 he became much more confused; he was completely disoriented and his speech was quite incoherent. He heard gun shots in his room; he said there were dead bodies there and that his wife was sleeping in the hospital with other patients. He attempted to jump from a window, and it was necessary to place him in restraint pending his transfer to a mental hospital.

On arrival at the mental hospital, he was found to be heavily sedated with paraldehyde. After emerging from the effects of this, he was restless and constantly responded to both auditory and visual hallucinations. When asked where he was, he replied that he was at "Mom's and Pop's place." Upon being asked why he was in bed, he answered, "It seems to be a precaution to be parked here to smooch." He pointed to the bedcovers and said, "That's my wife there." He felt about the covers and remarked, "See that stone. It makes me G–d mad." He turned and shouted over his shoulder, "Well, come on, you might as well take it off. Sure going to get hell over that. What do you think of buying that place out?"

By October 26 the patient was more coöperative but still disorganized and restless. A physician introduced himself to the patient, who then said, "Yes, I heard about Hugh Pendleton. I better sleep pretty good tonight. He's got his offices at DeKalb and Jacoby Streets. Do you know it's him?"

On October 29 he knew where he was but gave the date as October 5 and had no recollection of having been in the general hospital. He stated that he had been depressed over his daughter's troubles and had taken triple bromides. For several following days there were periods during which he was noisy and restless and his verbal productions were incoherent and irrelevant. By November 9 his sensorium was fully clear and his apperception was intact. When asked about his experiences, he replied, "I must have caused considerable uproar at home with my antics. They thought I was drunk. I insisted I was not. I took it upon myself to take that bromide medicine for my nerves. My wife tells me I was in C. Hospital for four days. It's a blank wall. It seems I only really started remembering things from last Saturday, when my family saw me. My folks were telling me about some of the stuff that I did. I sure feel like an ass."

On November 10 the patient's blood bromide content had been reduced to 75 mg. per 100 ml. His convalescence continued without interruption and on November 20 he was discharged as recovered.

BIBLIOGRAPHY

General

Berg, D. F.: Extent of illicit drug use in the United States. Division of Drug Sciences, Bureau of Narcotics and Dangerous Drugs, United States Department of Justice, 1969.

Cameron, D. C.: Youth and drugs. A world view. J.A.M.A., 206:1267–1271, 1968.

Dole, V. P., and Nyswander, M.: Medical treatment for diacetylmorphine (heroin) addiction. J.A.M.A., 193:646–650, 1965.

Gossett, J. T., Lewis, J. K., and Phillips, V. A.: Extent and prevalence of illicit drug use as reported by 56,745 students. J.A.M.A., 216:1464–1470, 1971.

Hekemian, L. J., and Gershon, S.: Characteristics of drug abusers admitted to a psychiatric hospital. J.A.M.A., 205:125–130, 1968.

Kolb, L.: Drug Addiction: A Medical Problem. Springfield, Ill., Charles C Thomas, 1962.

Krantz, S.: Deterrents to drug abuse. The role of the law. J.A.M.A., 206:1276–1279, 1968.

Mason, P.: The mother of the addict. Psychiat. Quart. Suppl., 32:189–199, 1958.

Rado, S.: Narcotic bondage: A general theory of the dependence on narcotic drugs. Amer. J. Psychiat., 114:165–170, 1957.

Report on drug addiction. II. New York Academy of Medicine, Committee on Public Health. Bull. N.Y. Acad. Med., 39:417–473, 1963.

Rubin, E., and Lieber, C. S.: Alcoholism, alcohol and drugs. Science, 172:1097–1102, 1971.

Seevers, M. H.: Psychopharmacological elements of drug dependence. J.A.M.A., 206:1263–1266, 1968.

Vaillant, G. E.: A twelve year follow-up of New York Narcotic Addicts. III. Arch. Gen. Psychiat., 15:599–609, 1966.

Wikler, A. (ed.): The Addictive States. Proc. Assn. Res. Nerv. Ment. Dis., 44, 1968.

World Health Organization: Technical Report Series, No. 407, WHO Expert Committee on Drug Dependence. Sixteenth Report. Geneva, 1969.

Opium, Its Alkaloids, and Related Synthetics

Editorial: Narcotics addiction: Where will it end? J.A.M.A., 215:1661, 1971.

Freedman, A. M.: Clinical studies of cyclazocine in the treatment of narcotic addiction. Amer. J. Psychiat., 124:1499–1524, 1968.

Gearing, E. R.: Evaluation of methadone maintenance program. Int. J. Addict., 5:517–543, 1970.

Jaffe, J. H., and Senay, E. C.: Methadone and δ-methyl acetate: Use in management of narcotics addicts. J.A.M.A., 216:1303–1305, 1971.

News and Comments: Narcotic antagonists: New methods to treat heroin addiction. Science, *173:* 503–506, 1971.

Preble, E., and Casey, J. J.: Taking care of business —the heroin user's life on the street. Int. J. Addict., *4:*1–24, 1969.

Amphetamines and Other Psychostimulants

Bell, S. S.: Comparison of amphetamine psychosis and schizophrenia. Brit. J. Psychiat., *3:*701–707, 1965.

Connell, P. H.: Clinical manifestations and treatment of amphetamine type of dependence. J.A.M.A., *196:*130–135, 1966.

Espelin, D. I., and Done, A. K.: Amphetamine poisoning. Effectiveness of chlorpromazine. New England J. Med., *278:*1361–1365, 1968.

Hallucinogens

Ackerly, W. C., and Gibson, G.: Lighterfluid "sniffing." Amer. J. Psychiat., *120:*1056–1061, 1964.

Cohen, S.: Suicide following morning glory seed ingestion. Amer. J. Psychiat., *120:*1024–1025, 1964.

Frosch, W. A., Robins, E. S., and Stern, M.: Untoward reactions to lysergic acid diethylamide (LSD) resulting in hospitalization. New England J. Med., *273:*1235–1239, 1965.

Jackson, B., and Reed, A.: Catnip and the alteration of consciousness. J.A.M.A., *207:*1349–1350, 1969.

McGlothlin, W. H.: LSD Revisited. Arch. Gen. Psychiat., *24:*35–49, 1971.

Schultes, R. E.: Hallucinogens of plant origin. Science, *163:*245–254, 1969.

Taylor, R. L., Maurer, J. I., and Tinklenberg, J. R.: Management of "bad trips" in an evolving drug scene. J.A.M.A., *213:*422–425, 1970.

Barbiturates and Other Sedative Drugs

A.M.A. Committee on Alcoholism and Addiction: Dependence on barbiturates and other sedative drugs. J.A.M.A., *193:*107–111, 1965.

Matthew, H. (ed.): Acute Barbiturate Poisoning. New York, Excerpta Medica Foundation, 1971.

Smith, D. E., and Wesson, D. R.: A new method for treatment of barbiturate dependence. J.A.M.A., *213:*294–295, 1970.

Wikler, A.: Diagnosis and treatment of drug dependence on the barbiturate type. Amer. J. Psychiat., *125:*758–765, 1968.

Cannabis Sativa (Marihuana and Hashish)

Dornbush, R. L., Fink, M., and Freedman, A. M.: Marijuana, memory and perception. Amer. J. Psychiat., *128:*194–197, 1971.

Halikas, J. A., Goodwin, D. W., and Guze, S. B.: Marihuana effects: A survey of regular users. J.A.M.A., *217:*692–694, 1971.

Marijuana and health: A report to the Congress. Amer. J. Psychiat., *128:*189–193, 1971.

Meyer, R. E., Pillard, R. C., Shapiro, L. M., and Mirin, S. M.: Administration of marijuana to heavy and casual users. Amer. J. Psychiat., *128:* 198–207, 1971.

Tennant, F. S., Preble, M., Prendergast, T. J., and Ventry, P.: Medical manifestations associated with hashish. J.A.M.A., *216:*1965–1969, 1971.

Chapter 28

"By human caring is meant that feeling of concern, regard, respect one human being may have for another. Its biological roots lie in the maternal and paternal behaviour of all living things, and it is reinforced by environmental circumstances. Most important of these is the presence of caring in another human being.

"Upon it, along with aggression, rests our survival."

David E. Sobol

Behavior Disorders of Childhood and Adolescence

This and the succeeding two chapters describe the personality disturbances recognized during childhood and adolescence. Described here are the behavior disorders in which the major etiologic factors depend upon weaknesses and deficiencies in the developmental process, particularly the transactions between the growing child and the parents or parental substitutes. Those special symptoms which bring children to the attention of physicians and psychiatrists—the speech and learning disturbances, tics, and disorders of sleep, alimentation, and evacuation—are described in the Chapter 29. Chapter 30 is devoted to mental retardation, including the various causes of impairment of cognitive development dating from the earliest period of human life.

EXAMINATION OF THE CHILD

The treatment of children's psychiatric disorders differs in many respects from that of adult psychiatric problems. In large measure this is because the child is living through the most active phase of the developmental process. His personality is less structured and formed, and from one stage of growth to another he shows rapid modifications in behavior.

Those who work in the field of child psychiatry must have a knowledge of the ever-changing patterns of healthy behavior at the various age levels as a means of evaluating the existence of disturbance. Again, the environmental pressures leading to disordered personality functioning in the child may usually be discovered in the present or recent past. They contribute a continuing influence in the life of the child. Since at this age the child is dependent upon his parents emotionally and in all aspects of his living, one must deal directly with the parents in the course of arranging the treatment and in determining future management. The child seldom comes to treatment on his own; he is brought in by the parents or referred by community agencies such as schools or courts.

Still another difference is evident in the practice of child psychiatry. This has to do with the means of obtaining information and evaluating the problem of the child. Of necessity, much of the history must be obtained from the parents and from others who are related to the child in his school environment or in other aspects of his training. Inferences in regard to his emotional reactions and relations with others, particularly in the younger age periods, are derived from psychological testing and from play therapy, wherein the child acts out his fantasies. Because of the necessity of obtaining information from parents and social agencies and through psychological examination of the intellectual and emotional life of the child, the work of the child psychiatrist must be actively supplemented by the skills of the clinical psychologist and psychiatric social worker. Furthermore, in prescribing treatment, consideration must be given to the significant persons in the child's environment as well as to the child. The outcome of a particular problem depends to a great extent upon the family structure from which the child comes. There are some symptoms that are fostered by the family. In such circumstances, efforts directed toward understanding and modifying the behavior of the child remain unsuccessful unless the significant family members also come into therapy.

Although in recent years the tendency has largely been to consider the majority of behavior disorders as emotionally determined, there is a growing recognition of the great extent of brain injury consequent to childbirth as contributing to many of these disturbances.

While the specific problems of the brain-injured, epileptic, and mentally defective have been discussed in foregoing chapters, their recognition and significance in the developmental interactions of the child were not then especially considered. There is now a general appreciation that one must attend to those behavioral sequences which characterize emotional stability, attentiveness, integration of action, and all forms of sensory reception and perception at differing periods of maturation, rather than the simple aspects of sensorimotor and reflex functions tested in the ordinary neurological examination, if one is to assess the existence of brain dysfunctions or delay in maturation. Whatever the type of disturbance or its etiology, it must be recognized that troublesome trends in the development of the growing child make it difficult for him to be accepted comfortably by those who care for him. The difficult and asocial responses of the child, as well as the parental figures, should be understood in this context rather than from that of moralistic disapproval.

Sources of Referral

Today, in the United States, schools, more than any other source, refer children to psychiatrists for examination owing to behavior disturbances. The other important referral sources in this country, in order of frequency, are physicians, social agencies, courts, guidance clinics, and parents. The types of behavioral problems in children referred tend to vary, depending upon the source. From the schools come largely the children who are difficult to manage in the classroom—the trouble makers—as well as those with academic problems arising from the reading and learning disorders. Physicians send in largely the children with psychosomatic complaints and those in whom the behavioral response to impairing illness, either acute or chronic, is considered abnormal. For the most part social agencies request consultation for those children orphaned and neglected. With their very extensive responsibility in caring for such children, the patients they refer tend to have the most serious problems. The court referrals to psychiatrists generally consist of children charged with delinquent acts or neglected or abused children whose parents are charged as responsible. Guidance clinics have need from time to time of special diagnostic studies or wish placement of their patients in residential or day care centers staffed by psychiatrists. Parents may refer children for any of the aforementioned reasons; the fact that others prove to be the main sources of referral suggests the perceptive limitations of parents for the social functioning of their children.

The Examination

The diagnostic process differs greatly from child to child and confronts the examiner with overt behavioral problems much more frequently than in the conduct of clinical assessment of the vast majority of referred adults. Depending on the problem, the child will be seen initially, briefly or at some length. Physical and neurological examinations are in order if they have not been performed previously. Psychological tests are desirable in many instances but in some cases are not necessary. In general, the parents, if they are available, will prove the major source of information, but that provided by the sources of referral is clearly of importance. When families and the referring agency are not ready informants, a social worker's evaluation will be necessary.

For the examiner there is a necessity to be able to relate to those children who are brought in frightened and resistive, and to learn to accept with patience whatever they may do in their initial visit: whether they scream, kick, bite, or tear and grab things from others; whether they are inattentive or aggressively social; whether they are silent, sullen, or stubborn and unwilling to communicate in any way.

The clinical examination of the child is more important in his assessment than the history. This is so, because the child is unable to provide the history made available by adult patients, and that given even by parents will be incomplete as only the patient records his experiences and the suffering these induce in him. Consequently the overt behavior and the inferences one may make from it take on significance in the diagnostic process. It is not surprising that such processes as play rooms and play therapy, as well as other means of eliciting overt behavior of the child, have evolved and become so important in the diagnostic process.

Diagnostic Information

The child psychiatrist will seek from the diagnostic study information on the child's behavior as it relates to the following points:

1. His motility and speech, including his spontaneous productions and play.

2. His relationship behavior with others as demonstrated and related in the interview and during spontaneous play.

3. His affective behavior, including that toward the examiner.

4. His attitudes toward family members, school, and playmates.

5. His stated interests and motivations toward them.

6. His own evaluation of the problems for which he is referred, as well as his perception of problems.

7. His temperament, which will include the examiner's evaluation of his general activity, intensity of reaction, tendency to approach or withdraw, adaptability, attention span and persistence, distractability, and threshold of responsiveness to various sensory stimuli.

To examine young children it is necessary to make available a situation offering the opportunity for attracting the child's attention and providing pleasure and the potential for eliciting his repertoire of behaviors. The office furnishing most likely to provide this situation will include a play table; blocks; water colors; crayons; clay and plasticene; dolls representing adults, children, and babies in costumes attractive to children of the area; toy furnishings of various rooms of a home and school, including bathrooms; a punching bag; balloons; and some simple craft utensils.

For older children and adolescents the diagnostic exchange alone may be sufficient to elicit the desired information. Variations with questioning, story telling, and play have been found more suitable for some.

Psychological Testing

Those tests in general use are described in Chapter 8. The use of psychometric scales, widely applied in western countries, preceded that of the development of generalized tests of personality functioning. Interest in mental testing developed in the latter half of the nineteenth century, with contributions of such workers as Sir Francis Galton and J. M. Cattell. In 1905, Binet, a French psychologist, and Simon, a psychiatrist, the former's associate on a commission appointed to study the matter of instruction of defective children, published the first scale of intelligence for school children. They drew up a set of graded problems constituting a progressive scale arranged in steps of increasing difficulty, which, in 1908, was revised to include age levels. These problems constituted tests of imagination, attention, comprehension, suggestibility, logical memory, language functions, common information, and ability to discriminate concepts, detect absurdities, and solve problems. These tests, first introduced into the United States in 1910 by Henry Herbert Goddard of the Training School for Feeble-Minded Children at Vineland, New Jersey, were devised after studying the abilities of children of all ages up to 16 years, after which age it was found that there was little increase in native intelligence as distinguished from knowledge.

The Binet scale was restandardized in the United States in 1916 by Lewis M. Terman of Stanford University, who first used the term "intelligence quotient" (I.Q.) for the relationship of mental age to chronological age, which in 1911 had been suggested by Stern as a more constant quotient than the developing mental age. This Stanford test was revised in 1937, when some of the previous shortcomings were eliminated, new problems were introduced, and the scale was extended for both the higher and the lower mental ages. The two forms (L and M) of the 1937 revision were combined into a single improved scale in 1960 (Form L-M).

In the application of the test, the patient is given a standardized series of graded groups of tests, each successively more difficult than the preceding. The tests are grouped according to the age at which they are usually passed. Each succeeding group should be solved by a child one year older than the child who solved the preceding one. One group of the series, for example, should be successfully solved by a child of six, and the next most difficult group in the series by a child of seven. The mental age of the person examined is the average of the series of tests which he can successfully pass, the lowest age group used in determining the average being that one in which all the problems were successfully solved, and the highest one being that in which at least one problem was solved.

INTELLIGENCE QUOTIENT. In earlier forms of the Stanford-Binet scales, an intelligence quotient (I.Q.), as the index to relative intellectual brightness, was arrived at by dividing the mental age of the patient by his chronological age (after 13 years, increasing fractions of successive chronological age increases were disregarded, until age 16, after which 15 was used for all adults) and multiplying the quotient by 100 so as to eliminate decimals. In the latest revision (Form L-M), however, this ratio method has been corrected for deviations occurring at various ages and for the fact that recent retest findings indicated that mental growth as measured by the test extended beyond age 16, contrary to earlier assumptions. For adults, the chronological age of 18 is now used. The resulting standard score I.Q.s are presumably directly comparable at all age levels. Because of the difficulties with the "mental age" concept as applied to adults, many authorities prefer use of the Wechsler scale for evaluating adolescents and adults, because on it I.Q.s are determined by separate norms for each of the age levels through old age. Nevertheless, the Stanford-Binet scales are often considered preferable for children, particularly in evaluating mental deficiency.

It should be remembered that, because intelligence tests are expressed in terms of numerical findings, their apparent definiteness is apt to be misleading. It should be remembered, too, that an adult who is, say, 10 years old mentally but 40 years old chronologically is a very different person from a child of 10. He may not be able to do any more with his intellect than a 10-year-old child, but he has had 30 more years of experience in living, and his emotional experiences, conditionings, and maturity may be very different. The results of these tests will therefore be modified somewhat by the home environment and social status of the subject. Qualitative features of the subject's limitations may offer the experienced clinician information on the role that cultural deprivation may be playing in his difficulties. They are useful as guides to educational policy and, to some extent, to the complexity of the social and occupational situations to which adjustments may be expected. If the subject's score gives him a mental age of less than 10 years, it is not to be expected that he will be both self-supporting and capable of an unsupervised adjustment in an urban community. Although we can scarcely identify the various attributes and qualities that enter into what we call intelligence, yet there appear to be a number of more or less distinct components in mental ability, each of which can be measured by appropriate tests. Aptitude tests have been devised to discover evidence as to one's fitness for certain types of professions or occupations, but any conclusions based on them must be accepted with great discretion.

Not infrequently in medicolegal matters the question arises as to the responsibility of an alleged feeble-minded person. In general it may be said that no limitation of responsibility should be recognized if the offender has a mental age exceeding 10 years.

The various intelligence tests fall, also, into two groups insofar as technique of application is concerned. Some, like the Stanford test, must be given to one person at a time. Others, like the Army Alpha or the Kuhlman-Anderson, can be administered to groups. The advantages of the individual examination rest in better rapport, and the potential for examining and stimulating motivation and assessing cultural influences on responding.

ETIOLOGY

The child is a changing personality, and in order for his emotional growth to proceed in a natural and spontaneous way it is necessary that he receive affection, understanding, security, and discipline and be stimulated by achievement and social acceptance. It is necessary, too, that he feel satisfaction in his relation with his parents, that he develop a feeling that he is lovable, that his individuality be respected by his parents, and that he have confidence in his own strength and capacity as a person in his own right. The maladjustments of childhood sometimes originate from a single cause, but more frequently they arise from the combined action of several types, particularly emotional and situational ones. Also, in some instances, they arise from intellectual and perhaps other constitutional causes. Although care must be exercised not to oversimplify the problem and explain it by one formula it is perhaps reasonable to assume that in many maladjustments of childhood human relationships have, through their influence upon the developing personality, acted as a significant etiological factor. Of all these relationships, that of parent and child is the one in which the problem is most frequently rooted.

Disturbances and distortions in the personality growth process result in undeveloped phases of the child's personality. The undeveloped phases may have arisen through such factors as the striving of the mother to hold her child as an undifferentiated part of herself. Thus the child does not obtain the natural love, guidance, and direction necessary for his development into an independent personality, with fulfillment of his individual potentialities and responsibilities. Again, the failure of the personality development, with resulting inadequate capacity of the child to deal efficiently and realistically with the business of living, may result from the fact that he struggled to protect his dependency status against the demands of growth, against giving up his infantile relationship to the mother, and against an independent organization of his own powers and capacities. According to this point of view, the child has been delayed or blocked in some aspect of his growth toward a normally functioning self and cannot handle his feelings in a way that permits those growing relationships with others that are essential for his development.

The affective state of well being, induced and maintained through consistent and interested maternal care, so well described by Sandler, may be interrupted at any stage of growth by deprivation, loss, or even the fantasied loss of those on whom the child is dependent. Its interruption leads the child to a subjective sense of loss, which may be of such a magnitude that the child responds with behavior characterized by helplessness and passivity, perhaps denoted best as *childhood depression*. Depression in the infant and child then does not necessarily relate to feelings of aggression toward the lost parent or parent surrogate. According to Sandler, the growing child responds to the distress of deprivation in one of the following ways: by angry protest and aggressive unacceptance; by denial through passivity; by reversal in clowning; by direction of the distress against himself; or by presenting psychosomatic symptoms. If deprivational states are worked through, normal growth and development can follow. The psychopathology of childhood depression is described later in this chapter under the section on Neuroses.

In Chapter 4, Personality Development, there were described the transactional processes of general significance at various stages of growth. In Chapter 7 were described many variables which pathogenically interrupt those processes which establish the progressive sets of well being and health on which successful

maturity rests. The succeeding paragraphs will mention other pathogenic factors that were not emphasized earlier.

Early Mothering Experiences

Observation of infants seems to show that the need for mothering, sensory stimuli to skin and mucous surface, and instinctual emotional gratification is present from the time of birth, and that the lack of these may result in inhibition of personality development. Sudden weaning or attempts to establish toilet training at too early a stage of the child's development may indicate parental attitudes that pave the way for later emotional and behavioral disorders. At about the beginning of the third year, the necessity for growing into relationships with other people and accepting their values becomes definitely greater.

Other factors that may distort the parent-child relationship and disturb personality development are neurosis, psychosis, or psychopathic, antisocial, or aggressive tendencies on the part of the parent. The psychological fate of the child is to a considerable extent determined by the emotional health of the parents and by the complex forces interacting within the family group. Many faulty parent-child relationships are related to the parents' own personality structure, their emotional conflicts, biases, and past experiences. To secure a clear picture of the influences to which the child is subjected, one should know how the parents feel unconsciously about the child, what conflicts disturb the parent-child relationship, even what conflicts have existed between the parents and their parents, and how these have affected the ability of the parents to relate themselves to the child. The emotional reaction of the parents to the behavior of the child should not be overlooked. Occasionally the behavior of the parents is a result of the child's behavior rather than the cause of it.

Early institutional care or other interruptions in the continuity of parent-child relationship are harmful and lead to defects in personality development expressed as emotional apathy or inadequacy in forming relations with others, inability to accept obstructions, failures, and separations, as well as perceptual, intellectual, and language disturbances.

Bernard and Crandell, from their examination of the available research on adoption and foster homes, give strong evidence of the necessity to avoid repeated disruptions for children through changing foster homes. The ultimate health of a child who is not to remain with his own parents may depend mostly on the later ameliorative mothering by the adoptive or foster parent or on his trauma-reinforcing attitudes than on the original parental separation. The latter has its major impact at that time in early life (from five to six months of age) when the infant is developing attachment behavior. Impermanence of care through repeated transfer from one foster family to another, as well as congregate foster care, provides a less effective means of preventing psychiatric and social disability among those children who lose parents.

Relations to siblings may be the source of personality problems. Parental favoritism and a feeling of being supplanted by the birth of a younger sibling may arouse abnormal sibling rivalry and jealousy. It should be remembered that it is particularly difficult for some children to share an adult (especially a parent) with another child.

Parental instability with resulting shifts of attitude on the part of the child may prevent identification, one of the most important mechanisms in shaping character. Death of a parent, or more frequently desertion or divorce, preceded, usually, by a long period of domestic unhappiness, may be important in the production of personality disorders. Attitudes experienced by the stepchild or the foster child may create personality maladjustments. Many school experiences are important in giving rise to personality problems.

Failure in school and the factors that contributed to the failure, such as mental retardation or unhappy home conditions, faulty handling by teachers or difficulties in relations with classmates, often are sources of personality difficulties. Sometimes poverty and privation operate to produce neurotic traits or behavior disorders. In such a case, the deprivation has some special meaning to the child.

Belonging to a social group regarded as inferior or alien to the major environmental one with the resulting conflicts in identification with one's own family group in ideologies and in accepted culture may create many emotional problems. Difficulties in language and lack of social and educational privileges and experiences also contribute to the problems. The child who feels rejected is often insecure and anxious, as a result of which he is hyperactive, emotionally unstable, has difficulty in concentrating, feels resentment toward the person who denies him the love he wants, and expresses his hostile feelings by temper tantrums and disobedience. He may cover up his need for affection by an air of bravado and attack. Students of child delinquency report that generally the delinquent has had an unhappy childhood characterized by feelings of rejection, inadequacy, and guilt and by lack of affection.

The attitude of the parents toward the child is greatly influenced by the degree of satisfaction and contentment they have been able to achieve in their own lives. Frequently the mother carries over into her relationship with her child the unresolved conflicts that arose in her relationships with her own parents. Hostilities and resentments from such a source may enter a disturbing relationship with her child that has a harmful effect on its social and emotional growth and development. Conflict over hostile feelings is common in parents, and much of the behavior expressed in troublesome parent-child relationships derives from that source.

Parental oversolicitude is much more frequent than neglect and is equally pernicious in its results. Such overprotection in every phase of the child's life, including dress, health, food, play, and association with other children, prevents the development of independence, responsibility, and maturity of personality essential for successful adaptation. Such children, shielded from all the ordinary hazards of life, are rendered dependent, infantile, and frequently hostile. They lack the satisfying pleasures of childhood and are usually whining and deceitful. Oversolicitous parents, in their anxiety to protect the child against imaginary harm, usually nag, scold, and constantly admonish him. As he grows older, they continue to treat him as a child rather than as a responsible, or at least partially responsible, person.

Maternal overprotection is more frequent than is paternal oversolicitude. It may be manifested in the case of both the wanted and the unwanted child and for various reasons. With the unwanted child, the fact that the prospective arrival of the child was unwelcome may have made the mother feel guilty for having entertained such a thought. A smothering oversolicitude then represents the denial and disguise of a hostile rejection of the child—a device for the denial of hate. The defensive reaction to her unconscious hostility to the child may lead her to extravagant measures of protection resembling an obsessional neurosis. Perhaps her marriage proved frustrating and she finds in her child a solution of her own emotional needs. Overprotection may take the form of continuing such activities as feeding, bathing, nursing or dressing the child long past the usual time. It may be shown, too, by the mother's practice of sleeping with the child even in his teens, or by a desire to have the child constantly in her presence. Usually, also, there is oversolicitous protection against physical danger, illness, or the "bad influence" of other children.

In her training of the child, the overprotective mother is either indulgent or dominating. The child of the indulgently overprotective mother continues his infantile demands and expectations long after they should have been outgrown. He is often a disciplinary problem, and his behavior may be characterized by disobedience, impudence, tantrums, an aggressively demanding attitude, and varying degrees of tyrannical behavior. He may be selfish, conceited, and a show-off. His bossy and demanding attitude betrays the fact that maternal indulgence has stimulated the development of aggressive components of the child's personality. Feeding problems are common in the child of the indulgent, apprehensive mother. The problems of the dominatingly overprotective mother's child are largely of anxieties, fears, shyness, and submissive behavior. In both cases, the overprotection operates against outside influences that make for growth in social adaptation. The child may use neurotic symptoms to control the mother and retain the infantile advantages of the emotionally intertwined mother-child relation.

Many instances of the overprotective relationship arise from the mother's insatiable hunger for love, a hunger based on a severe privation of love in her own childhood. To this impoverishment in the child of all those positive feelings implicit in parental love—recognition, security, affection and sympathy—Levy gives the term "affect hunger."

The emotional influences in a particular family are never identical for any two children. Probably, too, a mother's psychology is such that no two children can bear for her the same emotional meaning. Occasionally a mother may entertain a hostility toward a particular child, arising, perhaps, from a hatred that is directed primarily toward her husband and then transmitted to a child who resembles him. Again, disappointment concerning the sex of the child may create a maternal attitude that is traumatic to it.

The overstrict, punitive father may arouse disturbing tensions and such emotional reactions as fear, anxiety, resentment, and hostility, with consequent personality or behavior disorders. The tension of actively aggressive impulses evoked by the severity of a father who represents an object of frustration and fear may cause the boy to erect defenses against his aggression, perhaps in the form of an obsessional character or an obsessional neurosis.

Handicaps and Overambition

The child who is so retarded mentally that he cannot compete with his peers, the one who is small for his age but strives to compensate through his readiness to fight, the child who is deaf or who has suffered from a prolonged physical illness or from encephalitis may react with emotional or behavior disturbances. The brain-injured child must not be forgotten, either. Beneath this child's disturbed behavior there may be a rich and troubled inner life marked by anxiety, regression, and frustration. Neurological or orthopedic handicaps, obesity, or other physical abnormalities that attract attention require special consideration.

Other factors that stimulate self-consciousness or an exaggerated feeling of difference in relation to those about the child also act as potentially pathogenic factors. Overambitious educational expectations sometimes evoke emotional and behavior reactions of a neurotic nature.

One must not forget the emotionally deprived child who appears to be retarded in every field of personality development, including even intellectual functioning. Such children are most frequently found among those who were reared in institutions during infancy.

FORMS OF PSYCHIATRIC PROBLEMS

The deprivation states and conflicts of childhood leading to depressions and anxieties are often expressed as transient symptomatic reactions related to some current situation or emotional conflict.

Although the child may present a variety of manifestations of these affects, one or another symptom is seen as most disturbing. When the child suffers from prolonged and definitive disturbances of the psychotic, neurotic, or defective type, these are to be discriminated from the forms of psychiatric problems classified under the Adjustment Reactions of Infancy or Childhood.

ADJUSTMENT REACTIONS OF INFANCY

Those transient disturbances in infancy, such as undue apathy, undue excitability, or disturbances in feeding and sleeping that take place on a psychogenic basis and are unassociated with physical disorder are usually classified under the nosological term mentioned. In most instances it will be found that as a result of the infant's interaction with the mother, or a mother surrogate, or because of a deprivation of such a relationship, these disturbances take place. An example of the types of disorders which one might classify as adjustment reaction to infancy are those symptomatic responses of the infant to separation from the mother.

Disturbances of behavior due to isolation or maternal deprivation in children reared in institutional homes during the first two years of life have been known for the past three decades. Schlossman coined the term "hospitalism" in 1926 to designate the condition. Levy defined the genesis of the condition in his paper, "Primary Affect Hunger," in 1933, and Spitz has more recently studied experimentally the withdrawal of the infant, his apprehension on the approach of others, weepiness, sadness, loss of appetite and of weight, and insomnia that take place in the periods between six and twelve months as a consequence of separation from the mothering one. The child may show a retardation of development, with inability to walk, delayed reaction to external stimuli, slowness of movement, and stupor if the separation is continued for a period of time. If the mother returns, there is a rapid disappearance of the evidence of disturbance and behavior. Illness, tension, or anxiety in the mother may also lead to similar, though usually less severe, disturbances in the behavior of the infant. Prolonged maternal deprivation is productive of severe personality maldevelopment, as described elsewhere in this chapter.

ADJUSTMENT REACTIONS OF CHILDHOOD

These are manifested in such simple repetitive activities as nail biting, thumb sucking, enuresis, masturbation, and temper tantrums. One group of these disorders concerns the manipulations of certain parts of the body. Here we find such conditions as thumb sucking, nail biting, nose picking, and tongue sucking. These conditions are generally differentiated from tics; they are felt to occur at a high level of awareness, are intermittently present, are variable in duration, intensity, and course, and the action in itself seems to be pleasurable. If they are interrupted at any stage of a single performance, they are recognized by the patient as actions for which he is responsible and that are subject to his control.

THUMB SUCKING. One of the earliest forms of body manipulation, this is usually either the consequence of deprivation in the early sucking activities of the infant or, in older children, a regressive act during periods of tension or fatigue. Levy, from his observations, concluded that in the majority of the infants thumb sucking is a result of insufficient lip movements or incompleteness of the sucking phases of the feeding act, regardless of the type of feeding. Thumb sucking results not only from difficulties in feeding the infant and expressions of anxiety in the mother, but also from faulty techniques of nursing. Probably of greater concern are those anxieties in the parents related to the presumed effects of thumb sucking. In the past, various statements were made to the effect that distortions of personality as well as malformations of the jaws and palate resulted from thumb sucking. The management of this adjustment reaction is to be directed to the parental attitude rather than to the thumb sucking of the infant.

NAIL BITING. This is probably the commonest of the forms of habitual body manipulation occurring in both children and adults. It is usually first seen around the fifth year of life and increases in its occurrence up to the tenth or twelfth year, when children gradually relinquish the habit. Threatening efforts to prevent the child from carrying out this act are usually unsuccessful. The condition is now recognized as an expression of tension. Its removal may be attempted through understanding and relieving the source of the underlying anxiety.

MASTURBATION AND OTHER MANIPULATIONS. Masturbation, commonly practiced by children, requires treatment only if the parental or adult attitudes toward the act have instilled in the child anxieties and fears that affect his personality development adversely. More frequently the problems of masturbation in a child involve clarifying misconceptions of the ill effects of the procedure in the minds of the parents and preventing radical efforts to prevent the act.

The other varieties of body manipulation, aside from hair pulling (trichotillomania), are relatively of little importance. Hair pulling calls for more careful attention and may be associated with serious problems within the family.

ADJUSTMENT PROBLEMS OF ADOLESCENCE

Considering the complexity of the developmental tasks which confront the adolescent, it is surprising indeed that there are not more demands for assistance in adjusting during this period of life. Where psychiatric and/or psychological counseling is available and accepted, as in many colleges in the United States, up to 20 per cent of the student body at one time or another request aid. The vast majority come for problems other than those described in the preceding chapters concerned with general psychopathology, but many do have neurotic and psychotic conditions.

The adolescent must not only adapt to the rapid physiological changes taking place within himself which herald his biological and sexual maturity, but must also acquire those social skills which will insure him the capacities for both intimacy with another as well as those needed to effectively establish himself in groups. Also, he is brought to face those personal decisions which will determine his future career. In this task a determination and persistence are needed once the decision as to his life work is made, and in the daily competition of life he must be free to use his aggressive drives along socially acceptable lines without paralyzing guilt or fear.

Adolescence is the period when exploration, trial, and effort are made in seeking the eventual decisions which establish the individual adult identity. Today in the affluent western societies where increasing numbers of adolescents and young adults are supported through college and graduate schools or are able through family support to postpone these decisions which were forced in earlier generations, the period of adolescence tends to be prolonged—the potential for commitment as an independent and self-sustaining adult is delayed in this moratorium.

Doubtful and anxious as he attempts differing tasks at home, school, or work; frightened over his pent-up rage at those in authority in any of these settings; guilty, ashamed, or filled with despair in his sexual explorations; accepted or rejected and accepting or rejecting others; envious of the success of his friends or alarmed at their demands upon him, he often seeks help today. The expressions of his maladaptation are usually those of anxiety with tension, restlessness, and

insomnia, occasionally compounded by minor depressive symptoms and the physiological expressions of these treatment affective states.

With the rapidly changing value systems in our society expressed in the more permissive attitudes toward sex and personal liberties, many are concerned over the defiant responses of the adolescent expressed in his dress, his speech, and his clothes. The experimentations with drugs, sex, and violence and the "hippie cultures" are to be recognized in large part as indicative in the adolescent of his struggle for identity.

When these forms of acting out carry the adolescent to acts and associations imperiling himself, the justification exists for his referral for study and possible treatment. Not all, but many of the more persisting and destructive forms of adolescent acting out will be discovered to be neurotically determined and deserving of treatment as described in other chapters. However, often the offensive behaviors of the adolescent are aggravated by parental efforts at correction through authoritarian dominance. In such instances, parental counseling or family treatment is in order.

BEHAVIOR DISTURBANCES OF CHILDHOOD AND ADOLESCENCE

Hyperkinetic Reaction

It was the description of the overactive behavior of children who had suffered definitive brain damage early in life that led to the definition of this syndrome. Unfortunately, owing to this history, hyperactivity in children is too generally equated with the existence of brain damage—even though minimal. Other children, without such damage, may also express themselves through overactivity.

The affected children are reported by parents and teachers as being excessively active. Their restlessness, garrulousness, and impulsivity often disrupt classrooms and irritate their elders. Their short attention and concentration spans and subsequent distractibility make it impossible for them to maintain continuing direction or focus on the tasks or objects before them. Those who contact these children may refer to them as spoiled, undisciplined, badly mannered, or odd. Secondarily such children may react to their social disability by such other behavior as clowning, negativism, withdrawing, or avoiding.

In those children with the minor signs of brain damage there will be found evidence of impairment of fine movements and coordination, deficits in attention and affect; perceptual, intellectual, and memory faults; and central sensory impairment. In approximately 50 per cent of the affected group the electroencephalogram is abnormal. Not necessarily all, but often only a few of these "soft" neurologic signs are used to support the contention of minor brain damage.

History of birth injury, encephalitis, or some other encephalopathic disturbance would support the contention of maldevelopment of the central nervous system with subsequent impairment in integrative function. In evaluating the symptoms it is important to determine if the hyperactive child's problem is due to attentional or perceptual deficit or to a combination of the two. In others the activity is due to impulsivity or failure to retain events well.

Treatment today is best effected by combining the pharmacologic approach with therapy of the child and parental guidance. In the treatment the physician must come to know the nature of the handicap, its source, and the capacities and limitations which are imposed on the child. The parents, too, must come to know and accept his condition. Eventually both parents and child should recognize where he may compete with peers equally, may be required to limit participation, or may best act as an observer. The progress of treatment of those with limitations caused by brain damage are so arranged as to allow the development of the child's best personality characteristics and assets.

It has been found that many hyperactive children respond favorably to prescription of the central nervous system stimulants, particularly methyphenidate. Initially, it may be given in 0.25 mg. per kg. daily in divided doses before breakfast and lunch. This dosage schedule may be doubled during successive weeks of treatment up to a level of 2 mg. per kg. If a change in behavior occurs, the drug should be continued for several months. It may be withdrawn slowly to determine if its continuation is required.

Other children may respond better to dextroamphetamine. When the stimulants do not work, a trial of a phenothiazine or chlordiazepoxide is indicated.

Withdrawing Reaction

Traits of seclusiveness, shyness, and sensitiveness characterize the overinhibited; traits which are probably most commonly overlooked. Worrying, apathy, and undue submissiveness also are the expressions frequently noticed in this syndrome. The majority of the overinhibited are reared in families where punitive or critical suppression of activity is the general frame of transaction. Many of the children have some physical deficiency or inadequacy. Their affective life is one of shame or guilt for presumed failures in meeting the ego ideal or the superego demands.

Such children indulge in daydreaming. There is an absence of close friendships as well as affective relations of all kinds. Often they have been deprived or suffered in their relations with parents and others and in reaction formation have turned to fantasy and social isolation. If withdrawal continues, impairment will follow in their capacity to effectively evaluate reality.

The sources for the child's frustration in human relations may stem from maternal ill health in the form of psychosis or neurosis, or a personality disorder. In other instances the child may suffer from a debilitating or crippling physical illness or react against the neglect given through paternal or familial sources.

Treatment requires the development of an emotional relationship with the child which allows him to express and be drawn away from his life of fantasy. From that relationship his further socializations may be encouraged.

Overanxious Reaction

Those youngsters whose predominant symptoms are persistent anxiety, excessive or overdetermined fears, restless sleep, nightmares, and psychophysiologic symptoms are classified as suffering the overanxious reactions. Continued into later life the sources of such symptoms will establish the basis for the well-recognized anxiety states and neuroses and some of the psychophysiologic states.

Children suffering these symptoms are seen often by parents as worriers, sensitive, shy, and aspiring. They feel inferior, are submissive to others, and cry easily. They are anxious to meet the expectations of others and to avoid criticism, as their major drive is to maintain security through pleasing. Often the mother is herself ridden by anxiety, is fearful, and nags the child to meet social expectations. Frequently these children are found in ambitious middle class families who promulgate high standards of achievement. The children come to recognize that their acceptance within the family is conditioned on their continued outstanding performance, thus establishing for themselves strict superego and aspiring ego ideals.

Treatment for these children is best done by uncovering techniques along the psychoanalytic model. In such treatment, the sources of the driving effects of guilt and shame are alleviated by uncritical revelation of the child's anxiety and rage in relation to the parental figures and identifications with the less punitive figure of the therapist.

Runaway Reaction

In this group the predominant feature is the running away from home. Such children often steal at home before running away. Often seclusive and apathetic, they admit their unhappiness at home. Parents complain, too, of their staying out at night. Frequently they seek their solace in peers whom they perceive as stronger than themselves and as accepting of them. Some, through their passivity, are engaged in homosexual behavior, and others drift into companionship with various adolescent gangs, including the delinquent and antisocial groups. Such children, however, are generally deficient in the sense of loyalty necessary to establish them as acceptable members of well-knit adolescent groups, as often they are deceptive.

The family transactions of these children have been such that they feel rejected through the processes of unusual severity or inconsistency. Often physically slight, they are incapable of development of an aggressive adaptation to living. Their growth is associated with a derogatory self-image and a deep lack of self-confidence and esteem. Only children and illegitimate children often fit into this behavioral pattern.

Treatment of the home is necessary if change is to occur. When this is unlikely, the children are best placed in a foster home or a treatment facility to gain the necessary corrective socializing experience.

Unsocialized Aggressive Reaction

This is diagnosed in children with assaultive tendencies; they start fights, are cruel to other children and animals, defy authorities, and are maliciously mischievous. These actions are performed without guilt feelings. The youngsters come from rejecting parents who provide limited opportunities for association and through their indifference or absence fail to offer the needed warmth and support which establish healthy identification and development of superego and ego ideal.

Socialized Delinquent Group

These children may be identified by the existence of several of the following overt behaviors: gang activities, bad companions, coöperative and furtive stealing, habitual truancy from school, and staying out late at night. Here the family pattern is one of negligence and the environment allows exposure to delinquent influences. Each child gains his security through group identification and support. Many of these early behavior disorders represent transformations or reactions to aggression. Aggression may play a part in the very symptoms that at first sight seem to bear no relation to it. Frequently, in fact, the troublesome behavior of the child is not of such a nature as to suggest its real source. The conduct disorder may be an adaptation to submissiveness or may result from an effort to obtain substitute or compensatory satisfactions for those not received at home. Again, the conduct disturbance may represent the child's attempt to bolster up feelings of inadequacy or inferiority, an effort to make himself feel courageous and superior by overemphasizing his independence in the form of aggressive and disturbing behavior. Sometimes it serves as defiance of authority or as a means of controlling the mother or of tyrannizing the household. Some forms of conduct disorder represent efforts to escape from anxiety-ridden situations. In others, the behavior disorder arises as a consequence of a desire for punishment created in response to marked feelings of guilt.

In Chapter 25, Personality Disorders, the etiology suggested by Johnson and Szurek for such antisocial conduct disorders as firesetting, truancy, stealing, and unacceptable sexuality as it occurs in some children is discussed. Here the source for the antisocial behavior is believed to be in the parent's unwitting sanction or indirect encouragement of the child's behavior. In these instances, the child is healthy, not deprived emotionally or exposed to cultural patterns that encourage the pattern, but comes from an apparently "good" family. In such instances, the parent appears overtly to interdict the act that is the source of complaint. However, study of the parent-child interaction in the course of collaborative treatment has demonstrated that, through unconsciously driven behavior, the parent or both parents communicate their permissiveness to the child. The approval is often expressed in nonverbal forms by undue attention to the child's disturbing behavior, by the lack of consistent firmness, and in its management through unwitting and sometimes suggestive remarks, smirks, or encouragement. In such instances, change in behavior requires treatment of the permissive parent, who obtains a vicarious gratification from the child's misbehavior that acts out the parent's repressed impulses.

A 7-year-old boy was referred for psychiatric consultation from the Board of Education because of his inability to make a satisfactory adjustment in his class room. The teacher reported that he was constantly aggressive toward other children and that much of his behavior seemed bizarre. He had been discharged from a class the previous year because of similar disturbances of behavior. The mother reported that she had had difficulty in controlling him at home. To her he seemed very restless, blinked his eyes frequently, and masturbated constantly. She summed up her problem in one sentence, "I can't seem to get through to him." She dated the change in his behavior to the age of 2½, when he first was observed to be tense and seemed to joke about everything said to him. When the boy was examined, he was found to be pale, stocky, but well developed, and with a husky voice. He frequently asked what would happen to him when he would return to the class room. He seemed anxious concerning the possibility of bodily injury and became very apprehensive when feeling the cutting edges of carpentry tools in the play room. He did not talk spontaneously and was evasive in his replies. There was evidence of poor motor coördination and little patterning in what he did. Psychological tests showed him to be hesitant, suspicious, and interpretive of all remarks as hostile. He frequently evaded by apparent misunderstanding or not hearing what was said to him. It was felt the child needed assistance in a residential hospital setting.

In the discussion of the problem with the father, it was learned that on many occasions the father had beaten the boy severely. It seemed evident that the father was competing with his son in many ways, and he remarked in regard to games with him, "He can't lose, he wants to win the games we play. I usually win. It's hard for him to beat me. If he loses, he loses legitimately!" The father also indicated his resentment toward the son and spoke of his son's interest as silly. He expressed favoritism for a younger child. The mother was found to be an immature, dependent, and self-centered person, limited in her fantasy life and depressed in mood.

When the boy was brought to the hospital, he first expressed much concern about "who is boss" on the ward. He frequently insisted that he was "the boss" and often attempted to engage in power struggles with other children and the doctor. He remarked, "Well, if you are strong, how come you haven't killed me yet?" Frequently he talked of his own strength or expressed desires of being killed. In play sessions, he acted as the father and behaved in an impatient, angry, and cruel way to a doll. The game often ended with the doll killing all other little dolls and destroying the furniture and the parents. With continuing treatment, he became destructive and aggressive in the hospital. This behavior subsided when he was provided an interpretation that apparently it was his wish to provoke the psychiatrist to respond as would have happened at home. He then made efforts to seek closeness to the psychiatrist.

Additional history disclosed that the patient was a planned child, and his early development had been quite normal. The mother reported that bowel training had been difficult and that she had had a constant struggle with the child. She stated that she had beaten him if he failed to excrete properly and admitted being constantly frustrated and angry in caring for him.

In the course of the treatment of the child, it became apparent that the problem was one of a hateful struggle for control between the boy and his chronically distressed mother. His only conception of existence seemed to be in fighting and attaining the position of "the boss." The father contributed to the child's hostility through his competitive feelings and his hostile aggression toward the child. The boy's behavior slowly but gradually improved in the protective milieu of the residential treatment center and with play therapy sessions in conjunction with special schooling. After 18 months he was discharged home. By then his parents had received some understanding of their problems through psychotherapeutic treatment.

Neuroses

DEPRESSION.   As mentioned earlier, childhood depression does exist. It is reactive to deprivation of or loss of affectional attachment, most often owing to adverse family relations. Those children so suffering appear sad or unhappy, often are withdrawn socially and, if questioned, speak of being unwanted or unloved. The depressed children most frequently conceive of themselves negatively. Verbally they describe themselves as "stupid" or "mean" or use some other derogatory application expressing badness, failure, or disgust. Often there is evidence of difficulty in control of their aggressive drives. Many of the children display this in fighting, biting, or other destructive actions against persons or physical objects. Subtle expressions occur, too, in the form of teasing others. Public defecation or enuresis may accompany the depression, as do insomnia and excessive autoeroticism. Psychosomatic symptoms have been considered as depressive equivalents.

The study of depressed children by Poznanski and Zrull found that the parents, too, have personality difficulties expressed in outbursts of anger, temper tantrums, or criticism as well as differing degrees of emotional distancing from the children. Physical abuse is common as a form of punishment in the family, and some of the mothers indulge in punitive measures of weaning and toilet training. Scapegoating and bullying by both parents and older siblings occur. Divorce or separation is frequent in the families in which these depressed children were raised.

PHOBIAS.   These disorders, of a transient variety, are common in childhood, particularly fears of heights, the dark, animals, and other frightening figures. To be considered pathological, the response to the feared object must be over-determined and leads to gross disturbance of behavior, with anxiety or panic. Children who have been harmed by animals or by adults may be expected to have a generalized overreaction to them. In these instances the reaction may be thought of as a conditioned response. In other children, however, the phobia represents a displacement of fear to some other object and derives from aggressive drives directed toward one or the other parental figure. The dynamics of these phobic states are described in Chapter 24.

The *school phobias* are probably misnamed. In most instances, the anxiety reaction on going to school is due to response to separation from the mother —a form of separation anxiety. A therapeutic regimen that directs the prompt return of the child to school has a high chance of success, particularly with younger children. Such techniques have been described as successful by many over the years.

A highly successful method for rapid resolution of acute school phobia has been reported in detail by Kennedy. The method is effective, without relapse over time in those children brought in with the first episode of refusal to attend school. This refusal usually follows a weekend of physical illness. The child expresses concern about death. The mother's health has been in question. Such children are usually weak students. The parents communicate well, are well adjusted in most living areas, and are perceptive emotionally, but the father may be competitive with the mother in household activities.

Kennedy states that the treatment procedure necessitates the following: working relations with the school, the avoidance of interest in the child's physical complaints, structured interviews with the parents, interviews with the child, and forced school attendance. Provided the history reveals at least a predominance of the above features, the parents must be brought to the therapist together, and the father is directed to take the child to school. The mother may be advised that she can go with the father or visit the school during the day—but not remain. The principal or teacher must participate by keeping the child in the classroom. In the interviews with the parents the therapist must be confident, optimistic, and firm, advising the parents that they, too, are to avoid all discussion of the issue of school attendance with the child until such time as it is required. They must be firm and matter of fact in preparing him for attendance in spite of complaints. After three or four days of

being conducted to school, the child usually goes alone, without complaints or symptoms.

Such a method has been ineffective when failure in treatment has occurred several times or when the onset is insidious and not on the first day following a physical illness.

Older children with school phobia usually are found in families with highly disturbed parents who are incapable of mastering their own anxiety over aggressiveness and providing the firmness necessary to face the complaints of the child. Oftentimes parents of older children who have failed to enter school due to phobia are themselves severely neurotic or psychotic. Here therapy for the parent is necessary to effect change.

Pittman and his colleagues report that in 9 of 11 cases of work phobia in adults the patients had histories of overt school phobias or reluctance to attend school in childhood. Work phobias must be differentiated from the success phobias described in the earlier chapter on Neuroses. In the work phobias the anxiety is related to concern over surrendering dependence and leaving home, in contrast to the success phobias in which inhibition of action results from anxiety over repression of aggressive assertion and success in competition.

OBSESSIVE-COMPULSIVE TRAITS. In the past, doubt has been expressed over the existence of neurotically fixed obsessive-compulsive symptoms in children. Judd's study discovered such states in a group of children averaging about seven years of age. Often the symptoms appeared with dramatic suddenness in intellectually superior children. Never were there single compulsive acts. The most common were handwashing and touching compulsions or bedtime rituals, while the associated obsessional ideations usually were related to contamination or infection, right or wrong, or fears of harm and danger. A considerable number of symptoms invariably led to the child's conflict with his social environment. As with adults with an obsessive-compulsive neurosis, the children so affected seemed rigid, with an overmoralistic superego, fearful of defying rules, and overcompliant to parental authority. Yet these children often had an active fantasy life. Within the family one or both parents were compulsive; the early history of bowel training was not punitive. Such children commonly were ambivalent, but with open aggression usually expressed toward one or both parents. They also often had transient phobic symptoms. These states are differentiated from the compulsiveness usually found in healthy children, in whom it is not perceived as incongruous and does not require efforts at resistance.

The healthy child is able to give up the ritualistic behavior or play and also carries it out with pleasurable affect; nor does it disrupt his ordinary relations or activities.

The outcome of such childhood obsessive-compulsive states is as yet not well documented. Some respond well to psychotherapy.

CONVERSION REACTION. Children exhibit conversion reactions as do adults. The symptoms are usually grossly evident and present as convulsive seizures of the tonic-clonic type, astasia-abasia, urinary retention, hemiparesis and/or hemianesthesia, aphonia, and blindness. Often the conversion symptoms may be associated with various psychophysiologic expressions of anxiety conversion. As in adults, it may not be directly related to the existence of a hysterical personality structure.

Looff suggests from his study that families of children with conversion reactions encounter difficulty in verbal expression of affects as related to sexual maturation and functioning. On the other hand those with children expressing essentially the physiologic symptoms of anxiety were exhibited in expressing this intense concern over separation.

These reactions and their developmental history and dynamics are discussed in detail in Chapter 24, The Neuroses.

Psychoses

These are described under the appropriate headings in previous chapters.

THERAPEUTIC MEASURES

The treatment of personality difficulties of the child must vary with the individual and his problems. The principal emphasis, however, is on "the child's needs, strivings, and growth tendencies in a social and cultural background." The fundamental objective is a healthy reorganization of the personality and an improved emotional adjustment. Many of the child's behavior problems and neurotic difficulties arise from emotional handicaps sustained through earlier relationship experiences that were not conducive to healthy emotional growth. One seeks, therefore, to acquire an understanding of the forces that have been operating in the early life of the child. Although the child cannot, of course, develop beyond the limits of his constitutional potentialities, it is the aim of therapeutic measures to remove or reduce his persistent and crippling emotional difficulties and to aid him in reorganizing those emotional attitudes and patterns of reaction that have been governing his personality functioning. In this way, growth of the patient's personality toward new and more spontaneous and satisfying patterns is made possible.

A growth-promoting therapeutic relationship must be substituted for the previous ones that produced insecurity, abnormal aggression, or hostility and that reinforced infantilization and prevented growth in the direction of self-reliance and social maturity. Into this relationship the child brings his resentments, anxiety, fears, and guilt, and the fantasies that have arisen from such feelings. The first essential is for the psychiatrist to establish a friendly, interested, and satisfactory relationship between the child and himself. He accepts the child as an equal and as a person in his own right. He neither stresses nor ignores the difference in age and maturity but assumes it as a matter of course and does not assume an artificially childish language. In the therapist the child finds someone who can help him as he is. The therapeutic approach must be a gradual one. To hasten it may defeat the relationship and cause the child to withdraw into evasion, indifference, or falsification. Any early reference to behavior disorders may stimulate hostility or tension. Early discussions may therefore deal with the child's interests and activities and in direct questioning about neutral matters. With the therapist-child relationship satisfactorily established, the patient may, in this friendly atmosphere, verbalize his conscious conflicts, opinions, ideas, and feelings, which can then be discussed. In another way, too, the therapist-child relationship may be of value.

Through this relationship, the child projects his anxiety and hostility onto the personality of the physician. By projection the child may make use of the therapist to symbolize an unacceptable part of himself as he moves toward freeing himself of the unacceptable aspect. The child may also project onto the therapist desirable qualities that he hopes to attain. The therapist will not be critical of the child's behavior and will take his ideas seriously and as worthy of attention and consideration. He will seek to feel and understand just what problems the child is trying to solve when by that very effort he is creating the problems that have brought him to the psychiatrist. His attitude will not be one of condescension. Within the security of the dependent relationship with the emotionally more mature therapist, whom he trusts and imitates, the child relives his emotional conflicts. The physician will aim to have the child feel that the therapist is a kindly adult, a helpful, protective father who understands his feelings and is helping him.

Occasionally with older children and adolescents, if the problem is a simple and largely environmental one, talks with the patient concerning situations that are troublesome may be not only a direct but also an important treatment. The patient may have reacted to a situation with confused apprehension and undesirable behavior because he did not understand the chain of circumstances that produced a given result. One must not, however, by merely attempting to have the child see what is wrong or undesirable about himself, expect him to relinquish his old ways or control them more effectively. Even with simple problems there must usually be a reorganization of emotional attitudes and patterns of reaction. To secure this the patient must not only have wholesome compensations and outlets but, through an acceptable and gratifying, and therefore therapeutic, relationship with the psychiatrist, gain a stimulus toward new ways of feeling, i.e., to change, to grow.

Family and/or group therapies are important in enhancing ego growth in many instances. The physician may wish to make use of *group therapy,* consisting of clubs, camps, dancing classes, boarding schools, or other activities, to enable the patient to make contacts with others and develop interests of his own. In some cases, separation for long periods of time from an overprotective mother may be desirable. In younger children, play techniques involving psychoanalytical principles are largely used.

Parental Therapy

Since, as already indicated, the child's problem usually arises from the living relationship between himself and a parent and is interwoven with a parent's attitude, modification of parental attitudes toward the child is necessary to effect change. This is particularly so with the younger child.

Usually a series of interviews either with both parents or with the mother is desirable before the child is examined in order to discuss the problem that the latter presents. The physician, by giving the mother—but sometimes both parents —an opportunity to express and relieve her perturbation and anxiety, gains her confidence, often secures revealing information about personality characteristics of the parents, and assists the mother in seeing the child's trouble in a truer perspective. She may like to explain the child's behavior as a result of heredity, but the therapist will usually discover that the mother's neurotic conflict has entered the child's handling. Her expressions of guilt, accusations, hostility, anxiety, and excuses may betray the nature of interpersonal relations that have been a source of difficulty.

Inquiry should be made as to the onset of the child's difficulty, the mode and circumstances of its first appearance, and its development. The interview will presumably, too, assist the physician in securing desirable information concerning the child's cultural background, the family's ways of living, its intelligence, its beliefs and problems, the relationships between father and mother, and the child's group relations. Through a knowledge of the parents' past and present attitudes toward the child, the psychiatrist learns much as to what situations the child's behavior is an adjustment. As previously indicated, it will often be found that the mother is carrying over into her relationship with her child the unresolved emotional problems that arose in her relationships with her own parents. The aim is to uncover a dynamic picture of the experiences and emotions of the child in relation to those surrounding him.

The problem may have arisen from the father-child relationship, but more frequently it arises from that of mother and child. If, as is probable, the problem has arisen from the relationship between the child and the mother, both require therapy. They are not, however, interviewed together. The psychiatrist and social worker collaborate in helping parents and child to resolve difficulties that have arisen through living together.

Through visits, the mother acquires a new understanding of her relation to the child and a realization that she has a part in the child's therapy. The simultaneity of these appointments, usually held weekly and 45 minutes in duration, assists mother and child to realize that the problem requiring help does not exist solely in the child or in the mother but in the relationship between them. As previously indicated, the parents' psychological problems are usually one of the most serious obstacles to a resolution of the child's problem. It is the task of the therapist to assist the mother to a better understanding and an emotional acceptance of herself in her relation to the child.

If the mother's feeling for her child is one of rejection, treatment of the latter's problems is often difficult. The mother, burdened with anxieties and fears, cannot emotionally accept or understand a direct interpretation of her unconscious feelings or her personality patterns. By indirect methods, therefore, the mother is helped to objectify the problem, to formulate her thinking, feeling, and behavior in relation to the child, and to allay her guilt and anxiety. She is assisted in establishing a normal and satisfying relationship with the child that will permit a progressive and wholesome growth of her personality. No attempt should be made to make the mother recognize that she is coming for treatment for herself as a patient. If a favorable rapport is established with the therapist, the mother accepts this relationship as a search for causes for the child's difficulties, and in examining the family life, she may begin to examine herself. The mother's influence and behavior in relation to her child are partially dependent upon her own self-understanding. She may be helped to see family members in their respective relationships and, knowing their life experiences, may begin to find new meaning for their behavior. In this manner her understanding of, and her relation to, the problem child may become clearer. Any necessary manipulation of the environment will be carried out by the social worker.

Play Therapy

It is well recognized that free association is a valuable technique with adults for the investigation of significant psychological material below the level of consciousness. In children, however, play is a more normal mode of expression than is one limited to verbal forms. Play technique consists of introducing a child to a group of toys and permitting him to use them freely while the observer looks on. The toys given him represent all the common interests of childhood—animals, building blocks, and other objects of a creative type. Dolls often represent members of the family. Play being the medium in which the child expresses himself most freely, the use which he makes of the toys reveals his fantasies, offers insight into his mental mechanisms, and gives clues regarding his unconscious. In the child, play may be regarded as the speech of the unconscious. He may use the imaginary characters of his play to express his own disturbed feelings. Being a projective technique, play may show human relations and problems arising out of them. It therefore sheds light on the family relationships as no other medium can. It illuminates the relation both of the child to his parents and of the parents to the child. Hiding behind the anonymity of a doll, he may tell of death wishes directed toward a parent or sibling. The child should be permitted to choose the toy and use it spontaneously, since he will select the medium of expression best suited to himself and therefore best adapted to express his immediate problem or situation.

In play, therefore, we find an excellent projective technique for the diagnosis of hidden aspects of the personality and for a study of the emotional life of children. We know that the child's emotional life revolves primarily around his mother, father, and siblings. Since play provides a feeling-projecting medium, we find in it a readily available means of investigating the child's emotional attitudes toward the family. These, it will be found, are often ambivalent. We have already seen that the child's problems often arise from the interpersonal relationships in the family. Play, therefore, is often used by the child as a spontaneous projective technique for expressing the nature of the relationship in which his problem is rooted. He brings into his play the reactions and feelings connected with this problem. Drawing and painting may also be used as projective techniques, not only for securing clues as to the child's problems and psychic dynamics, but also as therapeutic adjuncts. In his art sessions, the child may attribute various imaginary roles to parent or sibling and may use his products as a channel of release.

There are many interesting phenomena in play technique comparable to those observed in psychoanalysis. For example, the child may show an anxious care in excluding some toy from his play, or on approaching some aspect of the play that he seems to find unsafe, not permissible, or unsatisfactory to the point of discomfort, he becomes upset and is unable to go on playing in peace. This is strikingly similar to the signs of emotional disturbance present when, in free association, conflicts and anxieties push too near the surface. In this way, the psychiatrist may secure clues to the sources of the child's difficulties. To be able not only to interpret the disruptions or interruptions of play such as those just described, but also to interpret the symbolic gestures and words that the child constantly presents, is of great aid in ascertaining the source of his difficulties. To do so, however, requires experience, insight, and imaginative vision on the part of the psychiatrist. Gardner has devised an effective elaboration of play therapy to assist the child in communicating his problems through the use of mutual story telling.

Pharmacological Therapy

Pharmacological treatment with the amphetamines and the tricyclic antidepressants is indicated particularly in those children with the hyperkinetic syndrome so often associated with evidence of brain damage or maturational lags. Amphetamine has a so-called paradoxical effect in such children, acting as a sedating agent particularly for those who are overactive, with a limited attention span, impulsivity, emotional lability, and erratic behavior. The drug has been reported as more effective in children who have no abnormalities in their electroencephalograms than in those in whom defects are found. Yet even the latter often improve with its administration. Similarly, the tricyclic antidepressants have been used in similar behavior disturbances. Methylphenidate (Ritalin) has proven effective when administered to children with the hyperkinetic syndrome, including some with abnormalities in the electroencephalogram and "soft" neurologic signs.

BIBLIOGRAPHY

Beck, L., Mackay, M., and Taylor, R.: Methylphenidate. Results on a children's psychiatric service. New York State J. Med., 23:2896–2902, 1970.

Bernard, V. W., and Crandell, D. L.: Evidence for various hypotheses of social psychiatry. In Zubin, J., and Freyhan, E. A. (eds.): Social Psychiatry. New York, Grune and Stratton, 1968.

Bowlby, J.: Attachment and Loss. Vol. 1. New York, Basic Books, Inc., 1969.

Burks, H. F.: Effects of amphetamine therapy on hyperkinetic children. Arch. Gen. Psychiat., 11: 604–609, 1964.

Chess, S.: An introduction to Child Psychiatry. New York, Grune and Stratton, 1969.

DeAjuraguerra, J., et al.: Le Choix Therapeutique en Psychiatrie Infantile. Paris, Masson et Cie., 1967.

Finch, S. M.: Fundamentals of Child Psychiatry. New York, W. W. Norton & Co., Inc., 1960.

Gardner, R. L.: Therapeutic Communication with Children. The Mutual Story Telling Technique. New York, Science House, Inc., 1971.

Jenkins, R. L.: Varieties of children's behavioral problems and family dynamics. Amer. J. Psychiat,. 124:1440–1445, 1968.

Johnson, A. M., and Szurek, S. A.: Etiology of antisocial behavior in delinquents and psychopaths. J.A.M.A., 154:814–817, 1954.

Josselyn, I. M.: The Happy Child. New York, Random House, 1955.

Judd, L. L.: Obsessive compulsive neurosis in children. Arch. Gen. Psychiat., 12:136–143, 1965.

Kanner, L.: Child Psychiatry. 3rd ed. Springfield, Ill., Charles C Thomas, 1957.

Kennedy, W. A.: School phobia: Rapid treatment of fifty cases. J. Abnorm. Psychol., 70:285–289, 1965.

Knobloch, H., and Pasamanick, B.: The developmental behavioral approach to the neurologic examination in infancy. Child Devel., 33:181–198, 1962.

Levy, D. M.: Maternal Overprotection. New York, Columbia University Press, 1943.

Levy, D. M.: Primary affect hunger. Amer. J. Psychiat., 94:643–652, 1937.

Levy, D. M.: Capacity and motivation. Amer. J. Orthopsychiat., 27:1–8, 1957.

Lippman, H. S.: Treatment of the Child in Emotional Conflict. 2nd ed. New York, McGraw-Hill Book Company, 1962.

Looff, D. H.: Psychophysiologic and conversion reactions in children. J. Amer. Acad. Child Psychiat., 9:318–331, 1970.

Millechap, J. G.: Drugs in management of hyperkinetic and perceptually handicapped children. J.A.M.A., 206:1527–1530, 1968.

Pittman, F. S., Langsley, D. G., and De Yoeng, C. D.: Work and school phobias. A family approach to treatment. Amer. J. Psychiat., 124:1535–1941, 1968.

Poznanski, E., and Zrull, J. P.: Childhood depression. Clinical characteristics of overtly depressed children. Arch. Gen. Psychiat., 23:9–15, 1970.

Rada, R. T., Meyer, G. G., and Krill, A. F.: Visual conversion reaction in children. I. Diagnosis. Psychosomatics, 10:23–28, 1969.

Redl, F.: Controls from Within. Glencoe, Ill., Free Press, 1952.

Redl, F., and Wineman, D.: Children Who Hate. Glencoe, Ill., Free Press, 1951.

Sandler, J., and Joffe, W. G.: Notes on childhood depression. Int. J. Psychoanal., 46:88–96, 1965.

Schlossman, F. E.: Zur Fragedes Hospitalismus im Sauglingsaustalten. Ztschr. f. Kinderheilkunde, 42:31–38, 1926.

Shaw, C. R., and Lucas, A. R.: The Psychiatric Disorders of Childhood. 2nd ed. New York, Appleton-Century-Crofts, 1970.

Sobel, D. E.: Human caring. Amer. J. Nurs., 69: 2612–2613, 1969.

Sommerschild, S., and Kreyberg, P. C.: Prognosis in Child Psychiatry. Baltimore, Williams & Wilkins Company, 1968.

Spitz, R. A.: Anaclitic depression. The Psychoanalytic Study of the Child, 2:313–342, 1946.

Szurek, S. A.: Comments on the psychopathology of children with somatic illness. Am. J. Psychiat., 107:844–859, 1951.

Chapter 29

Special Symptoms

In addition to the varieties of behavior disturbance described in the previous chapter, many children are referred for psychiatric examination by parents or other interested persons as the result of social difficulties encountered by them owing to very specific abnormalities in development. The common complaints center about speech expressivity, ability to learn to read and write, various tics and other psychomotor difficulties, sleep disturbances, and failures in development of excretory control such as enuresis and encopresis. If uncorrected, some symptoms may continue into adult life or influence adversely healthy personality development through continuing persistence of anxiety with arousal, secondarily, of pathological characterological or symptomatic defenses.

SPEECH DISTURBANCES

Disorders of speech are reflected in phonation, speech sound articulation, fluency and rate, or symbolic representation. They may result either from physiological disturbances in the organs of phonation, their innervation or the brain processes concerned with speech or as the result of interference through emotional instability. Wendell Johnson concludes that 4 per cent of children in the United States have significant problems. The majority of these lisp, about 16 per cent stutter, slightly less have speech defects associated with hearing loss, and the remainder have impairment owing to voice problems, fluency and rate problems, retarded speech development, complications of cleft palate and lip, those of cerebral palsy, and other neuromuscular defects. Usually considered to have a significant relationship to emotional disturbance is stuttering.

STUTTERING. This disturbance customarily has its beginning in childhood and, when persistent, seriously impedes the child's social adaptation and development. It must be recognized that short periods of stuttering may take place between the second and fourth years, when the growing child's efforts at expression exceed his capacity to verbalize. Parents who have themselves been stutterers or have been related to a stutterer often become overly anxious and tend to emphasize the child's defect by their efforts at control through admonitions to speak more slowly and by their evident preoccupation with the speech difficulty. It is not surprising that many stutterers are made anxious by silence. Silence seems to "freeze them" and they may have difficulty commencing speech. Gould and Sheehan suggest that silence may become the conditioned cue for arousal of anxiety and therefore stuttering.

The persistent stutterer is considered to have a conflict between passive and aggressive drives, which is reflected in his speech. Such a child often tends to show other compulsive and ambivalent traits. His speech expresses his obstinacy in his forcing others to wait while he completes his efforts.

LEARNING DISTURBANCES

Approximately 12 per cent of all children in the United States fail to learn to read as well as the average. Although these children have better than normal intelligence and their social and vocabulary development is excellent, as well as their vision, they suffer from dyslexia, occasionally but not always associated with left-handedness and with difficulty in converting to right-handed writing. This disability manifests itself in a variety of ways: sometimes as confusion of one consonant with another, such as b's for d's, p's for q's, or t's for f's, or as a reversal of the syllables, words, or entire sentences as mirror writing, with a complete failure to recognize words.

Another group of children suffer from an inability to learn as a consequence of the newer methods of teaching reading. By these methods, children are taught to read whole words, phrases, and sentences, with the analysis of individual words into phonic sounds and letters undertaken only secondarily. Because of their particular perceptual capacity, some children are unable to learn to read or spell by this method of pedagogy. In such children the emotional expressions of fear and anxiety, caused by failure to meet the standards of the family or class and by hostility resulting from feelings of rivalry and jealousy, tend to imbue concepts of personal inferiority and encourage behavior disturbance.

These children first have a reading disability which, in time, becomes a learning disability. Early in life, if properly tested by psychologists, they show evidence of perceptual-motor and visual-motor weaknesses as compared to other children of their age. By adolescence many of the signs of such lags in ego functions have disappeared, and the early and often severe hyperkinesis has improved greatly. These children appear to have compensated, as they have an adequate intelligence and may read very well. Yet there are residual signs of reading disability. Their spelling capacity is very poor owing to inability to retain verbal visual configuration. Handwriting is not rhythmic, and their organization of their school papers is poor. On multiple-choice examinations their performance is often good, but essay examinations reveal their weaknesses. They are customarily inarticulate, and language is not used well in their communication. Their written compositions are unimaginative. Metaphors are understood poorly, and when they are asked to define them concrete responses are given—not, however, the egocentric and loose replies of the schizophrenic. The boys are often able in mechanical efforts and in sports. Emotionally they are usually explosive and have a limited tolerance for frustration. With proper tutoring these youngsters are often able to proceed in school. Later they do better in technical or business colleges than in the formal academic institutions.

Many behavior disorders founded on such a basis disappear rapidly with improvement in the reading. The important element in treatment is recognition of the underlying incapacity to learn. Here the use of a remedial teacher is often the effective technique to bring about a satisfactory modification of the behavior disturbance. The following case illustrates this problem.

O. E. was an 8½-year-old boy referred for evaluation and for possible treatment of emotional problems involved in his inability to read. The school teacher and psychologist felt that the patient had an emotional block that prevented his learning to read. The child was restless and unruly in school and a difficult problem in management. Physical examination was negative except for confusion in handedness. Past history was free of gross emotional disturbances. He was well liked by his many friends and had many interests. His parents had high academic aspirations for him and were distressed by his poor scholastic performance. He was compared unfavorably with his very bright 10-year-old brother.

During the psychiatric interview he appeared friendly and cooperative and fully understood the reasons for his being in the doctor's office. He said, "I can't read and it gets me worried." He handled a pencil very poorly in either hand, and in printing reversed several letters and words. He could not read. Psychological tests revealed an average intelligence. He could not be tested in reading achievement, because this was so defective. Bender Gestalt designs were below his age level, but he showed difficulty in integration of the designs. A diagnosis of learning disability was made. It was felt that the problem of anxiety was secondary. A remedial reading teacher was engaged. Parents and teachers were encouraged to let him progress and learn at his own speed. He did well under special instruction, progressing slowly but quite satisfactorily in reading. His restlessness, tension, and disobedience subsided quickly.

K. de Hirsch points up the differentiations of these children, usually boys, from the group of scholastic underachievers whose difficulties stem from poor reading comprehension owing to preoccupation with their fantasy life, phobias, or depressive inability to focus attention. These children, in contrast to the previous group, are often highly verbal and their abstract competence is good. Later in school they do poorly, however, as they lack persistence and attentiveness. Usually rather schizoid, they develop learning difficulties in the context of conflicts over control of aggressive impulses, associated with anxiety and depression. Their major need is for psychotherapy rather than for tutoring in remedial reading.

TICS

Tics occur as involuntary but apparently purposeless movements of interconnected muscles. They frequently involve the muscles of the eyelids, with blinking or squinting, but also occur as repetitious, frowning, grimacing, sniffing, grunting, swallowing, head twisting or shaking, coughing, grunting, or explosive verbalizations. *Gilles de la Tourette's* disease or *maladie des tics* is a tic syndrome involving the upper body, including the face, shoulder, and arms. It may be associated with coprolalia and sometimes echolalia and echokinesis. Often, tics are first noticed in childhood; they then disappear, only to recur at a later date at the time of some conflict.

Frequently it will be found that the tic was first noticed after a frightening experience leading to a fear of injury and that it represents a defensive muscular withdrawal response of small muscle groups appropriate to the expected trauma. Although initially the defensive muscular contraction may have involved many muscles, the tic represents a rudi-

mentary response of small muscle groups. Because of the persistence of the response beyond the particular time of the injury, the tic-like movement becomes inappropriate and involuntary. The use of the small muscle groups develops as a consequence of parental prohibition for the full movement. The tic then represents both the fear of injury and the attempt to maintain gratification by complying with parental wishes.

Children with tics are often restless, self-conscious, sensitive, or spoiled, or may be overambitious and overconscientious. Easy excitability and fatigability are observed. There are other children who are shy, seclusive, and embarrassed. The tics of psychogenic origin are to be differentiated from those that occur as a result of encephalitic disease affecting the basal ganglia. Treatment of the latter is difficult.

A six-year-old boy was brought to the clinic by his mother, who complained that he jerked his head and blinked his eyes frequently. She stated that he had begun this habit about four or five weeks previously. When the habit spasm began, she paid little heed to it, but later she slapped him in the face for it. At first she thought it might be caused by disease of his eyes. She became annoyed when he began to open his eyes with his fingers. The boy reported it was his feeling that his eyes were closing on him when the lids were heavy.

The mother went on to describe her son as restless, unable to sit in a chair, and very fidgety. She also reported that he had occasional headaches and had begun to suffer from asthma at 17 months of age. His last attack had taken place 12 months previously. Early in life he had played with younger children, but now he played only with those of his own age. The boy had been breast fed for six months and bottle fed until 1½ years. At five months of age, he had been able to sit alone and had stood up and taken some steps at 9 months. At the end of the first year, he had said a few words. She indicated that his bowel and bladder training had been completed in less than a year. The mother had dressed the boy until a year and a half ago and said that he wished her to dress him even now. It was only at this time that he had begun to wash himself. The story of his schooling showed that he had entered the first grade at 6, had done very well, and was advanced several classes. He was, at the time of examination, the youngest child in his class. It was the mother's impression that he felt uneasy. The father was described as a happy-go-lucky person who enjoyed his children. The mother thought of herself as being well. There were three children, the patient being the eldest. A sister was two and a half years younger and a baby was 18 months old.

When the boy was seen, he was found to blink, roll his eyes, and grimace about his mouth. He said that the trouble with his facial muscles came on after he had arrived home from school some weeks before and done his homework. He felt he could not stop the movements once they started. He also reported that he had been unable to sleep well and admitted some recent worries about masturbation. He saw himself as a sickly boy and described his fear of playing rough games with others. The matter of the boy's masturbation was discussed with the mother, who became overtly anxious in dealing with this subject. On returning home, she was able to talk to her son on the subject without threatening him. The mother discontinued bathing him and allowed him to go to bed later. During several additional hours, the matter of the sexual interests of the son was brought up for discussion by the mother. The physician worked with her and the boy, with gratifying results. The facial tics disappeared following a series of four visits. Treatment for the asthma was continued for several years.

Simple tics have a good outlook for spontaneous disappearance, but the prognosis for the complex conditions such as Gilles de la Tourette's disease is less favorable. The parents and others must be assisted in their efforts to correct the child in attempts to suppress the movements, and to desist from other punitive and oppressive efforts at training. In treatment the effort is made to uncover the original fears and anxieties that generated the tic as well as the reactive impulse often symbolized in its continuance. There are some reports suggesting that the butyrophenone and phenothiazine drugs relieve the more severe tic-like syndromes.

DISORDERS OF SLEEP

Many children are referred for psychiatric care by mothers complaining of problems in their patterns of sleep. The most common complaints center around restlessness, talking in sleep, nightmares, irregular sleep habits, night terrors, and sleepwalking. The majority of these complaints do not signify existence of psychiatric disorder but rather the anxiety of the parent and her difficulty in establishing a satisfactory milieu conducive to induction and maintenance of steady sleep.

There are wide variations in sleeping patterns during the developmental period. While premature babies sleep almost continuously throughout the day and night, the sleep time of the infant gradually diminishes in relation to the waking time as he ages. The majority of the simple problems in relation to sleeping occur as the result of ineffective patterning of sleeping habits within the family. Babies who are regularly rewarded when they cry out by being quickly picked up and carried elsewhere, those who find they can terminate separation from the mother through their activity, restlessness or crying when placed in bed, or who are visited frequently by parents during the night are those who develop patterns of restlessness, delay in initiating sleep, or restlessness in sleeping.

Late napping prevents others from falling asleep at night. Sleep difficulties in older children usually reflect some anxiety as the result of insecurity in the family or school relations. Once poor sleep habits are established they are difficult to modify. Early advice to the mother is important then in preventing those continuing disturbances which present into adulthood.

RESTLESS SLEEP. In most children with marked restlessness, history generally discloses that they are equally overactive and excitable during the day. However, there are some active during the day hours who achieve quick and deep sleep easily. Specifically, the complaining mother may report jerking, rolling, and turning during sleep, periodic awakening, or rhythmic movements such as rocking or head banging. The latter expressions of restless sleep may represent either conflict with the mother, related to overdependence, or the existence of brain damage or retardation.

TALKING SLEEP. The majority of children express themselves occasionally at some time through sleep talking, heard as a few words or phrases. Sleep talking may indicate more serious and persisting anxiety, particularly if continued and associated with other manifestations of behavior disturbance. Teeth grinding (bruxism), too, may start in childhood.

NIGHTMARES AND NIGHT TERRORS. In contrast to the frightening dream, the child experiencing a nightmare (incubys) cries out in his sleep and awakens with the expressions of an acute anxiety attack. He is perspiring and breathing heavily. His pupils are usually dilated and his facial expression terrified. He may complain of tightness or heaviness of his chest. He is, in fact, overbreathing. With a frightening dream the child awakens, but is not in an acute anxiety or panic attack. Repeated frequently, the child may become fearful of going to bed. The majority of frightening dreams and nightmares occur physiologically during REM sleep. The child may be able to recount the contents of the nightmare or dreams. If so, inferences may be made as to the sources of his fright and anxiety. From these preventive advice or therapeutic plans may be derived to correct the stimulating source of these sleep disturbances.

Night terrors, referred to sometimes as *pavor nocturnus,* are severe panic reactions associated with frightened crying out and sometimes frenetic motor activity. Much less common than the frightening dream or nightmare, they have been observed, at the earliest, commencing at age two. In contrast to the nightmare, the suffering child cannot be consoled and appears to remain throughout in a semi-sleeping disoriented state from which he cannot be aroused. After ten or fifteen minutes he then falls alseep to awaken later with a complete amnesia for the occurrence. The etiology of pavor nocturnus has been much discussed. Speculation suggests that its source may be epileptic or hysterical. Many children with this condition have severe behavior disorders. Fisher states that the most

severe nightmares occur during Stage 4 sleep. His description of cases of this kind suggests that they represent pavor nocturnus rather than the ordinary nightmare or dream. To him there occurs eruption of deeply repressed and intense anxiety to account for such states.

SLEEP PARALYSIS. This condition is sometimes referred to as a nightmare but differs from it as an occurrence taking place when the sufferer falls off or awakens from sleep. There is much anxiety during this episode in which the sufferer cannot move, talk or shout, even though trying to do so. Partially awake and also partially somnolent, he attracts attention to himself by moaning. Some try to break the paralytic attack by forcing a leg or arm off the bed. A touch generally leads to arousal. Frightening hypnagogic hallucinations accompany many attacks. The sufferer feels as though there is a heavy load on his chest and may speak of "someone sitting there." Sleep paralysis is thought to be different from narcolepsy and cataplexy. It differs from pavor nocturnus and nightmares in the sleeper's awareness of his location, his recollection of the event, and the paralysis.

SOMNAMBULISM. Sleepwalking in childhood may be perpetuated into adolescence or adulthood. It appears to be related to a maturational defect in which action-oriented activity with imagery occurs during deep sleep in contrast to the fantasy noted with dreaming sleep. It is now known that somnambulistic incidents take place in stage 3 and 4 sleep as described in Chapter 3. Continuous electroencephalography during sleep shows that somnambulistic episodes commence shortly after a sudden burst of high-voltage slow-wave activity (S frequency). This type of cortical activity is found in the electroencephalographic records of 95 per cent of infants between the ages of six and 11 months. By the age of ten years only 3 per cent of children still show such activity during sleep. In contrast, sleep talking, like nocturnal enuresis, bruxism, and head banging, accompanies dreaming (REM) sleep.

Somnambulism is unrelated to specific personality organization, may occur with any level of intelligence, and often occurs in those with little evidence of emotional unrest. In many respects it appears related to psychomotor epilepsy.

As described earlier in this book, sleep disturbance may arise during later life as symptoms of more profound personality disorder. This symptom, however, may be the complaint that brings the patient to medical care. Also, the sufferer may medicate himself and become drug dependent by attempting to relieve this disruptive symptomatic expression of his illness.

TREATMENT. In the case of children, the psychiatrist will explore the ways in which the child has been trained and attended by the mother as regards his sleeping behavior. Also, he will attempt to discover in the child's thinking the possible reasons for his abnormal sleeping behavior. Usually there will be found anxiety over separation from the mother, of being harmed, of dying during sleep, or of losing control of bladder or bowels, so causing criticism or punishment later by the mother.

In those instances in which the sleep disturbances appear to be an expression of inadequate or anxious training on the part of the mother, she should receive appropriate counseling.

If the problem is one of bad dreams or nightmares, their content may reveal the sources of the anxiety in the daytime relations of the patient, thus allowing the psychiatrist inferences as to the treatment method most likely to alleviate the source of the nighttime disruption.

Pharmaceutical control of sleep disturbances may be necessary if the preceding methods fail in relief. In the instances of severe disturbances with interruptions by nightmares or pavor nocturnus the choice of hypnotic or other drug may best be determined after electroencephalographic analysis of the child's sleeping pattern.

The Kales suggest as treatment for the primary insomniac encouragement of physical activity during the day but no exercise near bedtime. Exercise several hours before sleep increases stage 4 sleep. The adult patient should be urged to regulate his day and night schedules. If, however, he does not fall asleep, he should be advised not to remain in bed if unable to sleep. Thus, he is to condition himself to go to bed when sleepy. Also, before bed he is advised to avoid stimulating mental activities, including games.

For difficulty in falling or staying asleep, the Kales recommend flurazepam. When insomnia is associated with depression, a tricyclic antidepressant medication should be given throughout the day—these agents increase stage 4 sleep and maintain sleep.

The REM suppressant drugs (the barbiturate hypnotics, glutethimide [Doriden] ethchlorvynol [Placidyl], methyprylon [Noludar], methaqualone diphenhydramine [Benadryl]) are useful, particularly in those psychosomatic conditions in which sleep arousal with REM cycles is associated with symptom expression such as pain of duodenal ulcer or nocturnal angina pectoris. Glutethimide is perhaps the best, owing to its long duration of action and continual suppression of REM. With the improvement of the patient these drugs must be withdrawn very slowly to minimize the REM rebound phenomenon.

Those drugs which suppress stage 4 sleep and do *not* suppress REM sleep (chloral hydrate, flurazepam hydrochloride [Dalmane], methaqualone [Quaalude], chlordiazepoxide hydrochloride [Librium], and diazepam [Valium]) are indicated for somnambulism and pavor nocturnus.

FEEDING DISTURBANCES

PICA. The craving, chewing, and eating of non-nutritive and sometimes poisonous substances is a frequent behavior pattern in children. It requires supervision over time by parents to bring about the discrimination required to direct the growing child's innate drive to mouth objects of all kinds so that he eventually chews and ingests foodstuffs only. Pica may be understood as the continuance of the infantile pattern of mouthing and thus may be regarded as a developmental immaturity, a fixation or regression to an infantile level of behavior. In other instances the mouthing continues as an expression of deprivation of parental supervision—a neglect of either attention or food or both. On occasions the behavior is determined as a familial or cultural expression, the child mouthing a specific object also chewed upon or mouthed by older family members or those in the community. Pica has been reported as occurring in about 20 per cent of populations of children seen in mental health clinics.

Since the etiologic factors leading to this mouthing disturbance are multiple, the primary sources will be found only in careful assessment of the child, his developmental state, and the family and cultural environment in which he has been raised. Hunger, neglect, brain damage, mental retardation, or cultural factors may singly or jointly be causative. One of the most serious consequences of pica, mentioned earlier in this book, is lead poisoning, in which children chew and eat objects covered with the old lead-containing paints.

Treatment must be directed to correction of the underlying forces leading to pica. In cases of neglect or retardation, training is necessary under constant but interested supervision of those capable of establishing a warm human contact.

ENURESIS

This disturbance, the involuntary passage of urine, occurs commonly and is frequently referred to the child psychiatrist. In some psychiatric clinics, enuresis is the problem for which the majority of children are seen. At the age of two years, some 80 per cent of children have ceased to wet themselves. By the end of three years, the average child is usually able to keep his clothes and bed clean and dry. Enuresis occurs twice as frequently in boys as in girls; it is unrelated to intelligence, and in the majority of instances has been persistent. There is a group of children in whom the habit disappears only to recur at a later date during a period of tension.

By far the most frequent variety of enuresis is the nocturnal type, although diurnal enuresis and combinations of both have been noticed.

In the majority of instances, no physical disturbance of the nervous system or genitourinary apparatus is found on examination. Enuresis may occur as a matter of inadequate training, resulting either from parental attitudes or because of lack of opportunity for adequate training. In some infants, the mother is overprotective, and the child's continuing inability to maintain himself dry is accepted by her on the basis that he is too small or weak for training. The child is thus infantilized and retains an infantile lack of control. Lack of opportunity for training as a causative factor occurs only in children reared in rural homes or in crowded urban areas, where toilet facilities are inadequate and the child is not expected to visit the bathroom under conditions of cold or crowding. In other instances, enuresis occurs as an expression of revenge in which the child wets, a reaction to too rapid and punitive training.

A common type of enuresis is the regressive. In children suffering from this form of enuresis, wetting occurs as a means of again obtaining the gratification of maternal contact. Very frequently regressive enuresis may be seen as a consequence of the birth of a younger child, with the loss of the mother's attention. The child now wets in order to obtain the care and personal attention and affection he misses because of the mother's preoccupation with the newborn. In such instances, the proper parental reaction conducive to change is to allow the youngster more attention for a time in order that he may grow beyond his childish needs. Punishment seldom leads to modification of regressive enuresis.

The series of studies by Margaret Gerard suggests that two-thirds of the enuretic children have failed to identify with the parent of the same sex. The failure of sexual identification seems to take place in families in which the parent of the opposite sex has a passive personality, whereas the parent of the same sex is feared as more strict and rigid. Enuretic boys consequently tend to be passive and unassertive youngsters who are unable to compete actively, whereas girls with the wetting problem are found to be tomboyish and aggressive.

It is well to recognize that enuresis is often symptomatic of anxiety-arousing problems in the family. The symptom is often severe, prolonged, and not easily modified by therapy. It leads, if continued, to many additional conflicts in the growing child, depending upon the attitudes of people with whom he is in contact. As a result of punishment and shaming, the enuretic child develops secondary feelings of inadequacy. Many suffer from sleeplessness in their attempts to control the bladder. These children have feelings of embarrassment and lack of self-confidence that restrict their capacity to form easy relationships with others, as well as feelings of helplessness resulting from their inability to control the habit. They are often told repeatedly that they suffer from "weak bladders" or "weak kidneys," their personal conviction of physical weakness and disability thus being deepened. Exposed to the consequences of teasing when sent to camp or to school with other children, their sense of social inadequacy is again magnified.

The newer physiologic and pharmacologic knowledge has expanded the opportunities for treatment of enuresis. Enuresis usually takes place during deep sleep unassociated with rapid eye movements and their typical electroencephalographic recording of REM. Ritvo reports that about 40 per cent of enuretic periods take place during stage 2 sleep and over 40 per cent during stages 3 and 4. Two thirds of all wettings seem to be preceded by electroencephalographic arousal. Ritvo states that one may distinguish waking, arousal, and nonarousal type of enuresis. He concludes that when enuresis persists beyond age three or four, the symptom may form a nucleus around which other neurotic formations occur. Ritvo found that children with arousal and waking enuresis had a history of sporadic wetting, and several other neurotic symptoms but no family history of enuresis, although the families exhibited much concern over the patient. The group of children with "nonarousal wetting" came from families with history of enuresis. The children had a history of regular wetting and were indifferent to it. The mother is then instructed to awaken the child and have him evacuate the bladder. Regular repetitions of this act with avoidance of bed wetting often lead to inhibition of wetting.

A number of clinical trials with imipramine (Tofranil) have shown that this tricyclic compound with anticholinergic properties, will interrupt enuresis in from 70 to 80 per cent of children. The drug may be given before the noon meal and prior to bedtime in 10 mg. doses for younger children and 25 mg. doses for adolescents. After a year of being dry, approximately a third of the children treated continue to be nonenuretic. If enuresis recurs on withdrawal of imipramine, resumption of the drug usually relieves the symptom once again.

In those children refractory to such measures, psychotherapy should be attempted. The following is a case report of a child effectively treated in this manner.

A 12½-year-old girl was brought to the pediatric psychiatric clinic by her mother, who complained that she wet her bed, was very nervous and restless, bit her nails, and screamed while playing with other children. The mother recounted that her daughter had been enuretic since infancy. Initially, she wet her bed every hour or so during the night; at this time, she wet it once or twice a week. The mother waked her up twice during the night.

She stated that if the children got her daughter to laugh in the day time, she occasionally wet herself. The mother stated that the daughter had slept with her for two years in the same bed. Her daughter always liked exciting things and was admired by everyone around her, but she did not care for work about the house and wished to be a lady; nor did she wish to learn anything. When asked to help with the housework, she argued and became angry.

The daughter was the only child. The mother felt that the pregnancy was quite normal. The child was breast fed for 14 months and walked at one year but was slow in beginning to talk. Her dentition was completed at seven months, and bowel control at three years. The mother continued to feed the girl until the age of 8, since she would not take a spoon in her own hand. Her mother bathed her until she was 11 years old and reported that her daughter had dressed herself only for the past six months. She first allowed her daughter to cross the street alone within the same period of time. The explanation of this was that the mother had seen another child run over some time before. The girl had had no unusual illnesses, but was sick with teething and vomited a great deal at that time. Her school work was good. She began school at six and a half and was regularly promoted with her class. On psychological testing, she was found to have an I.Q. of 113.

The mother described the father as a nervous man whose hands shook and who was preoccupied with palpitation of the heart. He was seen as impatient and easily upset. The mother considered herself a fairly healthy person but nervous since an operation for appendicitis the previous year. She spoke of crying quite easily and complained about her marriage, stating it had not been happy in the early years as her husband was attached to his mother.

When the daughter was seen, she was found to be a tall, gangling, very talkative, "smart alecky" girl, rather restless, walking about uneasily. In discussing the problem of bed wetting, she stated that she used to have difficulty in sleeping because "I was afraid I couldn't wake up in time and then I couldn't get to sleep; then I would worry because I couldn't sleep and I wouldn't." She said she had slept better since her parents did not put her to bed so early. In discusssing her parents, she said, "They have to love me, I'm the only one." She described her mother as "treating me like a baby. She won't let me go to the movies alone." She volunteered that she did not want to grow up but preferred to remain the same age as she is now. "It is more fun."

In subsequent treatment hours with the mother and child, it was learned that the daughter had been unwanted but always overprotected, the mother believing that some harm would come to her. Initially she was a shy child but later developed many friends, mostly among older children. Although she was at first distant with her father, she had become quite close to him since the mother became ill and was not available to do everything for her. She stated that her father was a mother to her. The child and her mother were seen only intermittently over the following three years, as they lived at a distance. She did better at school but continued to be enuretic, although with diminished frequency. After three years, the enuresis disappeared, but there was occasionally frequency of urination at night or during the day. In the meantime, the child worked out many of her conflicting feelings in regard to her dependent relationship with her mother and ambivalent attitude toward her father.

ENCOPRESIS

Much more uncommon but more disturbing to parents and those associated with children is the persistence of fecal soiling. This condition is usually evidence of serious psychopathology when its existence is unassociated with anatomical or physiological defect. Its presence indicates a more severe disturbance than enuresis.

Encopresis is to be differentiated from fecal incontinence the latter referring to soiling caused by a physical disorder such as Hirschsprung's disease, defects of the rectum or anal sphincter or impairment in neurologic control to the cerebral, spinal, or lower motor neuron disease. Encopresis denotes incontinence with constipation.

Encopresis should be reserved for children who continue to soil after the usual age for establishing bowel control; over 90 per cent achieve this control by age 3. Any child who continues to do so frequently following the fourth year should be considered as possibly having this condition in the absence of demonstrable physical defect. The majority with encopresis will be found to be mentally retarded; others are brain damaged or psychotic.

Children with this behavior may soil continuously or episodically. The former have not been successfully trained to bowel control, whereas the latter usually have undergone such training but regress to soiling later. The two varieties of this condition generally occur with about equal frequency. In studies of large series of patients seen in psychiatric clinics, approximately 3 per cent presented this symptom.

In the instances of secondary or regressive encopresis, onset usually occurred following some family incident threatening the future patient's closeness to the parents. Such precipitating incidents have been birth of a sibling, the mother's going to work, parental separation, entrance of the child into school, or punishment.

Most of the children with this symptom tend to be passive and often appear depressed. In the Bellman study 15 per cent of the fathers and 1.3 per cent of the mothers had a history of encopresis between ages 7 and 14, whereas almost 10 per cent of the brothers had the same symptom.

One group of children soil from inadequate parental training, sometimes owing to parental guilt and passivity over their own earlier conflicts in learning bowel control. In the regressive group soiling may be regarded as a counteraggressive act against loss or aggression on the part of parents or siblings. In some instances soiling takes place when children are withholding defecation and represents fecal overflow around an impaction—a condition denoted as psychogenic megacolon. In this condition the soiling is sometimes mistakenly considered a diarrhea.

Treatment is usually difficult in those children brought to psychiatrists. Since the symptom is expressive of a family conflict, the parents must be involved as well as the child. Help is needed to bring the parents to avoid expressions of critical disgust toward the child which gives him the power to use the symptom as a counteraggressive expression to them. So, too, the family conflict or deficiencies in training inducing the symptom must be discovered and efforts made to bring about its correction. The mother must be discouraged from emphasizing the symptom by recourse to use of laxative and enemas. She must be assisted to bring the child to toilet regularly without recrimination or disgust, leaving him alone in the bathroom. Before doing so, the child should be given by mouth a peristaltic stimulant such as lemonade.

When the symptom has existed for years, it is usually necessary to separate the child from the family. This is best done in a child psychiatric unit where a staff is available to manage. Encopresis seldom presents beyond puberty.

FIRE-SETTING SYNDROME

Through its sometimes frightening and destructive consequences, fire-setting behavior in children and adolescents is a symptom complex of importance which demands immediate attention. Watching fires and learning to light fires and extinguish them are exciting and pleasurable for most children, perhaps more so for boys than girls. Usually first experienced under supervision by parents and adults at an early age, many youngsters indulge in preparing, setting, watching, and extinguishing fires. This playful activity is not pathological. However, when the individual child indulges repetitively and his actions take on destructive overtones, the motivations are usually neurotically determined.

Fire-setting occurs infrequently even among seriously disturbed children. Bender found only 60 instances among 1755 disturbed children under 15. The vast majority of fire-setters are boys. The fire-setting child or adolescent is usually reported to have expressed other antisocial behavior; generalized aggression, stealing, and truancy are common. Also, he may have a learning disability or some physical handicaps.

Fire-setting occurs among younger children and in adolescents, but the two groups are not distinctive, as some of the young child fire-setters once again indulge in adolescence. In the younger group the act often has as its dynamic aggression as revenge directed against some significant person. Among adolescents the same motivation exists but also complicated by sexual motivations, as well as fantasies of union or reunion. The majority of fire-setters are diagnosed as psychotic or borderline.

In the younger group the fire-setters usually show evidence of acute anxiety. They have frightening nightmares and fantasies. Many seem to come from homes where the father is involved with making or maintaining of fires; others have close associations with firemen. These children set fires near their homes and do so in association with fantasies of burning some family member who has seemed to reject them or to displace them from a favored role with the parents.

Among adolescents the act is more complex and the fires set often are dangerous and seriously destructive, thought through, and planned in advance. Often the fire-setting is carried out by a pair of adolescent boys. One is the organizer and director and the more dominant; the other is passive. Between the two there exists a homosexual bond. Once started, the fire-setter almost always remains to observe the fire and may assist those attempting its extinction. During the period of watching, they report sensing excitement, pleasure in power, sometimes sexual arousal, and discharge. Dreams of fire were noticed by Freud to occur in the enuretic, and enuresis has been noted as frequent in the history of fire-setters, suggesting among analysts that fire-setters be regarded as urethral erotic.

As Macht and Mack emphasize, fire-setting should be regarded as a complex syndrome in the adolescent with different motivations attaching to various segments of the behavioral sequence. For the most part the adolescent fire-setters were schizophrenic and mentally retarded. In all their cases the acts occurred when the patient's father was absent, arousing yearning, rage, and frustration owing to that absence. The patient identified with the father or his surrogates in fire departments, thus determining fire-setting as a preferred act. Observing and extinguishing the fire, set to relieve anxiety related to the aggressive drive, seems to serve as a means of alleviating the guilt attached

to that drive, mastering and controlling it. Both dependent and sexual frustration underlay the need to express aggression through fire-setting. Impulse control may be viewed for the act through identification with the absent parent.

TREATMENT. Because of the seriousness of this symptom and its potential harmfulness to both the child or adolescent and the community, immediate decision should be made to bring the individual into treatment. Initially hospital treatment is indicated. Removal from the home usually brings about cessation of the fire-setting.

M. L.,* a 16-year-old, female high school student and only child, entered the hospital after having set five small grass fires in a park. One year prior to her admission, the patient's father, a merchant seaman who served as a fireman in the engine room aboard ship, had suddenly left home on a sea voyage. He had not been to sea in many years and had held fireman jobs (working in boiler rooms, stoking furnaces, etc.) on land. The patient had favored his going back to sea and had taken his side against her mother in the discussion leading up to his leaving. Subsequent to his leaving, Mrs. L. became depressed and withdrawn and developed intractable vomiting. The mother spent two weeks with a friend during which time the frightened girl lived alone at home. When Mrs. L. returned, she was still suffering from vomiting and the patient was forced to take care of her. This continued for some six months, during which time the patient became more anxious and unhappy. When Mrs. L. failed to improve and the patient continued to worsen, they decided to move in with the paternal grandparents. Both mother and daughter rapidly improved and two months prior to admission they moved into an apartment of their own near that of the grandparents. The patient became progressively more anxious, especially at night. Frequently, she would ask Mrs. L. to stay with her in her bed, which the mother would do. She began to attend school erratically, preferring to stay at home with her mother, who at the time noted that M. L. was becoming increasingly angry at Mrs. L. for reasons of which the mother was unaware. The anniversary of the father's leaving on his voyage coincided with Mrs. L's receiving a letter saying that he would be home in a month's time for a short visit and would then return to sea. The patient felt happy

---

* This case is quoted, with gratitude for permission to use it here, from the paper by Lee B. Macht, M. D., and John F. Mack, M.D., as given in the Bibliography under the Fire-Setter Syndrome.

at first that he was coming back, and then dis-
appointed, angry, and despondent that he would
be leaving again shortly. She talked at length with
a girlfriend, felt very close to this girl, and was
relieved. However, upon leaving her, she suddenly
felt the urge to set a fire. She set five small grass
fires in a park and then turned in the alarm and
stayed to watch the firemen put them out. She
told her mother of this behavior in hopes that
Mrs. L. would have her hospitalized, but Mrs. L.
did not believe her. Two days later she set fire to
her coat sleeve, after which she was hospitalized.
She was seen in intensive psychotherapy, two or
three times a week, over the next several months in
the hospital, and then as an outpatient for a total
of two years.

Her past history contained the following pertinent data. When the patient was 5 years of age,
Mr. L. (with whom the girl always spent a great
deal of time and was very close) left for his first
sea voyage since her birth. The mother observed
that as soon as the father left, the patient became
"extremely clinging and cried a great deal and
was very sad." Mrs. L. stated that the patient would
even follow her to the toilet and would not allow
her to be out of sight. She noted that the patient
"demanded to sleep in the same bed" with her,
which was allowed. Mr. L. returned after an absence of three months, and the patient immediately
"calmed down and was just like she was before"
(according to the mother). The father did not go
away again until the time we have already noted.

The patient recalled observing several fires
during the years from 8 to 12. In particular, she
recalled seeing a large grass fire while on a walk
with her father. She remembered enjoying the
scene and she remembered her own and also her
father's excitement at the fire. She later recalled
that he told her of lighting fires when he was a
boy. Mr. L. corroborated his early history of fire-
setting, saying that he had set several "small fires
in the woods as a teenager." He alluded to the
fact that he still "loves fires" and will go out of
his way "to see a good fire."

Observation of the patient's behavior when her
mother and father visited on the ward was striking.
The mother sat placidly watching as father and
daughter paraded around the hospital arm in arm.
She was virtually ignored—as was almost everyone
else—by the twosome. This corresponded to interview material with the patient at that time having
to do with wanting "to be with him and always
close to him." She said she planned "to join him
and live with him in Japan after his next trip."
She added as an afterthought, "Mother will come
along too, of course."

Mr. L. left for the sea again rather suddenly.
The patient, who had been more outgoing on the
ward during his visit, became quite withdrawn.
She later described feeling progressively more and
more "anxious and angry." She felt "like explod-
ing, like setting a big fire or something." She asked
a female attendant with whom she had been
speaking to call a doctor to talk to her (she knew

there was a male doctor on call). During the time
she waited, she tried to play cards with some
female patients but found she was "becoming
more panicky" with them. She then tried to read
but felt no better. Finally, in desperation she
took a cold shower but still felt the same. She
remarked that she "needed to cool off." Then, "as
all else had failed," she set the shower curtain and
some window curtains on fire and immediately
"felt relieved." When the doctor arrived, she was
already calm and in excellent control.

Interview material almost a year after the fire in
the hospital revealed that she had felt "furious at
him (father) for going again, and leaving me with
Mother. I couldn't stand that again, it hurt too
much. I like my mother, true, but be alone with
her . . . and have to take care of her . . . I'm sorry,
that would have been too close." She continued,
"I wanted him home. . . . I couldn't stand his
going away again. I would have done anything to
get him to stay. But he loved the sea . . . more
than me and I hated him for that. I think I hated
him so much that I wished he were there . . . in
the fire."

* * *

Eight months later the patient wrote to the
therapist from a distant city saying she wished to
correspond with him. She reported that she was
well and self-supporting but that she felt "ikky."

* * *

To our knowledge, she has not resorted to fire-
setting since the hospital episode.

BIBLIOGRAPHY

Speech Disturbances

Barbara, D. (ed.): The Psychotherapy of Stuttering.
Springfield, Ill., Charles C Thomas, 1962.
Gould, E., and Sheehan, J.: Effect of silence on
stuttering. J. Abnorm. Psychol., *72:*441–445, 1968.
Johnson, W.: Problems of impaired speech and
language. J.A.M.A., *170:*2102–2103, 1959.

Learning Disturbances

de Hirsch, K.: Two categories of learning diffi-
culties in adolescents. Amer. J. Orthopsychiat.,
*33:*87–91, 1963.
de Hirsch, K., Jansky, J. J., and Langford, W. S.:
Predicting Reading Failure. New York, Harper
& Row, 1966.
Johnson, D. J., and Myklebust, H. R.: Learning
Disabilities. New York, Grune & Stratton, 1967.

Tics

Bruch, H., and Thum, L. C.: Maladie des tics and
maternal psychosis. J. Nerv. Ment. Dis., *146:*446–
456, 1968.

Gerard, M. W.: The psychogenic tic in ego development. Psychoanal. Stud. Child., 2:133–162, 1946.

Mahler, M. S., and Luke, J. A.: Outcome of the tic syndrome. J. Nerv. & Ment. Dis., 103:433–445, 1946.

Disorders of Sleep

Broughton, R. J.: Sleep disorders: Disorders of arousal? Science, 159:1070–1078, 1968.

Fisher, C.: A psychophysiological study of nightmares. J. Amer. Psychoanal. Assn., 18:747–782, 1970.

Kales, A., and Kales, J.: Evaluation, diagnosis and treatment of classical conditions related to sleep. J.A.M.A., 213:2229–2235, 1970.

Schneck, J. M., and Fuselli, H.: Nightmare and sleep paralysis. J.A.M.A., 20:725–726, 1969.

Zung, W. W. K.: The pharmacology of disordered sleep: A laboratory approach. Int. Psychiat. Clin., 7:123–146, 1970.

Feeding Disturbances

Cooper, P.: Pica. Springfield, Ill., Charles C Thomas, 1957.

Enuresis

Drooby, A. S.: A reliable truce with enuresis. Dis. Nerv. Syst., 25:97–100, 1964.

Gerard, M. W.: Enuresis: A study in etiology. Amer. J. Orthopsychiat., 9:48–58, 1939.

Mariuz, M. J., and Walters, C. J.: Enuresis in nonpsychotic boys treated with imipramine. Amer. J. Psychiat., 120:597–599, 1963.

Oppel, W. C., Harper, P. A., and Reder, R. V.: Social, psychologic and neurologic factors associated with enuresis. Pediatrics, 42:627–641, 1968.

Ritvo, E. R.: Contributions of sleep research to understanding and treatment of enuresis. Int. Psychiat. Clinic, 7:111–122, 1970.

Encopresis

Bellman, M.: Studies on encopresis. Acta Paediat. Scand., Suppl. 170, 1966.

Silber, D. L.: Encopresis: Discussion of etiology and management. Clin. Pediat., 8:225–231, 1969.

Fire-Setting

Macht, L. B., and Mack, J. F.: The firesetter syndrome. Psychiatry, 31:277–288, 1968.

Chapter 30

Mental Retardation

Definition

There exists a large group of individuals whose personality limitations rest essentially upon failure to develop sufficient intellectual capacity to cope with the demands of their environment and thus to establish an independent social existence. This lack of intellectual capacity derives from an innately imposed limitation in cerebral development, is the result of disease or injury to the brain suffered before, during, or in the immediate period after birth, or is the consequence of impaired maturation due to insufficient environmental stimulation from familial and cultural sources.

In the early years of developmental impairment, the rate of maturation or the acquisition of various sensorimotor activities most frequently provides the evidence for the diagnosis of mental deficiency. Thus delays or failures in the sequential evolution of motility, language, control of evacuation of the bladder and bowel, and ability to interact with other children provide the clues. Inability to acquire and retain knowledge as the result of experience is an indication of a deficiency in *learning ability* and is best observed during the child's school years. If the mental defect is mild, the child may show little evidence of it until he enters school. Social adaptation becomes important as an indicator of mental retardation, particularly at the adult level, but is reflected earlier in the individual's capacities to relate to parents, teachers, and peers.

In terms of intellectual functioning, the mentally retarded appear to have difficulty in retention and recall and thus in the acquisition of information. These lacks, in turn, limit their capacity for analysis and synthesis of information and for other than relatively simple efforts at problem solving. Under circumstances in which their intellectual capacities are overtaxed, whether these involve clear-cut intellectual tasks or a complex including emotional and social factors, these individuals appear inept and deficient in planning and judgment. When not taxed beyond their capacities, provided their emotional development has been healthy, they perform well in accustomed social and vocational settings.

Prevalence

Owing to the differences in criteria for the diagnosis of mental retardation, as well as the varying cultural tolerances for and demands upon the subnormal and also the individual's capacity to relate to his peers, comparative estimates of prevalence are difficult to assess. Thus, 1 to 4 per cent of the population are considered educationally subnormal in different countries, and another 6 to 9 per cent are so impaired intellectually that they require special education within the school system. In the United States various estimates have shown that 3 per cent of the children born annually will never achieve the intellect of a 12-year-old, 0.3 per cent will fall below the level of the 7-year-old, and 0.1 per cent will be so impaired in their intellectual capacity that they will remain completely helpless throughout their lives, incapable of caring for themselves in any way.

In Great Britain, where registers of the mentally retarded have been kept by local health authorities commencing with the Mental Deficiency Act of 1913, the rate of subnormality may be drawn well for specific population groups. Susser reports that in the industrial town of Sulford this rate was 44 per 1000. A similar rate was discovered in rural Anglesey.

When the age and sex of the mentally subnormal are examined as to distribution from such local register reports, it becomes clear that the rates for both young and old are very low when compared with the excess figures for the adolescents and young adults. Susser states that permanent biological attributes present at birth could produce such a distribution. His conclusion is that *recognized* mental retardation must be a social attribute. Furthermore, recognition is determined by the social roles demanded of individuals at each stage of life. Although the capacity to fulfill such roles rests upon the biological inherited structure of each individual, the complexity of the social roles determines the stress of those roles for each individual. In modern societies education and training are necessary to undertake many of the new roles, and in consequence the standardized school system makes it impossible for many to achieve the skills and aptitudes necessary to succeed. A new type of retardation has come into being.

The more physically impaired an individual is born, the earlier his social limitations will be recognized. The low grade defective or idiot scores less than 20 on intelligence tests, the medium grade or imbecile will have I.Q.s from 20 to 50, and the high grade or feeble-minded over that level. In an approximation of distribution between these groups about 10 per cent will be found in the low grade category, 40 per cent in the medium grade, and 50 per cent in the high grade. It is the latter who are discovered in adolescence and early adulthood when confronted by the complex social roles

of modern society. Those severely retarded owing to obvious biological deficiencies are discovered early in life as they fail to keep pace with other infants and children in their growth and development. The medium grade become conspicuous as their weaknesses are exposed during schooling. In the Susser analysis only 1 in 20 of the middle grade had been detected by five years, seven of ten by 15. Thirty per cent of this group were not recognized until after leaving school.

The vast majority of the retarded live in local communities, and many make satisfactory social adaptations. Others require special training in order to allow them to perform simple tasks and care for their own needs. The remainder require institutional care. While in the past it has been estimated that one bed per 1000 population should be provided in institutions for the mentally defective, the nature of those admitted has been changing in recent years. Thus, in the United States, there has been an increased admission of those with lower grades of defect associated with brain damage. The shift in the population of defectives in public institutions remains unexplained. There are those who relate it to increased survival at birth due to more effective prenatal and natal care. Others have suggested that the increase of special facilities in local communities has allowed the local management of the higher-grade retarded.

Today some point out that civilization tends to preserve the unfit and that therefore a general decline in physique and intelligence is to be feared. Penrose, an outstanding English investigator of mental deficiency, is of the opinion that the number of defective and subnormal individuals is not steadily increasing. He concludes that propagation of the unfit is not a danger to the community because such persons tend to propagate less efficiently. In his opinion, decisions about segregation or other disposition of high-grade defectives should be based solely on medical, psychological, and social grounds; he maintains that the equilibrium with respect to biological fitness and intelligence level will be retained. Probably the only areas where the average intelligence is falling are certain small rural communities in which there has been inbreeding of poor mental stock and a rapid emigration of better stock. The incidence of mental defect, particularly at the moron level, is distinctly higher in rural than in urban areas.

DETERMINATION OF INTELLECTUAL RETARDATION

In order to determine whether a child who is suspected of being mentally retarded really is, and in order to outline constructive treatment, one should study the many factors which led not only to his intellectual defect but to his unique personality pattern. If one or both of the child's parents are known to be defective, it may be found that heredity has been an important factor. It should be kept in mind, however, that intellectually retarded parents contribute not only defective genes but usually a home atmosphere deficient in intellectual, social, and personality-forming influences, restricting the potentiality of mental growth.

In many of the severely subnormal there is some evidence either of a general biological inferiority or of the sequelae of former traumatic or inflammatory processes in the central nervous system. Other evidences of a biological inferiority are anomalies of the skull, such as microcephaly, oxycephaly or tower-shaped skull, hydrocephalus, the spherical skull of the mongoloid, and asymmetry of the skull. Low frontotemporal hairline, asymmetries of the face, malformations of the external ear, anomalies of the eye and its appendages, uncomeliness of the nose, thickness of the lips, receding or protruding mandible, imperfectly formed or irregular erupted teeth, and malformation of the palate are much more frequent in mentally defective individuals than among persons of average intelligence. For those who wish to consult an atlas demonstrating extraordinarily well through color photographs the many varieties of physical deformity encountered among those with severe mental retardation, the writer recommends the one prepared by Gillis and Feingold and published recently by the United States Government Printing Office. In addition to the physical deformities often seen in the severely retarded, electroencephalography frequently reveals abnormality in both standard and sleep recordings.

In most severely retarded children there will be a history of delay in the development of physiological, psychological, or social functions. In the newborn, early indications of deficit are shown in weakness or absence of the sucking, Moro, and grasping reflexes, and of crying in response to painful stimuli, closure of the eyelids, and contraction of the pupils. The infant shows apathy, difficulties in sucking, and, later, delay in commencing to use his motor apparatus at the customary stage of maturation.

The healthy child smiles by the second month, and crying is now accompanied by tears. The head and eyes turn toward sounds. At the fourth month, the child usually begins to hold up his head; two months later he should be able to sit for several minutes. At this time, he should begin to crawl, may grasp for objects, holds up his arms to be taken, and distinguishes people. At the tenth month, he should stand, and at one year he should take a few steps, say "Mama" and one or two other words and recognize toys. At 18 months, he should be walking well. Delay in the acquisition of these motor skills suggests impaired cerebral development.

There exists an important relation between intelligence and the capacity for development of correct and distinct speech. The degree of intelligence is closely indicated by the age of acquisition of speech; by the character of articulation, i.e., whether the articulation is clear, slovenly, slurring, or jerking; by lalling, or the substitution of one consonant for another; and finally, by the extent of vocabulary, since this measures rather well the stock of ideas. Usually the normal child should be speaking a few words at one year and should articulate clearly between the ages of three and four.

A more valuable indication of the presence or absence of defect than either the history of school progress or an examination in school work is the practical knowledge and general information possessed by the individual. Here we find that the ability for breadth and accuracy of observation, and the capacity for comparison, planning, and discrimination essential for the successful solution of the practical problems connected with occupation and the business life, are inadequate in the mental defective. His range of knowledge, too, concerning common objects and events in his environment is limited. The defectives often vary in their ability to apply their intelligence to concrete life situations.

In considering the field of social history and behavior, it should be kept in mind that social incompetency does not necessarily mean social delinquency. Such chronic social problems as poverty and recidivism are associated not so much with mental defect as with a population of borderline intelligence. The extent to which criminality is a result of mental defect is usually overestimated. Studies by English psychiatrists show that the percentage of criminals who are retarded mentally is about 3.5. Probably the percentage in the United States is about the same. The percentage of criminals of borderline intelligence is doubtless higher. Although acquisitive crimes occur most frequently both among the feeble-minded and those of normal intelligence, it is estimated that serious sexual offenses are nearly ten times as common among defectives as among ordinary criminals.

Individual psychological as well as social factors contribute to delinquency among the feeble-minded. In the borderline defective, especially, it will be found that the precipitating factors of his delinquencies are emotional ones. Some be-havior disorders may represent a rebellion against, or a flight from, a difficult environment. If the feeble-minded child is rejected by his home, feelings of hatred and resentment may be stimulated and transferred to all parental surrogates. Again, aggressive and destructive behavior may represent a compensation for an underlying sense of inadequacy. Some defective individuals, through their wish to gain recognition, are easily led into delinquency by stronger, dominant personalities. Because the defective person obtains thrills and satisfactions so quickly, he is apt to follow those who show evidence of bold and vicious behavior.

Degree of Retardation

In Chapter 28, Behavior Disorders of Childhood and Adolescence, the methods of examination of the child were described, including the various psychological tests now used to determine mental functioning. From such tests as the Wechsler-Bellevue may be derived an Intelligence Quotient, which, as stated there, must be recognized as representing only the current functioning of the individual at the time the test was administered. The term *borderline intelligence* is often used for those with I.Q. scores consistently in the 70 to 90 range.

Since general intelligence tests are valid only if they measure overall capacity to solve mental problems, in recognition of the limitations of all presently available tests, the American Association for Mental Deficiency has proposed a *behavioral classification* of deficit which consists of the two dimensions of *measured intelligence* and *adaptive behavior*. Thus the measured intelligence dimension is scaled into five levels in terms of Standard Deviation units* which describe the distribution of test scores in the general

---

* A statistical unit which expresses the dispersion from the mean of a range of measurements in a sample.

population. The adaptive behavior dimension classifies four levels of behavior in the two areas of degree: to function and maintain oneself independently and to meet satisfactorily the culturally imposed demands of personal and social responsibility. This scale is given in the accompanying table.

Additional scales should be used to supplement the clinical judgments. For example, the Vineland Social Maturity Scale is useful at the preschool level and may be supplemented by items from the Gesell Developmental Schedules, the Cattell Infant Intelligence Scale, and the Kuhlmann Tests of Mental Development.

TERMINOLOGY. There is a tendency to discontinue the use of the descriptive terms idiot, imbecile, and moron. Since, however, they are still occasionally used,

their definition, as adopted in 1934 by the American Association on Mental Deficiency, may be quoted: "An idiot is a mentally defective person usually having a mental age of less than three years, or if a child, an intelligence quotient less than 25. An imbecile is a mentally defective person usually having a mental age of three years to seven years, inclusive. A moron is a mentally defective person usually having a mental age of eight years or upwards, or if a child, an I.Q. of 50 or more." As for the I.Q., the Association stated: "As a rule the upper limit for a diagnosis of mental deficiency should be an I.Q. of 69, but this limit should not be adhered to in cases where medical, social, and other factors clearly indicate that the patient is mentally defective."

*Adaptive Behavior Classification**

	PRE-SCHOOL AGE 0–5 MATURATION AND DEVELOPMENT	SCHOOL-AGE 6–21 TRAINING AND EDUCATION	ADULT 21 SOCIAL AND VOCATIONAL ADEQUACY
Level I	Gross retardation; minimal capacity for functioning in sensori-motor areas; needs nursing care.	Some motor development present; cannot profit from training in self-help; needs total care.	Some motor and speech development; totally incapable of self-maintenance; needs complete care and supervision.
Level II	Poor motor development; speech is minimal; generally unable to profit from training in self-help; little or no communication skills.	Can talk or learn to communicate; can be trained in elemental health habits; cannot learn functional academic skills; profits from systematic habit training. ("Trainable")	Can contribute partially to self-support under complete supervision; can develop self-protection skills to a minimal useful level in controlled environment.
Level III	Can talk or learn to communicate; poor social awareness; fair motor development; may profit from self-help; can be managed with moderate supervision.	Can learn functional academic skills to approximately 4th grade level by late teens if given special education. ("Educable")	Capable of self-maintenance in unskilled or semi-skilled occupations; needs supervision and guidance when under mild social or economic stress.
Level IV	Can develop social and communication skills; minimal retardation in sensori-motor areas; rarely distinguished from normal until later age.	Can learn academic skills to approximately 6th grade level by late teens. Cannot learn general high school subjects. Needs special education, particularly at secondary school age levels. ("Educable")	Capable of social and vocational adequacy with proper education and training. Frequently needs supervision and guidance under serious social or economic stress.

* Reprinted from Sloan, W., and Birch, J. W.: A rationale for degrees of retardation. Amer. J. Ment. Def., *60*:258–264, 1955-1956.

Among these severely retarded, the expectations for life are less than for the general population. Losses from this population are less than in the past; as medical care has improved, their survival time has been prolonged. Thus in the group with Down's syndrome (mongolism) alone, prevalence has risen from 1 per 4000 in 1929 to 1 per 1000 in 1958. There exists a controversy at present as to whether more new cases are added to this population owing to better general medical care than in the past, or whether this care has, in fact, reduced the number.

As for those with mild retardation, it is of interest that in the Salford studies, reported by Susser, in adulthood two-thirds of these persons were no longer carried in the local register as impaired. In terms of their social functioning they had improved! Such findings have been reported from other countries, as well, where many later are found well employed, married, and with families.

The groups who fail socially in adult life are those who have been detained for antisocial behavior, because of either delinquency or transgressions of the sexual codes. The majority come from broken homes or severely disrupted families known to social agencies. Their failure to adapt derives essentially from the deficiencies in the family structure which establish the capacity for affective ties, and inculcation of the necessary superego standards and ego ideals upon which depend much of successful adult adaptation.

APPARENT DEFECT. Several writers, notably Kanner, have called attention to a group of children who have often been neglected. This is composed of those who may be described as apparently feeble-minded or pseudo-feeble-minded. In many cases persons have been declared feeble-minded solely upon the basis of their intelligence quotient. Although usually the I.Q. correctly measures a person's intellectual capacity, at times conditions may mask a child's intellectual potentialities. Among such conditions are blindness, deafness, spasticity, specific reading or numerical disability, or emotional blocking, with consequent inhibition of intelligent behavior or of responses in psychometric tests.

The child with sensory defects often leads an isolated existence, full of frustrations and confusion and deprived of certain necessary types of stimulation and information, with the result that he may not demonstrate his real intellectual potential. Sometimes a learning difficulty actually caused by emotional retardation may be mistaken for an organic deficiency. Occasionally the awkwardness of the examiner stimulates a negativism that prevents an accurate assessment of intelligence. The author is familiar with the case of a child whose admission to the public school system was refused because of his alleged imbecility as demonstrated by psychometric tests. The boy's parents, knowing that he was not feeble-minded, sent him to a private school where he soon demonstrated that he was of superior intelligence. At the usual age he entered a university, from which he graduated with honors.

The "idiot savants" are an uncommon subgroup among those of subnormal intelligence who often amaze by their highly developed intellectual capacity in some isolated area of functioning. One such patient seen by the author accurately and rapidly added six-digit numbers presented quickly to him. He could stand at a railroad crossing and add the numbers painted on the sides of successive cars in trains made up to over seventy units. In the recent pair of "idiot savant" twins studied by Horwitz et al., these brothers demonstrated a phenomenal capacity as calendar calculators. They have a remarkable memory for dates. Given a remote date, they are capable of instantly replying with the weekday of the date requested. Of the hypotheses put forward to explain this unusual incongruity in intellectual behavior, suggestions range from the existence of an unusual eidetic imagery, of mechanisms utilizing memory and repetition as substitutes for usual learning, or the existence of computer-like mechanisms in the brain. In the twins studied by Horwitz et al., the conclusion was reached that the subjects memorized a conventional calendar—one mastering a range of 400 years—an effort to which they devoted 15 years and in which they were assisted by a photographic memory. They were observed from the age of six spending hours looking at an almanac which contained a perpetual calendar, and later their father gifted one with a "perpetual" calendar with which they played for hours and hours.

ETIOLOGY

Mental deficiency, then, is a symptom associated with a large number of disease entities which affect the organism in its earliest stages of growth and development. It is not a clinical entity itself. The group of mentally retarded is by no means homogeneous; it is marked by wide dissimilarities in etiology, clinical phenomenology, and pathology linked only by the common criterion of subnormal intellect. To be excluded from the group are those instances of impairment of intellect which occur as the result of brain damage after adolescence and to which is applied the term dementia.

In the past it has been the custom often to classify the mental deficiencies in terms of the temporal relationship of the impairment factor to birth. From a clinical standpoint, it is convenient to divide them into those operating prior to birth, those resulting from injuries at birth, and those resulting from injuries or disease occurring after birth but before mental development has been fully attained.

The American Association on Mental Deficiency recently has recommended an etiologic classification of mental retardation with supplementary qualifications to indicate the existence of a genetic component, secondary cranial anomalies, impairment of special senses, and motor dysfunction. Since both classificatory systems are in use, a brief statement is provided of the etiologic factors recognized

to function in the *prenatal, neonatal,* and *postnatal* periods. Later, specifically defined entities are to be described under the suggested etiologic headings of the American Association on Mental Deficiency.

CAUSES ACTING BEFORE BIRTH. It is often difficult to determine whether a mental defect was caused by factors inherent in the genes or whether toxic, infectious, endocrine, traumatic, nutritional, and other prenatal pathogenic factors operating on the germ cell or within the pregnant mother tended to weaken or distort developmental capacity of the brain. Among prenatal factors may be pertussis, mumps, and other viral infections, particularly the virus of rubella, which late in the first trimester of pregnancy may pass through the placenta and damage the brain. Anomalies of various organs often coexist with the defect.

Other causes may be toxoplasmosis, Rh incompatibility (usually if the fetus is Rh-positive and the mother Rh-negative), the influences responsible for the chromosomal nondisjunction causing mongolism, and also damage to the fetus by therapeutic doses of roentgen rays. Fetal oxygen deficiency as a cause of brain damage and subsequent mental defect usually occurs during labor but may happen earlier also. The mental deficiency of cretinism may be caused by thyroid deficiency at a very early prenatal age or may be coincidental with the hormonal defect rather than caused by it. Toxic, anoxic, and infectious states which, in the adult nervous system, may be reversible or completely recoverable can produce permanent changes in the fetal neural structures, leading to impairment of developmental potentiality. There are doubtless many possible causes for a failure of, or for accident to, neural evolution in intrauterine life, but they are inadequately understood. The extent to which feeble-mindedness is caused by congenital syphilis is uncertain but probably does not exceed 1 per cent. It is now a much less frequent cause than formerly.

Premature births, particularly those with birth weight less than 2500 gm., and maternal malnutrition are associated as well with the birth of a greater number of children with mental defect than average.

Probably from 50 to 65 per cent of the cases of feeble-mindedness arise from poorly understood causes existing prior to birth. It is now agreed that hereditary transmission of mental defect plays a much less important role than was previously believed.

CAUSES ACTING AT BIRTH. Birth trauma resulting in either mechanical injury to the brain or asphyxia with resulting anoxia may be a cause of mental defect. In recent years the surgical removal of subdural hematomas has prevented some degree of mental defect which would otherwise have followed birth injury. The most frequent immediate causes of cerebral hemorrhage at birth are prematurity and difficult labor. Asphyxia at birth is a common cause of mental defect. If the resulting anoxemia exists sufficiently long, it will produce permanent degeneration of the ganglion cells of the cerebral cortex, with resulting impairment of mental capacity. It is estimated that about 8 per cent of the mental defects result from causes acting at birth. Probably, however, 50 per cent of the children showing clinical evidence of brain injury are not mentally defective.

CAUSES ACTING AFTER BIRTH. The various forms of viral and bacterial encephalitis and of meningitis are the most frequent factors acting after birth in the production of feeble-mindedness. Although head trauma with brain damage in infancy or early childhood occasionally results in feeble-mindedness, this is much overemphasized by the laity. In institutionalized mental defectives, it will be found that the defect in about 1.5 per cent of the inmates is the result of postnatal cerebral trauma. Toxemia and vitamin deficiency in infancy and early childhood may, if long continued, produce irreversible changes in the cortex with varying degrees of mental retardation. Convulsive disorders often accompany mental defects resulting from organic disease of the brain.

In the congenitally blind and deaf, the reduced number of stimuli received from exteroceptors results in a certain degree of mental defect unless compensatory training is provided. It is generally agreed, too, that retardation in intellectual development may be caused by emotional factors without organic defect. Probably from 25 to 30 per cent of the cases of feeble-mindedness result from causes acting after birth.

ETIOLOGIC CLASSIFICATION

DUE TO INFECTION

Although there remains controversy as to whether maternal infections cause congenital brain damage without direct infections of the growing fetus, there is much evidence to show that in many conditions a direct fetal brain infection does take place. At times this infection may occur without clinical evidence of illness of the mother.

Cytomegalic inclusion body disease is a mild or subclinical virus infection in the mother which causes fetal brain damage, hepatosplenomegaly, erythroblastosis, and jaundice. It is recognized by inclusion bodies in the urine, cerebrospinal fluid, and other tissues of the infant.

Congenital rubella, associated with illness of the mother in the first trimester of pregnancy, causes mental deficit and other congenital anomalies such as deafness, cataract, and cardiac malformations. It has been found that there is a direct relationship between the period of the maternal infection and the frequency of occurrence of abnormality in the infant. Approximately 50 per cent of live-born children are abnormal if the mother is infected in the first month of pregnancy, 15 per cent in the second month, and 10 per cent in the third month.

Influenza contracted by the mother during pregnancy has been associated with mental deficiency consequent to malformation of the infantile brain.

Congenital syphilis is diagnosed on the basis of maternal infection with positive serologic tests for syphilis and the various signs of congenital syphilis in the child, including Hutchinson's teeth, interstitial keratitis, choroidoretinitis, and pupillary abnormalities. Juvenile paresis, another form, is discussed in Chapter 13.

Toxoplasmosis is due to infection *in utero* from the mother with the protozoan-like organism, *Toxoplasma*. At birth, or shortly thereafter, the infant may show wasting, convulsions, spasticity, choroidoretinitis, hydrocephalus, or microcephaly.

Finally, other infectious processes incurred by the fetus, such as meningococcal meningitis and equine encephalitis, can cause mental deficiency.

DUE TO INTOXICATION

Bilirubin encephalopathy (kernicterus) may follow any condition which produces jaundice with a high level of serum bilirubin in the newborn. Since kernicterus may now be prevented by exchange transfusions, recognition of the potential danger of high levels of bilirubin in the first few days of birth is highly important. It is now widely accepted that a value of 20 mg. of bilirubin per 100 ml. of plasma is indication for such transfusion, even though there is wide variability in the occurrence of this encephalopathy when correlated directly with plasma levels of bilirubin.

Stern has found that phenobarbital administered to expectant mothers during the last weeks of pregnancy will lower the newborn infant's serum bilirubin. He has recommended that such treatment be started in Rh immunized mothers in the thirty-second week of pregnancy. Infants with diabetic mothers or those infants with prenatal distress or those badly bruised with excessive red cell breakdown have been given the drug for the first five days of life in doses of 8 mg. per kg. per day. Such infants cleared bilirubin from the blood, the action taking place by the drug enhancing the liver's glucuronide-forming capacity. Exposure of infants with neonatal jaundice to sunlight also lowers the serum bilirubin level by converting bilirubin to its water-soluble derivatives which do not cross the blood-brain barrier and are readily excreted. Infants so exposed seem to be protected from kernicterus. In many patients this exposure appeared to eliminate the need for exchange transfusion.

The cause of the increased bilirubin levels in the blood is related to insufficiency in glucuronide formation in the newborn period due to a reduced amount of liver glucuronyl transferase, the enzyme responsible for conjugating bilirubin, as well as a deficiency in the donor substrate, uridine diphosphate. Often it is due to Rh incompatibility between the fetus and the mother, but it also may result from other blood incompatibilities, including those between A, B, and O types.

In the absence of blood incompatibility, kernicterus is associated often with prematurity and neonatal sepsis. The early stages of kernicterus are difficult to determine, but the condition may be assumed in the presence of drowsiness, poor feeding, unstable body temperature, a high-pitched cry, and alterations in the Moro reflex. Opisthotonus, loss of the Moro reflex, and ocular signs are indicative of marked damage. Mental defect, choreoathetosis, and deafness are the common late sequelae.

Pathologic studies of the brain show yellow staining with bilirubin in the basal ganglia, cerebellar nuclei, hippocampus, and medulla, and, when severe, loss of cells, glioses, and demyelination are noticed.

Encephalopathies, caused by lead or carbon monoxide or following the post-serum and post-vaccinal encephalitides, are other more frequent causes of retardation due to intoxication. Lead poisoning has been discussed in Chapter 18.

DUE TO TRAUMA OR PHYSICAL AGENT

Difficulties of labor, such as those occurring with malposition or malpresentation of the child or disproportion between the head of the child and the pelvis of the mother, can cause damage to the infant's brain at birth. Common lesions with birth injury are meningeal tears and rupture of blood vessels and brain substance, often with intracerebral bleeding. Considerable hemorrhage leads later to brain softening and cyst formation, particularly after difficult forceps delivery. The falx cerebri or tentorium may be torn, resulting in subarachnoid or subdural hemorrhage. With time the structural evidence of acute injury at birth is supplanted in the process of repair with such nonspecific tissue changes as glioses, cavitation, and areas of defective myelination.

The *diagnosis* of severe injury at birth may be immediately inferred with pallor of the infant, inability to make sucking movements, respiratory distress, high-pitched feeble cry, tense or depressed fontanel, nystagmus, and retinal hemorrhage. At later stages of growth, the brain-injured child may be overactive or underactive and show fluctuations of muscle tone, impaired associated movements, primitive reflex activity, difficulties in convergence, and trouble with posture.

The growing child finds himself at a disadvantage in learning *complex motor skills* such as walking, climbing, skating, and cycling, even though there may exist few or none of the classical neurological signs of damage to the motor system. *Perceptual processes* are impaired, and normal responses to stimuli are limited. The child with injury of the visual portion of the brain may discriminate with difficulty foreground from background or may show an inability to remember sounds, localize their source, and discriminate pitch; he also may present incapacity in perceiving and understanding spoken language. Some children have an inability to discriminate tactual stimuli.

The development of *social behavior* is deviate due to confusion and frustration, and although the most frequently encountered tendency is toward hyperactive aggressive behavior, other children may be passive and withdrawn or show ritualistic and compulsive activity. The symptomatic picture in an individual patient is highly specific, depending upon the locations, extent, and degree of the brain injuries. Thus there does not exist a universal clinical picture, and the clinician will make the diagnosis without the presence of the full range of sensory-motor or behavioral disturbances.

Mental deficiency of this type is caused as well by asphyxia at birth due to interference with the placental circulation, overdosage with anesthetic agents or drugs depressing respiration, or, much more rarely, by prenatal irradiation of the uterus.

DUE TO DISORDERS OF METABOLISM, GROWTH, OR NUTRITION

Perhaps in no other area has so much new understanding accrued from research in the past decade as in that concerned with the abnormalities of brain development due to the inherited specific metabolic defects. This group of conditions may be separated into those due to abnormalities in lipid, carbohydrate, and protein metabolism. The early recognition of many of these defects is highly important, since the institution of proper dietary measures may prevent or appreciably reduce the amount of brain damage and subsequent impairment of mental function.

Lipoidoses (Sphingolipoidoses)

There are four forms of rare lipoidoses, each characterized by varying organ accumulations of different fatty acid derivatives of the base sphingosine. Thus in amaurotic family idiocy (Tay-Sachs disease), ganglioside accumulates in the central nervous system; in Niemann-Pick disease deposits of sphingomyelin exist in the nervous system as well as in the reticuloendothelial system and in parenchymal cells; in Gaucher's disease the cerebroside, kerasin, collects in the nervous system only in the infantile form of the disease but regularly is found in excess in phagocytic cells in the spleen, liver, lymph nodes, and bone marrow; while in metachromatic leukodystrophy sulfatides accumulate in the white matter of the nervous system as well as in the liver, spleen, and kidney. These substances are normally present in all tissues but are present in greater amounts in the nervous system. The metabolic dysfunction which leads to their abnormal accumulation and their relationship to the impairment of brain function remains unknown.

Of the lipoidoses, the infantile form of Tay-Sachs disease is the most common. The condition is transmitted by a single recessive gene. Thus, although both parents may appear healthy, if both are carriers, the probability exists of one out of four children suffering the disease. Marriages producing affected children represent an increased occurrence of consanguinity. The majority of cases are from Jewish families, but non-Jewish are also affected.

At birth the infant seems normal, but within the first year the child's development is impeded. He becomes apathetic, appears to have muscular weakness, cannot hold his head steadily, and regresses in his ability to grasp objects. There is advancing visual deterioration, and ophthalmoscopic study of the retina shows a typical "cherry-red spot" in the macula. The course is progressive, with death ensuing in one to three years. In a late infantile form of the disease (Bielschowsky's disease) the onset is in the second or third years and it is more common in non-Jewish families.

Prenatal diagnosis of Tay-Sachs disease is now possible through culture of the cells of amniotic fluid obtained by transabdominal amniocentesis as early as the sixteenth week of pregnancy. In high risk pregnancies marked reduction is found in the enzyme hexosaminidase H in the amniotic fluid, in both cultured and uncultured cells from that fluid. Such diagnosis has allowed termination of pregnancy before birth of the affected child.

Within the nervous system pathologic changes are found in the brain, cord, and sympathetic system. Swelling and distortion are seen in the ganglion cells; their cytoplasm is often vacuolated and some are necrotic.

Niemann-Pick disease, transmitted as an autosomal recessive, manifests itself symptomatically by the time the infant is six months old. There is usually a regular progression to a fatal termination by the third year. Abdominal enlargement due to splenomegaly and hepatomegaly precede the indications of intellectual retrogression which ends in amentia, and is associated with such neurological signs as spasticity, abnormal movements, tremor, and convulsions.

Vacuolated leukocytes may be found in the blood of some patients with Niemann-Pick disease. Similar leukocytic vacuolation has been found in some unaffected parents and siblings of the patients, perhaps indicating that they are heterozygous carriers.

In the infantile form of *Gaucher's disease,* consisting of about one-third of the cases, the clinical picture is very similar to that of Niemann-Pick disease. The course is rapidly downhill. Diagnosis may be made by bone marrow aspiration. Plasma acid phosphatase is often elevated.

Metachromatic leukodystrophy is a familial condition, found in many countries, in which the affected child develops well during the first year or two but then becomes incoördinated and shows muscular weakness. Progressive impairment of brain function takes place, with both neurological and intellectual deficits leading eventually to death between the third and sixth years.

Chemical analysis of urinary sediments from a 24-hour collection for individual glycosphingolipids from affected patients with the illnesses will allow the differentiation of the specific glycosphingolipid through its abnormal accumulation. In the case of many of these conditions the diagnosis has been made by discovering that the level of activity of the respective enzymes is markedly reduced in preparations of the patient's leukocytes.

The only existing form of treatment for lipoidoses consists in nursing and maintenance of general health.

Aminoacidurias

Within the past decade there have been discovered a sizable number of specific defects in amino acid metabolism that cause mental deficiency. All are transmitted through a recessive autosomal gene. While these conditions are rare, their early diagnosis becomes increasingly important as some dietary regimens have been devised which prevent the evolution of brain damage and subsequent mental deficiency.

PHENYLKETONURIA. This is the most frequently encountered and most thoroughly understood of the specific metabolic disorders of protein. The condition was recognized in 1934 by Fölling, a Norwegian biochemist. Since the associated mental defect in this condition, as with other disturbances of protein metabolism, may be prevented by diagnosis shortly after birth and treatment with proper diet, early recognition is highly important.

This form of familial mental deficiency is inherited as a rare autosomal recessive. Since each parent is a heterozygous carrier, a quarter of the children will have the illness, one-half will be carriers, and a quarter will be healthy noncarriers. For each pregnancy the chances are one in four of having a phenylketonuric child and three in four of bearing a normal child. Approximately one case of phenylketonuria occurs in 25,000 births; in insti-

tutions 1 per cent are estimated to have this condition.

As Yu and O'Halloran report, there is a high rate of retardation among the children of mothers with phenylketonuria. In their series all of 12 children born of such mothers were retarded; ten were heterozygotic for the disease and two had a typical phenylketonuria. As serum phenylalanine levels are high in pregnant heterozygous women and this and other amino acids are readily transported across the placenta, Yu and O'Halloran recommend that measures be taken to reduce the occurrence of mental retardation in the nonphenylketonuric children of affected mothers. Such mothers should not nurse their children. Also, pregnancies should be planned and the diets of such women should be low in phenylalanine some weeks before conception. When pregnancy ensues and the mother has high serum levels of phenylalanine, consideration should be given to therapeutic abortion.

Heterozygous carriers may be detected through the use of the phenylalanine tolerance test. Four hours following the oral ingestion of L-phenylalanine in a dose of 0.1 gm. per kilogram of body weight, the blood level of such carriers will be in the neighborhood of 20 mg. of phenylalanine per 100 ml. A considerable proportion (5 to 15 per cent) of parents of these patients represent cousin marriages.

Diagnosis. Clinically, retardation in motor and mental development is observed before the end of the first year, and it is thought that all damage to the nervous system takes place within the first two years of life. Although most untreated patients learn to walk, few speak; a quarter have grand mal convulsions, and electroencephalographic abnormalities are even more common. The mental defect is severe, with the intelligence quotients usually below 50. Less than 10 per cent develop normal intelligence or only mild mental defect. The children usually have fair hair and blue eyes, and there is frequently an associated dermatitis. The stature is somewhat dwarfed, head measurements are less than normal, and the incisors are widely spaced. Accompanying the marked mental deficiency and the metabolic error are neurological manifestations generally regarded as an extrapyramidal syndrome. The posture of the patient is usually that of general flexion, with bent head and body; both flexor and extensor muscles are rigid, the deep reflexes are active, and many patients show hyperkinetic or dyskinetic manifestations, such as tremor and athetosis. Encephalograms suggest that the extrapyramidal signs may be referred to cortical atrophy of the frontal lobe.

The urine has a penetrating, musty odor and contains abnormal amounts of phenylalanine and its derivatives, phenylpyruvate and phenylacetate. Phenylpyruvic acid can be easily detected in the urine by adding a few drops of ferric chloride to an acidified specimen. An intense green color develops in the presence of phenylpyruvic acid. Other conditions and substances may lead to a false-positive test. For this reason the serum level should be examined, as the amino acid phenylalanine is found in increased amounts in the blood, spinal fluid, and perspiration. The blood levels reach 30 to 50 mg. per 100 ml. While the blood phenylalanine level is elevated within a day after birth, the urinary excretion of the amino acid and its derivatives does not occur for at least the first week of life. It is now recognized that a significant number of infants with elevated blood phenylalanine levels do not have the disease. Thus, to establish a firm diagnosis in the early weeks of life, both a positive blood test and a positive urine test should be obtained. This confirmation is needed because the early treatment by dietary restrictions, which carries with it the potential for inducing serious nutritional handicaps, should not be undertaken lightly.

All infants should have their urine tested for this condition between the third and ninth weeks. For siblings of a phenylketonuric, tests should be repeated every two weeks until the tenth week if serum phenylalanine levels cannot be obtained.

A few normal children show elevations of serum phenylalanine during the first six weeks of life.

According to present knowledge, the defect is caused by a blockage in the conversion of phenylalanine into tyrosine due to a deficiency of the enzyme phenylalanine hydroxylase, as shown by Jervis. Thus the unmetabolized amino acid accumulates in the body fluid and large amounts of its deaminated products— phenylpyruvic, phenyllactic, and phenylacetic acids—are excreted with it in the urine. The metabolism of the amino acids tyrosine and tryptophane is affected secondarily. The mechanism by which the defect in metabolism leads to failure in cerebral development remains unknown.

Pathologic findings consist of a diminution in brain size, glioses of the white matter, and retardation of myelinization. In brains of those dying later in life degenerative changes have been reported in the cortex and basal ganglia. There is a marked failure of myelinization of the nervous system.

Treatment. Treatment with a diet restricted in phenylalanine appears to both prevent and greatly limit cerebral damage, particularly when commenced before the child is 15 months of age. There is now available commercially an acid hydrolysate of casein with phenylalanine removed but supplemented with additional amino acids, minerals, and choline. It may be given at the level of 2.0 to 2.5 gm. per kilogram of body weight, with additional fats and carbohydrates to meet caloric requirements. The casein hydrolysate is supplied as Lofenalac, and the manufacturer provides full instructions for the diet. The phenylalanine levels of the blood serum should be maintained below 10 mg. per 100 ml. during the first year of life. How long the dietary restriction must be maintained in order to insure full cerebral maturation remains undetermined.

MAPLE SYRUP URINE DISEASE. This specific inherited defect in amino acid metabolism was described in 1954 by Menkes; it received its name from the characteristic maple syrup-like odor of the urine. Within the first week of life, the infant appears spastic, loses the Moro reflex, and then undergoes progressive cerebral deterioration, with death in a few months. Studies of the urine show marked increase in excretion of the branched-chain amino acids leucine, iso-leucine, and valine as well as methionine, but cystine and other amino acids are abnormally low. In this disease transami-nation of methionine and the branched amino acids occurs normally, with forma-tion of ketoacids, but further degradation is blocked, with accumulation of these four ketoacids and amino acids in the blood owing to absence of the enzyme that catalyzes decarboxylation. There also appears to be a secondary disturbance of tryptophan metabolism. Therapeutic studies with diets low in these acids are encouraging but require further evalua-tion.

Cystothioninuria, anginosuccinuria, ci-trullinuria, aspartylglycosaminuria, and histidinuria are other aminoacidurias dis-covered in a few mentally defective pa-tients. All these conditions are inherited, probably as autosomal recessives. They are diagnosed by chromatography. There are several conditions in which the body metabolism is normal but a defective renal reabsorption leads to overflow and loss of amino acids. The familial *Hartnup* disease is a generalized aminoaciduria associated with a pellagra-like rash, cere-bellar ataxia, and often mental deficit. Other patients have been reported to have little mental deficit but personality dis-turbances and dermatitis later in life.

Hereditary hyperammonemia, caused by an enzymatic defect in the liver at the ornithine transcarbamylase step of the urea cycle which impedes conversion of ammonia to urea, is of interest in that the brain astrocytic structure is transformed to Alzheimer II type. This cell type is found in the brain of adult patients with chronic liver disease.

Hyperuricemia in infants is associated with mental retardation in boys only. This condition, known as Lesch-Nyhan syndrome, is sex linked and is charac-terized by deficiency of hypoxanthine-guanine phosphoribosyltransferase, lead-ing to increased purine synthesis.

The child born with this condition demonstrates an extraordinary aggressive-ness toward his own body and toward others. The symptoms become apparent about the age of four months when the affected children develop spasticity, choreoathetotic movements and compul-sive self-biting of the mouth area and fingers. Later on this aggressivity may be directed toward others through hitting, punching, and biting. The condition is associated with elevation of the serum and cerebrospinal fluid uric acid. Treatment with probenecid or allopurinol diminishes the uricosemia.

A prenatal diagnosis may be made by study of cells obtained through transab-dominal amniocentesis. Amniotic cells from affected infants fail to take up hypoxanthine in the absence of the en-zyme. Termination of pregnancy may be undertaken if such prenatal diagnosis can be made.

It is of interest that hyperuricemia, diagnostic with gout in adults, has also been found by Anumonye and his associ-ates to be associated with the capacity of drive and a wide range of activities in business executives.

Defects in Carbohydrate Metabolism

GALACTOSEMIA. Galactose diabetes, a specific metabolic defect of carbohydrate metabolism inherited as an autosomal re-cessive trait, is productive of profound disturbance in growth and development and leads to mental retardation unless recognized early and properly treated. It appears that galactosemia represents a single block in the formation of the enzyme, galactose-l-P-uridyl transferase which leads to collection of galactose-l-phosphate in cells. The eventual effects of galactosemia relate to the amount and duration of galactose consumption and are reversible by removal of this substance from the diet.

The infant born with galactosemia seems to be normal for several days but shortly commences to show difficulty with feedings, vomits, and may develop diarrhea. If milk feeding is continued, there may occur jaundice, enlargement of the abdomen because of ascites and hepatomegaly, nuclear cataracts, and the indications of mental defect in delay in standing, walking, and talking. Sugar is present in the urine, which is nonfermentable with heat.

The condition may be diagnosed just after birth by incubating erythrocytes of cord blood with galactose; in the galactosemic blood, galactose-1-phosphate accumulates in the cells. Galactose tolerance tests are abnormal, and the cephalin flocculation is elevated. If milk is eliminated from the diet and soybean of casein hydrolysate substitutes are utilized in its place, the symptoms subside. Early diagnosis, with proper treatment, may prevent permanent cerebral damage.

Mental deficiency may also accompany *glycogenosis* (von Gierke's disease), which is associated with deposition of glycogen in various organs and sometimes involves the brain. Transient hypoglycemia with later retardation has occurred in the children of hypoglycemic mothers.

Gargoylism

This condition, also known as a lipochondrodystrophy, is characterized by deposits of mucopolysaccharides in the organs and connective tissues of the body. In the brain there are extensive deposits of gangliosides in neurons, giving rise to intracellular structures known as zebra bodies because of their appearance under electronmicroscopy. It is now recognized that there exist several variants of this condition. The most widely studied are the Hurler, the Hunter, and the Sanfilippo syndromes, but others exist as well (Scheie, Maroteaux-Lam, and Morquio types). A major difference between the

Hurler and Hunter syndromes is the mode of transmission; the former is carried as an autosomal recessive, and the latter is sex linked. Thus in the Hunter syndrome women, the carriers, transmit to their sons but not to their daughters. The Sanfilippo variant is also an autosomal recessive, characterized by severe mental retardation but few general physical defects.

At birth the infant's head may be enlarged, joint movements are limited, and later the cornea appears clouded. At three months the upper lumbar vertebrae and long bones show deformities by x-ray, and kyphosis is evident. The characteristic features are protrusion of the forehead out of proportion with the stunted body, saddle nose, bushy eyebrows, coarse features, and a deep crease between the thick lips and chin. Abnormal bodies are found in the leukocytes, and there exist both hypermucopolysacchariduria and hyperaminoaciduria. Later in life there develop wedging of the vertebrae, shortened and flexed deformity of the hands, flexion deformities at the hips and knees, and enlargement of the liver and spleen. Most children die in their teens. No treatment is known.

Diagnosis of these conditions is established by finding a secretion of mucopolysaccharides chondroitin sulfate B (CSB) and heparitin S (HS) in the urine in amounts in excess of 15 mg. daily. In the Hurler syndrome CSB exceeds HS in excretions by 2 to 1; the ratio is equal in the Hunter syndrome. Mostly HS is excreted in the Sanfilippo syndrome. Fibroblasts cultured from the skin of these patients show signs of accumulation of mucopolysaccharides. Toluidine blue staining of lymphocytes discloses mucopolysaccharide inclusions in high proportions of these cells. It is now possible to diagnose these conditions by withdrawing amniotic fluid before birth and examining the cells contained therein for such accumulations. This prenatal test has been used successfully for prenatal diagnoses in mothers who have previously given birth to afflicted children and thus allowed the termination of pregnancy by abortion.

The evidence suggests that the muco-polysaccharide accumulations are the result of failure in the degradation process. The absent enzymes for the Hurler syndrome exist in the Hunter cells and vice versa.

Hypothyroidism

This condition, either congenital or acquired, may lead to retardation in mental growth. Sometimes recognizable at birth, it usually is not manifest until later months when it may be noticed that the infant is dwarfed, particularly with failure in growth of length. The subcutaneous tissues are thick so that the features are coarse, the skin dry and cold. The child appears dull and puffy. The tongue protrudes and the lips are thick. The forehead may be wrinkled, the hair is thin, and the anterior fontanel is widely open. There is often abdominal distention with associated umbilical hernia, slow pulse, and such neurological signs as ataxia, rigidity, and hyporeflexia. The basal metabolic rate varies from -20 to -50, the protein-bound iodine value of 4 to 8 μg. per 100 ml. is much below values found in healthy subjects, and the uptake of radioactive iodine is reduced. Usually after the age of two the blood cholesterol is elevated, and x-ray studies show recurrent development of ossification centers and epiphyseal union.

In areas where goiter is common, the congenital type may be the consequence of maternal iodine deficiency. The congenital type also includes those cases with absence or hypoplasia of the gland and those with a genetically determined enzyme defect causing inadequate synthesis of thyroxin (biochemical hypothyroidism). In the latter cases, the thyroid appears to be morphologically normal, although a goiter may develop later. However, the degree of mental retardation found in each individual is related as well to the familial occurrence of low, average, or high intelligence and opportunities for education.

Treatment consists in establishing a euthyroid state as early and rapidly as possible without the induction of cardiac decompensation. Desiccated thyroid is as effective as thyroxin and triodothyroxin. The dosage of these agents must be carefully regulated in order to protect the heart from damage. In young infants a daily dose of 15 to 30 mg. of desiccated thyroid is indicated initially. Every two or three weeks this dose may be elevated by 15 mg. Daily doses of 45 to 60 mg. are adequate to maintain the euthyroid state at ages below one year. Between 1 and 3 years of age 75 to 120 mg. is needed daily, and at later ages 150 to 180 mg. Studies have shown that approximately half of those with the most severe types of cretinism commencing before birth and apparent in the first months of life, if treated before the age of six months, attain nearly average intelligence quotients, and less than one-fifth of the group have persisting moderate retardation. Delay in beginning treatment is less disastrous for those with an insidious onset commencing from birth and not clinically recognized until they are over one year of age. It has been suggested that there exists a critical period of brain development in the prenatal or early postnatal life, when irreparable failure may occur as the result of thyroid deficiency.

The neuropathologic findings are reduction in the number of cells in the cortex; failure in myelinization and delays in maturation of fiber tracts and neurons has been reported. The electroencephalogram shows low amplitude and slow alpha rhythm; these are reversible with thyroid medication.

DUE TO NEW GROWTHS

Tuberous Sclerosis

This clinical form of feeble-mindedness, sometimes known as epiloia, is characterized by epilepsy, mental defect, and a butterfly-shaped rash of cutaneous nodules resembling sebaceous adenomas but really consisting of hyperblastic connective and vascular tissue. The disease results from a congenital blastomatous malformation involving the neuroectodermal system. The brain shows diffuse disturbances in cytoarchitecture and localized neoplastic glial formations.

It is transmitted by a dominant gene with reduced penetrance. Neurofibromatosis, inherited in a similar way, and trigeminal cerebral angiomatosis (Sturge-Weber-Dimitri disease), which is characterized by the "port-wine stain" or cutaneous angioma of the face, may both be associated with cerebral defect and mental retardation.

DUE TO CHROMOSOMAL ABERRATIONS

Down's Syndrome

This frequent variety of mental deficiency is perhaps most widely known as mongolism, because the physiognomic features are suggestive of those normally exhibited by the Mongolian race. It is estimated that three to four infants will be mongoloid of each thousand births and that 5 to 10 per cent of all defectives fall into this category.

Clinically the patient is characterized by short stature and a small, round skull, with a flattening of both the occiput and the face. The hair is scanty and coarse. The palpebral fissure is narrow and oblique, with the inner end lower than the outer; a fold of skin continued from the upper eyelid over the inner angle adds to the resemblance to the Asiatic countenance. The tongue is large and fissured, with its papillae hypertrophied, and it is often constantly protruded and withdrawn through the open mouth. The nose is short and broad, with a depressed bridge; the hands are large and stubby, the fifth finger being particularly short and often incurved. The joint ligaments are lax, and the muscles are hypotonic, giving the joints an unusual mobility. The palate is often deformed, the abdomen is large, and the genitalia are underdeveloped. The palm and finger prints are characteristic, as the two main creases across the palm are replaced often by a single crease (simian line). In a tenth of the patients, a congenital heart defect is found. The mongoloid's good disposition and tendency to imitativeness often conceal at first the seriousness of his mental defect. Most mongoloids have an I.Q. between 15 and 40, with an upper limit in the 50's.

There are no distinctive pathologic changes in the bodily organs. The brain tends to maintain the embryonic convolutional patterns and to have a disproportionately small cerebellum and brain stem. The ganglion cells of the third cortical layer are sparse and irregularly dispersed. Abnormal changes are reported in the pituitary, thyroid, and adrenal glands, and the heart and arterial systems are poorly developed.

Hyperuricemia is the rule in this condition, and many develop diabetes. Blood serotonin is abnormally low in those with Down's syndrome according to Tu and Zellweger. These observers also found that there exists a lack of response to 2-tryptophan loading as well as a fall in blood serotonin level after administration of dl-penicillamine. The latter may be corrected by administration of pyridoxine. These findings suggest a depression of decarboxylation of 5-hydroxytryptophan in Down's syndrome.

Cytogenetic studies by Lejeune in 1959 showed that the somatic cells of patients with mongolism have 47 chromosomes instead of the normal 46, owing to a trisomy of chromosome 21. It is suggested that, during miosis, nondisjunction persists, with the mongoloid receiving the undetached segment. Since then there have been reported a number of cases with a normal chromosome count of 46 but an excess of genic material attached to chromosome 21 or another chromosome (usually 15 or 22) due to a translocation. In this latter form of mongolism, now recognized as constituting approximately one-fourth of the cases, one of the parents,

usually the mother, carries the translocation. She has only 45 chromosomes, but
one holds excess genic material usually
found in two chromosomes in the healthy.
Mosaicism, in which there exist differing
chromosomal aberrations between the
skin and blood cell, occurs in some with
the syndrome. It is of interest that a
chromosomal trisomy has been found in
a chimpanzee resembling the Down condition.

Late maternal age long has been related to the birth of children with this
syndrome. It now appears that the form
due to nondisjunction, in which there are
47 chromosomes, is more typically related
to births occurring in older women. The
form due to translocation, on the other
hand, characterizes births in younger
mothers. The cause of both chromosomal
nondisjunction and translocation remains
a mystery. Radiation exposure, autoim-
mune reactions, and vascular deficiencies
in the ovary all have been suggested as
etiologic for these chromosomal aberrations.

The higher incidence of chronic myelo-
cytic anemia in those with Down's syndrome no doubt is due to the fact that
a translocation or delection defect of
chromosome 21 or 22 occurs in this blood
disease.

Treatment. By tissue culture of leukocytes and subsequent chromosome counts,
it has been possible to establish the diagnosis within a few days of birth. However,
specific therapy is unknown. For purposes
of prevention, potential mothers may be
advised that the risk of bearing a child
with this condition increases with age:
between the ages of 35 and 39 this risk is
1 in 280; ages 40 to 44, 1 in 70; 45 to 49,
1 in 40. For mothers with a translocation
defect and only 45 chromosomes, the risk
is one in three.

Klinefelter's Syndrome

This condition, found in males only,
with a mental defect in approximately
one-fourth of those affected, is associated
with an anomaly of the sex chromosomes.

Those affected are tall, lean individuals
with breast enlargement (gynecomastia)
and small or underdeveloped testes.
There exist aspermia and increased secretion of follicle-stimulating hormone;
cytologic examination shows chromatin-
positive nuclei. Men and adolescent boys
with this condition have limited sexual
drives. They often feel inferior owing to
the delay in achieving physical maturity
and react to the body image conflict with
resulting personality disturbances. Thus,
in addition to mental retardation, there
have been observed schizophrenic, passive-dependent, and antisocial personality
disorders with this genetic abnormality.

It is now known that clinically un-
distinguishable cases may have different
cell karyotypes. A little over a half have
47 chromosomes with the count due to
an XXY arrangement rather than the
normal XY sex chromosomes. In some
there have been observed XXXY or
XXXXY sex chromosomes. In all such
cases cytogenetic studies show one or
several extra chromatin-positive bodies,
depending upon the number of X chromosomes. In less than half the cases
various mosaic patterns are found in the
somatic cells, a condition in which two
types of cells are found due to a nondisjunction considered to take place in
mitotic division after fertilization.

Turner's Syndrome

This condition, also due to nondisjunction, occurs in females and is associated
with the presence of one X chromosome
and the absence of Y. It is called the Xo
variant. Such females lack secondary sex
characteristics and show, in addition to
mental defect, other congenital abnormalities, including short stature, "webbed"
neck, deafness, and aorta malformation.

DUE TO UNKNOWN
PRENATAL INFLUENCE

Conditions for which no definite etiology has been established are those associ-

ated with various cranial and cerebral anomalies. *Craniostenosis* of various types, hydrocephalus, and hypertelorism fit into the first group. Among the relatively small number of feeble-minded persons who exhibit distinctive characteristics of the skull or general bodily conformation, or of brain structure, that entitle them to recognition as clinical varieties are the *microcephalics*. Arbitrarily those defectives, mostly imbeciles or idiots, whose skulls on completion of development do not exceed 17 inches in circumference, are designated as microcephalic. Those of this clinical variety show a peculiarity not only in the size of the head but also in its shape, which is characterized by a receding forehead and a flattening of the occiput. The hair, which is wiry in texture, extends low on the forehead. The scalp is greater in amount than is necessary to cover the cranium, with the result that the excess becomes arranged in corrugations. The chin is usually receding and the stature is short. As might be expected from the limited cranial capacity, the brain of the microcephalic is markedly underdeveloped. Histological defects are the rule, and gross anomalies besides those of size are common.

PSYCHOSOCIAL DEPRIVATION

Among the group of mild retardates are those in whom the disorder derives essentially from deprivation of the necessary experiences in the local culture or subculture to allow the development of their potential for social adaptation. This condition usually is recognized in school children, or slightly beyond, with I.Q.s in the range of 50 to 80. No pathologic findings are discoverable on extensive physical, neurological, and laboratory studies, nor is there history of brain or metabolic disturbance. Generally the father will be found to be a manual or blue collar worker, and the older siblings, if any, will be discovered in the higher levels of secondary education, including the advanced technical schools. In other instances the child from a minority group doubtful of the advantages of academic or technical education or speaking a language other than that used in the public schools will have lacked the motivation to perform in the prevailing local school system. The condition is most common in boys and also in children from larger families. Often more than one child in the family is so classified. As mentioned earlier, many persons diagnosed in adolescence or early adult life as retarded are among those in whom the deficit rests upon failure of development owing to educational deprivation in a cultural system which fails to motivate the youngsters to learn.

When the family is intact and stable the outlook for effective social adaptation is favorable. When parents have been lost or the parental relations are broken or pathological, the later social history often reveals erratic work records and frequent transgressions of the law. Children from such families are at high risk for longterm confinement in institutions for the retarded.

Treatment requires special schooling which motivates toward acquisition of reading and simple numerical skills, as well as the teaching of attitudes to others and employment and the development of technical abilities that allow acceptance socially. Schooling should be more prolonged than for other children, to make allowances for the existing slowness in learning. To allow such schooling, the family's attitudes must often be influenced by their involvement and by persuasion from the teaching services.

Screening and early detection of the school populations bring to light such backward children. It is among this high risk group for whom the special programs should be made available early, in order to prevent the social consequences of late adolescent or early adult failure with the consequent deleterious effects in further damaging mental health.

PSYCHOSES WITH MENTAL DEFICIENCY

It is generally agreed that most of the mental disorders that afflict persons of normal intelligence may also afflict the mentally defective. Sometimes, also, defectives suffer from psychoses of an acute transitory nature, presenting episodes of excitement with depression, paranoid trends, or hallucinatory experiences. The psychoses are often situational in origin.

TREATMENT

Although the limits of development of those aspects of the organism that we call intellectual are for the most part fixed, to a narrow extent intelligence grows by use and atrophies by disuse. It has been found that if identical twins are separated soon after birth and one is provided with educational opportunities definitely superior to the other, he will develop an I.Q. higher than the one placed in a less favorable environment. Even though the intellectual capacity cannot be materially increased, the social capacity can be improved in individuals in whom it is most needed, viz., in the higher-grade defective. It should be remembered that the development of a normal personality requires not only a certain native intellectual endowment but also such emotional essentials as affection, security, social recognition, achievement, and new experiences. So too, the retarded or defective child should be led to feel that he is loved, approved, and wanted as a member of the family and of groups outside the family. Surrounded with affection, handled with devoted patience, and psychologically stimulated through fondling and play, such a child should acquire the feeling of significance and security essential to the development of a stable personality.

Emotional Problems

The emotional problem created for the parents by the retarded or defective child may be a difficult one, and the manner in which it is met has much influence upon future development. The knowledge that one's child is not developing normally often comes slowly, and the mother may refuse to face the situation and develop a sense of personal shame, failure, and even guilt. Her tearfulness and the father's angered disappointment may leave the child confused, frustrated, and isolated. Again, if he is rejected, emotionally deprived, coerced, and perhaps beaten, the child is restless, insecure, aggressive, and hostile, and perhaps becomes delinquent. Feelings of frustration and futility are more common among parents of the mentally retarded child than among parents of the physically handicapped. The latter can often experience a feeling of compensation in the child's intellectual and emotional growth. Since such satisfactions are lacking in the case of the mentally arrested or retarded child, the underlying problems of the parents are intensified and often expressed in their attitude toward him, with the result that he develops hostility and behavior problems. Many, perhaps most, defective individuals, like normal individuals, have conflicts regarding their hopes, fears, anxieties, and frustrations. The manner in which these are met by parents and teachers will have much influence on their behavior and social adjustment. Many mentally defective persons are more incapacitated by their emotional difficulties than by their intellectual deficit. As with children of normal intellectual endowment, frustrations, humiliations, ridicule, anxieties, emotional deprivations, and insecurities may be expressed in delinquent behavior.

Education and Employment

In the field of education, teachers should concentrate from the start on those abilities and aptitudes with which the child is most fully endowed. Perhaps nothing is so devastating to the mental health of a defective child as to be offered lessons that are beyond his powers of comprehension.

The social training of retarded children is of immense importance and of far greater significance to them than mere educational attainments. The extent to which they are accepted as agreeable individuals by and in a community is directly proportionate to their social adjustment. This attitude of the community has a direct relation to the mental health of the growing child. If he is accepted, he will feel that he has fulfilled his main ambition of being somebody in the eyes of others. If he is not accepted, he has a feeling of failure and frustration, or grievance and ill will against society, all of which breed discontent and unhappiness, leading to emotional difficulties and maladjustment and perhaps even to delinquency and crime.

Lack of intelligence is not by any means a bar to gainful employment. In many unskilled occupations, what counts in obtaining and retaining a job is not so much skill, literacy, or information as steadiness, reliability, honesty, and the ability to get along well with workmates and the foreman. With happiness will come mental health; and a child who has good mental health, even if he is intellectually defective, is an asset to the community.

It should be considered an obligation of the state to discover, classify, and provide suitable education for all retarded children as early in their careers as possible. In some states an attempt is now made to meet this obligation by requiring an examination of all public school children who are retarded three years or more in their classes and by directing that special classes be provided for such children. Probably with most of these defectives it would be better if they were discovered and assigned to special classes earlier. By assignment to a special class, the child is removed from too difficult a curriculum in which he has no interest, from critical classmates, perhaps from an antagonistic teacher and other humiliating conditions that create feelings of inferiority, destroy

a sense of security, and lay the foundations for the easiest method of defense, that of overt, unsocialized behavior and socially maladaptive compensations. Since the child in the special class can compete with his fellows, the undesirable reactions mentioned are not only not stimulated but there is created a feeling of security, self-reliance, satisfaction, and success that has great constructive value in personality formation. Approbation, attention, and praise afford great satisfaction and, within reasonable limits, may produce a desirable, stimulating effect on the individual's effort to fit into a world that is always going to be beyond him. Feeble-minded children should be encouraged to take part with normal children in all those games in which the defective child can compete on equal terms with the normal one.

Institutional Care

In many ways, the first persons who should be selected for admission to the institutions for feeble-minded are children of the moron level for whom special classes are not available or who are deficient in social adaptation. Among the beneficial results of institutional training are an improvement in attitude, stabilization of emotions, and development of habits of industry. It is especially desirable that young mentally defective children who are beginning to form antisocial habits should be placed in an institutional school before these habits become fixed, particularly if the home environmental influences cannot be modified.

Provision should also be made in the institutional schools for the training of those children of the lowest mental levels. The number of persons who have been trained in the state institutions and placed in the community as useful, often self-supporting, members of society has increased in recent years. It is now estimated that 50 per cent of those admitted to the state schools can be returned to the community socially improved. Such institutions should therefore be looked upon as important parts of the public educational system. There are many who cannot be prepared for living successfully in the community, and yet in the routine, protected life of the institution these individuals become useful citizens.

The problem of treatment of those with moderately severe mental defects is simple and consists largely of physical care and custody. In those with moderate impairment, efforts should be directed at training the child to dress, undress, and bathe himself, to improve his habits of feeding himself, and to curb destructive tendencies, and in teaching him to avoid ordinary dangers, to associate common objects with their names, to pronounce a few easy words, and to express simple wants. At best the object can be merely so to train the child that his care will be less burdensome. Whether this simple training will be undertaken at home or in an institution will depend on many factors, such as the capacity of the mother for training, the size of the family, its economic status, et cetera. In the case of these defective children, the efforts of the mother may usually be more profitably devoted to the rearing of her other children, to the duties of the home, or to such other activities as may contribute to the welfare of her community and the development of her own personality.

With institutional care of the moderately defective child, the family is usually able to make a better economic and social adjustment. From a community point of view, these defective individuals do not constitute an important problem. Their number is small compared to that of individuals with the higher degrees of mental defect, and many die at an early age. They do not constitute a eugenic problem, since the defect is rarely of familial origin, and very few ever procreate.

Some institutionalized defectives are noisy, overactive, aggressive, and destructive. In such cases the phenothiazine derivatives often exert a desirable sedative effect.

Sterilization

Opinions as to the value and wisdom of sterilization of the intellectually retarded are varied. Suggested as a means of preventing feeble-mindedness, its eugenic value is much more limited than was at first appreciated. Probably too little is known about the inheritance of mental defect to apply sterilization in any but the lower grades of that condition, in which, in fact, the likelihood of procreation is the least. The legal provision for sterilization applies in most states to those committed to public institutions, but experience shows that a large proportion of high-grade defectives, who of all defectives are most frequently afflicted with a familial disease, are not committed to institutions. In these, too, the social adjustment is determined fully as much by social and family influence and environment as by the intelligence. Experience has thus far shown that, even when the law provides for their sterilization, only a few of the retarded who are supported by their families are subjected to this operation. Those in the upper levels of the subnormal group are the most highly reproductive.

Contrary to the opinion of many, most high-grade defectives are not prolific. Statistics show that only a very small percentage of male defectives who are committed and subsequently discharged ever marry or have children. Experience indicates that a majority of the detrimental behavior on the part of mental defectives is not their sexual irregularity and reproduction but vagrancy, dependency, and delinquency. The mortality rate among the retarded is so high that danger from their unrestrained propagation is limited. It is now recognized, too, that society does not need protection from the retarded girl as much as the retarded girl needs protection from society.

Many retarded couples will live a successful, happy life if not burdened with the financial, physiological, and other strains incident to rearing a family, yet many suffer social and economic collapse if obliged to assume these burdens. Much neglect and ill-treatment of children would be forestalled if persons intellectually or emotionally unfit to rear children could be sterilized, but such a measure can scarcely be determined solely on the basis of the I.Q. Its usefulness is more individual than social.

Finally, sterilization as a general policy is a superficial method of approaching the problem of retardation, since it ignores the need for special investigation and research as to its cause and prevention.

BIBLIOGRAPHY

GENERAL

Association for Research in Nervous and Mental Disease. Vol. XXXIX. Mental Retardation. Baltimore, Williams & Wilkins Company, 1962.

Birch, H. G., and Gussow, J. D.: Disadvantaged Children. Health, Nutrition and School Failure. New York, Grune & Stratton, 1970.

Bruton, J. L., Corsellis, J. A. N., and Russell, A.: Hereditary hyperammonaemia. Brain, 93:424–434, 1970.

Feinberg, I., Braun, M., and Shulman, E.: EEG sleep patterns in mental retardation. Electroencephal. Clin. Neurophysiol., 27:128–141, 1969.

Gesell, A., and Amatruda, E. S.: Developmental Diagnosis. New York, Paul B. Hoeber, 1949.

Gillis, S. S., and Feingold, M.: Atlas of Mental Retardation Syndromes: Visual Diagnosis of Facies and Physical Findings. U.S. Department of Health, Education & Welfare, Division of Mental Retardation. Washington, D.C., U.S. Government Printing Office, 1968.

Heber, R.: Epidemiology of Mental Retardation. Springfield, Ill., Charles C Thomas, 1970.

Horwitz, W. A., Deming, W. F., and Winter, R. F.: A further account of the idiot savants, experts with the calendar. Amer. J. Psychiat., 126:412–415, 1969.

Penrose, L. S.: The Biology of Mental Deficiency. 3rd ed. New York, Grune & Stratton, 1963.

Susser, M.: Community Psychiatry. Epidemiologic and Social Themes. New York, Random House, 1968.

DUE TO INTOXICATION

Diamond, I., Lucey, J., and Schmid, R.: Prevention of hyperbilirubinemia and kernicterus by exposure to light. Studies in newborn guinea pigs and premature infants. Trans. Amer. Neurolog. Assoc., 93:70–71, 1968.

Stern, L., Khanna, N. N., Levy, G., et al.: Effect of phenobarbital on hyperbilirubinemia and glucuronide formations in newborn. Amer. J. Dis. Child., 120:26–31, 1970.

DUE TO DISORDERS OF METABOLISM, GROWTH AND NUTRITION

Aminoacidurias

Anumonye, A., et al.: Plasma uric acid concentrations among Edinburgh business executives. J.A.M.A., 208:1141–1144, 1969.

Boyle, J. A., Raivio, K. O., Astrin, K. H., et al.: Lesch-Nyhan syndrome. Preventive control by prenatal diagnosis. Science, 169:688–789, 1970.

Cunningham, G. C., et al.: Phenylalanine tolerance tests. Amer. J. Dis. Child., 117:626–635, 1969.

Dunn, H. G., Perry, T. L., and Dolman, C. L.: Homocystinuria. Neurology, 16:407–420, 1966.

Holt, L., Jr., and Snyderman, S. E.: Disturbances of amino acid metabolism. Bull., N.Y. Acad. Med., 36:432–450, 1960.

Hsia, D. Y. Y., et al.: Atypical phenylketonuria with borderline intelligence. Amer. J. Dis. Child., 116:143–157, 1968.

Michener, W. M.: Hyperuricaemia and mental retardation. Amer. J. Dis. Child., 113:195–206, 1967.

Yu, J. S., and O'Halloran, M. T.: Children of mothers with phenylketonuria. Lancet, 1:210–212, 1970.

Defects in Carbohydrate Metabolism

Neufeld, E. F., and Fratantoni, J. C.: Inborn errors of mucopolysaccharide metabolism. Science, 169:141–146, 1970.

Zelson, J., and Dekaban, A. S.: Biological behaviour of lymphocytes in Hunter-Hurler's disease. Arch. Neurol., 20:358–361, 1970.

Lipoidosis

Desnick, R. J., et al.: Diagnosis of glycosphingolipoidosis by urinary sediment analysis. New Eng. J. Med., 284:739–743, 1971.

O'Brien, J. S., et al.: Tay-Sachs disease. Prenatal diagnosis. Science, 172:61–64, 1971.

DUE TO CHROMOSOMAL ABERRATION

Down's Syndrome

Benda, C. E.: Down's Syndrome. Mongolism and Its Management. New York, Grune & Stratton, 1969.

Kaufman, J. M., and O'Brien, W. M.: Hyperuricemia in mongolism. New Eng. J. Med., *276:* 953–956, 1967.

Lilienfeld, A. M.: Epidemiology of Mongolism. Baltimore, Johns Hopkins Press, 1969.

McClure, H. M., et al.: Autosomal trisomy in a chimpanzee. Resemblance to Down's syndrome. Science, *165:*1010–1011, 1969.

Penrose, L. S., and Smith, G. F.: Down's Anomaly. Boston, Little, Brown & Company, 1966.

Tu, J. B., and Zellweger, H.: Blood serotonin deficiency in Down's syndrome. Lancet, *2:*715–716, 1965.

Klinefelter and Related Syndromes

Beeker, K. L., et al.: Klinefelter's syndrome. Clinical and laboratory findings in 54 patients. Arch. Int. Med., *118:*314–321, 1966.

Swanson, D., and Stepes, A. H.: Psychiatric aspects of Klinefelter syndrome. Amer. J. Psychiat., *126:*814–822, 1966.

Chapter 31

Psychotherapy

Psychotherapy may be defined as the treatment of emotional and personality problems and disorders by psychological means. Although many different psychological techniques may be employed in an effort to relieve problems and disorders and make the patient a mature, satisfied, and independent person, an important therapeutic factor common to them all is the therapist-patient relationship, with its interpersonal experiences. Through this relationship, the patient comes to know that he can share his feelings, attitudes, and experiences with the physician and that the latter, with his warmth, understanding empathy, acceptance, and support, will not depreciate, censure, or judge him no matter what he may reveal, but will respect his dignity and worth.

Since the patient goes to the physician for help and the latter offers this to him, the patient usually brings a positive transference attitude to the therapeutic situation. This positive transference attitude is found in the vast majority of patient-physician relations that exist in medicine. It underlies the expectations for recovery and explains many magical cases of cure. Its psychogenesis derives from man's long period of dependent development in which his early pains and fears were frequently and repeatedly alleviated and relieved by the attention, interest, and strength of his parents and those they brought him to for aid. This learned expectancy of help from the early support of parents is transferred to the physician as a professional and forms the fulcrum for all successful psychotherapeutic ventures.

It must be recognized that not every patient brings to the therapeutic situation the hopeful expectancy that characterizes the positive transference. Pervasive attitudes of distrust, suspicion, and hatefulness may make it impossible for the patient either to come himself or to accept under pressure contact with the physician, whether he is in need of medical or psychological treatment. Patient attitudes of this kind, which prevent the early establishment of an effective psychotherapeutic relationship, usually are found in those deprived of parents in early life, frequently shifted from one institution or foster home to another, or brought up in a home situation limited in loving support and encouragement by too demanding or rejecting parents. For individuals whose development has taken place under these circumstances, the opportunity has been limited to learn and ingrain the important ego attitudes of hopefulness and trust. Thus those whose growth has taken place under conditions of severe deprivation of early healthy mothering may be expected to enter psychotherapy with an initial impediment in the central focus of the psychotherapeutic relationship—the hopeful and expectant contact between patient and physician. In such patients, the effort to overcome the initial distrust—the initial resistance—may consume many months of contact. There is theoretical reason to believe that some individuals have undergone such serious deprivations in mothering at critical periods during early infancy and childhood that the patient-physician relationship necessary for forms of individual psychotherapy may never be capable of establishment.

Types of Psychotherapy

Types of psychotherapy fall into two general groups. One may be described as genetic-dynamic, the other as supportive, suppressive, nonexploratory, or nonspecific. In the former are included both psychoanalysis and a variety of brief psychotherapeutic techniques. No single psychotherapeutic method, approach, or technique is desirable for all patients or for all kinds of emotional difficulties. The types of psychotherapy must be determined by such factors as nature of the patient's problems, dynamic diagnosis, age of patient, intelligence, emotional maturity, family and social situation, the goals of treatment, the effectiveness of the technique in achieving these goals, and the specialized training and skill of the therapist.

The therapist, regardless of the type of therapy he employs, must have certain qualities. He should have a liking for people, possess a warm capacity for projecting himself into the situations and feelings of others, and be able to understand human motivation. He should possess few personality characteristics that are defensive in nature. Both therapist and patient must relate meaningfully each to the other.

GENETIC-DYNAMIC THERAPIES

Psychoanalysis and the dynamic psychotherapies have in common the assumption that the patient's emotional or personality difficulty had its genesis in significant psychological experiences and developed in accordance with the dynamic processes that determine psychopathology. Both assume that the patient's present attitudes and modes of reaction to life experiences are largely governed by reactions and attitudes to experiences in the past, by patterns of behavior laid down in the brain systems through prolonged learning and through experiencing pain and pleasure, aversion and reward, in the stream of family and social life. Yet these therapies vary significantly in their theoretical assumption and their technical application.

Since the theory and practice of psychoanalytic therapy have been most intensively studied and clearly defined, *its assumptions and methods form a convenient model* against which other treatment methods and variations in technique may be examined. For this reason, psychoanalytic treatment is here described first.

PSYCHOANALYSIS

It should be borne in mind that the term psychoanalysis is used in two very different senses. Freud originally applied the word to a particular therapeutic method, but it is now employed also as the name of a system of theoretical psychology. The psychoanalytic techniques may be used both for the investigation and the treatment of mental and emotional disorder.

Value and Indications

Psychoanalysis has elucidated many aspects of human behavior that had baffled interpretation and has led to a deeper understanding of the factors that have been responsible for personality development and patterns. Through psychoanalysis it has been learned that phenomena in adult life that are seemingly unintelligible take on meaning when understood in terms of chronologically earlier experiences. It has, too, been of immense value in bringing into awareness the unconscious roots of the problem of the mentally ill.

The application of the increased knowledge of the mind secured through psychoanalysis has, moreover, been of great therapeutic value. As a system of psychotherapy, it aims to establish its methods on the general principles and knowledge of the dynamics of emotional life. Psychoanalysis makes possible a study of deeply repressed psychological forces and attempts to demonstrate how certain inner situations and roles persist and result in attitudes and motivating mechanisms that lie behind consciousness but may determine the whole course of life. It emphasizes, more than other psychological theories, the role of infantile experience in determining adult behavior. Probably many psychoanalysts underestimate the influence of later experiences in life. Often these are of more precipitating significance.

It is an etiological, uncovering, or insight type of therapy, in contrast to the supportive, nonexploratory types described in a subsequent section. Doubtless the most important discoveries of Freud in relation to psychotherapy were those of free association as a means of exploration of the patient's mind, the study of resistance, and the analysis of the transference. Psychoanalysis should not be undertaken except by one who has had systematic training in its techniques. The goal of psychoanalytical therapy is the uncovering and modifying of unconscious psychological forces. Through the analysis, the patient should discover the influences of these unconscious forces upon the pattern of his daily life and upon his relationship to other persons.

Theoretically, psychoanalysis is the choice of psychotherapy if the goal of treatment is a thoroughgoing modification of the personality. The analyst seeks to bring about changes in personality structure by undoing the unfavorable patterns established in earlier years. Psychoanalysis aims to explore the hidden forces determining the behavior which brings suffering to the patient, with the hope that thereby he may acquire a maximum of self-knowledge and effect an alteration in the structure of his personality by undoing and reorganizing the unfavorable patterns that were established in an earlier period.

PREPARATION OF THERAPIST. It is now generally agreed that an analytical psychotherapist should have a personal analysis as a basic preparation for analytical therapy. In this analysis, the prospective therapist undertakes a penetrating psychological study of himself. With the aid of his analyst, he is expected to explore thoroughly the unconscious realms of his mind, trace his personality development back to the formative experiences of his childhood, and arrive at a fuller knowledge and a more realistic appraisal of himself. Such an analysis helps the therapist to recognize his own impulses, wishes, anxieties, and defenses and reduces the danger that they will interfere with the therapeutic relationship with the patient, or that the physician will be rendered anxious by a hostile patient because of arousal of his own hostile or sadistic impulses. As in all patient-physician relationship types of psychotherapy, the therapist must avoid treating the patient as a projected part of himself. The personal analysis enables the therapist to avoid many problems that may otherwise arise out of countertransference, discussed later. Also, the personal analysis is extremely helpful in acquainting one's self with the technique of an experienced analyst. The future therapist should also receive a long period of supervised clinical work before undertaking psychoanalytical therapy without the guidance of a trained therapist.

USE IN NEUROSES. Psychoanalysis finds its greatest therapeutic usefulness in the psychoneuroses, character disorders, and some cases of incipient schizophrenia. The greatest success obtained in these disorders is characterized by a greater potentiality for transference than exists in other neuroses. In the psychoses, the usefulness of psychoanalysis is limited.

Even though the nature of his neurosis would indicate that a patient is a suitable subject for psychoanalysis, certain other elements may contraindicate any therapy of this nature. Unless the patient sincerely wishes for relief from the neurosis and is prepared to undertake the therapy seriously and resolutely, no attempt at psychoanalysis should be made. Since a person cannot profit by such therapy unless he has a well-developed capacity for introspective understanding, the analysis of a person of subnormal intelligence cannot be successfully undertaken.

Rarely can much be accomplished by the analysis of persons over 45 years of age, although more depends upon the plasticity and receptivity of one's personality pattern than upon chronological age. Psychoanalytic therapy is unlikely to be successful in highly dependent individuals, those who demonstrate through their life history little evidence of self-reliance or efforts to gain a personal independence away from parents or parental substitutes. Where the life history shows that the patient has made efforts to give up his infantile attachments to the parents, even unevenly and irregularly, the potential for success is enhanced.

Principles and Technique

Psychoanalytical therapy involves, among other psychological principles, such important ones as *unconscious content, free association, resistance, transference, countertransference, interpretation,* and *analysis of dreams.* These are discussed briefly, but no attempt is made either to present them in detail or to examine the many problems that arise in the actual employment of the technique.

The analyst should have had considerable experience with both psychotic and neurotic patients, and be well acquainted with the principles of dynamic psychology. Interviews are held five or six days per week for periods extending from 45 minutes to one hour. From one to three years are usually required for an analysis. It is generally considered desirable that the therapist and the patient should not have been previously acquainted, also that their relationship continue to be a strictly professional one, free from social contact. In order that free association may be facilitated, the patient usually reclines during the interview, relaxed on a couch, while the analyst is seated a little behind and to one side of him. The analyst can observe the patient, but as the latter cannot see the analyst, he is not constantly looking for signs of the therapist's response. In some instances the patient and therapist may conduct the analytic process seated when this posture seems more effective in facilitating free association.

Free Association

Although dream analysis and other techniques are employed as supplementary means, the principal method is that of free association. To obtain such consciously unguided association, the therapist asks the patient to say whatever comes to his mind and warns him against changing the sequence of his undirected thoughts and against withholding anything because it seems irrelevant or distressing. There should be an uncensored, uninhibited verbalization of everything and anything that comes to mind.

The permissive atmosphere of the therapeutic relationship facilitates free association. Opinions and feelings are expressed with a minimum or no guidance by inquiry. As material through the free association process emerges, often in symbolic form, from the consciously inaccessible portion of the mind, it becomes conscious. That it may be used therapeutically, however, it is necessary that the patient's repressed material be made conscious and also that interrelations and implications of the material be recognized.

It is essential that the therapist be exceedingly guarded and discreet in pointing out connections among the material produced by free association or suggesting interpretations of it. The meaning of the material, as pointed out elsewhere, must be largely discovered by the patient himself. Through the free association process, the patient explores early memories, recreates significant experiences and the feelings contingent on them, reactivates relations with parents, siblings, or other persons, and tries to bring into consciousness feelings and ideas about himself and his attitudes as they existed in childhood. The purpose of the analysis, however, is not in any way to secure a history but rather for the patient, through free association and his interpretation of its products, to discover the tendencies, motives, desires, and other influences that have led to his personality problems and his defenses against anxiety and have constituted dynamic forces in his life.

Gradually, as associations increase in number and in their richness of material from the unconscious, what has appeared irrelevant and meaningless to the patient begins to assume significance to him. As previously indicated, the therapist seldom provides interpretations of material replete with symbolic disguises, and the patient is advised to discover for himself the meaning of his associative products. This does not mean that comment or carefully restrained aid in interpreting these products is not permissible, but that the associations must be purely of an autogenous nature and that the patient must, insofar as possible, discover this significance for himself and come to appreciate that his symptoms bear a relation to some deep-seated personality problem. Because of the great degree of self-revelation that it makes possible, free association is perhaps the most valuable of all methods in disclosing psychodynamics.

Resistance

Free association does not, however, assure smooth and easy passage of all repressed memories and emotions into consciousness. Although the patient's trust in the analyst and the confidence that he is not being judged by the therapist aid him in facing emotional constellations with which he could not deal in the past, as certain repressed and forgotten experiences and emotions are about to be brought within the scope of immediate observation, an opposition to their complete awareness or an aversion to facing the unconscious basis of his motive, appears. This opposition, known technically as *resistance,* may be manifested by sudden silences, denials, block-ings, forgettings, evasions, embarrassments, and strong emotional reactions. It derives from the patient's transference distortions of the therapist as a punitive, critical, or punishing replica of some significant person in his own past life experiences.

The dynamic significance of the repressed material may be estimated by the degree of resistance to its emergence, and by the severity of the defensive reaction. By noting the occasion and the topics that evoke the patient's defensive resistances, the analyst secures clues as to the nature of the repressed material. Usually the patient's inflection or sudden change of subject indicates that the nucleus of a conflict is being approached or that he is unwittingly attempting to avoid recognition of an unconscious motivation.

Again, the resistance represents an unconscious effort to evade memories or insight. The analyst seeks to detect and bring to the patient's attention a recognition of his deep-rooted and repressed feelings and drives. This tends, however, to lead to an unconscious resistance to therapy. The resistance serves, of course, as a defense mechanism against the anxiety that would be aroused by a threatening self-knowledge of repudiated feelings and impulses. Care is taken not to probe too deeply or too rapidly in the early stages of an analysis so as not to arouse too great anxiety.

Recently Sandler and his colleagues outlined the various forms of resistance. Thus there is *depression-resistance* that emerges when impulses, memories, or feelings arise against which the patient must defend himself in order to escape conscious distress. *Transference resistance,* sometimes regarded as the most difficult obstacle to analysis, occurs when the patient struggles against revealing his innermost thoughts and feelings as regards the therapist—many of course revelatory of infantile and childish desires. Another important resistance is that which would expose the gain or value of the illness, the secondary gain in the advantages derived from being cared for, gratifying aggressive, domineering, or revengeful impulses toward caretakers, or satisfying masochistic trends. *Id resistance* refers to the unwillingness to change well-established behavioral patterns derived from one basic drive. Here the patient must "work through" his resistance. *Superego resistance* is that aroused when the patient feels threatened by guilt unconsciously perceived as the analytic work tends to loosen his rigid inhibitions in expression of his aggressive sexual or dependency drives, producing what is designated as the "negative therapeutic reaction." Resistances may evolve as the changes in the patient produce difficulties in important interpersonal relations; by fear of detachment from the analyst as the treatment approaches its ending; by threat to his self-esteem through need to expose infantile behaviors which induce shame; and by the potential of having to give up well-established character traits which sometimes have taken on an autonomous gratifying existence.

Transference

What is perhaps regarded as the most significant concept in psychoanalytical therapy, and one of the most important discoveries of Freud, is the emotional reaction of the patient toward the analyst, known as the *transference*. Transference is usually defined as a repetition in the patient's present life, and particularly in his relationship to the analyst, of unconscious emotional attitudes developed during childhood within the family group and especially toward the parents. It represents a carrying over, and attaching to the therapist, of the friendly, hostile, or ambivalent attitudes and feelings that the patient formerly entertained in relation to the parent or other meaningful person of the past who played a significant role in his life. The patient reacts toward the therapist as if the latter were this person. He projects upon the therapist the significant images of those to whom he was related in the past.

The significance of the transfer is that it throws light upon the patient's relationship with the individual whom the therapist represents. The patient comes to react as if the therapist were actually the other person and therefore interprets the behavior of the analyst in conformance with his concept of the person toward whom he originally had the reaction. Important unconscious factors are therefore revealed, not only by free associations and dreams, but also by transference behavior. In the resulting reaction, often referred to as the transference neurosis, the original pathogenic conflicts of the early family relationships are repeated with lesser intensity in relationship to the analyst. This may lead to extreme anxiety, illogical hostility with paranoid implications, clinging affection, or serious acting out of impulses in order to invite the therapist's punishment.

The therapist must not be surprised or disturbed by a hostile or critical attitude of the patient toward him. Rather does he objectively study those feelings with the patient, point them out to him, and seek to trace them to their origin. An effort is made to make it clear to the patient how his feelings really arose out of earlier relationships. The patient's reliving of his original conflict in the transference situation is used by the therapist as an important therapeutic experience. The sudden discovery of the transference distortions reveals to the patient with major impact the means by which he has frequently misperceived and misjudged his relations with those during his recent life.

By encouraging the patient to retrace his memories to early childhood, he may find the source of these feelings. In so doing he is relieved often of the pathological anxiety, guilt, or shame that he has suffered neurotically as he discovers and understands the emotions and events originally felt toward other significant persons in his past experience transferred during therapy to the physician.

One aspect of the transference situation that may arise is the tendency of the patient to repeat in relation to the therapist a pattern of dependent emotional relationship such as the one that hampered his emotional adjustment and personality development in the past.

Countertransference

A phenomenon that accounts for many mistakes and failures of psychotherapy is that known as *countertransference*. This consists of such negative attitudes of physician to patient as anger, impatience, or resentment. These and similar attitudes are almost certain to interfere with the therapeutic effectiveness of the physician. For the most part, the countertransference reactions arise in the therapist as a result of the patient's influence on the physician's unconscious feelings and have their origin in the latter's irrational projections and identifications. The therapist must not permit his own unconscious feelings and attitudes aroused during phases of treatment to intrude in his relations with the patient.

It should be added, however, that just as countertransference can account for failure in therapy, so it can also in the hands of a skillful therapist be put to good use diagnostically and therapeutically. For instance, a patient, not intending to do so, may nevertheless arouse annoyance in the therapist. The latter perceives this as an index of the patient's hostility. The therapeutic task is then to find out, first, why the patient is afraid to express overt hostility, and second, what the patient's hostility represents.

Interpretation

Another technique, especially important in its relation to therapy, is *interpretation*. This is the process whereby the therapist helps the patient to understand the meaning of his mental phenomena and behavior—usually mental phenomena the existence of which he is not aware. As the therapist perceives connections between the experiences revealed by the patient through his free associations and the behavior and symptoms of which he complains, he offers tentative explanations as interpretations. From these interpretations the patient is brought to insight as to the dynamic motivations leading to the persistence of his impairing social behaviors.

Often when such interpretations are correct but arouse the anxiety of the patient, he will respond with evidence of that anxiety in denial, anger, or other manifestations of resistance. However, usually the reaction formation against the interpretation is followed by further verifying free associations, which lead the patient to an insight gained through his own later convictions.

Timing of interpretations is important. The more experienced the therapist, the more likely that his guidance through interpretation will occur at those moments when they may be most useful to his patient. Frequency of interpretation is important as well. The inexperienced therapist is likely either to remain too passive or to impede the patient's own growth by interrupting too frequently to offer his interpretive remarks. Intellectually able patients with the ego assets of courage work well at analysis with minimum need for such interpretative assistance.

Cautious interpretations are necessary in order that the patient may acquire an understanding of the significance of transference phenomena. As is to be expected, the patient, through his need for protection against anxiety, will manifest a resistance to the therapist's interpretations. An added task for the therapist is to assist the patient through interpreting his resistance. The therapist never confronts the patient with a blunt interpretation of the meaning of his symptoms. The more obvious their meaning, the more cautious he must be in explaining them. It has been correctly said that whenever the patient cannot see the obvious it is because he needs his blindness. The therapist does not impose his own interpretations. The patient is likely to gain more insight into his problems and behavior through making his own associations, or at least in being merely guided and helped to draw his own conclusions and fully assimilate his interpretations into his psychology.

REPRESSION AND ANXIETY. The efforts of the therapist and patient should lead to an undoing of repression in order that the repressed may be brought to consciousness and its critical judgments. Thus a rational decision can be made if all the facts are at hand instead of having only part of them available as was previously the case when some were unconscious. One aim of analysis is to bring about such a state that the conscious ego, with its reason, logic, and critical abilities, may assume control when it is confronted with unrealistic, pleasure-seeking, infantile demands that cannot be satisfied by reality.

In every neurotic individual there is overt anxiety when the repressed material approaches consciousness. This anxiety then causes the ego to renew its efforts to secure repression, often through the aid of other defense mechanisms. In the analytical transference situation, the patient allows himself to experience the anxiety without renewed efforts at repression by the ego. This the patient can do, since he identifies himself with the analyst who is there to help him and will, he is confident, protect him from danger. Thus, over a period of time, there is a fractionizing of the anxiety, a gradual exposure of the repressed, until finally the reasonable, judging portion of the ego recognizes that what was repressed is not appropriate in the present life of the patient.

Dream Material

Another important method employed by psychoanalysis for rendering contents of the unconscious available for conscious scrutiny is the examination of *dream material*. The dream is no longer regarded as an accident of our psychic life but as a phenomenon directly connected with it. Since presumably it represents a product of the patient's thinking that lacks the directing and inhibiting forces exercised by awareness, the material it presents for examination discloses more clearly than does consciously directed thinking the underlying strivings of the personality. Tendencies that may not be expressed in the presence of clear consciousness work freely in dreams. They serve as a convenient disguise for the patient's unacceptable, rejected emotions. In them the analyst finds a symbolic expression of the patient's inner tensions and clues to his repressed thoughts, feelings, childhood memories, and experiences. When a dream persists in memory or is repeated, it has special significance because it specifically fits and reveals something constant and basic in the forces that make the personality.

Freud divided the content of thought of dreams into two categories. One he called the *manifest content*—the content as it appears to and is recalled by the dreamer. The recollected or obvious content is not, however, the significant element, which is contained in what is known as the *latent content*. The latent content, were it to appear in its naked form, would be too disturbing and painful and is therefore distorted and disguised so that its recollection will not disturb the dreamer. The disguise of mental material, the repression of which suffers nocturnal relaxation, is brought about by the mechanisms of displacement, condensation, symbolization, dramatization, and elaboration. The joint activity of these mechanisms is known as the *dream work*, a process by which the latent dream content is transformed into the manifest content. By condensation, two or more ideas, wishes, or persons are fused into one, emphasis on significant mental material is displaced, and the content is dramatized and filled out by a deceptive secondary elaboration.

As a result of the dream work, the manifest content may appear to be merely an irrelevant, confused product, yet it really represents the symbolic expression of inner tensions and of other important psychic material, the hidden meaning of which must be interpreted in terms of the total life situation of the individual. It will be noted that the mechanisms that in the dream work cause the latent content of the dream to assume the form presented in the manifest content are the same ones that are operative in producing many neurotic symptoms. Such symptoms are in their dynamics identical with dream processes. In both, one notes the operation of the psychological laws of the unconscious.

In psychoanalysis the dreamer is encouraged to report to the physician any recent or recurring dream. Starting from the manifest content of the dream, free associations are employed. The patient is requested to report all that comes into his mind in regard to the various objects, actions and affects revealed in the manifest dream content. The latent or underlying significance of the symbolic imagery in the manifest content is brought to light. There arises here, of course, the same problem of symbolization and interpretation as in free association, and the analyst must in the same way encourage the patient to discover the meaning concealed in the manifest content of the dream rather than impose the arbitrary acceptance of fixed symbols. It should be remembered, however, that the object in dream interpretation is not so much the translation of certain symbols as the discovery of the ideas and motives that are dynamic in determining the patient's reactions in his waking life. In addition to the analysis of dreams, the skilled therapist will recognize in the patient's reporting of unusual interest in particular passages of books or dramatic productions or art forms a possible symbolic representation of some conflict situation within the patient. Gifts proffered by the patient also contain this potential. Therefore, the therapist seizes these spontaneous opportunities to bring the patient to free-associate to the objects of interest that he has brought into the analysis. The analytic work here is similar to that with dreams; its result is equally or even more revealing than the analysis of the latter.

Personality Reorganization

To be successful, psychoanalysis should so thoroughly reveal to the patient his underlying strivings and problems that, with the assistance of the therapist, he can reorganize the forces of his personality, redirect his affective energy into constructive channels, and prevent its further dissipation in dissociation, substitution, and other evasive, neurotic ways. It aims to give the patient freedom from disabling fears, distress, and inhibitions and to enable him to achieve insight sufficient to handle ordinary conflicts and reasonable reality stress. In psychotic patients it is usually too difficult to overcome resistance or to establish transference to a degree that will permit extensive personality reorganization, but much has been accomplished with many such patients.

Modified Psychoanalysis

Because of the time required for an analysis, and therefore the relatively few persons who can be treated thereby, various brief and modified psychotherapeutic techniques now are employed which utilize psychoanalytic understanding. Many psychiatrists combine selected features from psychobiological, supportive, and psychoanalytical therapies. Franz Alexander, although making use of psychoanalytical principles, sought to make psychoanalysis less time-consuming. He believed that prolonged, uninterrupted, daily interviews may favor the development of a too dependent relationship and consequently postpone recovery. He therefore reduced the contact with the patient as much as possible, gave the patient more independence, and discouraged regressive tendencies. Even in those modified psychoanalytic therapies, the therapist seeks to bring his patient to recognize the significance of his patterns of behavior and their relationship to early environmental and cultural influences or to interpersonal relationships and experiences.

Outcome

Although there exist reports of numerous studies of the effectiveness of psychoanalysis and other psychotherapies, there is now a widespread recognition that for the most part the research, design, and conduct of these studies leave much to be desired. There is, in fact, little in the literature to suggest that we have scientifically validated outcome studies of effectiveness of any of the therapies reported in this chapter. Comparisons between forms of therapy are, at best, tenuous, because most reporters have failed to specify the goals of the treatment before its application. Obviously a treatment directed to personality reorganization and prevention of further disturbance attempts an achievement much more complex than one directed to symptom alleviation.

Effective designs for evaluating treatment should state the theoretical basis for the treatment to be examined and the goals in behavioral changes. Also, such reports should state the details of the treatment, including the setting. The patient population should be defined by age, sex, sociocultural, diagnostic, and symptomatic classification. The measuring devices need description, standardization in various populations, and evaluation, and should be performed by others than those providing treatment. Such studies should include a design which compares the psychotherapeutic effectiveness of two or more treatments. Decisions must be stated as to whether the controls will be sought within the behavior of the patient over time or by comparison groups, both methods presenting considerable weaknesses. For a thorough discussion of the design of research on effectiveness of psychotherapy and a body of information useful in assessing reports on outcome now in the literature, the article by Fiske et al. is recommended as the best extant.

Weber, Elinson, and Moss have presented a recent, highly sophisticated study which meets many of the requirements outlined previously as regards evaluative study and compares changes in behavior over time in 1329 patients treated by the psychoanalytic method and a briefer psychodynamic psychotherapy. Using as indicator of change an ego balance scale in which the coders quantitated modification of behavior in nine areas of functioning (dependency, pleasure, sex, affects, defense, emergency emotions, guilt pathology, social), they report that the length of time patients are in treatment bears a direct relationship to the improvement recorded. With both forms of treatment there occurred a rising rate of improvement over time. With the less intensive psychodynamic psychotherapy, this improvement reaches its maximum in six months to a year and then levels off. Patients in analysis did less well during the initial year than those in psychotherapy, but a greater number improved over the succeeding years and achieved higher levels of functioning than those in psychotherapy. Analytic patients showed significantly greater net improvement on the sex, defense, and pathology of balances than the other group over one to two years. The changes for the better on the dependency balance were equal for both groups.

As for patients in the different diagnostic groupings, psychoanalysis proved most effective for those with neurotic character disturbances. The psychoneurotic and psychotic did about equally in both forms of treatment.

OTHER PSYCHOTHERAPIES

PSYCHOBIOLOGICAL THERAPY

Although many other phases and differences characterize the techniques of the two therapies, it may be said that in psychoanalysis, problems and their genesis are ascertained by an exploration of the unconscious through free associations, and that in psychobiological therapy these problems are approached largely at a conscious level and discussed directly in the form of an ordinary conversation, with attention directed toward definite situations and the patient's reactions to them. Psychobiological therapy does not recognize nor does it systematically use the patient-physician relationship, the transference, to explore the genetic dynamics of the patient's behavior. In both forms, the therapist seeks to modify the unhealthy attitudes that have prevented the patient from carrying on his daily tasks without disturbing his relations with others or creating anxiety within himself. The therapist aims to assist the patient in establishing a more rational, more constructive, and therefore healthier pattern of living.

Because of the principles involved, Adolf Meyer characterized as distributive analysis and synthesis the technique of psychotherapy known as psychobiological therapy. Guided by the therapist, the patient analyzes or critically examines one by one and in their relative importance the various factors and situations and his personality reactions thereto that, in the light of his symptoms and complaints, may have been of dynamic importance in producing his emotional problem or pattern of behavior. Then by inductive reasoning and by discussion with the therapist, the patient, from the material secured through analysis, reconstructs his difficulties and formulates how the understanding acquired thereby may be used constructively to modify emotional reactions and established patterns of behavior and a wholesome integration of the personality be thereby achieved.

Some physicians also use word association tests, Rorschach's ink blot test, dreams, and even free associations for securing material that may be used as topics for discussion. If the patient has the intelligence and personality maturity to participate in analysis and synthesis, it is often helpful in psychoneuroses, affective disturbances that are of reactive origin, immaturity reactions, mild paranoid reactions, and psychosomatic or somatization reactions.

Attention is directed more to actual situations and circumstances than to the discovery of unconscious attitudes and mechanisms. The therapist does not, as in psychoanalysis, attempt to have the patient relive early experiences but to have him understand the present meaning of them and his present attitude toward them. The physician's interested and receptive attitude and his noncritical acceptance of the patient's problems, feelings, and fears help him to recognize his own emotions and to understand himself better. As in psychoanalysis, one must be careful not to overwhelm the patient with interpretations and thereby cause him to build up his defenses and resistances.

The discussions aim to help the patient trace genetically the origin of his complaint in past experience, both in that of which he is aware and in that which has been excluded from memory. Such a biographical analysis includes a study of somatic factors, drives, and activities and a survey of the patient's psychosexual development. It emphasizes human relationships in general, including difficulties with others and social successes and failures.

The therapist asks questions frequently, not so much for the purpose of securing an answer as for promoting a study by the patient himself of his modes of reaction to life experiences. The patient is asked to analyze past experiences and to study them for factors involved. His conclusions are subject to a critical review and are made a topic for therapeutic discussion.

After various experiences, situations, and symptoms have been discussed and analyzed, the patient may be asked to reformulate them into a dynamic life story with its motivations in order that thereby he may as nearly as possible reproduce the origin and development of his problem and understand the means whereby he attempted to meet it. Great care must be exercised lest any interpretations to which an effort is made to guide the patient be made too early, without fact, or in terms not acceptable to him. Usually the therapist makes use also of other appropriate measures, such as reassurance, guidance, persuasion, desensitization, and ventilation.

Brief psychotherapy of this type has been used with success, particularly in clinic practice, for some years. In some instances the therapist sets a time limit for the treatment. Frank emphasizes that the results in these treatments bear a strong relationship to the expectations of both the patient and the therapist. When both are expectant of improvement and change, the outcome is usually gratifying. Clearly outcomes which rest upon the expectations of the patient derive from the infantile experiencing of constancy of dependency and trust.

In such treatment, following the initial diagnostic assessment, the effective therapist generally formulates for the patient the nature of his problem and the goal or goals toward which the psychotherapeutic work will be directed. Also, the patient is advised clearly what he should attempt to do in the treatment sessions. He is sometimes given the termination date and requested to state his willingness to accept the treatment arrangements. As Mann describes the course of time-limited brief psychotherapy, the initial sessions are characterized by magical expectations that all will go well. During the middle phase the patients express in their behavior their desire to avoid that which they have disliked confronting in the past. In general this relates to separation without resolution from a significant but "ambivalently experienced person." In the end phase the therapist actively interprets the conflict situations. Transference interpretations are limited to the last session.

Brief psychotherapy seems indicated for patients who have had no prior treatment, with a disturbance of recent origin, absence of physical complaints, and a referral by a physician. The selection of patients doing well in time-limited treatment correlates well with the high responders for termination of time-unlimited treatment as found in the Terminator-Remainer tests devised some years ago, as well as with their high scoring on the Bass Social Acquiescence Scale.

CONFRONTATION TECHNIQUE

From what has been stated earlier, in terms of the need for caution in interpretation, confrontation would seem largely undesirable as a psychotherapeutic technique. Yet it has been employed in brief therapies and as an aid to interpretation in the longer dynamic expressive treatments.

Garner has most clearly defined a confrontation technique which he employs in his psychotherapeutic approach. His goal is problem solving in contrast to the permissive dynamic psychotherapeusis of the coercive suppressive approaches. Recognizing a crucial problem within the patient vaguely perceived by him, the therapist clearly states the issue to him. Moreover, he suggests a realistic solution. Garner does so in an exaggerated manner to illustrate the needed action. Finally, he provides a statement of the repetitive conflicts derivative of the status quo to emphasize that lack of gratification in its continuance. The patient's thoughts and feelings in regard to the confrontation are then sought.

OTHER PSYCHOTHERAPEUTIC TECHNIQUES

In addition to the genetic-dynamic therapies, in which group psychobiological therapy and psychoanalysis may be included, there are various other psychotherapeutic techniques. These may be classified in numerous ways. The following classification seems, however, to be a logical one: (1) superficial expressive therapy; (2) suppressive therapy; and (3) supportive therapy. Although classical psychoanalytic techniques are not employed in these forms, they are often to some degree psychoanalytically oriented.

SUPERFICIAL EXPRESSIVE THERAPY

In the discussion concerning psychoanalysis, attention was called to the fact that free association and an observation of its sequence of ideas, dreams, and the associations to them (transference phenomena and defensive reactions, such as resistances) served as means both of exploration and of expression of unconscious material. In the superficial expressive therapies, various techniques, sometimes with associated adjunctive devices (such as drugs that alter the level of consciousness), are employed for the purpose of exploring and securing expression of the preconscious and other relatively superficial mental content. Among the superficial expressive therapies would be included narcosynthesis, ventilation, and abreaction.

Narcosynthesis

In this form of therapy, the patient is given an intravenous injection of pentothal sodium or sodium amytal to the point of thorough relaxation but not of sleep. In this state, censorship is less active, and suppressed or repressed material emerges. Conscious control is obliterated and inhibitions removed. The patient's subconscious is revealed relatively rapidly and with the minimum of psychic trauma. Positive or negative feelings may be overtly expressed and trends disclosed.

The technique is of considerable value when the patient has recently been subjected to severe traumatic experiences that stirred impulses and anxiety to a degree that they could not be handled without repression and symptom formation. Under these circumstances, abreaction often contributes to the therapeutic process. The greatest usefulness of narcosynthesis is in acute anxiety states, early traumatic neuroses, conversion hysterias, and the dissociative amnesias and fugues. It is not satisfactory in obsessive-compulsive states or in chronic neuroses. The technique not only breaks down inhibitions but favors the establishment of rapport, puts the patient in a suggestible frame of mind, and appeals to him because it uses a physical means of approach, which he usually accepts more readily. Resistance, or an unconscious effort to evade memories and insight, is reduced by the narcosis and interpretation is thereby facilitated.

Ventilation

Ventilation is an expressive type of therapy in which the patient's anxiety is relieved to a greater or lesser degree by his being given an opportunity in a tolerant, empathic setting frankly to "talk out" and discuss with the therapist personal problems and "worries" that he ordinarily would not discuss with others. The physician, with an attitude of understanding and encouragement, interrupts the patient as little as possible, although occasional questions may be necessary to keep the thread of the story in meaningful channels.

Among topics that may require ventilation may be doubts, impulses, conscious anxieties, family problems, and feelings of guilt. Some phases of the material expressed often represent confession of thoughts or actions considered intolerable and for which relief from guilt or shame is needed to alleviate anxiety. Others may consist largely of "blowing off steam" regarding resentments. Frequently a joint discussion of present conflicts and past life situations as they seem to relate to emotional or psychosomatic symptoms may bring relief to troublesome aspects of the patient's life. Perhaps in this way the patient may discover a linkage of events and feelings with present reactions and symptoms.

An occasional question may help the patient to find the meaning of his symptoms himself. A correction of misinformation regarding personal problems may result in some diminution of the patient's anxiety. The patient-physician relationship adds to the therapeutic effect of ventilation. Ventilation may at times be supplemented by a superficial psychotherapy based on a knowledge of psychodynamics.

Abreaction

There is a superficial expressive type of psychotherapy in which anxiety is lessened by an emotional reliving of the stress situation which produced the neurosis. A therapeutically beneficial discharge of dammed-up emotions associated with the recall of a repressed memory occurs. The existence of a high degree of emotional tension is the basic indication for abreaction. It often tends to produce a desensitization, i.e., a reduction of emotional tension related to a repressed psychological conflict. The emotional reactions discharged are usually those of grief, rage, or fear. Sometimes the abreaction may include an expression of hostility toward the therapist.

Abreaction, with its beneficial effect in bringing about a reliving and possible working out of the emotional aspects of a stressful experience, may be spontaneous, suggested under hypnosis, or facilitated with barbiturates.

SUPPRESSIVE THERAPY

Suppressive psychotherapy aims to strengthen repression and other usual defenses or to lessen the intensity of a disabling symptom by such means as dogmatic assurance, persuasion, suggestion, and hypnosis. It makes no search for, or any effort to solve, the actual dynamic problem. If, therefore, it produces any relief, the problem still remains and may readily return under any stress or strain.

Persuasion

Persuasion as a form of psychotherapy is particularly associated with the name of Paul Dubois of Berne. This therapy is based upon the principle of intellectual explanations and moralizing discussions. It is explained to the patient how faulty intellectual and emotional attitudes on his part were reactions to certain diffi-culties; also how such tendencies led to undesirable habits and unhealthy emotional and mental conditions. According to Dubois, an important method of therapeutic approach is through self-criticism and through reasoning as to the nature of the symptoms and as to the false ideas and bad mental habits that led to the symptoms.

In persuasion the emphasis is on rationalism and on moral suasion, on an appeal to "reason" and to will rather than on an understanding of the personality and the dynamic factors in its formation. By means of persuasion, the therapist seeks to create, convert, or strengthen certain impulses and to remove or diminish others, to create or strengthen some inhibitions and to free the patient from enslaving ones. It is the aim of the physician, through reasoned argument, to implant in the patient's mind the conviction that his symptoms will disappear. Persuasion probably overestimates the potency of rational processes in any attack upon the products of emotional factors.

Suggestion

In suggestion the therapist seeks to aid the patient by subtly, often indirectly, implanting or inducing the idea or belief that unpleasant or disabling symptoms are being relieved. The successful use of suggestion requires that the physician manifest an attitude of assurance, professional authority, and sympathy. The patient, because of his respect for and confidence in the physician, tends to accept the idea presented. His critical ability is lessened and his mood is influenced. His attention becomes narrowed. In his state of expectancy, he comes to believe that the results predicted will actually take place.

The best results in suggestion therapy are secured when there is no deep-seated disturbance of the personality, as in hysterical conversion symptoms of recent and superficial origin, or in anxiety states following accidents. The employment of electricity, massage, or manipulation in conjunction with suggestion is not advisable, since the patient may attribute the recovery to external agencies. In such cases, the recovery is frequently not permanent and at best is only the disappearance of a symptom and not a cure. In the event of a probable recurrence, the same agencies must be employed in exactly the same manner and frequently by the same person.

Suggestion does not, of course, give the patient any understanding of the cause or dynamics of his disability, and in hysteria, it tends to fix even more firmly the usual propensity to receptivity so characteristic of that disorder. It tends to restrict rather than increase insight. Even though a symptom is relieved by suggestion, the problems and psychological needs that produced it remain unchanged and their evasion may soon be sought by some other symptom. For this reason, the use of suggestion should be accompanied by some kind of reëducation.

INDICATIONS AND APPLICATION. In spite of the limitations of suggestion, its use may be considered permissible in children, in persons of limited intelligence, and in immature, hysterical personalities.

Assuming, for example, that the symptom to be removed is a hysterical conversion symptom, such as a recent paralysis, the physician deals with it by direct suggestion accompanied by some explanation as to the nature of the paralysis. His attitude must be one of conviction and certainty, and the patient must have confidence in him. The physician demonstrates that the capacity for passive movement still exists. He informs the patient that no organic disability that can interfere with function is present. In referring to the patient's disability, the physician comments as to what a nuisance the former's disability must be to him. At the same time he instructs the patient to move the extremity naturally and without forced effort. The patient is apt to make the mistake of attempting the movement by a strenuous effort that leads also to an innervation of the antagonist group of muscles, resulting in a rigid immobility.

The interview with its atmosphere of conviction must continue until voluntary exercise of the function is restored, even though an hour or two be required. The physician, through the very full life story he has obtained from the patient and through a knowledge of the circumstances under which the disability occurred, must be able to convince the patient not only of the meaning and purpose of the symptom but also that the loss of function has persisted because he believed it to be a real loss. The restoration of function is not a matter of attempt to exercise it on the part of the patient, not a matter of "will," but a matter of belief that it is possible.

The physician must be careful both in word and manner not to create the impression that he considers the patient to be either feigning or exaggerating his inability. Anything that will tend to offend the patient's self-respect must be avoided. Ross emphasizes that the atmosphere of the interview during which the physician attempts removal of the symptom must be one of reasoned logic and of scrupulous avoidance of dramatic demonstration or of artful deception. The patient would prefer to believe that manipulation or some agency outside of himself removed the disability, but he must be made to see that no external interference was instrumental. The patient must be convinced that the disability disappeared because he recognized its purpose and unreality.

The loss of the symptom is at first accompanied by a feeling of relief and pleasure, but unless he fully recognizes the sequence and relation of events and feelings, the patient may suffer a relapse when again confronted with the same problem or unpleasant situation from which the symptom had unconsciously provided an escape. In that case, the sense of relief is followed by anxiety, sleeplessness, mild depression, physical distress, and perhaps by disability. A frank discussion of the situation with the patient may enable him to make an emotional adjustment to it; again, if the problem springs from the environment, a removal from the source of the difficulty may be wise. Unfortunately, the presenting symptom is often not an isolated affair but an expression of characterological tendencies that are apt to lead to difficulties of adjustment unless a thorough reconstruction of the personality occurs.

Hypnosis

Hypnosis has been defined as an induced state of dissociation produced through suggestion. Some have considered the trance state as a condition of hypnosis, a special state of consciousness in which the subjects are more responsive than others to suggestions for anesthesias, amnesias, age regression, and hallucinations. In recent years this view has come under question through the work of a number of experimenters. In an exhaustive review of the trance state, Barber has proposed that a better explanation for hypnosis and the hypnotic state is that certain individuals, more responsive than others to suggestions, respond appropriately when their attitudes, motivations, and expectancies to the situation are positively inclined.

Without using the trance induction technique customarily applied by hypnotists, Barber and others have been able to induce all the characteristics of the hypnotic trance in groups of unselected men and women simply exposed to brief "task motivational instructions." He found among these unselected groups of individuals as much response to the task motivational instructions in bringing about body immobility, aggression, hallucination, analgesia, and amnesia as among another unselected group exposed to the usual trance induction techniques.

As an analogy to the hypnotic trance state, Barber suggests that of a member of an audience viewing a staged dramatic presentation in which he projects himself to identify with the affects, actions, and communication of the actors. In so doing his attention is diverted from the initial awareness that the performance is contrived and that he is a passive viewer. He enjoys the emotional experiencing into which he has projected himself. The hypnotic state may be considered a behavioral change based upon the patient's hopeful preconceptions of that state and of the therapeutic interpersonal relationship. The therapist is perceived as an authority.

Clearly the selection of patients—those responsive individuals amenable to rapid behavioral change through induction of hypnotic trance—is an important precondition of the decision to use hypnotic technique. Hilgard and others have devised various methods to identify the trance-responsive or highly suggestible individual. Spiegel's method of eye-roll levitation rapidly identifies the subject likely to respond. Spiegel and Shainess are of the opinion that those identified as highly suggestible among patient populations and who in largest numbers will be found among the hysterical, anxiety, and depressive neuroses are the least likely to profit from long-term intensive psychotherapies. If corroborated by others, the importance of identifying easy responsivity to suggestions becomes of major clinical import on decision-making as regards appropriate selections of treatment method for the individual patient.

TECHNIQUE. Through monotonous and repetitive verbal suggestions, the therapist diverts the patient's attention from all other stimuli and directs it to the therapeutic procedure. The patient's range of conscious perception narrows; he becomes increasingly drowsy and enters a trance-like sleep. By the psychiatrist's suggestions, the patient is motivated to carry out instructions and to accept the belief that in the hypnotic state he is capable of activities unusual for him otherwise. In this state of semiconscious suggestibility, inhibiting psychological defenses may be bypassed, at least temporarily. Suggestions given during hypnosis may be acted upon after its termination or even at a suggested period after its termination. These posthypnotic suggestions have great therapeutic potential.

INDICATIONS AND VALUE. Although there is much prejudice against its use, hypnosis occupies an important and valuable place in the therapeutic armamentarium of the psychiatrist. Its greatest value is to modify conversion symptoms, recover amnesic defects, and examine childhood behavior through suggestion of age regression, and as an anesthetic means in dentistry, obstetrics, and certain surgical conditions.

Marks et al. compared the hypnotic techniques to the desensitization variant of the behavior therapies in treatment of phobias, each patient being exposed to 12 successive weekly treatments by the differing methods. Both treatments brought about equally significant improvement but not complete relief of disability. It seemed that the hypnotic techniques were superior with the most anxious and desensitization with the opposing groups in whom habituation was more rapid and counterconditioning occurred readily.

Although a symptom may often be made to disappear dramatically through hypnosis, the factors that produced it are merely repressed and the fundamental personality problem is unchanged. Another reason why hypnosis is not a measure that is permanently successful when used alone is that suggestions lose their effect after a time. It also has the disadvantage that, when the patient's symptoms are suggested away, he may become dependent on the hypnotist instead of developing an ability to solve his problems independently. For these reasons hypnosis should be supplemented by an insight-producing and constructive form of psychotherapy. Any real cure requires a knowledge of the underlying factors that produced the symptoms.

Hypnosis may be of value when painful experiences have been repressed and have given rise to symptoms. The memory of the traumatic experience may be revived by hypnosis and the symptom made to disappear with an accompanying abreaction, in which the patient goes over and over the traumatic situation, crying and sobbing or showing other expression of pent-up emotions.

Mention has already been made of the fact that hypnosis may be used as a means of investigating aspects of the patient's mental life beneath full awareness. Under hypnosis, forgotten experiences may be revived, and the patient can discuss material about which he cannot or does not want to talk in the waking state. The use of intravenous barbiturates as a means of recovering repressed memories is more certain and requires less time than does hypnosis. It does not, moreover, involve the emotional dependence often prerequisite to successful hypnosis.

SUPPORTIVE PSYCHOTHERAPY

Support is particularly useful as a therapeutic technique in cases in which some immediate measures must be taken to relieve a patient, about whom little is known, with unmanageable anxiety. Thus it is an important technical procedure for management of acute personality disturbances when time must be gained for further study and selection of more appropriate therapeutic approaches. For some patients in whom psychotic ego fragmentation is likely, it is often the only and most appropriate therapeutic method. Support may be regarded as a means of maintaining anxiety at a level at which the patient may successfully face his emotional problems.

TECHNIQUE. Through direct verbal statements of reassurance of the absence of danger and the ready availability of help and authoritative statements as to a plan for treatment, the hopeful expectations of the patient are enhanced. Sympathetic statements by the psychiatrist of his recognition of the patient's distress as he recounts his disturbing symptoms or experiences are helpful in fostering a sense of understanding and emotional relatedness, as sometimes do statements that reflect the physician's recognition of the patient's rationalizing defenses to protect him from anxiety. Verbal appreciation of the patient's constructive actions when he decries himself and of his past actions forms still another mode of bolstering the ego. As for other measures of support, the establishment of a regular system of therapeutic visits or other contacts by telephone or letter often forms the basis for a sense of constant reassurance.

Supportive psychotherapy is not based on genetic and dynamic considerations but aims to reduce the tensions of anxiety or of other incapacitating tensions by supportive techniques. Care must be taken, however, not to disturb important and acceptable personality defenses. The techniques employed are of a simple type, and the choice of selection will be determined by many factors, such as the personality characteristics, age, life situation, and the nature of the patient's emotional problem or illness. Among the measures employed will be reassurance, use of authority, permissive attitudes that relieve guilt, reasoning, encouragement, counseling, explanation, advice, and manipulation of environment, including, perhaps, an attempted alteration of attitudes of key persons in the patient's life situation. Little attempt is made to bring about an adjustive personality change but rather it is attempted to help the patient to maintain or improve his ability to face and handle his reality at his best integrative level.

Although supportive therapy consists essentially of strengthening old, but socially acceptable, defenses and cultivating new but related ones, the therapist should usually not be satisfied with the exclusive use of such mechanisms, but as circumstances permit, he should try to work beyond the symptoms and aid the patient in acquiring at least some insight. In employing supportive therapy, the physician should bear in mind the danger that he may thereby encourage dependence and a regressive passivity in the patient. Support should be accompanied by efforts to promote maturity of personality. In both genetic-dynamic and supportive therapy,

only limited results can be expected if there are harsh environmental pressures from which the patient cannot escape.

BEHAVIOR THERAPY

From the methods devised by Pavlov, Watson, and others to produce conditioned reflexes in animals, as well as from the various studies on reinforcement theory by American psychologists, commencing with the studies by Thorndike and elaborated by Hull, Skinner, and their colleagues, approaches to treatment of specific symptoms have been developed. These treatment methods are designated as behavior therapy. The behavior therapies are founded on the premise that all social behavioral expressions, healthy or maladaptive, are learned or represent distortions or deficits in the learning processes of the growing human. Therefore, they are considered to be subject to modification through processes which extinguish the original learning experiences that led to the establishment of a repetitive pathological response or, where deficits in behaviors are considered the cause of the abnormality, more effective behavioral responses are engendered by exposure to new learning experiences. Such experiences must be associated with arousal of emotion in the form of gratification (pleasure) or aversion (pain). Mowrer provides a historical review, a critical commentary, and a significant bibliography on the subject.

Perhaps the major difference between the conduct of behavior therapy and that of psychoanalysis and the dynamic therapies is the emphasis placed on the control of behavior through "its consequences," rather than its origin in antecedent experiences and preëxisting sets to repetitive psychodynamic response. In the recent controversies between those espousing one or another approach there has been a failure on the part of both to examine the operations of the several methods of treatment to determine the similarities and differences. H. Hunt and Dyrud provide the best critical appraisals of the relations between the several approaches. The emphasis in behavioral analysis as a means of identification of ongoing and current factors maintaining pathological behavior represents a major clarification in conceptualizing treatment approaches to patients, because it demands more extended and careful scrutiny of the continual rewarding or aversive social controls to which the patient is exposed. Thus, clearly the role of the relationship of the patient to the therapist or others in the environment as rewarding or aversive must in the future be recognized by behavioral therapists. Such precise analysis of the social forces currently influencing patient behavior goes unstated in the psychoanalytic theory; yet it may be recognized that Harvey, Sullivan, Fromm, and others have emphasized the influence of culture and society on the patient. Nevertheless they did not specify in their teaching of psychotherapeutic technique the necessity or the ways or means of modifying the immediate contingencies influencing behavior. The patient was required to bring about changes within himself so as to effect his response to and relationship with the outside world.

But as Hunt indicates, in practice behavioral theories are so general that they, too, often fail in assisting the behavioral therapists in the very task necessary to conceive of treatment plans needed to assure the desired behavioral change. Some of the difficulty rests in the obscurity of the subtle rewards offered in the social environment and in the lack of importance attached to the internal rewarding or aversive systems of the individual contained in the development of his ego ideals and superego. These recognitions come from psychodynamics. The emphasis from learning theories upon "behavior as maintained and controlled by its consequences" is now influencing the development of newer treatment methods which recognize and utilize the constructs and methods of both therapeutic procedures.

Hunt is of the opinion that those behavior techniques which rely upon extinction are confronted with serious difficulties and is of the belief that eventually the more successful procedures in behavioral therapy will be found in those directly strengthening desirable or constructive behaviors as substitutes for the undesirable.

Indications

Precise recommendations for the prescription of behavior therapy remain obscure. At present it may be said that the method of desensitization is successful in treating phobic states. In a study reported by Gelder and his colleagues, patients with phobic symptoms who were treated with nine months of weekly desensitization sessions showed more improvements than a comparable series treated by individual psychotherapy once a week for one year. There were, however, more dropouts from the behavioral therapy group. Symptom substitution did not occur over a two-year period, and patients who showed improvement in symptoms also reported similar changes in their adaptation with others both at work and during leisure. Wolpe and Lazarus, particularly, report the successful use of the method in a variety of neurotic conditions, including compulsive states and sexual aberrations, and include in their series patients treated without success by other individual psychotherapies.

Operant conditioning methods have been tried with some success in improving the verbal performance of mute, autistic, and mentally defective children, stutterers, and enuretic children. They have been used to mold constructively the socially deficient behaviors of regressed and nonproductive schizophrenics. Through the use of specifying clearly the treatment goal and utilizing reinforcement in the form of "token economies," by exhibiting the desired behaviors the patients are rewarded with a token which they are free to exchange for food, bed, hospital privileges, and small luxuries. Under such treatment programs it has been reported that many long-term hospital patients increase their self-care and group activities. Whether these effects will generalize further to produce the ego organization required for extra-hospital adaptation remains a matter for future assessment.

Treatment Techniques

The therapist directs his attention particularly to the patient's overt behavior, ignoring the subjective aspects of the patient's life. He attempts to define the identifiable life conditions which control and perpetuate the undesirable behavior. No effort is made to identify the underlying precursors in experience, the associated subjective symptoms, or the presumed motivating forces. In contrast to other psychotherapeutic procedures, little attention is paid to the patient-therapist relationship and transference phenomena. The aim of treatment is modification of symptoms rather than personality characteristics.

Through a careful history the therapist notes the patient's complaints, their expression in overt behavior, the situations in which they are expressed, and particularly the preceding associated situations and the succeeding behavior of the patient. Analysis of this information by the therapist is utilized to decide whether the symptom represents a conditioned response to an isolated fear-arousing situation, a response aroused through generalization of the initial emotionally charged situation, or a response that is perpetuated through its social consequences. It is then necessary for the therapist to devise a series of experiences capable of easy manipulation by him that may be applied to modify the antecedent emotionally arousing stimuli. Such experiences or techniques now are commonly referred to as (1) *desensitization,* (2) *reciprocal inhibition,* or (3) combinations of the two. If the analysis of the behavioral response indicates that the behavior is maintained as the consequence of the social relationships after the act or as a deficit in experience, methods are arranged of *positive* and *negative reinforcement, aversive control,* or *extinction.*

In the *desensitization technique* the patient is repeatedly exposed to stimuli similar to those inducing the abnormal response (phobias) but at such low intensity that arousal does not occur. Over time the intensity of the exposure is increased by slight degrees until the patient is able to expose himself to the original stimulating situation without responding inappropriately. The *reciprocal inhibition* technique exposes the patient to a situation in which the original emotional inducing response is elicited but in competition with another competing emotion of greater intensity. Thus stimuli directed toward muscular relaxation may be provided simultaneously with the original anxiety-inducing stimuli. Wolpe and Lazarus have been the major proponents of techniques combining the two methods just described. The reader is referred to their writings. For the treatment of those conditions in which the behavior is one of contact or approach to situations inducing antisocial action, such as homosexuality or abuse of alcohol or drugs, *conditioned avoidance* methods have been tried. These methods are not new and have been used with varying success for a number of decades. Here the physician pairs the pleasure-giving situation with an unpleasant response, such as the induction of vomiting with apomorphine or creation of a neurovascular response with Antabuse.

Reinforcement methods are those in which desirable behavior is rewarded on its appearance by the immediate provision of a pleasurable substance or response. In the case of nonspeaking children, as soon as the patient utters a sound, the therapist gives a candy. With successive trials and appropriate shaping of the sounds to words and later sentences, the reward is provided but not necessarily on a regular repetitive schedule. In animal experiments, schedules of intermittent reward have proved more effective in inducing learning than regular schedules. *Negative reinforcement* schedules also have been tried. Here an unpleasant or painful situation is established and the production of a wanted behavioral response is the signal for relief. *Social* conditions used in psychiatric hospitals, such as isolation through detention, or deprivations later mitigated upon good behavior, probably represent long-tried shaping techniques of this type. *Extinction* technique has been successful in some instances when the response to the undesirable behavior was reinforced by the obvious attention of family members or of hospital or clinic staff. Here, instructions that the patient's behavior be ignored have in some instances led to improvement. Another technique of value in the treatment of some patients has been that of *negative practice*. Here the patient is requested to practice the undesired behavior particularly at those times when he experiences the usual emotion inducing the behavior. The explanation for the value of this method is not clear in the theories of behavior therapy. Very likely it rests upon the personality trait of negativism, and the use of this technique is indicated when such a factor is clearly present. Here the reader is referred to Haley's "Strategies in Psychotherapy."

Behavior therapy demands both a careful analysis of the stimulating situation inducing or perpetuating psychopathology and also individualization of the learning situations to bring about change in the individual patient. As practiced today it consumes as much time as more traditional psychotherapies. Its rudiments will be found in the treatment of phobias by Freud and suggestion therapies for hysterical symptoms described by Ross. Undoubtedly the study of behavior therapy, and its successes and failures in the future, will demand examination of the personalities of both patient and therapist and therefore inclusion within the theoretical framework of much of the knowledge now available from the psychoanalytic study of ego identification, transference, and countertransference.

SOCIO-PSYCHOTHERAPIES

Contrasting with those therapeutic processes in which the patient is treated by an individual therapist—the dyadic transactions described earlier in the chapter—in which the goals are directed to changes within the individual personality, there are various sociotherapies or group transactions directed to the development of or alleviation of stresses and conflicts between the personality and the social system.

There are many existing variants of group treatments concerned with aiding the individual to cope more effectively with the social milieu. He may be in need of a clearer perception of the interrelations, modes of communications, emotional conflicts, and related defenses existing within his family. He may have been deprived of socializing experiences beyond the family, or may have projected his perceptions of the idiosyncratic social relations of his own family onto those relations beyond the family group.

The effective diagnostician will assess not only the individual pathology of the patient but also that reflected in his transactions within the social system in which he is a member. Through the use of one or several of the group processes available, he has at his command methods of effecting the social perceptivity and transactional capacity of his patient that in many instances seems more suitable and more effective in inducing social adaptation than the individual psychotherapies alone.

Perhaps the concept of the sociotherapies and their contribution is best realized in the context of contributions of the various psychotherapeutic disciplines to the ego development of the hospitalized patient. All of those working within a well-run and organized hospital, a therapeutic milieu, must be imbued with the concepts of acting as agents directed toward treatment of the admitted patient. They should constitute in their contacts the members of a therapeutic community. Thus Edelson describes the *work group* in a therapeutic community as functioning to give to the individual participant and his ego system an input, generating, maintaining, or restoring reality testing and mastery through improvement of his skills. Its organization contributes to goal orientation to directly validated measures of accomplishment. On the other hand the group in the activities program stimulates the individual's commitment to seek and enjoy, to accept gratification in esthetics, social transactions, and their attending excitement, thus reducing the affective sense of despair in deprivation. Such groups contribute to the expansion or restoration of the positive affective response within the personality. Patient governments or community councils motivate the participants to identify or achieve common and shared ends, thus establishing the value systems of acceptable or nonacceptable between members of the group. The contribution to the personality system here is to the superego. Finally, the small family group motivate to the respect of institutional values and assist the inclusion of daily experiences with the values and meaning, thus confirming the value system. In turn these groups influence the individual personality through development and support of the ego ideal.

One may conceive of the sociotherapeutic subsystem of the hospitals included in the various group experiences directed by occupational and recreational therapists, nurses, and social workers as assisting the patient's ego and superego development in mastering the social system through development of the skills and methods needed for adaptation.

GROUP PSYCHOTHERAPY

Group psychotherapy had its beginnings in the work of J. Pratt, who, in 1905, initiated the use of didactic discussion and inspirational group meetings to bring about a favorable change in the morale of physically ill patients whose activities were restricted. The first patients to be treated in such groups were the tubercular; later others with various psychosomatic conditions were treated. As experience has broadened through successive testing of this treatment technique for the psychoses, psychoneuroses, and the various behavior disorders of adults, adolescents, and children, there have evolved both theory and technique that are significant in understanding, recommending, and pursuing treatment. Since the number of patients that may be treated simultaneously by a single therapist is considerable as compared with individual treatment, those concerned with management of massive programs of patient care have encouraged actively the widespread dissemination of the various group psychotherapeutic techniques. However, presumed expediency is the least powerful argument for recommending group psychotherapy.

Indications

Group psychotherapy neither supplants individual psychotherapy nor necessarily offers itself as a substitutive treatment for those to whom other psychotherapeutic doors are closed. On the contrary, it is claimed that there are specific indications for its use. Slavson notes that certain patients manifest aversion to the individual therapies because of fear, competitiveness, distrust, or antagonism toward all authority figures. Individual psychotherapy is too threatening and the patient finds in the group the acceptance and support necessary for the examination of his problems. For such persons, group psychotherapy alone may be successful, or it may serve as a preparation for individual treatment. Patients lacking sibling experiences, having antagonistic sibling attitudes, living in situations without opportunities for participation, experiencing destructive family relations, showing character disorders, presenting evidence of generalized social maladjustment, or fearing homosexual involvement with an individual therapist are often selected for group treatment. Patients with dull intelligence may benefit more from group therapy in peer groups than from individual therapy. Generally, all children gain from group association, and it is believed that many children who need therapy are suitable candidates for the activity form of group treatment. Exclusive group treatment is frequently considered successful when feelings of inadequacy, sibling rivalry, and social maladjustments are the presenting problems in children. Analytical group psychotherapy is considered the treatment of choice for adolescent girls with confused sexual identifications.

Group psychotherapy provides an opportunity to relive and correct in capsular form many distorting experiences of earlier life which have arisen in the context of situations creating destructive sibling rivalry, anxiety-provoking separations, loneliness, excessive spoiling, or exploitation.

The Psychodynamics of Group Process

Perhaps the most significant consideration giving rise to the concept of group interaction as a method of psychotherapy is the sociodynamic pattern of human maturation. The development of the infant from helplessness and dependency to tempered autonomy and acculturation takes place through a continuing series of transactions within a family and a series of extrafamilial social relations. If maladjustments are caused to develop by inadequate or unwholesome group situations during the formative periods of life, it should be possible to undo and modify them by exposing the maladaptations to continuous, structured group action in a more adequate and more wholesome setting.

Within all groups, the emotional processes that take place over time are centered upon the leader. In psychotherapeutic groups, the therapist occupies this role initially. The patient members of the group are tied to each other through their common bond with the leader. The group functions unconsciously as a family, with the leader representing the parental role, usually initially that of a father, as an authority figure. Each member of the group then assumes the role of a sibling in relation to the other group members. Toward the therapist the various members project their transference expectations and fantasies, while toward their fellows in the group they find similar expectations derived from their family experiences or they live through processes of sibling interchange lacking in early life.

In the newly constituted group the patient members are individually dependent and submissive to the therapist. The formation of the group around the leader in an authoritarian position is enhanced when the members are anxious and unsure; thus patient groups more rapidly assume the regressive position in relation to the therapist than other nontherapeutic groups centered around some task orientation. Authoritarian leadership is considered to enhance the submissive dependent relationship and therefore is eschewed in the therapeutic group, where the leader allows a free interchange. In this interchange the group members are encouraged to respond to each other and the leader freely. Thus disagreement and criticism are possible, as is a new type of identification in which the critic may identify with the criticized. This opens to the individual patient in the group a new opportunity for personal evaluation and opinion.

In this treatment process the therapist may become a model for admiration and thereby a focus for a new ego ideal, a model for superego change or growth, or a source for identification through either love or fear. Similarly, the relation to other group members later provides opportunities for alternative identification.

In the therapeutic group the individual member may act out his ambivalent affects toward authority and his peers. In his revelations through both verbal and nonverbal communications within the group, the individual has the permissive support of the leader and his peers in assisting him to reveal himself. Also he is exposed to awareness of his verbal distortions and the unconscious meanings of his mannerisms through the interpretative comments of his peers, a process which creates much reality checking and reëvaluation of personal motivations. Some group members live through new emotional experiences within and through the group transactions and thereby achieve greater understanding of both personal and interpersonal reactions.

Experience with therapy groups has revealed that the principles of treatment employed in individual psychotherapy are applicable to groups. The relationship between each member and the therapist possesses the qualities of individual therapy, and in addition all the patient-members become, in a sense, auxiliary therapists, thus increasing the emotional interplay. The group setting is a continuous reality factor, which presents an ever-fresh stimulus and provocation to behavior that may be therapeutically directed. Although the group support diminishes individual anxiety, many group therapists feel that the amount and character of affective interactions may be increased and accelerated.

The group situation is such that mechanisms are mobilized for self-defense against real or imagined threats occasioned by the presence of others. In large part this is a result of *transference,* the avenue through which projections, displacements, and other mechanisms operate. While the entrance of this attitudinal force into the group work presents a barrier, it becomes the very focal point toward which therapeutic intepretations and insight formations are directed.

Systems of Group Therapy

From the early group techniques of inspirational lectures there evolved group and individual discussions with the leader following his didactic presentations. Simultaneously Trigant Burrow applied to the evolving group therapy theoretical principles derived from psychoanalysis while Kurt Lewin in Germany was working out his field theories and explanations of group dynamics.

From these early experiments in group treatment many variants have been developed. Thus S. R. Slavson, who pioneered analytic group psychotherapy in the United States, derived his conceptual schemes from his experiences in the study of group psychodynamics of children with behavior disorders, a form of treatment organized around manual activities which he designated *activity group therapy.* J. L. Moreno developed the procedures of *psychodrama* and *sociodrama.* In the former, one or more patients interact with each other but are instructed to act out differing roles; in the latter the patients are the audience.

In England during the 1930's Joshua Bierer initiated experiments in which, through group discussions, a passive therapist attempted with a circle of approximately 10 patients to bring about attitude change through impersonal discussion of interpersonal issues. S. H. Foulkes, the founder of the Group Analytic Society and the first to utilize psychoanalytic principles in group psychotherapy in England, initiated this treatment procedure at the Mandsley Hospital.

Other groups have been established with problem-centered approaches directed toward guidance. Among these may be included Alcoholics Anonymous, as well as those groups established for narcotic addicts and homosexuals and for parents of children with cerebral palsy or mental deficiency. In such groups ego strength is enhanced through identification and sharing with others and the growing awareness of and increasing ability to cope with common problems shared by the group members. Later, if such groups remain cohesive, they, too, bring into the open the conflicts and associated emotions as well as the early contributing parental transactions upon which the individual psychopathologies rest.

There now exist group therapies which are essentially nondirective and which have a psychoanalytic orientation, as well as others which rely on more directive procedures based upon didactic or educational principles.

To be separated from the above are the nonclinical groups which aim to improve understanding of the group process to assist in development of assets for leadership, management, counseling, or other roles.

Such "sensitivity," "encounter," training or "T" groups are widely sponsored now by industries, universities, social agencies, and other organizations. In contrast to the group psychotherapies, the conduct of the group process differs in that the leader or trainer initially and generally assumes a nonresponding role —the group is structured to appear leaderless. The members of the group struggle to effect group structure, including leadership, procedures, and task orientation, and in so doing, reveal to themselves and others their customary patterns of behavior in relating to others. The conduct of such groups often has been given to leaders or trainers whose psychological knowledge and training remain undefined. Nor, until recently, have there been efforts to screen those enrolled in the groups, many of whom have been participants on the basis of pressure from the organization in which they are employed. It has become apparent that a number of participants develop acute emotional disturbances during such encounters, and a few have become overtly psychotic. The incidence of such psychopathological reaction is currently unknown. Stone and Tieger surveyed 105 applicants for a church-sponsored "T" group experience and screened out 15 whom they considered to have evidence of psychopathology, while eight failed to attend. Even following screening, two had disruptive emotional reactions. In another study of a wide variety of encounter group experiences Yalom et al. report 16 casualties among 209 individuals participating in encounter group experience—a high rate of distur-

bance. Lack of structure, the lowering of psychological defenses, and in some, the encouragement of extra-group contacts, including the physical, seemed to have precipitated ego disorganization through emergence of unacceptable aggressive, sexual, or dependent striving.

To prevent such reactions it has been recommended that participation be voluntary and informal, that participants be screened, that leaders define the limits of permissible behavior and that those in need of psychiatric assistance be excluded.

In some instances group processes are used to modify attitudes for political purposes, as in "brainwashing" methods employed by certain political organizations. Religious revival meetings also rest upon principles of group interactions that influence individual behavior and attitudes.

Among the group psychotherapists and those concerned with the use of group processes for other purposes, there are controversies today as to whether the principles upon which both rest are similar and convergent. There are those who believe that the group process, with its aim of bringing awareness of the interactions for the benefit of the group as a whole, tends to diminish psychotherapeutic processes for the group members. Others, such as Durkin, stress that all groups are comparable as they have a dynamic basis in ego interaction.

Technique

When possible, it is considered desirable to convene interview groups in round table formation in esthetically pleasant surroundings with an informal atmosphere predominating. Activity therapies may require work tables and a meeting room constructed of especially durable materials. Because of extratherapeutic acting-out, which may limit group work or fragment the group, it is usually desirable to separate the sexes. Groups may meet at any time of day or evening on a rigidly scheduled basis. Except for the intensive therapies, the group convenes once a week for periods of 60 to 90 minutes. More frequent meetings are necessary for groups having deep insight goals.

The proponents of the analytical psychotherapies urge that the *group leaders* have had personal intensive psychotherapy and further training in psychopathology. It is believed that group psychotherapists should have special training in the therapies, including a broad didactic educational background as well as a penchant for this form of treatment. The personality and motivations of the group leader are of importance; it is felt that therapists who normally experience discomfort in groups should not undertake group therapeutic leadership. A competent therapist of either sex may be a group leader. When both group and individual therapy are required for a patient, the therapist must be the same person.

When leaders provide a preparatory session in which the group participants are advised as to the nature of group therapy in dynamic terms, it has been observed that there evolves the development of those transactions conducive to the goals of treatment. The therapists advise that the aim of the group work is toward fostering group and personal maturation. To effect change the members are to immediately express their feelings and thoughts in relation to the group interactions.

Many groups maintain "open" *membership,* allowing participants to terminate therapy when they wish to do so and permitting others to join at any time. As a rule, the deeper the insight goal, the less variable the group membership. Some groups set date limits, while others go on indefinitely for several years. Goals, number of participants, and systems of therapy vary according to whether the groups are composed of hospital or clinic patients. Group psychotherapy is used in mental hospitals, out-patient clinics, private practice, affiliate therapeutic agencies of educational institutions, family agencies, with relatives of hospitalized patients, and with children. Certain groups employ a totally permissive atmosphere without rules.

Some groups employ agreed-upon taboos relative to group work. Many leaders, for example, regard it as desirable to inculcate ethical principles in the group relative to privileged communication and to forbid physical acting-out during meetings.

Group homogeneity and the number of participants are still debated subjects. Too much unification of interest may present the therapist with a symptom wall used as a rallying point for group resistance in the form of monothematic ruminations. On the other hand, too little homogeneity causes scattered interest. Extreme heterogeneity, e.g., alcoholic patients mingled with symptom-neurotic patients, or psychotic persons with transference-neurotic patients, may engender name-calling and mutual distrust. The groups should be large enough for an adequate amount of interaction, yet not so large that members are neglected. In formation of groups for psychotherapy, experienced group therapists suggest that the patients selected be of the same sex, reasonably close to one another in intelligence, reasonably close in age, and fairly well balanced as to traits. Homogeneity of sex helps prevent acting-out. Similarity in intelligence is found to be important because misplaced retarded patients may delay group development. Closeness in age is significant because of the need for some uniformity in social values, outlook, and philosophical points of view. Group balance is needed in order to avoid overloading with a particular group of symptoms that may, as mentioned, serve as a wall of resistance against the therapeutic effort. Generally, groups fare well when they are made up of multiples of a basic triad of patients: the activator, the mollifier, and the passive recipient.

The criteria for denying patients admission to therapeutic groups depend largely upon the orientation of the therapy involved. Most groups suffer from the inclusion of acute psychotic, aggressive paranoid, regressed schizophrenic, and manic patients. Patients with psychoses tending toward depression or those with potential or overt perversion, suicidal behavior, psychopathic personality, involutional states with compulsive and obsessional drives, or hallucinated thought-life are generally excluded from analytical groups. Such patients tend to disrupt, dominate, and exploit the group. They may also stimulate pathological processes in a deleterious way in other patients. In general, it is the feeling among group therapists that patients must have some capacity to participate in groups and at least a minimal amount of social hunger to gain from a therapy group.

The most significant factors which lead to early *dropout* from group psychotherapy appear to rest upon such personality disturbances as inability to tolerate intimacy; shame resulting from maladroit self-disclosures; marked deviancy from the group norms (in terms of age, ethnic difference, or degree of pathology), or need to compete with the leader by setting up a competing subgroup or acting as the group provocateur. Other factors which lead patients to separate from therapeutic groups have to do with personal incapacity to share the leader, inadequate orientation to the group treatment procedure, conflicts engendered when the patient is simultaneously in individual psychotherapy, and various external reasons related to undue stress and anxiety in the life of the patient. Failure to continue in group psychotherapy bears no relationship to the individual's ability to profit from some other form of psychotherapy or treatment.

Group Dynamics

Group psychotherapy possesses a characteristic that contrasts it with individual therapy in that it more closely resembles actual life situations and ordinary social intercourse, thus endowing the process with continuous reality meanings. Whereas in individual psychotherapeutic situations all attitudes, conditionings, and transferences are isolated in the patient

and channeled into the one participant-observer, in group interaction there exist a multiplicity of targets and a dilution of transference. These have both positive and negative values. On the one hand, these factors reduce anxiety and fear activated by hostile and aggressive feelings toward figures of authority, and they allow for redirection or deflection of the hostilities and resentments toward fellow members. On the other hand, these factors may add an almost insuperable complexity to the production of insights. This is due to the multiplicity of possible emotional interrelationships.

MECHANISMS. Probably all groups traverse phases of development roughly approximating three periods: (1) a stage of *group unification* with the emergence of group identity; (2) a stage of *group interaction* with the observation of dynamisms; and (3) a final stage of understanding and *resolution of dynamisms* with the production of insights.

Therapy takes place at different levels according to group goals. The factors of mutual support and reliance engendered by group sanction parallel the formation of group esprit and contribute toward the establishment of morale, which may be all that is desired for some groups. Simple ventilation through the phenomenon of emotional release may relieve tensions in given situations. Popular superstitions and ignorance may respond to educative group reorientation, with the consequent lessening of fears and anxieties.

Analytically oriented group psychotherapies make use of the classical factors of catharsis, resistance, analysis of transference, interpretation, and insight formation. The leader plays an important role in interpretation when resistance must be overcome, also in the resolution of transference. The group setting offers opportunities for the manifestation of social mechanisms and dynamisms not ordinarily found in individual psychotherapy. In addition to those mentioned above, the following are a few commonly encountered.

Displacement. A variety of feelings

toward the therapist, which the patient may be afraid to express, are displaced on less threatening group members or on persons not present.

Escape. This is achieved by selective silence or by a change of subject.

Deflection. This may be used for escape by redirecting attention to another group member.

Catalysis. This dynamism represents the manner in which each member activates all the others. Frequently it is valuable, especially in institutional group psychotherapy, to transplant a particularly alert or well-indoctrinated member as a nuclear cadreman, around whom new groups may be built. Such a catalyst accelerates early group work.

Identification. This primary mechanism in personality development is the insigne of civilization and enters importantly into the therapeutic process.

Universalization. This is the term given the dynamism occurring in patients when they discover that other people have problems similar to their own, that others entertain the same forbidden thoughts or experience similar unacceptable impulses. This mechanism alone is considered by some to be therapeutic. It reduces guilt, heightens self-esteem, and diminishes emotional burdens.

ADVANTAGES. Frequently small groups not only have supportive value but permit the expression of hidden anxieties and conflicts. Also members, by seeing their unconscious motives in action in the ways the members feel toward each other and to the therapist, may gradually gain insight into their difficulties.

Since anxiety is reduced and transference modified in group psychotherapy, the depth of insight may be less than in intensive individual psychotherapy, although some therapists claim that a depth of insight comparable with that of individual psychoanalysis may be attained.

An important consideration of group therapy is the realization that in chronically aggressive children the very antagonisms and violent hostilities that consti-

tute their antisocial tendencies are factors common to such groups and tend to promote unit formation, while the nonneurotic elements of the ego respond to the persevering interest and patience of the group leader.

The mobilization of certain defenses may be all that is desired in the treatment of many psychotic patients. The group process often encourages re-repression of unconscious fantasies that present themselves clinically as delusions. As the psychotic mechanisms are removed from consciousness, more normal ego elements resume their supremacy and the patient may become eligible for noninstitutional life or individual psychotherapy.

Mention should be made of the ever-increasing senile segment of the population, with whom considerable group therapeutic work is now being done in some institutions. A significantly greater number of senile patients so treated are enabled to return to better levels of adjustment than is the case when group therapy is not employed. The group process appears to increase alertness, dispel confusion, bring affects toward normal, and improve memory and orientation. Often the amount of incontinence is found to diminish in many patients on this program.

Results of Group Therapy

The statistical evaluation of therapeutic results of group work, as in all the therapies, remains largely impressionistic. A recent study of 22 juvenile delinquents treated with interview and activity group therapy and of the same number of controls revealed statistically significant improvement in the experimental group as measured by psychometric tests, school achievement, and maturity tests as well as by Rorschach personality assessment technique. Also, neurotic depressions are said to respond well to group psychotherapy. Most therapists of well-constituted groups report results that compare favorably with those of individual psychotherapy.

FAMILY THERAPY

With the expanding awareness of the importance of the interactions between family members in shaping and maintaining behavioral patterns of the individual (the psychic defenses and adaptative processes), family therapy has emerged within the past decade as an important new therapeutic technique. Experience with individual psychotherapies in the correction of psychopathology revealed the difficulty of bringing about changes in symptoms or maintaining gains achieved when individual patients were treated separately from the family group and then returned to the still-existing pathogenic milieu in the home. Too, when individual psychotherapy succeeded in bringing about substantial changes in symptom expression and more effective social adaptation, sometimes there were observed shifts in family homeostasis that led to frank appearance of psychopathology in other family members and, at times, dissolution of the nuclear family. Several decades ago a number of psychoanalysts and child psychiatrists commenced experimentation with various forms of family therapy. In some instances members of the family were treated individually, the therapists meeting regularly to consult each other; in others married partners were treated simultaneously either on a regular basis or through spaced conjoint meetings with a single psychotherapist. Family therapy as it is practiced today is best represented in the efforts of N. Ackerman, D. J. Jackson, and their associates. In their practice the therapist meets regularly with the members of the nuclear family, significant relatives, or members of the extended generational family—that is, parents and grandparents.

Indications and Contraindications

Family psychotherapy has found its greatest application in the tretament of those neurotic, psychotic, and personality disorders in which individuals "act out." Thus indications for its use are aggressive behaviors leading to maladaptation of children or adolescents at school or in the community, the various addictive states in adolescents and adults, and marital disharmonies with their roots in the complicated transactional processes of an extended family. Where psychotic defenses in an individual are perpetuated or clearly aggravated by reëxposure to a conflict-ridden family situation, again family psychotherapy may prove the necessary adjunctive method to assist in establishing social rehabilitation.

Family psychotherapy is not advised for children or adolescents when one or both parents are known to have an established paranoid psychosis or have a history of a personality disorder with traits of dishonesty, deceitfulness, untruthfulness, or recurrent antisocial behavior. The existence of a threatening family secret or of fixed cultural or religious prejudices against such treatment contraindicates its trial as well. Treatment is inadvisable if there is a physical disease which precludes participation by one or more family members or if a family member has fixed rigid psychological defenses which, if stressed by the anxieties of the treatment, might induce ego disruption and a psychosomatic crisis or a psychosis. Again, family therapy should not be initiated if breakup or dissolution of the family by an irreversible conflict is imminent.

Family Theory

The family is the indispensable social unit necessary for the growth and maturation of its various members. Without the maturing protection from excessive emotional arousal and the learning processes so important to later social adaptations that take place in the family, the growing members suffer personality warp or even failure. The transactions within the healthy family determine the stability of the later social adaptations of its various members. Within the family, its members express both similarities and differences in their modes of interaction. Their individual character traits and talents supplement and complement each other or may be the source for frustration of needs and desires and thereby induce family conflict and fragmentation.

The complementary aspects of family transactions enhance the self-esteem of the individual members, satisfy their needs, support their defenses in the face of anxiety induced within or without the family, assist in their efforts at solution of conflict situations, and support the development and fulfillment of each member's personal abilities and drives.

As the capacities of the maturing individual change and his personality emerges, it is inevitable that conflicts should wax and wane within the family. Family conflict has potential for both assistance and restriction of growth of each individual within the group. As Ackerman points out, "Competition and coöperation in family relations are not necessarily opposites. The true opposite of coöperation is not competition but apathy and indifference."

When the differences within the family become threats to the individuals, instead of being perceived as valuable, then family conflict leads to splits, with family members aligning against each other or selecting one or several members as scapegoats. The family conflict organizes around the selected member, who may be ill or who may be the family troublemaker, pet, clown, or presumed most talented.

Family conflicts center over differences and their presumed perquisites, passivity versus activity, controlling domination versus pleasure seeking, obedient versus defiant behaviors, drives for positions of power and wealth versus their relinquishment or destruction. Various members of the family group may alternately or regularly play the domineering role, that of persecutor, scapegoat, or mediator.

Family conflicts may be resolved rationally through their clear perception by the involved members or through their

containment by various compensations while solutions are sought. When the family members misperceive or distort their relations with each other, then the conflict situation leads to such accretions of emotion that one or several members act out or become isolated in the special roles mentioned beforehand. The theories of Bateson and Jackson and of Johnson and Szurek, mentioned in earlier chapters, are most pertinent in the comprehension of family conflict as it relates to pathological behavior and defective communication. It is under these circumstances that family psychotherapy may assist in a solution of the family crises as well as of the pathology engendered in the family members.

Technique

The primary aim of the family therapist is the mobilization of a rational and effective communications system between the family members—one which brings to awareness the hidden and distorted expressions of emotion which pervade the disturbed family and adversely affect the sick member or members.

The family therapist must take the position of a participant observer within the family group. He initially invites the family to meet with him as a group to discuss the problem of the referred member. In the initial discussion he may see husband and wife, parents and children, or the extended group. It is considered preferable to meet with the group without prior effort at gaining a formal history of the family. The therapist notes how the family members enter the room and the seating arrangement they establish spontaneously. On successive treatment sessions he ascertains if repetitive patterns of association and communication exist between particular family members. He notes those who dominate the commentary, those who interrupt, coerce, deny, or express their reaction through such nonverbal communications as frowns, smiles, or other bodily movements or remissions or by withdrawal. It is then his function through clarifying questions and interpretations of behavior to assist the family to become more open in their communications, to reassay and reorganize their patterns of coercion and malalliance and resolve conflicts by exposing their emotional responses to the real and unreal differences they perceive amongst themselves. The therapist uses his own personality and requires that the family members express their transference perceptions of him. He must be active, questioning, and at the same time supportive of those family members who bear the brunt of family attack in the course of the treatment sessions.

Family psychotherapy differs from group psychotherapy in that the members of the family bring to the psychotherapeutic process various roles and patterns of interaction long since established. The therapist's role as a leader is less sharply perceived in the initial phases of family psychotherapy, whereas in group treatments that position is evident from the initial meeting. Futhermore, the aim of the therapist differs in that his hope is to bring about a change in the family as an ongoing social institution. The group psychotherapist uses processes that emerge in an artificially constructed group to assist the individual members in achievement of useful personality change, but is not committed to shaping that process for any permanent function.

BIBLIOGRAPHY

Psychoanalysis

Abraham, K.: Selected Papers on Psychoanalysis. London, Hogarth Press, 1927.

Adler, A.: The Practice and Theory of Individual Psychology. New York, Harcourt, Brace & Company, 1956.

Freud, S.: Collected Papers (5 vols.). London, International Psychoanalytical Library, 1924-1950.

Freud, S.: The Interpretation of Dreams. New York, The Macmillan Company, 1933.

Fromm-Reichmann, F.: Notes on the personal and professional requirements of a psychotherapist. Psychiatry, 12:361–378, 1949.

Fromm-Reichmann, F.: Principles of Intensive Psychotherapy. Chicago, University of Chicago Press, 1950.

Fromm-Reichmann, F.: Psychoanalytic and general dynamic concepts of theory and of therapy. J. Amer. Psychoanalyt. Assn., 2:711–721, 1954.

Glover, E.: The indications for psychoanalysis. J. Ment. Sci., 100:393–401, 1954.

Greenacre, P.: The role of transference. J. Amer. Psychoanalyt. Assn., 2:671–684, 1954.

Greenson, R. R.: The Technique and Practice of Psychoanalysis. New York, International Universities Press, 1967.

Kubie, L. S.: Practical and Theoretical Aspects of Psychoanalysis. New York, International Universities Press, 1950.

Sandler, J., Holder, A., and Dare, C.: Basic Psychoanalytic concepts: IV. Counter Transference. Brit. J. Psychiat., 117:83–88, 1970; V. Resistance. Brit. J. Psychiat., 117:215–221, 1970.

Silber, A.: A patient's gift: Its meaning and function. Int. J. Psychoanal., 50:335–341, 1969.

Weber, J. J., Elinson, J., and Moss, L. M.: Psychoanalysis and change. Arch. Gen. Psychiat., 17:687–709, 1967.

Weber, J. J., Elinson, J., and Moss, L. M.: The application of ego strength scales to psychoanalytic clinic records. In Goldman, G. S., and Shapiro, D. (eds.): Developments in Psychoanalysis at Columbia University. New York, Hafner, 1967, pp. 215–273.

Psychotherapy

Aldrich, C. K.: Brief psychotherapy. A reappraisal of some theoretical assumptions. Amer. J. Psychiat., 125:585–592, 1968.

Balser, B. H.: Psychotherapy of the Adolescent. New York, International Universities Press, 1957.

Durkin, H. E.: The Group in Depth. New York, International Universities Press, 1964.

Fiske, D. W., et al.: Planning of research on effectiveness of psychotherapy. Arch. Gen. Psychiat., 22:22–32, 1970.

Ford, D. H., and Urban, H. B.: Systems of Psychotherapy. New York, John Wiley & Sons, 1963.

Frank, J. D.: The influence of patient's and therapist's expectations on the outcome of psychotherapy. Brit. J. Med. Psychol., 41:349–356, 1968.

Garner, H. H.: Interventions in psychotherapy and confrontation technique. Amer. J. Psychother., 20:391–404, 1966.

Haley, J.: Strategies of Psychotherapy. New York, Grune & Stratton, Inc., 1963.

Haskell, D., Pugatch, D., and McNair, D. M.: Time limited psychotherapy for whom. Arch. Gen. Psychiat., 21:546–552, 1969.

Karush, A., and Ovesey, L.: Unconscious mechanisms of magical repair. Arch. Gen. Psychiat., 5:55–69, 1961.

Kolb, L. C.: Psychotherapeutic evolution and its implications. Psychiat. Quart., 30:579–597, 1956.

Mann, J.: The specific limitation of time on psychotherapy. Seminars Psych., *1:*375–379, 1969.

Ross, T. A.: The Common Neuroses. Baltimore, William Wood & Company, 1937.

Hypnosis

Barber, T. X.: Suggested (Hypnotic) Behavior. The Trance Paradigms Versus an Alternative Paradigm. Medford, Massachusetts, The Harding Foundation, 1970.

Hilgard, E. R.: Hypnosis. Ann. Rev. Psychol., *16:*157–180, 1965.

Marks, I. M., Gilder, M. G., and Edwards, G.: Hypnosis and desensitization: A controlled prospective study. Brit. J. Psychiat., *114:*1263–1274, 1968.

Orne, M. T.: Hypnosis, motivation and compliance. Amer. J. Psychiat., *122:*721–726, 1966.

Spiegel, H., and Bridger, A. H.: Manual for Hypnotic Induction. Profile, Eye Roll Levitation Method. New York, Soni Medica, Inc., 1970.

Spiegel, H., and Shainess, N.: Operational spectrum of psychotherapeutic process. Arch. Gen. Psychiat., *9:*477–488, 1963.

Behavior Therapy

Dyrud, J. E.: Behavior analysis, mental events and psychoanalysis. Sci. & Psychoanal., *18:*51–62, 1971.

Gelder, M. G., Marks, I. M., and Woolff, H. H.: Desensitization and psychotherapy in the treatment of phobic states: A controlled inquiry. Brit. J. Psychiat., *113:*53–73, 1967.

Hewett, F. M.: Teaching speech to an autistic child through operant conditioning. Amer. J. Orthopsychiat., *35:*927–936, 1965.

Hunt, H. F.: Behavioral considerations in psychiatric treatment. Sci. & Psychoanal., *18:*36–50, 1971.

Liberman, R. P.: Behavior modifications with chronic mental patients. J. Chronic Dis., *23:*803–812, 1971.

McConaghy, N.: Results of systematic desensitization with phobias re-examined. Brit. J. Psychiat., *117:*89–92, 1970.

Mowrer, O. W.: The behavior therapies, with special reference to modeling and imitation. Amer. J. Psychother., *20:*439–461, 1966.

Rashkis, H. A.: How behavior therapy affects schizophrenia. Dis. Nerv. Syst., *27:*505–510. 1966.

Wolpe, J., and Lazarus, A. H.: Behavior Therapy Techniques: A Guide to the Treatment of Neuroses. New York, Pergamon Press, 1966.

Sociotherapies

Ackerman, N. W.: Treating the Troubled Family. New York, Basic Books, 1966.

Ackerman, N. W. (ed.): Family Psychotherapy in Transition. Boston, Little, Brown & Co., 1970.

Edelson, M.: Sociotherapy and psychotherapy in social psychiatry. Publ. Assn. Res. Nerv. & Ment. Dis., *47:*196–211, 1967.

Jaffe, S. J., and Scherl, D. J.: Acute psychosis precipitated by T group experiences. Arch. Gen. Psychiat., *21:*443–448, 1969.

Jones, M.: The Therapeutic Community. London, Tavistock Publications, Ltd., 1952.

Kadis, A. L.: Krasner, J. D., Winick, G., and Foulkes, S. H.: A Practicum of Group Psychotherapy. New York, Harper & Row, 1963.

Kaplan, H. I., and Sadock, B. J. (eds.): Comprehensive Group Psychotherapy. Baltimore, Williams & Wilkins Company, 1971.

Semrad, E. V., and Arsenian, J.: The use of group processes in teaching group dynamics. Amer. J. Psychiat., *108:*358–363, 1951.

Slavson, S. R.: Analytic Group Psychotherapy with Children, Adolescents and Adults. New York, Columbia University Press, 1950.

Stone, W. N., and Tieger, M. E.: Screening for T groups: The myth of health candidates. Amer. J. Psychiat., *127:*1485–1490, 1971.

Whitaker, D. S., and Lieberman, M. A.: Psychotherapy Through the Group Process. New York, Atherton Press, 1964.

Yalom, I. D.: A study of group therapy dropouts. Arch. Gen. Psychiat., *14:*393–414, 1966.

Yalom, I. D., Houts, P. S., Newell, G., and Rand, K. H.: Preparation of patients for group therapy. Arch. Gen. Psychiat., *17:*416–427, 1967.

Yalom, I. D., and Lieberman, M. A.: Encounter group casualties. Arch. Gen. Psychiat., *25:*16–30, 1971.

Chapter 32

"We must recollect that all our provisional ideas in psychology will some day be based on an organic substructure. This makes it probable that special substances and special chemical processes control the operation . . ."

Sigmund Freud

Pharmacological Therapy

Following the introduction in 1952 of the phenothiazine chlorpromazine as a potent new pharmacological agent for the treatment of the psychoses, numerous analogs and other new compounds have been synthesized, tested, and placed in clinical usage. The effectiveness of the phenothiazine analogs and certain antidepressant agents has altered particularly the management of the psychoses. Their widespread prescription has superseded to a large extent the various forms of shock therapy and the use of psychosurgery.

These agents have the capacity to modify affective states without seriously impairing cognitive functions. In the latter respect they differ from the sedative and hypnotic drugs previously available. Since it is expected that the able psychiatrist comes to practice fully knowledgeable from his previous medical studies of the well-known properties and clinical indications of the long-known central nervous depressants such as the narcotics, anesthetics, hypnotics, and intoxicants, as well as the stimulants, consideration is not given to these drugs in this text. Their skillful prescription, often in conjunction with that of the "neuroleptics," still is demanded in practice.

PHARMACOLOGICAL ACTION AND BRAIN FUNCTION

Both neuroleptic and antidepressant pharmacologic agents exert complex actions upon various neural systems and the neuron itself. These actions have been demonstrated through changes brought about in animal behavior (particularly through analysis of responses obtained under conditions imposed by classical and instrumental conditioning), through depth electroencephalography, and through electrophysiological and biochemical studies of synaptic transmission.

Much of the variation in effect produced by the differing agents is thought to depend upon their differing actions at the synaptic junctions within the brain, where both cholinergic and noncholinergic transmission is thought to occur. It is considered that the passage of a nerve impulse from activated neurons takes place across the synaptic junction by discharge into the synaptic cleft of the stimulating catecholamine, norepinephrine. That substance then activates the effector site of the postsynaptic neuron.

Whether norepinephrine alone or the catecholamine dopamine or the indole-amine serotonin also participate in synaptic transmission is not known. Epinephrine probably does not, as it exists in low concentrations in the brain. In the neuron norepinephrine exists in two forms: the labile form, capable of release by stimulation or by sympathomimetic drugs such as amphetamine, and that form contained in storage granules and released by reserpine. When released from the interneuronal structure the norepinephrine flows into the synaptic cleft and then is returned to the cell, where it is stored or oxidized by the enzyme monoamine oxidase. The monoamine oxidase inhibitors, such as iproniazid, increase the amount of intraneuronal norepinephrine, making more available. Reserpine depletes the intraneuronal amines, thus diminishing the amount available for activation.

Both the phenothiazines and the iminodibenzyls, such as imipramine, diminish cellular permeability. For this reason the released norepinephrine is partially prevented from returning to the neuron and its concentration in the synaptic cleft is prolonged over time. But the availability of the opposite site of the postsynaptic cell is decreased as well by the same pharmacologic agents. The principal action of the phenothiazines is to render the receptor sites less avilable so that the effect of the neurotransmitter is diminished. Imipramine and its analogs, on the other hand, prevent the resorption of norepinephrine into the activating nerve endings and thus increase the action of the neurotransmitter. Thus those drugs which deplete or inactivate norepinephrine in the brain usually produce sedative or depressive actions, while those that increase or potentiate it commonly bring about excitatory behavior and have antidepressant effects. Norepinephrine and serotonin are found in highest concentration in the hypothalamus. Dopamine exists in greatest concentration in the caudate and lenticular nucleus.

Such drugs exert their major effects upon the brain stem and limbic systems, the structures of which, as has been noted in Chapter 3, are principally concerned with systems modulating and shaping emotional behavior. The phenothiazines decrease the excitability of limbic structures, while reserpine does the opposite. While the iminodibenzyls stimulate limbic structures, the antidepressant monoamine oxidase inhibitors do not. The latter stimulate the reticular activating system, while the phenothiazines do not.

The explanations given for the varying effects of the various neuroleptic agents on synaptic transmission and on functions of limbic or reticular activating systems do not entirely explain their impressive actions in modifying affect in the major psychoses. The effect of each agent represents rather a little understood summation of its actions upon the totality of brain systems. What emerges from the pharmacological physiology is an appreciation of the differences of action of the various series of agents, a recognition that their functions vary, and therefore that the underlying neurohumoral constitution of the class of patients in which each is effective may well be idiosyncratic for that disorder. Constitutional differences may have origins in genetic differences, expressed in subtle variations in production, transport, storage, and metabolism of neurotransmitters within the brain. Both the effectiveness and the toxicity of drugs may be based as much on such variables as on dosage levels, routes of administration, and absorption.

NEUROLEPTIC AGENTS

The phenothiazine nucleus from which the various analogs have been synthesized consists of two benzine rings joined by a sulfur and nitrogen atom. By alteration of R_1 and R_2 in the formula, numerous derivatives have been developed (see accompanying table). From the attachment of a dimethylammopropyl side-chain at R_1 are derived chlorpromazine, promazine, and triflupromazine. Substitution of the piperazine side-chain in this position leads to the development of perphenazine, prochlorperazine, and trifluoperazine. The piperidine side-chain attached at R_1 results in thioridazin and mepazine. Compounds in the piperazine-substituted group are the most potent but also have the greatest tendency to produce symptoms of extrapyramidal dysfunction.

The general indications for the prescription of the phenothiazine derivations are the same as those for chlorpromazine. These drugs differ more in their toxic properties than in their abilities to modify selectively various "target symptoms."

Pharmacological experiments in animals show that the phenothiazines reduce conditioned avoidance responses. They do not inhibit escape, nor do they affect the response to conditional stimuli as do the barbiturates. They impair vigilance but not cognitive actions. Seizure threshold to both electroshock and convulsive drugs is unchanged. With large doses only there appear slow (5 to 6 per second) low-voltage waves in the electroencephalogram. Hypothalamically regulated activities are disrupted. Thus thermoregulation is impaired, adrenocorticotropic hormone (ACTH) secretion is diminished, and growth is diminished. Other endocrine effects are reduction in urinary gonadotropins. In animals, the estrous cycle and ovulation are suppressed by the pheno-

thiazines. The decidual reaction is prolonged by them and lactation is induced. Infertility occurs. These agents are well absorbed from the intestine (60 to 80 per cent) and widely distributed in the body tissues, where they remain bound for prolonged periods (6 to 12 months) after administration has ceased. They are metabolized in the liver through hydrolysis and glucuronidization.

ALIPHATIC DERIVATIVES

Chlorpromazine Hydrochloride

This is a synthetic drug, one of the series of alkyl, amine derivatives of phenothiazine, its full chemical name being 10-(3-dimethylaminopropyl)-2-chlorphenothiazine hydrochloride. It was developed in the Rhone-Poulenc Specia Laboratories in France during research on potentiating agents in anesthesia. The first clinical investigations with the drug were carried out in that country in 1952. In France, as in other European countries, it is marketed under the trade name Largactil. In the United States it is marketed under the trade name of Thorazine.

Chlorpromazine is a white crystalline

Phenothiazines

			TOTAL ORAL DAILY DOSAGE IN MG. (DIVIDED INTO 2-4 DOSES)	
R_1	R_2 U.S. TRADE NAME		OUTPATIENT RANGE	HOSPITAL RANGE
(Classified by side chain)				
Aliphatic				
Chlorpromazine	Thorazine		30-400	400-1600
Promazine	Sparine		75-200	200-1000
Triflupromazine	Vesprin		50-150	75-200
Levomepromazine	Levoprome		150-300	150-300
Piperidine				
Thioridazine	Mellaril		40-400	400-800
Mepazine	Pacatal		75-200	200-600
Piperazine				
Acetophenazine	Tindal		40-60	60-80
Carphenazine	Proketazine		25-100	50-400
Prochlorperazine	Compazine		15-60	30-150
Thiopropazate	Dartal		10-30	30-150
Perphenazine	Trilafon		8-24	12-64
Trifluoperazine	Stelazine		4-10	6-30
Fluphenazine	Prolixin; Permitil		1-3	2-20

powder that is readily soluble in water. Since only a small part of the drug is eliminated by the kidneys, most of it is presumably metabolized in the body, although the route is unknown.

PHYSIOLOGICAL EFFECTS. One of the early effects of the administration of chlorpromazine is a fall in blood pressure according to dose and individual reaction. Other effects are slowing of the pulse and of respiration, lowering of temperature and of basal metabolic rate, and transient leukopenia. Also, it frequently causes dryness of the mucous membranes and nasal congestion. It has an antiemetic effect as well. In large doses, chlorpromazine produces motor retardation, muscular hypotonia, and an unsteady gait. During the first two or three days of treatment, patients show varying degrees of somnolence but can be awakened without difficulty and are able to take food. However, as a rule, the increased need for sleep is reduced after a few days. Patients may complain of feeling faint, weak, cold, and drowsy, but the sensorium remains clear. The action of the drug is maximal at one hour after administration and appreciable effects continue for six hours. It potentiates the effects of barbiturates and of narcotics.

ADMINISTRATION. Chlorpromazine is available in 10-, 25-, 50-, 100-, and 200-mg. tablets, and also in 25-mg. (1-ml.) and 50-mg. (2-ml.) ampuls. There is no standard dose of the drug; this must be individualized. Chlorpromazine may be administered by oral or by intramuscular routes; however, it is so irritant that it should not be administered subcutaneously. Intramuscular injections should be given deeply in the upper and outer quadrant of the buttock, and when injected the solution supplied by the manufacturer should be diluted with physiological salt solution or a 2 per cent procaine solution and administered very slowly. Massaging the site of the injection for three or four minutes will help to reduce local irritation. Some physicians add hyaluronidase in order to facilitate absorption and prevent abscess forma-

tion. If quick action is desired, the patient may receive 25 mg. by deep intramuscular injection, and if this amount is not effective, an additional 25-mg. injection may be given within an hour unless contraindicated by marked hypotension. Subsequent intramuscular dosages may be increased gradually, even up to 400 mg. every six hours. The higher doses should be reached over a period of several days.

If, as frequently occurs, the acutely disturbed patient becomes quiet within 48 hours, oral doses (milligram for milligram or higher) may gradually replace intramuscular doses. Injections should not be continued for more than three or four days without being replaced with oral therapy. It will not usually be necessary to increase oral administration to more than 800 mg. a day, but if sedation is not secured, the dosage may gradually be increased up to as much as 1200 mg. a day. Usually this amount is sufficient for a maximum dose, although some psychiatrists give a maximum of 2000 mg. in 24 hours. Amounts up to 4000 mg. have been given, but large doses cause confusion and are not to be recommended.

As the patient begins to grow quiet, the dose may gradually be reduced over a period of weeks or months. If signs of returning symptoms appear, the amount should be increased immediately and additional parenteral doses should be given if necessary. When the patient is no longer disturbed, the dose may usually be reduced gradually and then continued for an indefinite period, the amount being the smallest that will control symptoms. Usually in the chronically disturbed patient this will be approximately 600 to 800 mg. daily. If there has been no improvement in symptoms after the patient has received these amounts daily for two months, the drug should be gradually discontinued.

In the less acutely agitated patient, treatment may be begun with 50 mg. given orally three times a day. This should be increased gradually until an effective and tolerable level is reached. Frequently doses of 100 to 400 mg. daily, if continued over a long period, will maintain sedation.

The most obvious response to chlorpromazine is somnolence, varying from slight drowsiness to deep sleep. The somnolence is most marked within 15 to 20 minutes after an injection; however, even when the somnolence is deepest, it is possible to rouse the patient easily. He shows little or none of the residual clouding of consciousness that follows comparable barbiturate sedation. Acutely agitated, restless, or excited patients show a greater response than do less disturbed patients. The tranquilizing effect does not seem in any way related to the underlying nature of the excitement: whether it is schizophrenic, manic, or confusional. If the patient responds well to the drug, he develops an attitude of indifference both to his surroundings and to his symptoms. He shows decreased interest in and response to his hallucinatory experiences and a less assertive expression of his delusional ideas.

INDICATIONS FOR USE. Chlorpromazine usually exerts a tranquilizing effect in a wide variety of disturbed psychiatric states —tension, psychomotor overactivity, agitation, impulsiveness, aggressive outbursts, destructiveness, and overtly anxious antagonistic, paranoid reactions.

It has a wide field of usefulness in *schizophrenia*, both in acute reactions and in overactive chronic reactions. The more destructive and aggressive the patient, the more likely is he to respond to chlorpromazine. In the acutely ill, schizophrenic hallucinations and delusional ideas frequently disappear within the first two weeks of treatment. The longer the schizophrenic patient has been ill, the less are his chances of attaining a moderate or marked improvement. Of schizophrenics who receive chlorpromazine (or reserpine) relatively early in their illness, more are able to leave the hospital and make adequate social adjustment than has been the case with any previous method of treatment. Among them will be many who, despite electroconvulsive or insulin coma and other forms of treatment, have shown no improvement. Chronic psychotic patients should be treated for extended periods (six to eight months) before the results are assessed. Best results are secured with patients who have not been ill for more than two years. Among these the results will depend largely on the clinical manifestations of the disorder, the degree of improvement being much greater in the overactive, disturbed patients.

Many patients previously so ill and preoccupied with the symptoms of their illness that they remained indifferent or hostile to attempts to alter their behavior, thinking, or emotional set become more amenable to therapy when taking chlorpromazine. Although many schizophrenics who have been hospitalized for years show some improvement, not more than 5 per cent of those hospitalized for five continuous years become able to leave the hospital.

From 30 to 35 per cent of the chronic schizophrenics who have long been hospitalized will not be materially improved by administration of chlorpromazine, yet the care of the approximately 60 per cent who do improve but are not able to leave the hospital is greatly eased. Delusions and hallucinations may persist but are usually no longer disturbing to the patient. The sullen, sarcastic, and antagonistic patient is less irritable and frequently becomes quiet, coöperative, and accessible, and there is a remarkable improvement in disturbed patients. Although the withdrawn, inactive, unresponsive, regressed schizophrenic patient does not usually improve sufficiently to leave the hospital, he frequently is able to modify his behavior, discontinue soiling, and no longer discard his clothing. The relief from the anguish, bitterness, hostility, and despair from which many patients suffer is of incalculable value. The chronic schizophrenic who improves should continue on a carefully determined maintenance dose for an extended period.

In *manic-depressive psychosis*, chlorpromazine is not a substitute for electroconvulsive therapy, but in the early stages of the manic phase it is a useful adjunct if the patient is overactive and unmanageable and the period required for recovery is usually shortened. It is often desirable to administer the drug by intramuscular injections for two or three days and then to continue it by mouth in 50 per cent larger doses. If the depressed patient is agitated, chlorpromazine will usually relieve, or perhaps more accurately mask, the agitation. However, reactive depressions do not respond particularly well to chlorpromazine.

The usually difficult problem of the restless or agitated patient suffering from *senile dementia* is often rendered much easier by the use of chlorpromazine. Sedation by means of the barbiturates may confuse him still further. Under chlorpromazine, in amounts of 25 to 50 mg. three times a day, he often becomes calm and manageable and can be cared for at home. Memory loss and disorientation are, of course, unaffected.

Chlorpromazine has proved of value in treatment of patients with the psychophysiologic disorders, including the pruritic dermatides, acne, rheumatoid arthritis, and asthma.

Occasionally, especially in institutions for their care, *epileptic patients* are subject to episodic or chronic disturbed states in which the patients may be hyperactive, noisy, hostile, aggressive, resistive, assaultive, destructive, and given to temper outbursts or furor states. A parenteral injection of 100 mg. of chlorpromazine is highly effective in quieting the acute, excited states. Most epileptic patients who exhibit chronic disturbed states are also quieted and relaxed by the drug. This may at first be given as 300 mg. daily and later reduced to 150 mg. Since chlorpromazine tends to potentiate the activity of barbiturates, it is well to reduce the dose of the latter drug during the administration of the former.

In relatively large doses, chlorpromazine is extremely helpful in the management of *acute alcoholic states*. It produces prompt control of motor excitement and

of nausea and vomiting, permits restful, relaxed sleep, and contributes to the relief of tension and anxiety. Its sedative effect hastens recovery in delirium tremens. It is definitely beneficial in nearly all short-lived mental disturbances of a delirious type. The use of chlorpromazine should supplement and not replace the administration of glucose solution, of insulin, and of vitamin B complex. It is not, of course, of value in the treatment of Korsakoff's syndrome or in the alleviation of chronic alcoholism.

UNTOWARD EFFECTS. Mention has already been made of some of the physiological effects of chlorpromazine. At times these side-effects are troublesome, but they rarely lead to serious complications. Occasionally the somnolence may become excessive and require a reduction of dosage. Usually, however, it disappears after the first or second week of therapy. Not infrequently an unpleasant taste and a dryness of the mouth and "stuffiness" of the nose result in discomfort. Tachycardia, palpitation, persistent constipation even to the point of fecal impaction, headaches, pyrexia, and pains in the legs or abdomen may occur. A pale and "pinched" facial appearance is common in patients receiving full intramuscular doses.

Both chlorpromazine and reserpine cause *hypotension* of the orthostatic type. This may lead to sensations of faintness or to actual fainting, especially on changing from a recumbent to a standing position. Both drugs should be given with great caution to patients suffering from atherosclerosis, cardiovascular disease, or other conditions in which a sudden drop in blood pressure may be undesirable.

Skin reactions occur in about 5 per cent of patients administered chlorpromazine. The urticarial, maculopapular, edematous, or petechial response takes place within one to five weeks after initiation of treatment. When drug administration is stopped, the skin clears and may remain clear even if the same treatment is resumed later. This is regarded as a hypersensitivity response.

Photosensitivity confined to areas exposed to sunlight may be produced by chlorpromazine. Usually this will result merely in redness and itching, but sometimes it will lead to edema and vesicle formation. Ordinarily interruption of the drug, the application of bland lotions, and the administration of antihistamines are sufficient treatment of the dermatological reactions.

Abnormal skin pigmentation, appearing as a gray-blue discoloration in areas exposed to the sun, has developed in some patients after prolonged high-dosage administration. Similar deposits of pseudomelanin have occurred in the cornea and lens, but only in rare instances have such deposits impaired vision. D-Penicillamine given in doses of 0.3 gm. three times daily for six days with mineral supplement substitution on the last day has been reported successful in reducing the pigmentation.

Jaundice, usually appearing from the second to the eighth week after use of the drug was started, develops in approximately 4 per cent of the cases, and its duration is variable. Since there is no evidence of damage to the hepatic parenchyma, the jaundice is undoubtedly cholestatic in origin. The total bilirubin content of the blood is greatly elevated, and the alkaline cholesterol is much increased, as is the percentage of eosinophils. However, there is little or no disturbance of the cephalin flocculation and thymol turbidity. The obstruction is within the intralobular canaliculi and a result of a pericanalicular lymphocytic infiltration.

If the patient's mental state is such that he can note and report his observations, it is well to ask him if there has been any change in the color of his urine or stools, also if he has been aware of pruritus. As a precursory symptom of jaundice, this has been known to occur within two days after the administration of chlorpromazine. Since it is simple and can easily be done at the bedside as a screening measure, some internists advise doing a sodium bilirubinate test twice a week for three weeks after beginning the drug. If jaundice appears, the drug should be discontinued and glucose administered intravenously, if indicated. Vitamins should be given, and also a high-carbohydrate, high-protein, and low-fat diet. It is often difficult to determine whether the jaundice is caused by the drug or by extrahepatic obstruction. Surgery for supposed disease of the biliary tract should be avoided. Liver function tests should probably be continued until they show that normal function has been restored. To what extent, if any, the liver will suffer harmful effects as the result of long-continued administration of chlorpromazine is as yet unknown. Although the jaundice is apparently related not so much to dosage as to a special sensitivity on the part of the patient, the drug may be resumed after normal function has been restored. The beginning dosage should not exceed 25 mg. given three times a day and should be increased slowly thereafter.

Chlorpromazine depresses the production of leukocytes. *Agranulocytosis* is fortunately of low incidence, probably less than 0.3 per cent, and it occurs within three to six weeks after the beginning of treatment. It is more frequent in women, particularly in those between 40 and 60 years of age, and its onset is sudden. Patients should be asked to report at once the sudden appearance of sore throat or of lesions in the mouth. Any rise in temperature should also suggest an immediate blood count. These cannot be relied upon as the sole criterion for agranulocytosis. In case blood dyscrasia develops, chlorpromazine should be stopped at once and penicillin and the broad-spectrum antibiotics should be given immediately. Corticotropin (ACTH) is also usually employed, and transfusion is often advisable. In spite of active treatment, the outcome is often fatal.

Parkinsonism appears in about 10 per cent of the patients receiving full doses of chlorpromazine. The clinical picture is the usual one of muscular rigidity, slowing of movement, festinating gait, sialorrhea, and at times a pill-rolling tremor. The condition is always reversible and may be relieved with benztropine methanesulfonate (Cogentin), 1 mg. twice a day.

Other *dyskinesias* which occur during the use of chlorpromazine (although much more commonly with the piperazine derivatives) are the akathisias and dystonias. Oral dyskinesias, sometimes persistent, have been noticed to occur following phenothiazine treatment. Neither their incidence nor the etiologic role played by the drugs in their induction is certain. Whether, in the elderly, the occurrence is associated with underlying basal ganglia brain disorder is unclear. Roxburgh reports successful control of this complication with treatment by thiopropazate hydrochloride in 30 to 60 mg. doses daily. Improvement occurs within 48 hours of administration of the drug. It has been suggested that the phenothiazine-induced extrapyramidal reactions are due to some genetic determinant.

A few cases of sudden death in the course of high-dosage phenothiazine treatment have been reported. It has been proposed that death was caused by ventricular fibrillation or asphyxia during a drug-induced seizure or by food aspiration.

Suicide attempts have been made with the various phenothiazines and the various antidepressants. Nevertheless these agents are much less toxic than the barbiturates or minor tranquilizers, and few of such attempts have been successful. With chlorpromazine as much as 30,000 mg. has been ingested with recovery. Following these attempts the vasopressor levarterenol is indicated. When convulsions occur, great care must be taken in attempting their control with barbiturates, as these drugs are potentiated by the phenothiazines.

Phenothiazines may lead to elevation of the cerebrospinal fluid proteins. Furthermore, immunological diagnostic pregnancy tests appear unreliable in women receiving chlorpromazine and other phenothiazines, as they yield a high incidence of false-positive results.

Miosis or blurring of vision is noted at times.

Occasionally nurses who administer chlorpromazine develop a troublesome contact dermatitis that clears when further exposure is avoided. The irritant qualities of the drug were dramatically illustrated in the case of one patient who rubbed an eye with a tablet of chlorpromazine. An extensive and violent inflammatory process resulted in loss of vision.

DISCONTINUANCE. It is not difficult to decide when the administration of chlorpromazine should be discontinued in the case of acute, confusional excitement or in the case of acute manic episode of manic-depressive psychosis. In the former, its use may be terminated soon after the sensorium becomes fully clear. In the latter, the dose may be reduced as the symptoms subside, and the drug may be discontinued after mood and motor activity have been entirely normal for two weeks. Experience thus far suggests that in chronic schizophrenia the drug should be continued indefinitely in optimal individual dosage. Although undesirable side effects of the drug usually appear within two months after its use is begun, the patient who continues on a maintenance dose after leaving the hospital should report frequently to a physician.

Withdrawal of chlorpromazine after prolonged administration should be carried out with deliberation. Sudden withdrawal, particularly in those patients who have been taking simultaneously an antiparkinsonian agent, may be followed by marked restlessness, insomnia, perspiration, and tremor.

SPECIAL THERAPEUTIC REGIMENS. *Rapid Tranquilization.* The immediate treatment of the acutely psychotic with the maximally tolerated dosages of phenothiazines is advocated by some to facilitate much ego reorganization and social adaptation. Such treatment seems to be particularly valuable when the patient is seriously confused and incapable of engaging in a meaningful verbal communication with others.

This method of treatment requires the quick establishment of a maximal daily dosage for each individual. Polak and Laycomb recommend that the patient be given an essential dose of 25 to 50 mg. of chlorpromazine orally and be observed closely for side effects for one hour. If none are noticed, the drug is prescribed in 50 to 200 mg. doses orally every hour for six to eight hours, depending upon his behavioral state. When the initial disturbed psychotic behavior has diminished within the first six hours—including as end points strong sedation or sleep—his dosage is arranged in successive days at two-thirds the total required initially. Each day thereafter the dosage is reviewed and modified, depending upon the observed behavior. In the first several days well tranquilized patients sleep a good part of the day. After the third day there generally takes place a considerable reduction of drowsiness. Often, side effects, too, diminish at this time. Only after this day is the total level of medication reduced.

If oral medication is refused, intramuscular dosages of one-third the oral may be substituted.

High Dosage Regimens. On the effectiveness of high dosage regimens of chlorpromazine (over 2000 mg. per day) against low dosage treatment among groups of chronic schizophrenics, Prien et al., reporting from the Psychopharmacology Research Branch Collaborative Group Study on 120 such patients, found that high dosages were significantly more effective when given to patients under 40, hospitalized less than 15 years, who had been receiving a nonpiperazine phenothiazine beforehand. There was little difference in high dosage and low dosage regimens in other patient subgroups. Those who had been on higher dosages beforehand were more likely to fail. For older patients high dosage caused a great increase in side effects. Dyskinesias occur in as high as 25 per cent of patients treated with high dosage regimens, particularly among the aged.

Long-Acting Agents. Fluphenazine hydrochloride has been found to retain its physiological activity longer than any other phenothiazine. This is probably due to its higher fat solubility than that of the other analogs. When combined with various acid esters (enanthic, deconoic, and lauric), its release from fatty tissue is further slowed. Thus the hydrochloride will demonstrate action for from two to six days in animals, whereas the ethanate acts for up to three to seven times that period and the deconoate ten times as long. In humans, their therapeutic action commences to recede after two weeks. The ethanate may be given at two-week intervals, the first dose, usually of 0.5 cc. (125 mg.), repeated and adjusted to individual need. Some patients do well on 24 mg. every four weeks; others require more.

Others start patients on oral fluphenazine, increasing the dosage to as much as 60 mg. daily in order to determine an effective dosage level without side effects. The intramuscular dose may then be half of the oral.

Promazine

This drug, sold commercially as Sparine, is identical chemically with chlorpromazine except for the absence of a chlorine atom on the ring structure. The general pharmacological properties are similar, also. Sparine has been recommended particularly for use for delirium tremens and in the treatment of the senile and arteriosclerotic brain syndromes, since it is claimed that it has less hypotensive effect than chlorpromazine.

Promazine is available for both oral and parenteral administration. The tablets for oral use may be given in doses of 25 to 200 mg. every four to six hours, the dosage being varied according to the response of the patient.

Triflupromazine

Marketed as Vesprine or Vespral, this neuroleptic may be administered orally, as well as in emulsion or intravenously. The emulsion is useful for those patients with difficulty in swallowing and those who retain tablets in the mouth, such as the catatonics and senile psychotics. The daily oral dosage range generally used is from 20 to 200 mg.

Methotrimeprazine or Levomepromazine

Sold as Levoprome in the United States and as Nozinan, Veractil, or Neurocil, this drug probably will receive wide usage as an analgesic. The drug is indicated for trial in patients with chronic and intractable pain syndromes. It is also reported to have antidepressive activity. It has been used successfully in the treatment of numerous chronic painful states, including posthepatic neuralgia, phantom limb pain, tabes dorsalis, and thalamic syndrome, and when given by injection it has been shown to be as effective as morphine in equivalent doses in acute postoperative and postpartum states. No addiction has been reported.

The effective dosage of levomepromazine for the chronic painful reactions ranges from 150 to 300 mg. daily. The drug is usually prescribed in 50-mg. doses three to five times each day. When relief of pain is obtained, the daily maintenance dosage often may be reduced. Levoprome is available only for parenteral injection.

PIPERIDINE DERIVATIVE

Thioridazine

This substituted piperidine derivative, marketed as Mellaril, has achieved wide usage, as it appears to be as clinically effective as other phenothiazines but produces fewer side effects and toxic manifestations. There have been reported disturbances in sexual function, such as decrease in libido, lack of orgasm, or delayed or inhibited ejaculation. In a few cases, however, it has led to a pigmentary retinopathy noted initially as diminishing vision, which has taken place between the twentieth and fiftieth days of administration.

The drug is highly effective in the treatment of the psychoses and has also been reported to relieve the symptoms of insomnia, fatigue, tension headaches, and anxiety associated with other psychophysiological reactions. The usual daily oral dosage is 300 to 800 mg. for the psychoses, and 20 to 50 mg. in the neurotic and psychophysiologic reactions.

PIPERAZINE DERIVATIVES

Perphenazine

This drug, known commercially as Trilafon, combines the phenothiazine and piperazine rings. It is said to have fewer side effects than chlorpromazine. Photosensitivity has as yet to be reported, and for this reason it is a useful agent for those who are exposed much to the sun. Perphenazine is supplied in tablets of 2, 4, and 8 mg., and is recommended in oral doses of 6 to 16 mg. daily, although an amount as high as 64 mg. has been given. It is said to be useful for tension headaches, intractable pruritus, certain neurodermatoses, and chronic painful conditions, as well as the psychotic states.

Prochlorperazine

This drug, sold as Compazine, is recommended for use in the treatment of various neurotic conditions for the relief of anxiety. It has powerful antiemetic action and is useful in the control of nausea and vomiting associated with drug or alcohol withdrawal. It has been administered usefully in treatment of numerous psychosomatic conditions. Compazine is usually given by mouth in doses of 5 to 10 mg. three or four times daily.

Trifluoperazine

Better known under the trade name of Stelazine, this agent is said to be particularly useful in activation of the chronically apathetic, withdrawn, or depressed schizophrenic, in contrast to chlorpromazine, which often aggravates these types of behavior. The drug is prescribed for the psychotic in initial doses of 5 mg. three to four times daily, this dosage being increased by increments of 5 mg. until the patient is receiving 40 to 60 mg. daily. For office patients, 1 to 2 mg. given twice daily usually proves an effective dosage.

Trifluoperazine has been prescribed with chlorpromazine in the treatment of patients who fail to respond to one or the other drug alone, where motor activation is desirable, or as a means of avoiding toxic effects of high dosages of either drug when given alone.

Fluphenazine

Fluphenazine (Prolixin, Permitil) provides a sustained action over time and therefore may be used effectively in a single or double dose throughout the day. It is a powerful antiemetic but does not prolong barbiturate hypnosis. For psychotic behavior, the initial oral dosage is 0.5 mg.; this is then increased to 10 to 20 mg. daily. In the psychoneuroses, the effective daily dosage range is usually 0.5 to 3 mg. daily.

Thiopropazate

Sold as Dartal, this drug is recommended for anxiety states, insomnia, anorexia, agitation, the psychophysiologic states, schizophrenia, manic-depressive reactions and the addictive states. It is prepared in tablets of 5 and 10 mg. The range recommended is from 10 to 120 mg. daily in divided doses.

Acetophenazine

Marketed as Tindal, this drug comes in 20-mg tablets. It may be given in doses as low as 40 mg. and up to 80 mg. daily. The indications and side effects are similar to those for other piperizine derivatives.

Carphenazine

This agent, known as Proketazine, is available in tablets of 12.5, 25, and 50 mg. Dosage levels have varied from 50 to 200 mg. daily.

URINE TEST FOR PHENOTHIAZINES

Recently a simple test for detection of chlorpromazine and other phenothiazines in urine has been described. To a small amount of urine (1 ml.) is added an equal volume of a solution containing equal parts of 10 per cent H_2SO_4 and 5 per cent $FeCl_3$. The mixture is gently shaken. The presence of phenothiazines is indicated by the development of a violet color.

RAUWOLFIA DERIVATIVES

Reserpine

For centuries the root of the plant *Rauwolfia serpentina* Bentham, indigenous to India and known there as the "insanity herb," was used in that country for the treatment of a wide variety of diseases, including mental disorders. In 1954 Dr. R. A. Hakim of Ahrnabad, India, was awarded a gold medal for the presentation of a paper on the cure of schizophrenia with a compound, the major ingredient of which was this drug. Reference to its sedative effect had, however, been previously made by many Indian writers. In 1943 note was made in the *Indian Medical Gazette* of its increasing popularity in the treatment of mental disease, and report was made of improvement following use of the drug in manic-depressive psychosis, schizophrenia, and other forms of mental disorder. In recent years reserpine and its analogs have been less frequently administered owing to their delay in action, their tendency to induce or intensify depression, and their association with gastrointestinal hemorrhage.

ADMINISTRATION AND DOSAGE. Reserpine (Serpasil) may be given intramuscularly or orally, and frequently in the early stages of treatment both methods are used simultaneously. However, the dosage must be individually adjusted in accordance with optimal results and the tolerance of the patient. Many recommend 5 mg. intramuscularly once a day for 10 days and 1 mg. orally twice a day. If necessary, the oral dose may gradually be increased to 10 mg. and continued indefinitely. The maximum dose should not exceed 15 mg. in 24 hours. Sometimes the dose must be reduced to 2 mg. or 1 mg. because of side effects. Reserpine acts more slowly than does chlorpromazine. In the effect produced, 10 mg. of reserpine is equivalent to about 300 to 400 mg. of chlorpromazine. As with chlorpromazine, a confusional state may develop in case of overdosage; the optimal level of the dosage appears to be proportional to the intensity of the emotional disturbance. If a patient shows no improvement after two months of treatment, it is probably useless to continue the drug, but if improvement follows, treatment should be continued for at least three consecutive months. As is the case with chlorpromazine, it is usually desirable to continue reserpine indefinitely for the chronic psychotic patient who has improved with its use.

CLINICAL EFFECTS. Even though the chemical structures of reserpine and of chlorpromazine are completely different, they are used for almost identical purposes and their clinical effects are strikingly similar. Although the psychological effects of these drugs are subject to quantitatively large individual variations, they both usually have a relaxing and quieting influence. Typically the patient receiving reserpine is somnolent and lethargic but is readily aroused and then seems quite alert. Studies of the effects of reserpine upon pathological activity suggest that these are less than were originally assumed, and that the apparent effects are a result largely of the increased somnolence during the hours of the day when the patient would normally be awake. Occasionally, from about two weeks to two months after beginning treatment, especially when receiving full doses of the drug, the patient may develop parkinsonism, usually of a more marked type than that produced by chlorpromazine.

Some patients receiving reserpine rapidly increase their tissue water, and this hydration may occasionally cause convulsions. Among other side effects occasionally observed are lactation in the nonpregnant woman and impotence in men. A serious drop in blood pressure occurs more frequently in the patient receiving reserpine than in the one receiving chlorpromazine. Reserpine also increases both the volume and acidity of gastric secretion and it is, therefore, contraindicated in patients with a known history of peptic ulcer. A rise of temperature occasionally occurs, as also does asthma. Clinical experience seeems to show that, in general, the side effects of reserpine are less hazardous than those of chlorpromazine, yet deaths have occurred because of sudden and excessive drop of blood pressure.

CLINICAL USE AND SIDE EFFECTS. Although reserpine is of value in other disorders, its greatest use is in schizophrenia. In acute schizophrenia with tension and anxiety or in milder chronic reactions, its use, as is true also of chlorpromazine, may shorten or prevent hospitalization.

Both reserpine and chlorpromazine may exert a highly desirable sedative effect on the overactive brain-injured child. It also often relieves the anxiety, fear, and restlessness frequently seen in the chronic asthmatic.

Reserpine may aggravate depressions and, in fact, has produced depression eventuating in suicide in the hypertensive patient. Such depressions are occasionally of such a severity that electroshock therapy is required for their relief.

There have been a few reports indicating that a combination of reserpine or chlorpromazine with electroconvulsive therapy may be dangerous.

BUTYROPHENONES

Haloperidol

The prototype of this series of agents, haloperidol, has been administered in Europe as Serenace for indications similar to those for phenothiazines. It has been particularly recommended for the manic and highly agitated. In some cases of Gilles de la Tourette's syndrome haloperidol has succeeded in control of symptoms. The analogs of haloperidol, methyperidol and trifluperidol, are under trial in the United States. The daily dosage range for haloperidol has extended from 2 to 25 mg. These drugs in high doses are associated frequently with extrapyramidal symptoms.

LITHIUM

The salts of lithium are now recognized worldwide as effective agents in the treatment of mania and hypomania. John F. J. Cade of Australia first tested the use of lithium in the treatment of such patients in 1949, extrapolating broadly from his experiments in animals in which he noticed that guinea pigs injected with the carbonate salt became temporarily lethargic.

Those who respond most effectively to the therapeutic use of lithium are patients with manic-depressive psychosis, manic or hypomanic, in whom these types of behavior predominate. Those with frequent alteration of manic or depressive attacks do less well. When there is impairment of thought processes with delusional or hallucinatory experiences, or the clinical picture is regarded as schizo-affective, the clinical response to the agent is generally less favorable than in the former categories of illness. Nevertheless, some 70 to 80 per cent of patients with manic or hypomanic behavior are effectively relieved of their aberrant behavior when treatment with lithium is properly carried out.

In comparison with the phenothiazines, there are a number of reports indicating that lithium is the more effective agent. The phenothiazines bring about a more rapid reduction in the abnormal behavior; yet lithium administration, which at times requires five to ten days to effect change, is often effective when the former agents fail. Generally treatment of the manic patients should be started with the phenothiazines. If control is inadequate or ineffective, lithium becomes the agent of choice. So, too, lithium may be used to maintain a behavioral steady state by continued administration, thus preventing recurrence of mania. Some patients have taken the agent for over 15 years. Its use to prevent depressive attacks has not been demonstrated. During treatment, leukocytosis and slowing of the electroencephalogram occur frequently.

In the United States lithium carbonate is now available commercially in 300 mg. tablets as Lithonate. The effective drug dosage by mouth will generally vary from 1800 to 900 mg. daily. It is necessary to maintain a serum lithium level between 1.0 to 1.5 mEq. per liter. For long-term control the serum levels are adjusted to remain between 0.6 and 1.5 mEq. per liter, which usually requires an oral dose of 300 mg. three times daily.

Lithium treatment does not impair intellectual activity, consciousness, or range or quality of emotional life. Patients taking the drug fully experience joy, grief, tenderness, sexual desire, and other affects. In this respect it also contrasts with the phenothiazines. Patients frequently speak of the drug as "putting a brake" on them. Those who have obtained a secondary gain from the sense of exhilaration and power in the license of hypomanic or manic attacks sometimes dislike the drug for this reason. Polatin and Fieve point out that in those with milder forms of manic-depressive illness, this factor, as well as the denial of illness and its chronicity, leads some to discontinue or refuse lithium carbonate both as continuing treatment and as a preventive of future recurrences. Less than optimal responses obtained in other patients or breakthroughs in hypomanic or manic behavior have been related by Aranoff and Epstein to crisis events in the lives of the patients under continuing treatment—the occurrence of family conflict, separations, or other intercurrent social distress. Also, they noted that in some manic patients the limitation of activity, which may be regarded as a behavioral defense, led certain patients to a shift in their defenses—some became more active, others depressed, and still others paranoid or disorganized.

Toxic Symptoms. In the years since its introduction into psychiatry as a therapeutic agent there have been very few serious complications. Toxic symptoms may occur above serum lithium levels of 1.5 mEq. per liter. Nausea, abdominal cramps, vomiting, diarrhea, thirst, and polyuria are the symptoms indicative of toxicity and suggest the need to reduce the dosage. If the drug is continued, central nervous system symptoms of marked lethargy, coarse tremors and muscular twitchings, ataxia, slurred speech, and convulsions ensue. Vomiting and diarrhea also occur. The patient may lapse into coma, and death may result from severe changes in electrolyte balance, with consequent cardiac and pulmonary complications. The drug is contraindicated in those with impaired renal, cardiac, or central nervous functioning.

The toxic symptoms may be reversed by prompt discontinuance of the drug and correction of the abnormalities in the fluid and electrolyte balance. When serious imbalance has occurred, correction has been brought about by ingestion or infusion of urea and alkalinization of the urine by infusion of sodium lactate, or administration of acetazolamide or aminophylline, which increase lithium excretion.

There is some question as to whether lithium treatment may induce goiter formation, but findings of an increased goiter incidence in patients with manic and hypomanic disease untreated with lithium, as well as the inability to detect any alteration in thyroid functioning in patients in treatment, suggest that the agent at best plays an inferior or secondary role in goiter production, probably only in those predisposed to dysfunction of this organ.

Lithium has not been implicated as a teratogenic agent. However, it should be given with caution throughout pregnancy.

Physiological Activity. Although lithium produces numerous changes in neuronal, biochemical, electrolyte, and endocrine functions, its exact mode of action in the manic-depressive psychoses remains unclear. It increases norepinephrine turnover rates in the brain, perhaps leading to a greater intraneuronal inactivation of norepinephrine. Synaptosomes, too, treated with lithium, take up norepinephrine which make less available at receptor sites. Lithium may alter membrane excitability, as it can replace sodium in the isolated nerve; its active transport out of the cell is much less than that of sodium.

Lithium administration in man leads to a generalized slowing of the electroencephalogram and has induced in some a seizure pattern. It increases cortisol excretion, suggesting a direct effect on the adrenal or a nonspecific effect on the pituitary adrenal axis. It modifies aldosterone excretion.

On electrolyte metabolism, lithium leads to diuresis, saluresis, and kaluresis immediately following its administration. Three days of administration reverses this picture and sodium retention commences. Like potassium but unlike sodium, it enhances metabolism in brain slices, suggesting that it may modify energy metabolism in that organ.

ANTIDEPRESSANT AGENTS

The antidepressant agents have proved useful in the treatment of manic-depressive reactions and are prescribed now as the initial form of therapy for the majority of patients suffering a depressive reaction. When delay in relief may be tolerated for several weeks and when suicidal drive is low, the antidepressants are preferable to electroshock therapy, with its impairment of memory function, its other complications, and the greater demand for special equipment and nursing care.

IMINODIBENZYL DERIVATIVES

Imipramine

Closely related to the phenothiazines, this drug, distributed under the name of Tofranil, was introduced for clinical use by Kuhn in 1957. It is similar to promazine, but a two-carbon chain replaces the sulfur in the latter. Imipramine is the prototype of the iminodibenzyl group.

PHYSIOLOGICAL EFFECTS. Imipramine reduces susceptibility to convulsions induced by either electroshock or Metrazol. It depresses the action of the reticular formation and evokes on the electroencephalogram a brain-wave pattern typical of sleep. Its action at the synaptic junction is described earlier in this chapter, in the section entitled Pharmacological Action and Brain Function. It has anticholinergic effects and thus atropine-like side effects. Unlike chlorpromazine, it does not modify the conditioned escape-avoidance response in animals.

The oral route is preferred in the administration of the drug, although it may be given by intramuscular injection. The usual initial dosage range is 25 mg. given three or four times daily, the amount being increased to a total of 200 to 300 mg. within several days.

INDICATIONS. Imipramine has been more effective in the manic-depressive reactions, particularly those with retarded depression, than in other conditions. With the agitated depressions, it has not been effective, even when combined with the phenothiazines. Depressive reactions with organic brain syndromes have responded well, but its usefulness is limited with the neurotic depressive reactions and hypochondriacal states. In some patients with chronic pain, recurrent psychosomatic complaints, and neurotic states, it has also been reported to be useful. Some of the apathetic patients with schizophrenia and catatonia have been mobilized with the drug, but, in general, it has not proved of value in the treatment of these reactions. Some physicians believe it is contraindicated.

The change in mood and behavior seldom becomes noticeable within the first week of administration, and maximum benefit accrues usually after two or three weeks of medication. Evidence of favorable response is shown with the patient first becoming less self-deprecatory and self-accusing and with reduction in his hypochondriacal complaints. Later there follow increased activity and socialization and improvement in general somatic functioning, including sleep.

Imipramine must be continued on a maintenance level after clinical improvement has taken place, as symptoms recur with its withdrawal. Many recommend that the drug administration be continued three to six months following satisfactory change in affect. The drug should be withdrawn gradually.

UNTOWARD EFFECTS. The majority of the side effects are minor, although they may impede acceptance of the drug by the patient. Dryness of the mouth is experienced by almost all who receive the drug and difficulties in accommodation in many. Perspiration is common, particularly about the head and neck, and by some it is thought to occur particularly in those who respond favorably. With it may occur flushing of the face. Dizziness, tachycardia, and postural hypotension are seen in the elderly and hypersensitive; thus the drug must be used with caution in patients with cardiovascular illness. With large doses, tremors may be induced. Impairment of urination has been observed. Photosensitivity occurs less frequently as a complication than it does with the use of the phenothiazines.

Insomnia is often noticed when the drug is first given. Later on, sleep tends to improve. The tricyclic antidepressants as a class tend to increase non-REM sleep while decreasing the percentage of REM sleep and the duration of each REM cycle. Thus the total number of REM interruptions during the night is increased. Hypomanic states have frequently followed its administration and require both its withdrawal and the use of a phenothiazine. Some patients suffer burning paresthesias in the forearms and hands and substernally. Rarely incoördination and convulsive attacks have been reported.

Although eosinophilia is common, leukopenia occurs much less frequently, and only a few instances of agranulocytosis have been seen. In the presence of glaucoma or urinary retention this drug and its analogs should be avoided.

Amitriptyline

Marketed as Elavil, this drug has similar actions, indications, and side effects as imipramine. The dosage range is 75 to 300 mg. daily, given by mouth. There is some evidence that its untoward actions are less than those of imipramine. Elavil has hypnotic actions that make it useful when sleep disturbance is a prominent expression of depression.

Nortriptyline

Sold as Aventyl, this agent is supplied in pulvules of 10 to 25 mg. The indications, contraindications, and side effects are similar to those for the previously described analogs. Some patients do better with Aventyl than with its precursors.

Dismethylimipramine

This agent (Pertofrane or Norpramine), stated to be produced in the body as an active metabolite of imipramine, also hopefully was considered to be therapeutically effective more quickly than its precursors. This claim has not been borne

out by double-blind studies. It is supplied in 25-mg. tablets and is usually effective in a daily dosage range of 150 mg.

Enhancement of Action of Tricyclic Antidepressants

Among the depressed group are patients who fail to respond to the tricyclic antidepressants even on high dosage regimens. Recently Wharton et al. have reported that when methylphenidate (Ritalin) is administered with the tricyclic compounds, the blood levels of the latter rise. Patients previously resistant to treatment with these compounds when administered alone have responded to the dual therapy. Methylphenidate is known to act as an inhibitor of hepatic drug metabolizing enzymes. It is suggested that its ability to enhance the therapeutic effectiveness of the tricyclics rests upon its inhibition of their metabolic breakdown. In this treatment the methylphenidate may be given in 10 mg. doses three times daily for several weeks in combination with the tricyclic antidepressant given in average or lesser dosage regimens.

Prang et al. and others have found that both thyroid-stimulating hormone and L-triiodothronine (T_3) enhance the therapeutic activity of imipramine and produce both a more rapid recovery and effective action in patients initially resistant to imipramine administered alone. The former appears the most potent. Coppen et al. report that the enhancing action of T_3 may be obtained only when administered to women. The explanation for the enhancing action of thyroid hormones is unknown, although it has been suggested that they sensitize the response of the receptors in the synaptic cleft to the action of the biogenic amines.

MONOAMINE OXIDASE INHIBITORS

The capacity of iproniazid to produce euphoria in some persons was observed during its early use in the treatment of pulmonary tuberculosis. It was found that the hydrazine iproniazid (Marsilid) had the property of preventing the breakdown of serotonin and epinephrine in the brain on administration of reserpine through its capacity to inhibit the enzyme, monoamine oxidase. Thus the cerebral levels of these amines rise.

The monoamine oxidase inhibitors potentiate the effects of many other drugs. Thus the amphetamines may prove excessively stimulating when given to patients who are taking iproniazid. They also potentiate the sedative-hypnotic actions of alcohol and barbiturates. Of most importance are their potentiating actions when given with the iminodibenzyls. When they are administered simultaneously the likelihood of serious hypotension, convulsions, and circulatory collapse is increased greatly. However, if they are cautiously administered with careful observations of blood pressure, their usage with imipramine and its analogs may enhance the therapeutic response in some patients.

Patients receiving the monoamine oxidase inhibitors should be warned to avoid cheese, wines, and chicken livers. These foodstuffs contain tyramine; its pressor effect is markedly enhanced by the monoamine oxidase inhibitors.

The therapeutic response to all is characterized by latent periods extending from days to weeks before relief of depression is discernible. They share in common the side effects of hypotension, expressed in dizziness, vertigo, and fainting. In the elderly, vascular collapse may occur when the patient is on high dosage. Constipation, vesical atony, peripheral edema, and such anticholinergic effects as dry mouth and blurred vision are seen. With central nervous activation there may occur hyperreflexia, tremors, insomnia, and restlessness. All may induce hypomanic episodes in the depressed individual when administered over time in high doses.

The agents described here are those now in general clinical usage and with limited toxicity in the prescribed effective dosage range.

Isocarboxide

Sold as Marplan, this drug is given by mouth in a dosage range of 10 to 30 mg. daily. It may induce hepatitis, blood dyscrasias, and skin disorders. It is as effective as iproniazid (Marsilid) but is regarded as less toxic than the latter, which has now been withdrawn owing to the large number of cases of toxic hepatitis apparently induced by its usage.

Phenelzine

Known commercially as Nardil, this drug is usually administered in the dosage range of 40 to 60 mg. daily. It is considered by many clinicians to be as effective as iproniazid and more so than nialamide and is said to cause fewer hypotensive symptoms than other monoamine inhibitors. Cases of liver toxicity have not been reported.

Nialamide

Known commercially as Niamid, this drug is prescribed in the dosage range of 75 to 450 mg. daily. Generally clinicians have found it less effective as an antidepressant in severe states than other compounds in this group. It may produce toxic hepatitis but seems less likely to induce hypomanic episodes.

Tranylcypromine

This monamine oxidase inhibitor differs chemically from those previously described, as it is not a phenylhydrazine. Marketed in the United States as Parnate, it is regarded as the most rapidly acting antidepressant in the MAO series, and is considered by many the most effective for the majority of patients.

The drug is available in 10 mg. tablets. The usual initial dosage is 20 mg. given in two doses, morning and evening. If little response is obtained within two weeks, an additional 10 mg. may be prescribed daily.

PARADOXICAL HYPERTENSION. In some patients severe occipital headaches develop on administration of Parnate. These may be accompanied by nausea and vomiting, pallor and sweating, pain and rigidity in the neck, or collapse—significant signs of paradoxical hypertension. Some develop photophobia. Ingestion of amphetamines or substances high in tyramine such as certain cheeses (Gouda, Stilton, Cheddar, and Limburger) potentiates the likelihood of this reaction. Onset of headache indicates the necessity for immediate withdrawal.

It is recommended that the monamine oxidase inhibitors not be administered with the tricyclic antidepressants. However, in depressed patients resistant to both series of drugs, some have cautiously and effectively prescribed combinations, carefully monitoring the blood pressure, pulse, and other physiological indicators.

With a hypertensive reaction, phentolamine (Regitine), 5 mg., or pentolinium (Rivolysen), 3 mg., should be given slowly by the intravenous route.

OTHER AGENTS

Meprobamate

Meprobamate, 2-methyl-2-propyl-1,3-propanediol dicarbamate, commercially sold as Miltown or Equanil in the United States, is known to synchronize selectively interneuronal electrical activity in the thalamic nuclei and to act as an anticonvulsant and muscle relaxant. In contrast to the previously described drugs, it is said not to affect activity of the autonomic nervous system.

It is reported to be of value in anxiety and tension states, phobias, tension headaches, psychosomatic disorders, insomnia, premenstrual tension, and neurodermatitis. It often produces relief of headaches that are the result of constant, almost unremitting contraction of the posterior muscles of the neck.

Continued ingestion of large doses of meprobamate can create physical dependence, manifested on abrupt withdrawal of the drug by hyperirritability of the central nervous system and convulsions. The type of addiction caused by meprobamate resembles that caused by chronic intoxication with excessive amounts of barbiturates or alcohol. Especial care should be exercised in prescribing meprobamate for alcoholics or narcotic drug addicts.

A wide variety of side effects and untoward reactions has been reported. Among them have been dermal hypersensitivity reactions and acute nonthrombocytopenic purpura. Large doses taken with suicidal intent may produce complete respiratory and vasomotor collapse. The drug is not as effective in the treatment of the psychoses in the seriously disturbed as the phenothiazine derivatives.

It is available in tablets of 400 mg., which may be prescribed three to four times daily. Blood and urinary changes and local disturbances have not followed its prescription. In a few persons, allergic reactions have been noted with urticaria, erythematous rashes, and rarely fainting spells and bronchial spasm.

Chlordiazepoxide

This agent, marketed as Librium, has tranquilizing properties similar to those of the phenothiazines and reserpine. It is a muscle relaxant and anticonvulsant but exerts no autonomic blocking action. It produces stimulation of appetite and, in large doses, lowering of blood pressure and bradycardia. It affects the electroencephalogram as do the barbiturates.

In the clinic it has been used for relief of anxiety and tension in a wide range of psychiatric and medical conditions. Prescribed in 10-mg. capsules, the drug is given in a usual dosage range of 20 to 80 mg. daily. Common side effects are drowsiness and limitation of spontaneity, with impaired concentration. Ataxia, dysarthria, hyperactivity, and headache have been observed as well as some acute overactive behavioral disturbances.

Diazepam

A benzodiazepam derivative (Valium), this drug has been found useful in anxiety states. It is useful, as well, as a relaxant of muscular tensions or tremulousness associated with anxiety, alcoholism, or central nervous system spasticity. It is useful in the treatment of the nocturnal "restless limb" syndrome. Its use may be associated with fatigue, nausea, dizziness, drowsiness, and ataxia. It has addictive properties similar to meprobamate and chlordiazepoxide, so that abrupt withdrawal is contraindicated. It is supplied in tablets of 2, 5, and 10 mg. and the daily dosage may be varied from 4 to 40 mg.

BIBLIOGRAPHY

Aranoff, M. J., and Epstein, R. S.: Factors associated with poor response to lithium carbonate: A clinical study. Amer. J. Psychiat., 127:472–480, 1970.

Brodie, B. B., Cosmides, G. J., and Rall, D. P.: Toxicology and the biomedical sciences. Science, 148:1547–1554, 1965.

Brophy, J. J.: Suicide attempts with psychotherapeutic drugs. Arch. Gen. Psychiat., 17:652–657, 1967.

Cole, J. O. (ed.): Symposium on Long-Acting Phenothiazines in Psychiatry. Suppl. Dis. Nerv. Syst., 31: Sept., 1970.

Dalessio, D. J.: Chronic pain syndromes and disordered cortical inhibition: Effects of tricyclic compounds. Dis. Nerv. Syst., 28:325–328, 1967.

Fieve, R. R.: Perspectives on the use of lithium in psychiatric illness. Int. J. Psychiat., 9:375–412, 1970–71.

Klein, D. F., and Davis, J. M.: Diagnosis and Drug Treatment of Psychiatric Disorders. Baltimore, Williams & Wilkins Company, 1969.

Morgan, L. K.: Restless limbs: Commonly overlooked symptom controlled by "Valium." Med. J. Austral., 2:589–594, 1967.

Murphy, D. L., Goodwin, F. K., and Bunney, W. E.: Leukocytosis during lithium treatment. Amer. J. Psychiat., 127:1559–1561, 1971.

Polak, P., and Laycomb, L.: Rapid tranquilization. Amer. J. Psychiat., 128:640–643, 1971.

Polatin, P., and Fieve, R. R.: Patient rejection of lithium carbonate prophylaxis. J.A.M.A., 218: 864–866, 1971.

Porter, I. H.: The genetics of drug susceptibility. Dis. Nerv. Syst., 27:25–36, 1966.

Prange, A. J., Wilson, I. C., Knox, A., McClane, T. K., and Lipton, M. A.: Enhancement of imipramine by thyroid stimulating hormone: Clinical and theoretical implications. Amer. J. Psychiat., 127:191–199, 1970.

Prien, R. F., Levine, J., and Cole, J. O.: Indications for high dose chlorpromazine therapy in chronic schizophrenia. Dis. Nerv. Syst., 31:739–745, 1970.

Roxburgh, P. A.: Treatment of persistent phenothiazine-induced oral dyskinesia. Brit. J. Psychiat., 116:277–280, 1970.

Schildkraut, J. J.: The catecholamine hypothesis of affective disorders: A review of supporting evidence. Amer. J. Psychiat., 122:509–522, 1965.

Wharton, R. N., Percel, J. M., Dayton, P. G., and Malitz, S.: A potential clinical use of methylphenidate with tricyclic antidepressants. Amer. J. Psychiat., 127:1619–1625, 1971.

Chapter 33

Shock and Other Physical Therapies

With the increasingly widespread usage of the pharmacotherapies and psychotherapies in psychiatric practice, the need for shock and physical therapies has diminished. The latter have proved more effective and more economical to administer for the majority of patients. In addition, their administration avoids either temporary or permanent damage to brain tissue and function. Nevertheless, the physical therapies remain important techniques in the therapeutic armamentarium. For the most part today their prescription occurs when a patient problem remains resistant over time to the psychotherapeutic and/or pharmacotherapeutic approach or, as in the case of the serious depressive psychosis, a prompt behavioral change is indicated to prevent either suicide or prolonged suffering.

ELECTROCONVULSIVE THERAPY

In 1938 Cerletti and Bini described a method of producing convulsions by electricity and began its use in the treatment of schizophrenia.

The apparatus operates on 100-volt, 60-cycle, alternating current and contains mainly a variable transformer, ohm, volt, and ampere meters, and an automatic timer. The combined voltage and time settings constitute the "dose." Applications may range from 70 to 130 volts continuing from 0.1 to 0.5 second. Usually one starts with 80 volts for 0.2 second. If this fails to produce a convulsion, the voltage may be increased to 90 or 100 volts and the period of application increased. If this does not result in a seizure, no further application should be made until the following day. Only generalized seizures are productive of desired results. The operator will find that the dose must be determined by the convulsive threshold of the individual patient. This threshold is higher in female than in male patients, and higher in middle-aged than in younger persons. The threshold is raised after the first seizure.

The patient becomes unconscious immediately after the current is applied, even if no seizure follows. He will have no memory of a "shock." The convulsion conforms closely to those of spontaneous origin, with a tonic phase continuing for approximately 10 seconds followed by a clonic phase of somewhat longer duration. The convulsion is accompanied by apnea.

Techniques and Responses

In addition to the usual physical examination, including blood pressure, before the patient receives electric convulsive therapy, a roentgenogram should be made of the chest and of the lateral aspect of the spine; there should also be an electrocardiogram. An electroencephalogram is recommended. If the patient is to be treated in the morning, he receives either no breakfast or a glass of fruit juice and one slice of toast two hours before treatment. The patient should void, and dentures should be removed before treatment. If the patient suffers from nausea follow-

639

ing the seizure, he may be given 50 mg. of Dramamine prior to the next treatment. He may receive the treatment either on a well-padded table or on a bed, the springs of which are supported by a board between spring and mattress. Compression fractures of vertebrae are occasional complications. Formerly it was believed that their frequency would be reduced if the spine was slightly overextended either by placing a firm pillow under the small of the back or by placing the patient on a Gatch bed during the treatment. This overextension is no longer generally recommended.

The patient is placed in a comfortable dorsal position, or the spine may be slightly flexed. The shoulders and arms are held lightly by a nurse to prevent extreme movements of the arms. Usually a restraint sheet is sufficient for the thighs, but if they are held, the control should not be too rigid lest fractures of an acetabulum or of a femur result. A padded tongue depressor or other resilient mouth gag is placed between the teeth to prevent biting the tongue or other injury. The assistant who holds the mouth gag in place holds the patient's chin firmly upon the gag so that the jaw cannot open too far and become dislocated. Electrode paste is rubbed into the skin on both sides of the forehead, and the electrodes, previously soaked in saturated salt solution, are applied to the prepared areas. The apparatus button is pressed and the patient instantly becomes unconscious. Following the clonic phase, there is a phase of muscular relaxation with stertorous respiration. It is well to roll the patient on his side to prevent inhalation of saliva. The patient remains unconscious for about five minutes, then slowly rouses during the next five to ten minutes.

After the treatment there is a period of confusion, during which the patient should be watched lest he fall out of bed. He should usually be permitted to lie for one-half to one hour after treatment. If left undisturbed, he may sleep an hour or more. In most cases there is no postconvulsive excited state, but a patient who is subject to this disturbance should receive 3¾ grains of sodium amytal intravenously just prior to application of the electricity.

Unilateral application of electrodes, in order to induce a focal seizure spreading from the nondominant hemisphere, has been recommended as a means of decreasing post-shock confusion, amnesia, and memory loss. In the study of the effects of this technique by Halliday et al., it was found that verbal learning was impaired selectively by electroconvulsive therapy when applied to the nondominant hemisphere and nonverbal learning by application to the dominant hemisphere. The latter loss seemed to persist longer after termination of treatment than the former.

In this technique of stimulation one electrode is placed midway across and 3 cm. above a line projected between the lateral angle of the orbit and the external auditory meatus. The other, or upper, electrode is placed 6 cm. higher than the lower and at an angle of 70° to the line. The placement is made over the nondominant hemisphere, dominance being determined on the basis of preferred skeletal muscular usage. The convulsive state induced by this method is exactly similar to that brought about by bilateral electrode placement, although occasionally contralateral (focal) convulsions take place.

Frequency

Treatments are usually given three times a week. The period for which treatment should be continued depends largely upon the results obtained and upon the nature of the disorder treated. In depressive reactions, the patient may have received the maximum benefit after five to ten treatments. In disorders in which the patient is slowly but definitely improving, treatment may continue to 25 or 30 applications, followed, if desirable, by maintenance treatments. Two treatments per day may be given for two or three successive days in the case of acutely disturbed patients who are threatened by psychotic exhaustion.

Indications

The greatest usefulness of electroconvulsive therapy is in depression. Its most frequent use, therefore, is in the treatment of involutional melancholia and of the depressive phase of manic-depressive psychosis. When depression is an associated symptom in other disorders, this form of therapy may be followed by beneficial results. It is frequently used as a substitute for insulin shock therapy in acute and subacute schizophrenia reactions. Its use as a "maintenance" treatment in chronically disturbed schizophrenics and in the manic phase of manic-depressive psychosis is discussed in another section.

Various "depressive scales" have been devised in recent years as a means of differentiating those patients likely to respond to electroshock. Clinical features which distinguish the therapeutically more responsive group are a good premorbid personality; lack of evidence of psychogenic precipitants to depression; weight loss; pyknic body build; previous depressive episodes; early morning awakening; nihilistic, somatic, and paranoid delusions; and ideas of guilt. Evidence of anxiety, hysterical features, and the blaming of others correlate with poor response to electroconvulsive treatment.

Induction of the convulsive state by unilateral parietal placement of the electrodes over the nondominant hemisphere, described previously in the section on Technique, is preferred by some for patients with associated organic brain disease such as senile or arteriosclerotic syndromes, those who depend heavily on memory functions in their vocations, and paranoid and phobic individuals who manifest increasing anxiety as memory impairment increases.

Contraindications

As experience with electroconvulsive shock therapy has increased, conditions regarded as contraindications have decreased. *Age,* in itself, is not considered a contraindication. The aged patient should, of course, be very carefully examined for physical abnormalities. Although the condition of the *cardiovascular system* should be carefully evaluated before electroconvulsive therapy is given, the strain of the convulsion on that system has probably been exaggerated. Hypertension, abnormal electrocardiograms, or a history of angina pectoris or of coronary thrombosis are not in themselves contraindications to treatment if the patient has a good cardiac reserve.

Cardiac decompensation usually debars electroconvulsive therapy. The presence of aortic aneurysm also excludes the use of this treatment. If hypertension is largely caused by emotional factors, it need not be a cause for rejection of treatment but, on the contrary, may be an indication for its use. Vascular accidents as a result of electroconvulsive therapy are exceedingly rare. The use of electroconvulsive therapy in the presence of myocardial disease depends upon its seriousness and the urgency of the need for treatment. If agitation is producing a constant strain on the heart, convulsive treatment may be used.

Generally speaking, *tuberculosis,* if there is a history of recent hemorrhage or evidence of high activity, excludes treatment, but the patient who is a feeding problem is often benefited through the resulting gain of weight. Latent tuberculosis is rarely activated. Except for recent fractures, *bone disease* is not a frequent contraindication to treatment. *Pregnancy* is not usually considered a contraindication. Electric shock is a safer form of therapy than insulin in the psychoses of pregnancy.

Complications

IMPAIRMENT OF MEMORY. Scarcely to be called a complication is the almost constant impairment of memory that accompanies electroconvulsive therapy. It may vary from a mild tendency to forget names to a severe confusion of the Korsakoff type. At first it tends to cover a long period prior to treatment, then gradually to diminish to events immediately before treatment. It is often distressing to the patient and may continue to some degree for several weeks or a few months following the termination of treatment. Full return of memory finally occurs. Psychological investigations indicate that electroconvulsive therapy is not followed by any intellectual impairment.

A recent careful analysis by Cronholm and Ottosson of the change in memory function which occurs after electroconvulsive therapy has shown that with the impairment of retention in memory function there simultaneously takes place improved capacity for learning. The fact that clinically improved patients complain infrequently of memory disturbance may be explained by the fact that they judge their response subjectively in terms of the greater capacity to learn and this experience dominates the impairment of retention due to the electroshock. One cannot accept then the subjective report of the patient relative to the effects of electroshock on his memory.

FRACTURES AND DISLOCATIONS. The most frequent complications in electroconvulsive therapy are fractures and dislocations caused by muscular contraction. The fracture occurring most often is a *compression fracture of vertebrae,* in the dorsal area between the second and eighth, usually the third, fourth, or fifth vertebra. Approximately 20 per cent of the patients suffer this injury, which occurs twice as frequently among men as among women. Apparently a majority of the fractures occur early in the course of treatment. They are not of major clinical importance and do not require special treatment. Many are found only on roentgenologic examination. Back pain may persist for a few days or weeks. Fractures of the femur, of the acetabulum, and of the neck of the humerus may occur. Dislocation of the jaw is frequent unless pressure is applied to prevent the opening of the mouth at the onset of the tonic phase.

APNEA. Apnea occurs physiologically in any general convulsive seizure, but in electroconvulsive therapy the respiratory arrest may be disturbingly prolonged. Some therapists use artificial respiration immediately after the convulsion as a safety measure. If apnea persists, artificial respiration should be continued. A metal airway should be available to prevent the tongue from falling back and to lead air through accumulations of saliva and mucus. Deaths as a result of electroconvulsive therapy are exceedingly uncommon.

In order to avoid fractures or dislocations and to diminish the risk in elderly or infirm patients, convulsions may be modified by means of drugs which inhibit the action of acetylcholine at neuromuscular junctions and often the muscular contractions.

Succinylcholine dichloride (Anectine) is the agent of choice for this purpose. It is best administered intravenously with atropine and methohexital or Pentothal. Pitts et al. have reported the induction of fewer cardiac arrhythmias with the former basal anesthetic than the latter. The optimal dosage of succinylcholine is 5.0 mg. per kilogram of body weight. The combination of drugs is injected intravenously slowly until the patient is unable to count or becomes unresponsive. At the end of the convulsion, oxygen under positive pressure is administered until the patient breathes spontaneously.

In approximately one in a thousand patients, prolonged apnea may occur after the use of succinylcholine. It has been suggested that those sensitive to this drug and its diethyl derivative, suxethonium, have inherited a less active variant of the enzyme pseudocholinesterase, which metabolizes the drug so that the drug action persists an undue length of time. It is now possible, through a rapid screening test, to disclose those whose serum contains the atypical cholinesterase incapable of breaking down the muscle relaxants. From Motulsky and Morrow's study, the gene frequency determining the existence of the abnormal enzyme is very rare among Negroes, suggesting that they are at very low risk for this complication in administration of electroshock therapy with succinylcholine.

Usually a period of controlled respiration will terminate the apnea. Coramine (1 to 2.5 gm. in 4 to 10 ml.) may be given intravenously to counteract excessive barbiturate. Artificial ventilation should be maintained until spontaneous respiration occurs.

Any patient responding with prolonged apnea after use of Anectine should be so informed. Neither he nor other family members should be administered this agent again unless careful quantitation is made of serum esterase activity.

Results of Treatment

In the depressions of involutional melancholia and of depressive psychosis the improvement following electroconvulsive shock therapy is striking. In 80 per cent or more of these disorders, five to ten treatments are followed by full or social recovery. Prior to the treatment of involutional melancholia by electric shock therapy, protracted depression, sometimes lasting for years, was the rule. Early treatment of this disorder and of the depressions of depressive psychosis by shock therapy will save many patients who would otherwise commit suicide.

Electroconvulsive shock therapy has no influence on the recurrence of manic-depressive episodes. Guilt and self-punishing, self-accusatory trends are usually rapidly alleviated. In less than half of the cases of the paranoid type of involutional psychosis is treatment followed by much improvement, even through the maximum number of convulsions is induced. Senile depressions are usually relieved unless arteriosclerotic or senile brain changes have been important determinants.

The results of treatment of the manic phase of manic-depressive psychosis are less favorable than of the depressive phase but have been greatly improved by the practice of giving treatments more frequently. Best results are secured by giving two treatments a day for the first

two or three days. These are usually followed by much confusion, but as this clears, the patient is found to be definitely improved.

The effectiveness of electroconvulsive treatment of schizophrenia has been the subject of much discussion. It is generally agreed that this form of treatment is beneficial in a large percentage of schizophrenics with affective features. It is also helpful in hastening a remission in early, acute forms of the disorder. It is of little value in hebephrenia or when the onset has been of a prolonged, insidious nature. The best results are secured in catatonic excitement. As with other shock therapies, this treatment is not followed by material improvement in the chronic, disorganized schizophrenic.

Electroconvulsive therapy is of little value in the treatment of psychoneuroses except in those manifesting depressive features and perhaps the anxiety states associated with gross stress reaction.

Ambulatory Treatment

For several years after the introduction of electroconvulsive therapy, it was considered essential that its application be limited to patients resident in a hospital. In more recent years there has been considerable relaxation in this practice. Whether, however, electroconvulsive treatments are administered to patients continuously confined to a hospital or to those who are not hospitalized, they should be given only by a qualified psychiatrist well trained in the technique. Many patients, particularly those suffering from mild depressions, continue to reside at their homes but periodically visit a psychiatric or a general hospital to receive shock treatments. Later in the treatment day, after consciousness has become fully clear, the patient returns to his home. The degree of knowledge, understanding, and responsibility of relatives, and their ability to exercise constant supervision of the patient in his home, must be carefully determined. If treatment is undertaken in a general hospital or in a private office, provisions for dealing with postconvulsive confusion and excitement or with respiratory or other complications must be made. The patient should remain in the hospital or in the physician's office until there is no longer any danger of undesirable after effects. He should never be permitted to return home unaccompanied, and there should be reliable and instructed persons there to supervise him during the entire course of treatment.

Mode of Action

The use of electroconvulsive shock is entirely empirical. Many theories, both psychogenic and physiogenic, have been suggested as explanations for its therapeutic action, but no one has offered a satisfactory explanation for the results obtained either by electroconvulsive or by insulin therapy. Some investigators suggest that cerebral anoxia, a result common to all the shock therapies, may somehow be the basis for the mental improvement. In both hypoglycemic and convulsive shock therapies, the brain is deprived of energy and oxidative metabolism to a degree that renders it inadequate to support cerebral function. The mechanisms producing these conditions are different, however. With hypoglycemia the brain is deprived of glucose and the cerebral metabolic rate is depressed. With electroshock, brain activity is raised to such a high pitch that cerebral function cannot be sustained by the oxygen and glucose coming to the brain in the blood.

Electroshock therapy modifies the sleep pattern profoundly in that it leads to increase in total sleep time, with diminution of rapid eye movement (REM) sleep. There seems, from animal experiments, no drive later to make up REM time in sleep. Electroconvulsive therapy, too, appears to produce a sustained increase in synthesis and utilization of norepinephrine in the brain. It appears, as well, to produce a short-lasting inhibition of brain protein synthesis.

In animals it has been shown that electroshock convulsions selectively obliterate conditioned fear reactions and other aversively controlled and learned behaviors. H. Hunt has shown, too, that this effect depends upon the occurrence of convulsion and is not the result of the impairment of memory functions. Some drugs enhance or attenuate the effect of electroshock on the *conditioned emotional response* (CER) in rats; whether these drug actions found in rats may be correlated with their clinical effects in man has not been established. Chlorpromazine given after electroshock to rats increases the CER. Meprobamate, on the other hand, decreases the conditioned emotional state even more. Curiously, Dilantin given simultaneously with shock enhances the effect of the shock, while phenyrone blocks out the convulsion and prevents the attenuating action of the convulsion.

Electrosleep, which is not to be confused with electroshock, has been used extensively in the USSR and is now under trial elsewhere. It is induced from a battery device passing a standard 100 pulses per second of pulse duration of 1 millisecond at levels of 1 milliampere for 30 minutes between electrodes placed over one eye and the related mastoid. The designation is a misnomer; many patients never fall asleep. No convulsions occur. Treatments are usually given five days per week for one or two weeks. The indications and therapeutic effectiveness of this technique are dubious.

INHALANT CONVULSIVE TREATMENT

Clinical trials have demonstrated that hexafluorodiethyl ether (Indoklon) given by a simple inhalation technique in doses of 4 to 6 ml. containing 0.05 of the agent per milliliter of solution is capable of inducing immediate convulsive responses. Recently Karliner has effectively administered Indoklon intravenously as a convulsant agent in association with succinylcholine and a short-acting anesthetic.

This convulsant may be used as effectively as electroshock therapy for the same therapeutic purposes and is accepted more readily by some patients. Thus it may serve as an alternative procedure to electroshock treatment.

INSULIN SHOCK TREATMENT

In 1928 Sakel, believing that the nervous hyperactivity occurring in morphine addicts during withdrawal of that drug was caused by an excess of epinephrine, expressed the opinion that the excitement might be relieved by large doses of insulin. Later the similarity of the abstinence symptoms to other excited states suggested to Sakel that the latter also might be influenced by the same drug. He accordingly administered insulin to excited schizophrenic patients. After a period of experimental clinical work, he published his results in 1933. The basic features in the method developed by Sakel are still regarded as most effective. At first Sakel tried to avoid the development of deep hypoglycemic states, but he soon observed that better results occurred if coma was induced. He then increased the dose with the avowed intention of producing insulin shock.

Neurophysiology

Unlike other organs, which can utilize carbohydrates, proteins, and fats for energy requirements, the brain is able to oxidize carbohydrates only. Since the rate of oxidation of carbohydrates is determined by the amount of insulin in the blood stream, the injection of a large amount of insulin into the body greatly reduces the sugar content of the blood. With a decrease in the amount of sugar available, the oxidative processes of the brain are so reduced that the effects are similar to anoxia of that organ, a condition known to lead to coma. The loss of consciousness in hypoglycemia is presumably caused by the fact that the brain cells are deprived of glucose, their principal fuel, without which the metabolic processes in the brain are progressively depressed.

According to the segmental-suprasegmental concept of evolutionary development of the central nervous system, there are ascending levels of integration both of structure and function. We may therefore think of successively higher levels, beginning with the lower medulla and culminating with the cerebral hemispheres. It has been shown that the rate of metabolism in each of the higher levels is greater than in that of the level immediately lower or older. The greatest susceptibility to low blood sugar exists, therefore, in the more complex and phylogenetically more recent areas of the forebrain. With the injection of large amounts of insulin, therefore, there is a step-like depression of function and there appear progressive neurological signs and symptoms corresponding to a phyletic regression or functional disturbance in the successively lower anatomical levels of cerebral cortex, diencephalon, midbrain, upper medulla, and lower medulla. There is a progressive dissolution of the functions of the brain, a dissolution that seems to turn back that organ through the path of evolution. As the blood sugar falls following the injection of a "coma dose" of insulin, various deficiency and release phenomena linked with functional patterns of different levels of the neuraxis become manifest in the signs and symptoms that characterize the successive stages of insulin coma. The symptoms and signs are listed in the accompanying table. The therapist must remember that the signs in Stage V are largely those of functional impairment of the cardiac, circulatory, and respiratory centers and therefore those of approaching danger.

All patients manifest in a general way the functional groups of signs listed in the table indicated. Each patient, however, presents an individual response, and there is often much overlapping of the stages. It is not uncommon, in fact, to see signs of various stages (such as II and IV) occurring simultaneously. This phenomenon is sometimes referred to as "irregular descent" and would seem to indicate that there is a variable resistance to hypoglycemia in various parts of the brain.

Preparation for Treatment

Although insulin shock therapy is a relatively safe procedure in the hands of a skilled therapist, most serious complications may occur with patients in whom an organic pathologic condition has been overlooked. In addition to careful and complete psychiatric, physical, and neurological examinations, such laboratory examinations should be made as will exclude the possibility of undertaking the treatment of a bad risk. It is generally agreed that there should be roentgenologic studies of the chest and of the lateral thoracic spine, a serological examination, urinalysis, blood count, and a determination of the fasting blood sugar. An electrocardiogram, especially in older patients, is highly desirable, even though the clinical examination is negative. It is advisable to discuss results and dangers with a responsible relative, and also to secure written permission for treatment.

Contraindications to Treatment

The presence of any organic disease must be individually evaluated and its seriousness weighed against the urgency for treatment. The following disorders, however, are usually considered as contraindications: (1) any active infection, or any chronic or subacute infection that may be "lighted up" by treatment; (2) serious heart, liver, or kidney disease; (3) diabetes or other endocrine disorder; (4) skeletal pathology; (5) lack of adequate superficial veins; or (6) age under 16 or over 45 years. Some therapists, however, have successfully treated patients who were pregnant or had epilepsy, myxedema, or allergy.

Technique of Treatment

The patient usually receives his dose of insulin at about 7 a.m. while still fasting. He remains under vigilant nursing observation from the time the drug is given until after coma is terminated and consciousness fully regained. Because of the danger of "after-shock" or other complications, the patient should be under competent nursing supervision during the succeeding 24 hours. A physician trained and experienced in insulin therapy should watch him constantly from the time he becomes unconscious until consciousness is fully restored.

The original method of Sakel, still very widely followed, begins with the intramuscular injection of 15 to 25 units of insulin, which is increased by 10 to 15 units daily until the desired depth of coma is reached. This is usually not reached until the dosage is between 80 and 275 units and from 7 to 15 treatments have been given. After coma dose has been reached, the dosage may usually be reduced somewhat in the hope that excessively deep reactions may be avoided, but it is adjusted daily for the remainder of the course of treatment. The dose of insulin required to produce coma is not related to the degree of hypoglycemia produced.

A technique in which rapidly increasing doses are administered was developed by Shurley and is often used. With this technique, the procedure begins with the administration to the fasting patient for five successive days of small doses of insulin increasingly graduated from 5 to 25 units. The purpose of this series of injections is to ascertain if the patient has a predisposition to allergic or hypoglycemic reactions. If there is no evidence of undue sensitivity, the course of treatment is begun.

The therapist seeks to produce the maximum physiological effect for the longest period of time permissible by the largest doses of insulin consistent with the patient's safety. Patients possess varying degrees of resistance to insulin. For

Hypoglycemic Symptoms
(Modified from Himwich)

STAGE	PSYCHOLOGICAL	MOTOR	SENSORY	AUTONOMIC

I
Depression of cerebral and cerebellar functions
	1. Gradually increased clouding of consciousness with defects in:
	  a. orientation
	  b. attention
	  c. understanding
	  d. perception
	2. Wild excitement, with or without psychotic syndromes
	3. Sleep
		1. Muscular relaxation (hypotonia)
		2. Tremors
		3. Imperfect voluntary acts (apraxia)
		4. Imperfect (incoherent) speech
			1. Visual disturbances	1. Parasympathetic overactivity
				  a. Watery sweat
				  b. Watery saliva
				  c. Bradycardia
				  d. Constricted pupil
				  or
				2. Sympathetic overactivity
				  a. Viscid sweat
				  b. Viscid saliva
				  c. Tachycardia
				  d. Dilated pupils
				3. Vital signs vary within normal limits —temperature dropping

II
Release of subcorticodiencephalon
	1. Loss of environmental contact, i.e., coma	1. Stereotyped (primitive) movements
		  a. Involuntary grasping
		  b. Involuntary sucking
		  c. Protrusion of tongue
		  d. Kissing
		  e. Snarling
		  f. Grimacing
		2. Motor restlessness
		3. Choreiform, athetoid, and hemiballistic movements
		4. Fine myoclonic twitchings → clonic spasms → convulsions (release of subcortical motor nuclei)
			1. Increased sensitivity to external stimuli (release of the sensory thalamus)	1. Sympathetic overactivity in waves
				  a. Tachycardia
				  b. Dilated pupils (react to light)
				  c. Exophthalmos
				  d. Flushing
				  e. Viscid perspiration
				  f. Viscid salivation
				  g. Increased blood pressure and perspiration (release of hypothalamus)

III
Release of the midbrain
	1. Deep coma	1. Loss of primitive movements
		2. Increasing hypertonus
		3. Spasm
		  a. Tonic (flexion of upper extremities with extension of rest of body)
		  b. Torsion
		4. Dissociated eye movements
		5. Pathological pyramidal reflexes most easily elicited
			1. Decreased sensitivity to external stimuli	1. Parasympathetic signs, which are overcome periodically by sympathetic signs with each spasm (dilated pupils do not react to light)
				2. Paradoxical pupillary dilation and hippus
				3. Vital signs variable

IV Release of upper medulla	1. Deep coma	1. Recurrent extensor spasm in all extremities 2. Magnus and de Kleijn reflex	1. Loss of sensitivity	1. Sympathetic signs with each spasm (pupils dilate but do not react)

V
Release of lower medulla
	1. Deep coma	1. Muscular flaccidity
		2. Depressed reflexes
			1. Loss of all sensitivity
			2. Loss of corneal reflex
				1. Parasympathetic signs
				  a. Pallor
				  b. Pinpoint pupils (do not react)
				  c. Slow heart rate
				  d. Depressed respiration

that reason, the initial treatment dose does not exceed 50 units of U 100 ordinary insulin given by deep intramuscular injection. This dose is doubled each day until a clinical response is secured or a maximum dose of 1600 to 2200 units is reached. Some patients are extremely resistive to insulin. If in such cases coma does not occur within the dosage range stated, the maximum dose may be repeated for five or six days or the dose may be "zig-zagged."

This procedure may be conducted in one of several ways. The most common method is first to give double the dose with which treatment was begun, the next day to give half the maximum dose, and on the third day to repeat the maximum dose. If a patient does not respond to this routine, larger doses may be given or the route of administration may be changed to intravenous. When a clinical response is obtained, the rate of dose increase is reduced from a doubling of the amount to one of 10 to 20 per cent. When sensitization occurs as manifested by a deeper coma on the same or a smaller dose, by an earlier onset of coma, or by a somatic crisis or other complication, the dose is reduced rapidly (by halves) until one just sufficient to produce the desired depth of coma is reached. Thereafter the maintenance dose must be determined daily as indicated by the patient's response. The depth and duration of each coma will vary in accordance with the opinion and experience of the individual therapist.

Some physicians believe that Stage II is sufficiently deep to produce beneficial effects. Others insist on various combinations of Stages III, IV, or even V. Many allow a maximum of two hours of coma per day, reckoned from the time of loss of consciousness. The coma should be terminated when Stage V is reached or if some complication develops. It is generally agreed that 15 minutes of Stage V is the extreme limit of safety. Few therapists permit the patient to reach this depth of coma.

Termination of Coma

Hypoglycemic coma is terminated by giving an adequate amount of carbohydrates by one of three methods: orally, by gavage, or by intravenous administration. In emerging from the coma, the patient ordinarily retraverses the phyletic stages through which he passed in developing coma. If he is able to drink, the patient is given eight ounces of a 50 per cent sugar solution. If he is unable to drink, the coma is terminated by tube feeding or by glucose given intravenously. Each method has its proponents. Probably, however, a gavage of 500 ml. of a warm 50 per cent glucose solution is preferable, especially if the patient has had a convulsion, has been uncoöperative upon waking, has inaccessible veins, or needs a reservoir of glucose during a prolonged coma. The intravenous method is always used in an emergency and routinely by many therapists.

When glucose is given intravenously, the patient receives from 20 to 50 ml. (sometimes more) of a $33\frac{1}{3}$ per cent solution. This method should be used also if the patient is not alert within 20 minutes after having received glucose by mouth. If he is suffering from simple hypoglycemia, he should respond to intravenous glucose within five minutes. If the coma is terminated intravenously, it is wise to give additional glucose by mouth lest there be a return of the hypoglycemic state. Following the termination of the coma, the patient should receive a substantial meal. It is important that he receive sodium chloride to replace that lost through perspiration.

Adjuncts to Treatment

Atropine sulfate ($\frac{1}{150}$ to $\frac{1}{75}$ grain) is given routinely with the insulin dose and again before electroshock if that is used in conjunction with insulin therapy, to decrease vagotonia. Vitamins B_1 and C are given to supplement the deficiencies resulting from the intake of large quantities of vitamin-poor carbohydrates. Diphenylhydantoin sodium (Dilantin), 4½ grains daily, may be given orally at the same time the patient receives insulin in order to prevent hypoglycemic convulsions. It should be gradually discontinued upon completion of the course of insulin therapy and should not be used if combined electroconvulsive therapy is employed. Postural drainage and the insertion of gauze wicks should be used to prevent aspiration of the excessive amount of saliva. Care must also be exercised to prevent aspiration of vomited material. Airways, oxygen, and artificial respiration may aid in preventing serious complications.

Some therapists use potassium chloride prophylactically to correct electrolytic balance and to prevent prolonged comas. Its value is still undetermined. Hyaluronidase, in doses of 75 to 150 turbidity-reducing units (T.R.U.) added to the insulin, has been found to be of value in reducing the amount of insulin required to produce coma, to increase the effective length of treatment levels, and to increase the number of therapeutically valuable reactions (comas). It is also said to diminish the frequency of aftershocks, as well as convulsions, restlessness, and exhaustion.

Duration of Treatment

Treatment is given five or six times a week for an average total course of 50 hours of coma. Although the number of treatment days may be somewhat smaller in acute cases and in those patients who have shown no benefit from treatment, the total number of hours should not be less than 30. More than 50 coma days are given by some therapists to patients who are continuing to show beneficial results. If a relapse takes place, it usually occurs within a month after discontinuance of treatment. The patient should therefore continue under observation for nearly that period of time.

Complications of Treatment

Since dangerous, and even fatal, complications may readily occur, it is essential that both physician and nurse possess sufficient experience and skill to enable them to recognize and deal immediately with emergency situations. Even though both possess these qualities, the mortality rate will be from 0.5 to 1 per cent.

PROLONGED COMA. Ordinarily there is a coincident termination of hypoglycemia and of coma following the administration of carbohydrates. Sometimes, however, the termination of hypoglycemia is not accompanied by a return to consciousness. If there is no evidence of returning consciousness within five minutes after intravenous administration of glucose or within 20 minutes after administration by gavage, one is confronted with a delayed awakening that may be the forerunner of prolonged or irreversible coma.

Treatment of delayed awakening consists of the intravenous administration of 100 ml. of 33⅓ per cent of glucose and 100 mg. of thiamine chloride. The latter stimulates the utilization of available glucose. If the patient has not already received intragastric glucose, he is given 500 ml. of warm 50 per cent glucose by gavage. If the patient does not respond within 15 minutes, it must be considered that prolonged coma exists. This is an emergency condition and accounts for over one-half of all deaths resulting from insulin coma. Persistent coma terminating in one to three hours is usually followed by complete recovery, but longer periods are dangerous.

Although not definitely proved, prolonged or irreversible coma is presumably caused by the nerve cells having become exhausted or otherwise irreversibly altered so that they are no longer able to utilize glucose, even though there is an ample supply present in the blood stream. In view of the marked diaphoresis that most patients manifest, there must be changes in water metabolism and also associated changes in electrolytic balance. The brain, following death from prolonged coma, shows either degenerative or hemorrhagic lesions together with cerebral edema. Even when prolonged coma is reversible, some patients are left with a permanent organic dementia. The hyperinsulinism brings about a state of anoxia even in the presence of an abundance of oxygen. Histological examinations show that the cellular changes are identical with those alterations residual to severe degrees of cerebral anoxia in cases of carbon monoxide poisoning or mechanical strangulation.

If the patient is in Stage II or III and shows signs of cortical irritability, 50 ml. of 50 per cent sorbitol or sucrose is given intravenously as a dehydrating measure. If there is no response within 15 minutes, or if the patient is in deep coma (Stage IV or V), 50 ml. of doubly concentrated human plasma are given intravenously. If the patient shows motor excitement, he should be restrained. Narcotics and sedatives should be avoided. Oxygen by nasal catheter, even in the absence of cyanosis, is usually advisable. If the patient's temperature is over 103°F., he should receive alcohol sponges or an ice water enema. Circulation and respiration should be supported by Coramine, 2 to 5 ml., given intravenously every three to four hours until the patient awakes. Epinephrine and caffeine are not recommended.

If the patient has not responded within 30 minutes after having received plasma, the coma may continue for hours or days. Normal blood sugar level should be maintained by 10 per cent intravenous glucose drip. Blood sugar content should be checked every two to three hours. The administration of sucrose and of thiamine chloride should be repeated every two or three hours. Other measures previously described should be repeated as indicated.

If treatment is begun again, it must be with a much smaller dose of insulin, since the patient will now be found to be very

sensitive to the drug. In those who recover from prolonged coma, the episode is often followed by a dramatic improvement in the mental state.

A much less serious complication is the not infrequent and sometimes unavoidable secondary hypoglycemia or *"aftershock."* In this condition the patient has emerged from the coma in a normal manner but within 12 hours again develops signs and symptoms of hypoglycemia. It is usually prevented by giving an adequate amount of carbohydrates at the meal following emergence from coma, with interval nourishment during the afternoon and evening. It is readily controlled by the intravenous injection of 50 ml. of 33⅓ per cent solution of glucose. This may be followed by sweetened fruit juice and other carbohydrates if the patient can be encouraged to coöperate.

RESPIRATORY COMPLICATIONS. These are second in frequency as the cause of death in insulin therapy. A moderate degree of salivation is usual in insulin shock but may be so excessive that pneumonia may result from aspiration of saliva. It is therefore important that the patient's head be kept turned to the side during treatment and that secretions be aspirated or absorbed by a gauze wick. A lung abscess may follow regurgitation and aspiration of feeding by tube or by a poorly given gavage. If symptoms suspected to be due either to pneumonia or to abscess appear, the patient should receive antibiotics. Pulmonary edema is usually of cardiac origin and should be treated accordingly. Laryngospasm may be helped by atropine. Edema of the glottis may require tracheotomy. Hiccough, usually due to disturbing changes in the medulla, should be regarded as a dangerous symptom. Here, as in other complications, the patient should receive intravenous glucose.

CARDIOVASCULAR COMPLICATIONS. Such minor complications as tachycardia, bradycardia, or arrhythmias usually respond to glucose alone. More serious complications, such as myocardial failure, cardiac dilation, aortic insufficiency, or general vasomotor collapse, require intravenous glucose, Coramine, strophanthin, and the usual supportive measures.

CONVULSIONS. There are two types of convulsions, the early and the late. The former are of a grand mal type and usually occur in Stage II. These are not dangerous and are successfully controlled by intravenous injection of glucose and subsequent prophylactic use of anticonvulsants. Late convulsions occur in Stage IV and herald a critical condition for life. The late seizure is usually abortive or atypical, with apnea and cyanosis. If not followed immediately by death, it frequently eventuates in a prolonged or irreversible coma. The patient should receive intravenous glucose at once, also a similar injection of 2 to 4 ml. of Coramine. If there is respiratory embarrassment, oxygen and artificial respiration should be employed. After either type of convulsion, there should be a rest period of one to several days, following which the dosage of insulin should be reduced 10 to 20 per cent when treatment is resumed.

ALLERGIC REACTIONS. These may be either local or general. The former reaction is more common and is manifested by an itching, burning sensation at the point of injection, which becomes indurated and painful. The erythema and induration disappear after a few days of local treatment. The generalized allergic reaction is exhibited in the form of urticaria with much itching. It is relieved by an injection of epinephrine or other antihistaminic agents.

Results of Treatment

As already implied, the use of insulin shock therapy is limited to the treatment of schizophrenia. There is complete agreement among therapists that there is an inverse ratio between the duration of illness and the recovery rate. The best results are obtained with patients who have not been ill for more than one year. After an illness of two years, the percentage of recovery or of improvement falls rapidly. The highest recovery or remission rate is among patients in their twenties who previously had well-integrated personalities, who have had a stormy onset of the illness, and have come to treatment within six months after its onset. Conversely, the results of treatment are poorer in the case of patients who have had limited personality resources, have long manifested schizoid traits, have had an insidious onset of their illness, and became overtly psychotic before 15 or after 40 years of age.

It is generally believed that patients showing tension or a mixture of affective and of schizoid features have a more favorable outlook for recovery, and also that patients who show a high resistance to insulin or fail to gain considerable weight during treatment do poorly. Much better results are secured with the paranoid and catatonic types of schizophrenia than with the simple and hebephrenic types, which respond very poorly.

There is admittedly a high rate of recurrence among schizophrenic patients treated with insulin therapy, but the remission or recovery rate for those who have been adequately treated with insulin is significantly higher than for a similar group of untreated patients. It has been said that over long periods of time recoveries are more stable in non-shock-treated patients than in those so treated. The use of insulin coma therapy is rapidly declining.

PSYCHOSURGERY

The operation of lobotomy, a surgical procedure consisting of a severance of the connection between the thalamus and frontal lobe, was developed by a Portuguese neurologist, Egas Moniz, and first performed by the neurosurgeon, Almeida Lima, in 1935. Moniz published his monograph in 1936, immediately following which the operation was introduced into the United States by Dr. Walter Freeman and Dr. James Watts. In 1949

Moniz received the Nobel Prize in Medicine for his work in prefrontal lobotomy.

Techniques

A variety of neurosurgical techniques were devised as a means of transecting the thalamofrontal fibers expanding from the dorsomedial nucleus of the thalamus to the frontal poles. As these procedures were tested, it became apparent that only limited transections of cortical white matter were necessary to bring about the desired therapeutic result. Thus division of the medial half of the white matter of each frontal lobe, the *bimedial operation,* has been found to bring about as much relief of anxiety, tension, and disorganization of behavior as the earlier extensive bilateral frontal lobotomies. The *topectomy* procedure, consisting of symmetrical removals of Brodmann's architectonic areas 9 and 10 of the frontal cortex, seemed also to bring effective therapeutic change without the unfortunate personality deficits of the earlier more extensive lobotomy procedures. Topectomy is now seldom performed, as postoperative convulsions occurred more frequently than with other procedures. The complicated thalamotomy procedure, in which the dorsomedial thalamic nuclei are destroyed by electrolysis, is seldom done. Blocking the frontal lobe by initial procaine and later alcohol injections has been tried.

Today, the few lobotomies performed usually are carried out through open craniotomies by neurosurgeons. Transorbital lobotomy, the closed procedure initiated by W. Freeman and conducted by some psychiatrists, generally has been abandoned.

Acute Effects of Operation

Immediately after prefrontal lobotomy, the patient loses his nervous tension and may appear stuporous or confused for a few days to a week. He remains indifferent to his surroundings, pays no attention to excretory functions, has to be fed and moved about in bed, is somnolent, and may vomit. He may confabulate and deny that he has had an operation. A few patients are noisy and manifest a repetitious, destructive overactivity. In many instances the success of the operation depends upon the supervision the patient receives for several weeks following. He must be forced out of bed, taken to the toilet at regular intervals, and made to bathe, dress, and feed himself. An excessive appetite is common and may result in a great gain in weight. In even the simplest matters the patient should be specifically instructed and guided for a considerable time. It is usually desirable that the patient go home as soon as possible after the operation in order that the constant social pressure of the home may stimulate more adequate social behavior. It is highly important that the operation be followed by an active rehabilitation program, which should include retraining and reëducational measures and a system of graded privileges.

The chief complication of lobotomy is the development of convulsive seizures. These are usually of the grand mal type and can be controlled by anti-convulsive medication.

Indications

Prefrontal lobotomy is a radical procedure that will be undertaken only after other forms of treatment, including tranquilizing drugs and some form of shock therapy, have failed. Its use since the introduction of the tranquilizing drugs has greatly decreased. Patients are selected for operation on the basis of symptoms rather than of diagnosis. The best results are secured in patients who show tension, agitation and distress, depression, worry, intractable pain syndromes, compulsions, hostility, and excited, impulsive behavior. Such symptoms as phobias, obsessions, hallucinations, and delusional experiences are relieved if they have not existed for extended periods, although the basic pathology of the thought process is not affected. Cruelty, avoidance of responsibility, and excessive use of alcohol before the development of the psychosis are contraindications.

In *schizophrenia* prefrontal lobotomy has no effect on the fundamental disease process, but in well-selected cases it may be followed by a great improvement in adjustment. The better organized the prepsychotic personality, the better the results, provided deteriorated, psychotic habits have not existed for several years. In general, lobotomy may be recommended after a two-year illness if the patient has, in the meantime, received active treatment with tranquilizing drugs, insulin, and electroconvulsive therapy without beneficial results. If the patient is a chronically deteriorated, inactive *hebephrenic* whose affect has been "burned out," little benefit is to be expected from operation. On the other hand, the behavior of the overactive, resistive, excitable, destructive, restless, unmanageable schizophrenic may be greatly improved. Such a patient may become quiet and somewhat sociable, and perhaps later he may be able to leave the hospital and even become self-sustaining. Not a few patients become free, cheerful, relaxed, interested in events of the day, and able to carry on a conversation on various topics. Sometimes activity may be so reduced that the patient sits about in a lethargic state.

Lobotomy is rarely undertaken in acute *manic-depressive* psychosis, since most cases yield either to electroconvulsive therapy or to tranquilizing drugs. It may be advisable in prolonged depressive states with tension that have not yielded to the variety of antidepressant drugs singly or in combination or to electroconvulsive therapy. It has not usually been of value in chronic manic states. Since the recovery rate in *involutional melancholia* following convulsive therapy is high, lobotomy is rarely used in this disease. There are, however, some cases of rut depression and rumination on

abnormal ideas, or cases with schizophrenic features that do not respond to convulsive therapy. In such cases and in the paranoid type of involutional psychosis lobotomy may be a beneficial procedure.

In severe obsessive-compulsive, obsessive-ruminative, and hypochondriacal types of *psychoneuroses* that have not been benefited by psychotherapy, the disabling tension and anxiety states may be relieved by lobotomy. Obsessive ideas may continue, but the relief from tension may permit the patient to pursue his normal activities. In general, previous conflicts remain, but the quantity of emotional charge is reduced. Probably the best results in lobotomy are secured in agitated depressions and in severe obsessive-compulsive reactions accompanied by so much tension that the patient is incapacitated. One should, however, be conservative in recommending lobotomy for the treatment of psychoneuroses.

The success of prefrontal lobotomy in controlling emotional disturbance and overactivity arising from it as seen in some chronic manic and schizophrenic states suggested that the operation might be of benefit in the treatment of severe behavior disorders following acquired brain disease or in pathological personalities. The results, however, have been poor and the operation is not considered justifiable.

Unpleasant Sequels

Observation of patients who have been subjected to prefrontal lobotomy suggests that the function of the "silent" regions of the frontal lobe is to elaborate and integrate affective responses with the other modes of response of the individual to the environment so as to secure an emotionally harmonious life. A change in personality with an accentuation of previous unpleasant traits is not uncommon but is by no means true in all cases. The patient's relatives must expect him to show an absence of self-consciousness, a facetiousness, and childlike pleasure in simple things. Sarcastic remarks and undesirable behavior must be overlooked. For many, the assumption of financial responsibilities is a dubious undertaking.

Even in cases in which results are otherwise good, the patient's sense of responsibility and his feeling for others may be impaired. Frequently there is a reduction in depth of feeling, in sensitivity, and in richness of inner life. Affect is more shallow than before the illness, and the patient usually lacks former sympathies and altruistic motives. There is an increase in self-esteem, tactlessness, and lack of self-criticism and of restraint. Imaginative foresight is usually less than normal. "He doesn't care whether school keeps or not." With less desirable results the patient may be lazy, tactless, suggestible, and childish, and manifest a silly euphoria. He may be unrestrained in word and action, careless in eating habits and personal appearance, and perhaps vulgar and profane. In the usual case, the outstanding change is in affect and not in intellect.

The careful long-term follow-up of Smith and Kinder on patients subject to topectomy has shown significant losses in their performance on various psychological tests. Some patients, particularly those schizophrenics who have led a purely vegetative existence without active mental conflict, may show no improvement and even exhibit an organic dementia also. Patients whose prepsychotic tendencies were characterized by active aggressiveness may, after operation, manifest an undesirable lack of restraint of these impulses.

Outcome

There have been published a number of reports of assessment of long-term outcome of patients treated by one of the varieties of lobotomy. Those reports vary because some represent the study of patients operated upon a decade or so past when lobotomies were frequently pre-

scribed, whereas others, such as that by Post, Rees and Schurr, present outcome on patients so treated more recently after all other methods of treatment had proved ineffective in establishing a social adaptation. This later report is most pertinent to the needs of the modern psychiatric practitioner. They found that a high proportion of the 52 patients with longstanding, continuous, and disabling illness other than schizophrenia, attained beneficial results. Thus 14 became socially well or symptom free, 14 benefited moderately, 15 benefited marginally, and nine were unimproved. These changes were maintained or enhanced over a three-year period of observation. The conditions so treated were psychotic depression, depressions with pain, depressions with obsessions, neurotic depressions, and obsessional and other neurotic states. Yet undesirable effects occurred in two-thirds, in terms of postoperative personality changes described earlier in this chapter. Those with chronic depressive symptoms were most likely to benefit, either as an isolated expression of illness or associated with other neurotic symptoms or the complaint of pain.

In general, in the bilateral sectioning of all white matter in suitable patients on whom operation has not been unduly deferred, approximately one-third will leave the hospital and make a tolerable or better adjustment. In some instances the degree of recovery is dramatic, the patient regaining a completely successful social, occupational, and economic adjustment. Another third will show a significant improvement. Some of them can be cared for at home, and the institutional adjustment of the remainder will be improved. A third of those operated upon will show no improvement.

All the recent studies of outcome suggest that the current tendency to avoid prescription of this procedure is unwarranted when other therapeutic measures have failed to bring about relief of distress and good social adaptation, particularly in the persisting disabling psychotic and neurotic disorders and in the other than nonreactive schizophrenic syndromes.

BIBLIOGRAPHY

Ballantine, H. T., Cassidy, W. L., Flanagan, N. B., and Mauno, R.: Stereotaxic anterior cingulotomy for neuropsychiatric illness and intractable pain. J. Neurosurg., 26:488–495, 1967.

Carney, M. W. P., Roth, M., and Garsile, R. F.: The diagnosis of the depressive syndrome and the prediction of E.C.T. response. Brit. J. Psychiat., 3:659–674, 1965.

Cotman, C. W., Banker, G., Zarnetzer, S. F., and McGaugh, J. L.: Electroshock effects on brain protein synthesis. Science, 173:454–456, 1971.

Cronholm, B., and Ottosson, O., Jr.: The experience of memory function after electroconvulsive therapy. Brit. J. Psychiat., 109:251–258, 1963.

Dolenz, B. J.: Indoklon: A clinical review. Psychosomatics, 6:200–205, 1965.

Freeman, W.: Frontal lobotomy in early schizophrenia. Long follow-up of 415 cases. Brit. J. Psychiat., 119:621–624, 1971.

Halliday, A. M., et al.: Comparison of effects on depression and memory of bilateral ECT and unilateral ECT to dominant and nondominant hemispheres. Brit. J. Psychiat., 114:997–1012, 1968.

Hunt, H. F.: Electroconvulsive shock and learning. Trans. New York Acad. Sci., 27:923–945, 1965.

Kalinowsky, L. B., and Hippius, H.: Pharmacologic, Convulsive and Other Somatic Treatments in Psychiatry. New York, Grune & Stratton, 1969.

Kety, S. S., et al.: A sustained effect of electroconvulsive shock on the turnover of norepinephrine in the central nervous system of the rat. Proc. Nat. Acad. Sci., 58:1249–1254, 1967.

Miller, A.: The lobotomy patient—a decade later. Canad. Med. Assn. J., 96:1095–1103, 1967.

Motulsky, A. G., and Morrow, A.: A typical cholinesterase Gene Ela: Rarity in Negroes and most Orientals. Science, 159:202–203, 168.

Pitts, F. N., Woodruff, R. H., Jr., Craig, A. G., and Rich, C. L.: The drug modification of E.C.T. Arch. Gen. Psychiat., 19:595–598, 1968.

Post, F., Rees, L. W., and Schurr, P. H.: An evaluation of bimedial leucotomy. Brit. J. Psychiat., 114:1223–1246, 1968.

Shobe, F. C., and Gildea, C. L.: Long term follow-up of selected lobotomized private patients. J.A.M.A., 206:327–332, 1968.

Smith, A.: Changing effects of frontal lesions in man, J. Neurol., Neurosurg. & Psychiat., 27:511–515, 1967.

Zarcone, V., Gulevich, G., and Dement, W.: Sleep and electroconvulsive therapy. Arch. Gen. Psychiat., 16:567–573, 1967.

Zinkin, S., and Birtchnell, J.: Unilateral electroconvulsive therapy: Its effects on memory and its therapeutic efficacy. Brit. J. Psychiat., 114:973–988, 1968.

Chapter 34

Psychiatry and the Law

Both psychiatry and the law—the former to a large degree, the latter to an important but lesser extent—deal with human behavior. Psychiatry seeks to ascertain the forces that result in behavioral deviations and how they may be redirected to lead to greater intrapersonal serenity and to more constructive and socialized purposes. The law deals largely with the social control of behavior. Although these two disciplines deal with two quite different aspects of behavior, they have many contacts, and since they approach problems of behavior from quite different points of view, it is not surprising that differences of emphasis and of opinion sometimes exist.

The psychiatrist is called upon to testify as to the propriety of civil commitment of persons to mental hospitals as a means of protecting the public and the individual from potentially dangerous behavior as the consequence of mental illness, and to effect treatment of the illness. Often he testifies as an expert witness concerning the mental competence of individuals alleged to be mentally ill to make those judgments that relate to the custody of property through civil actions such as marriage, divorce, and the making of wills and contracts. In many jurisdictions psychiatrists may be introduced in court to testify as to criminal responsibility. Undoubtedly their role in providing testimony in the last capacity is the one in which the most controversy exists between the legal profession and the specialty of psychiatry.

HOSPITALIZING MENTALLY ILL PERSONS

One of the important differences between the psychiatrist and the lawyer is in their respective attitudes toward the admission of the mentally ill person to a hospital. The psychiatrist urges that the dignity of the patient be respected and that the obstacles to his admission be no greater than those experienced by the physically sick person. The laws of many states still contain much archaic legal phraseology carrying connotations of criminal prosecution and guilt in their provisions for the hospitalization of the mentally ill. Since in many instances the mental patient does not recognize that he is ill, he does not seek treatment and may even resist measures designed to provide it, and since the Constitution of the United States provides that a person may not be deprived of his liberty without adequate notice and a chance to be heard, the law insists on a punctilious observance of what it regards as human rights.

A few years ago a special committee of the American Bar Association, in referring to the formal legal procedures of commitment of the mentally ill person, stated that these are "fundamental principles of justice which cannot be ignored. Without them, no citizen would be safe from the machinations of secret tribunals, and the most sane member of the community might be adjudged insane and landed in a madhouse." Although it is perhaps theoretically possible that a sane

656

person might be "railroaded" into an institution, it probably rarely occurs now in this country, certainly not in a public mental hospital. The lawyer should not be criticized too severely for his vigilant solicitude for the legal rights of the individual. The physician believes, however, that one's medical rights are no less fundamental than his legal rights, and that the sick person should not be subjected to heartless and harmful mental torture incident to commitment. Until very recently one state in the United States required that a mentally sick person must, except for temporary commitment, have a "trial by jury." (A jury trial is now optional.)

The vast majority of states have laws that permit a mentally ill person to apply for treatment in a public mental hospital. Such laws frequently state that the applicant must be mentally competent to make application and must give a certain number of days' notice in writing if he desires to leave. The extent to which persons apply for admission under the provisions of such a statute varies greatly among the states.

In addition to any laws providing for the voluntary admission of patients, every state has various laws governing the commitment of mentally ill persons. Frequently the patient with mental disorder caused by, or associated with, impairment of brain tissue function is not mentally competent to make application for his admission to a hospital. Among such persons may be those suffering from acute brain disorders associated with intoxication or infection, or from chronic brain disorders associated with cerebral arteriosclerosis or senile brain disease. The laws of a number of states wisely permit the legal guardian or close relative of such an incompetent person to arrange for his admission. "A person who is a fit subject for mental treatment should not be denied the easy method for admission merely because he may be too indecisive, weak-minded, or incompetent to sign his own papers."*

Many states provide for the emergency commitment of a patient. These commitments are temporary, and commitment for an indeterminate period must be completed before the expiration of the period for which the emergency commitment is permitted. The procedure to be followed in an emergency commitment varies greatly. In some states the law merely requires that a petition be filed with the hospital to which commitment is desired, together with a certification of one physician that the patient is in need of immediate hospital care.

In most states the law provides in general that when an involuntary commitment for an indeterminate period is contemplated, a petition for the patient's commitment must be filed with a judicial agency, that the patient be notified of the proposed judicial hearing on his mental state, and that he be examined by two physicians who will certify that he is suffering from mental disease. The judge presiding at the hearing is the committing agent, although in 21 states the hearing may be held before a jury if requested by the patient.

In a few states the law permits, without a judicial hearing or order, the superintendent of a mental hospital to receive a mentally sick person and detain him for an indeterminate period. Usually in such a case a relative or other responsible person submits to the superintendent a petition for the patient's admission. This petition contains a sworn statement setting forth reasons why the petitioner believes the patient is mentally ill. Accompanying the petition is a certification by two physicians that they have, within a prescribed period, examined the patient and that in their opinion he is mentally ill and in need of care and treatment in a hospital for the mentally sick. In one state most patients are admitted under the provisions of such a statute. It has been operative in practically the same form for over 70 years and has proved eminently satisfactory.

---

* Addendum, Law of Maryland, March, 1944, page 63, 34A.

British Mental Health Act, 1959

The laws governing commitment are, however, gradually becoming more liberal and reflect the need to preserve the psychiatrically ill from humiliating publicity and deprivation of their rights as well as to open more easily to them treatment on the same grounds as those with predominantly physical illnesses. Nowhere is this trend more advanced than in England, where a new Mental Health Act became law in July, 1959, and went into effect on November 1, 1960. Today in England nonstatutory admissions are allowed to the mental hospitals; the patient may enter informally if he so desires without the signature of papers by himself or others, and thus he receives treatment under the same circumstances as those with medical or surgical problems.

In cases in which compulsory admission is required to safeguard the patient or the community, this is recognized solely as a medical decision and not a civil or judicial one. The authorization for admission consists of the recommendation of two physicians, one of whom must be experienced in the treatment of mental disorders. In cases of emergency, the patient may be admitted and detained three days on the application of a mental welfare officer or any relative on the recommendation of one physician.

Discharge from the hospital also may be carried out informally on the decision of a physician, or at the request of the patient or relative on three days' written notice. When the patient is considered too disturbed to be discharged, he may be detained on medical recommendation, but he has recourse to appeal to the Mental Health Review Tribunals. Such tribunals are composed of legal and medical members as well as persons qualified in administration of social service. The tribunals are independent local bodies of skilled persons which evaluate the patient's mental condition and his need for continuing hospital care. If he is found to be without illness or unlikely to endanger himself and others, his discharge must be ordered. Each adult patient may apply to the tribunal once in the six months following his initial admission and once in each succeeding year of detention.

Special provisions are established for such groups as the psychopath. This act guarantees certain rights to the hospitalized patient. It establishes, as well, systems for the management of criminal cases. Thus the courts may order hospitalization instead of imprisonment for the convicted mentally ill persons who are suitable for treatment when facilities exist for such care.

To many, the British Mental Health Act of 1959 represents the penetration of a new frontier in the treatment of those with serious behavior disturbances. It reflects as well a profound concern with the development of community resources for their care. Its social pioneering may well establish the model for new humanitarian health legislation in other countries in the future.

The management of psychiatrically ill criminal offenders under the British Mental Health Act has taken a course unsuspected by the progenitors of this most liberal legislation. According to Rollin, it would seem that in the courts British psychiatrists are unusually optimistic as regards the effects of treatment in mental hospitals, even for the psychopathic, as against confinement in prisons. Accordingly more persons with criminal records, and many repeated recidivists, are entered into the British open hospital and community care system. As Rollin shows, under this method of management a greater proportion of those formerly entering the prison system now enter the open mental hospital system, which appears to be ineffective in providing the necessary management to modify the criminal tendencies and sustain public security. Here and there, when large numbers of those criminal mentally ill are entered in hospital, their easy escapes into the local community and their subsequent implication in further antisocial ills have produced adverse public reactions toward the modern mental health system in Britain and the forward-looking act.

In this respect those reports on the dangerousness of formerly hospitalized mentally ill persons assume significance. Rappaport has reviewed the literature and provided new data of his own. With Larsen he collected information on arrests for felonies (murder, negligent manslaughter, rape, robbery, and aggravated assault) committed by former hospitalized mental patients in the state of Maryland between 1947 and 1957 and compared it to the rate for the general population. The majority of offenses were contributed by discharged alcoholics and schizophrenics. According to this and other earlier studies, the hospital-discharged mentally ill have not been involved in criminal behavior to any greater extent than the general population. Both Rappaport and Larsen found that treatment did not reduce the later arrest rate, except among alcoholics. In their series an experience of psychiatric hospitalization tended to increase criminal activity in those with personality disorder of the antisocial type. In some areas of felony, notably robbery and rape, the psychiatric population was arrested more often than members of the general population.

What a modern system of law, cognizant of the special knowledge that psychiatrists have, should request of this specialty is a definition of the appropriate corrective management of an offender after his act has been judged and he found guilty by the jury. On the basis of a clinical evaluation, the psychiatrist, as expert, might recommend then either psychiatric treatment with attempts to modify pathologic affect through treatment by pharmacotherapy or other somatic therapies under professional care; or a prescription to attempt development of superego controls through emotional attachment and relearning in group and individual psychotherapies in a permissive but closed institution; for still others the recommendation given would be for a restrictive prison experience punitive toward his act when it is apparent that such exposure in earlier life was not gained by the offender.

Unfortunately neither the practice of law nor that of psychiatry has achieved sufficient understanding of the other, or of the potentials of the behavioral sciences, to the point that this appropriate use of psychiatric testimony be made in the courts today.

Model Act Governing Hospitalization of the Mentally Ill*

As previously indicated, each state has its own laws governing the commitment of the mentally ill. Because of this, there is great disparity among the states as to legal procedure in commitment. In many states, too, these procedures subject the patient to indignities and humiliations. For this reason, the National Advisory Mental Health Council in 1949 requested the United States Public Health Service to develop what might be considered as a model act. Very few states have enacted a law patterned on this "Model Act," but presumably, as states gradually modify their commitment laws, there will be a tendency to incorporate into concrete legal procedure the modern thinking reflected in the provisions of this suggested act. The act will not be quoted but attention is called to some of its most important features.

Voluntary Hospitalization

The proposed act is so drawn as to facilitate voluntary admissions but provides that upon the patient's written request he shall be forthwith discharged. If, however, in the opinion of the head of the hospital the release of the patient would be dangerous to himself or others, this official may notify the court and the

---

* A Draft Act Governing Hospitalization of the Mentally Ill, U.S. Federal Security Agency, Public Health Service, Publication No. 51, U.S. Government Printing Office, 1951.

patient's discharge may be postponed for as long as the court deems necessary for the commencement of proceedings for judicial hospitalization, but in no event for more than five days.

Involuntary Hospitalization

The draft of the proposed act distinguishes between involuntary hospitalization and compulsory hospitalization. Commitment proceedings may be involuntary in the sense that they are initiated by someone other than the patient himself, but the patient accepts the judgment of the physician and his family. In that case, there is no judicial hearing, and the commitment procedure consists merely of the filing of a request for the patient's admission and the certification of two qualified physicians that they have examined the individual and that in their opinion he should be hospitalized. It is presumed that most patients would be admitted on this medical certification, were statutes based on the "Model Act" adopted.

Compulsory Hospitalization

If the patient refuses hospitalization, a judicial hearing is necessary before the commitment may be made compulsory. In such a case, a petition for the patient's commitment may be filed with the court. This petition must be accompanied by a certificate of a physician stating that he has examined the patient and is of the opinion that he is mentally ill and should be hospitalized. Upon receipt of the application, the court gives notice thereof to the patient and appoints two physicians to examine him. If the examiners report that the patient is mentally ill, the court sets a date for a hearing at which the patient is afforded an opportunity to appear. If, upon completion of the hearing, the court finds that the patient is in need of custody and treatment, it orders his hospitalization for an indeterminate

period or for a temporary observational period not to exceed six months.

The "Model Act" also has humane provisions for the emergency commitment of a patient pending opportunity to initiate proceedings for an indeterminate commitment.

The proposed draft contains various provisions designed to promote the welfare and protect the rights of the patient requiring hospitalization. Among these is one that, pending his removal to a hospital, a committed patient shall not, except because of and during an extreme emergency, be detained in a nonmedical facility used for the detention of individuals charged with or convicted of penal offenses. As is already provided in many states, the "Model Act" would, except under unusual circumstances, permit the patient to communicate with official agencies inside or outside the hospital; to receive visitors and confer with counsel; to exercise all civil rights, including the right to dispose of property, execute instruments, make purchases, enter contractual relationships, and vote, unless he has been adjudicated incompetent. The act also greatly restricts the information that may be divulged concerning a patient except with the permission of either himself or his guardian.

Observation Commitment

Several states have legal provision whereby a person charged with, or under indictment for, a criminal offense, or if having been found guilty is awaiting sentence, may be committed to a public mental hospital for a limited period of observation. Following the examination of the prisoner, the hospital submits a report to the court. The hospital does not, of course, express any opinion as to the guilt or innocence of the prisoner. If he is found to be psychotic, commitment will usually be recommended. Frequently the report may include a statement as to whether or not the prisoner's mental condition is such that he is capable of conferring with counsel and preparing his defense. Some courts, especially juvenile courts, may, if the hospital has thoroughly investigated the social situation of the patient, welcome suggestions as to disposition of the prisoner. A juvenile court is, however, more an administrative than a judicial tribunal. Courts are, to an increasing extent, committing prisoners for observation before trial or sentence. Many criminal courts in large cities now employ a full-time or part-time psychiatrist. Occasionally a prisoner, while serving a sentence, develops a psychosis under the stress of confinement. He will then be transferred to a mental hospital, where he will remain until his recovery or until his sentence expires.

Commitment, Competency, and Civil Rights

Commitment does not in itself automatically adjudicate incompetency; in most states, in fact, a mentally ill patient is not by his commitment adjudged incompetent or deprived of his "civil rights." If, at the time of his commitment, the patient is formally adjudged as "insane" by judicial action, he is thereby rendered incompetent and deprived of certain civil rights. He may not buy or sell property or sign legal papers; he may not vote or hold office; it suspends his driver's license; it usually vacates his license to practice medicine, law, or other learned profession; it takes away from him the right to consent to or refuse to consent to the adoption of a child; it casts doubt on his right to make a will; and it impairs his right to marry, although usually, if he does marry while psychotic, the marriage will be valid unless specifically set aside. In most states he cannot start a divorce action.

The methods of erasing the adjudication and of restoring legal competency vary from state to state. Generally speaking, if commitability and incompetency are determined by separate procedures, then discharge (not leave-of-absence or parole) will vacate the commitment order but have no effect on the finding of incompetency. Another court action will be necessary to declare the patient competent and to discharge a guardian.

Habeas Corpus

A right that the psychotic person preserves, even though he has been legally adjudicated as insane, is that of applying for a writ of habeas corpus. This writ has for its object the speedy release by judicial decree. Under American and English law, this writ may be proclaimed on behalf of anyone who claims he is being restrained of his liberty illegally. Since a commitment may continue only so long as the patient needs care and custody, he may at any time petition for the issuance of such a writ on the ground that he is now sane and so entitled to release. At the hearing on the petition, the sanity of the patient is inquired into, and if the court finds him sane, he may be discharged. In some jurisdictions the court impanels a jury to determine the issue of sanity. In only a few jurisdictions are there any restrictions imposed on the frequency with which application for a writ may be made.

PRIVILEGED COMMUNICATIONS

In nearly all jurisdictions, a physician on the witness stand is not allowed, without the patient's consent, to disclose any information acquired in attending the patient in a professional capacity. It is generally held that the confidentiality of a patient's relations with his psychiatrist is peculiarly close, even more so than in ordinary medicine, and is not subject to violation even on a court summons. Usually courts have held that relations between a patient committed to a mental institution and a staff doctor are likewise of a privileged professional nature and are therefore protected from disclosure on a witness stand. The privilege has, in fact, been extended so far beyond the premise of protecting confidential communications that courts assume without argument that all statements of inmates to hospital doctors come within the rule.

Yet psychiatrists should be aware that the right of medical privileged communication exists only by statute. In some state jurisdictions, patients do not possess the right of privilege. It is therefore important that all psychiatrists ascertain the status of privilege in the state or states in which they practice. Where the patient does not have the legal right of a privileged communication and does not understand the consequences of waiving his right, it is imperative that the psychiatrist advise him of the legal limits of confidentiality and privilege in that particular community.

Physicians in public mental hospitals receive so many requests for information about their patients that they frequently forget the extent to which the hospital records are really of a privileged nature. They should therefore be guarded lest they divulge more information concerning patients than is permissible.

Marriage

In most states the criterion of legal capacity to marry is the ability to understand the nature of the marriage contract and the duties and obligations such a contract entails. The statutes are of little help in defining the degree of mental unsoundness that will suffice to void a marriage. If it is clear that if one party was so psychotic, drunk, or defective at the time of marriage that he or she did not understand the obligations assumed by the marriage contract, an annulment will usually be decreed. In general, however, courts are reluctant to declare a marriage void. Many states have laws forbidding mentally ill persons to marry. The objective of such laws is presumably to prevent the procreation of defective children. If

such is the case, the law is not based on any scientific proof of the inheritability of the disorder. Usually the courts will not annul a marriage on the grounds of fraud if a concealment of previous mental disease is the basis of the charge. Concealment of previous commitment to a mental hospital is not a ground for annulment on the basis of fraud unless the party concerned affirmatively stated that he never was in a mental hospital.

Divorce

In most states insanity is not a ground for divorce; however, in some states divorce will be granted if the insane spouse has been committed to a hospital for mental diseases for a period of years. The statutes in some states specify that the spouse must be "incurably insane." The psychiatrist is reluctant to testify that any mental illness is absolutely incurable. Perhaps he can say that in the light of present-day medical knowledge it is his opinion that the patient's disorder is incurable. He will remember that at the beginning of the present century he would have testified that general paresis, even in its early stage, was incurable. He certainly would not do so now.

Wills

A person's competency to make a will is known as testamentary capacity. This capacity must meet three criteria. The testator, or a person making a will, must (1) know that he is making a will, (2) know the nature and extent of his property, and (3) know the natural objects of his bounty. Expressed a little more simply, the person signing a will must know clearly what he is doing when he signs it. Although it is not necessary that he know the minutest details concerning his property, he must have a substantially accurate knowledge of what he owns. By "natural objects of his bounty" is meant the members of the testator's family, his warm friends, others to whom he feels especially grateful, or institutions or organizations in which he has felt an interest. Although he must know who are his living near relatives, the law does not require that he bequeath them anything. The failure of a testator to include a member of his family because of paranoid delusions of a psychotic intensity concerning the relative would probably render the will invalid, since the delusion would affect his understanding of the natural objects of his bounty. Statutes sometimes state that the testator must be of "sound mind and memory." This phrase means, in effect, that the testator must possess the testamentary capacity just described. The fact that the testator was psychotic or was committed to a hospital for mental disorders when he made the will does not necessarily mean that he lacked mental capacity to make a will, nor does it necessarily render it invalid. The psychiatrist must at all times bear in mind the three basic criteria as to testamentary capacity.

Since it is often difficult to draw a line between simple senility and senile dementia, the question of testamentary capacity of the elderly person may arise. Even though the testator's mental processes be slow, the courts will consider him competent if he can call to mind his property and the natural objects of his bounty. Senile persons may suffer not only impairment of mind and memory but also increased suggestibility and therefore be subject to undue influence. Many aged individuals are easy prey to the flattery of younger persons. The courts will hold invalid a will obtained by deception, threat, or the persistent suggestion of a domineering relative or of a flattering confidant.

Occasionally the psychiatrist will be requested to testify in court concerning the testamentary capacity of a testator, now deceased, at the time he made his will. In such a case the attorney will ascertain from witnesses every possible fact concerning the testator's behavior that will be helpful to the psychiatrist in forming an honest opinion concerning the testator's capacity on the day he made his will. These facts will be assembled in the hypothetical question describing the testator's behavior. At times a lawyer will request that his client be examined as to his competency at the time a testator prepares his will. The psychiatrist's examination will then be directed with special reference to the three basic criteria of testamentary capacity. He will secure from the testator a description of his property and its estimated value. He will ask the patient to name the members of his family and indicate their relationships. As he secures a description of each relative, the physician will note the nature of the emotional response evoked by the respective discussions concerning each. The physician's report to the lawyer should contain such verbatim statements made by the patient as will later suggest his testamentary capacity.

Competency and Contracts

Every person of legal age is presumed to be mentally competent, i.e., to have the mental capacity to carry on his everyday affairs. The burden of proof is, therefore, on one who would declare the adult incompetent. To determine that a person is incompetent, it must be shown that he has a mental disorder, that this mental disorder causes a defect in judgment, and that this defect in judgment renders him incapable of managing his property, the prudent making of contracts, or the taking of some other specific action.

The establishment of a mental disorder is not sufficient to warrant a finding of incompetency. It must also be shown that the mental disorder causes an impairment of judgment. No valid generalization can be made on the relationship of the various mental disorders to competency. The diagnostic label attached to the disorder is not as important as the degree to which judgment is impaired. Consideration must also be given as to whether the condition is static, progressive, or improving. A progressive organic disease of the brain is typically a disorder that renders a patient incompetent, but many patients suffering from psychogenic disorders, such as manic-depressive psychosis, schizophrenia, or paranoid disorders, suffer from such seriously impaired judgment that they are rendered incompetent.

If a person is considered incompetent and he has business affairs that require attention, a petition for the appointment of a guardian will be filed with the appropriate court. The issue of incompetency is usually tried before either a probate or a county court, without a jury. In several states a jury is still used. Usually a member of the patient's family is the petitioner, but anyone who has an interest in preserving the patient's estate may petition the court for the appointment of a guardian. Notice of a hearing on the petition must be given to the person, and in many states to certain others, such as his next of kin. A few states provide not only that the person is entitled to be present if he desires but that his presence is required. It must be shown, usually by medical evidence, that there is danger that in the absence of a guardian for the person's estate he will dissipate his property or become the victim of designing persons. Some courts require personal testimony by a physician, while others will accept a certificate of incompetency in lieu of personal testimony. If the person is declared incompetent, the court will decide whether his interests are best served by the appointment of a friend, relative, stranger, or corporation as the guardian. In some states the fact of commitment automatically adjudges the patient as incompetent. In such a case the appointment of a guardian is merely an administrative matter and requires no judicial hearing. Usually a guardianship obtains only in respect to the patient's estate and does not, unless so specified, include guardianship of his person.

CONTRACTS. Courts will usually rule that a contract or other legal transaction will not be set aside on the grounds of mental incompetency if the person had sufficient mental capacity to understand the nature and effect of the particular transaction. A higher degree of mental capacity may be required to understand a complex instrument or transaction than a simple one. The degree of judgment needed may vary greatly. It is sometimes claimed that a contract was executed during a lucid interval of a person admittedly disordered. Psychiatrists are inclined to question whether in most cases the patient's lucidity during such intervals was not more apparent than real. It is the prevailing theory that where the incompetency of one party was not known to the other party, where no advantage was taken of the incompetent, and where the contract has been executed and the parties cannot be put back *in status quo,* the contract is binding and cannot be voided on the grounds of incompetency.

Criminal Responsibility

The concepts of mind held by psychiatry and by the law are so disparate that it is difficult for the two professions to agree as to responsibility for behavior, especially criminal behavior. According to the concept held by law, the mind is dominated by reason and full will, and behavior results from a consciously determined intent. The law does not recognize partial responsibility, although to the psychiatrist responsibility does not have definable boundaries and degrees. Law confines its exploration of behavior to conscious data and assumes that a disorder of the cognitive faculty (knowledge) is the only basis for the determination of responsibility for behavior termed criminal. Psychiatry, on the other hand, assumes that mental processes are controlled by both conscious and unconscious factors, the latter playing a very important part; that behavior is an expression of the personality as a whole as determined by a multiplicity of complex factors, including the unconscious effect of early experiences, later pressures, and emotional needs. To the psychiatrist, the unlawful act may be not the result of a consciously determined "intent" but the surface manifestation of a more profound psychic disturbance, an indicator of breakdown in a system of psychic adaptive defenses erected to balance inner conflicts. The psychiatrist would go beyond the act itself and evaluate the total personality, both in its conscious and unconscious aspects. He recognizes the role of the intellect, but would give to emotions and the unconscious a greater weight in the balance of forces in mental life.

The difference in these concepts is a logical result of the gradual development of psychological knowledge. In ancient times lunatics were not regarded as suffering from disease but were believed to be possessed of demons and were beaten, kept in chains, and not uncommonly sentenced to death by burning or hanging. Even if the alleged lunatic had committed some crime, there was no consideration as to the offender's responsibility. Gradually, however, rules to determine criminal responsibility were formulated. Since American law is based largely on English law, it is of interest to note the early application of responsibility tests in the laws of England. In 1723 an English court declared that for an accused to escape punishment he must "not know what he is doing, no more than . . . a wild beast." This requirement, that to qualify for immunity the accused shall know no more than a wild beast, was altered and moderated somewhat about 1760 when the terms "right and wrong" were substituted for "good and evil." Slightly earlier, however, an accused person was executed after it had been determined that he had not shown a *total* want of reason."

The American law generally prevalent at this time stems directly from the famous M'Naghten case. In 1843 Daniel M'Naghten was tried for the willful murder of Edward Drummond, the private secretary of Sir Robert Peel. For several years M'Naghten had suffered from delusions of persecution. He had attempted to escape from his persecutors by leaving Scotland and going to England or to France. On many occasions he had complained to his father and to various public authorities. He became increasingly embittered and finally determined to right his imaginary wrongs by killing Sir Robert Peel. With this object in mind, he watched Peel's house. Seeing Drummond come out, he followed and shot him under the belief that he was shooting Peel. At M'Naghten's trial, his counsel entered a plea of "partial insanity." He was declared of unsound mind and committed to an institution for the criminally insane.

This case caused a great sensation in England, with the result that a few days after the trial a discussion took place in the House of Lords that proposed five questions to the 15 Judges of England regarding the law of insanity. The answers of the Judges can be reduced to two rules to determine the responsibility of a person who pleads insanity as a defense to a crime:

(1) "To establish a defense on the ground of insanity it must be clearly proved that, at the time of committing the act, the party accused was laboring under such a defect of reason, from disease of the mind, as not to know the nature and quality of the act he was doing, or if he did know it, he did not know he was doing what was wrong."

As a rule, the defendant "knows" the facts concerning the particular criminal act that he has committed, knows its harmfulness ("quality"), and its unlawfulness and consequences, but does not know the unconscious basis for it.

(2) "Where a person labors under partial delusions only and is not in other respects insane" and commits an offense in consequence thereof, "he must be considered in the same situation as to responsibility as if the facts with respect to which the delusion exists were real."

It should be borne in mind that the M'Naghten Rules are not a test of sanity and were not formulated as such. They are a test of responsibility in law for acts done. In many states the M'Naghten formula is the sole test of responsibility, and in others and in American Military Law it is still the main test supplemented by "the irresistible impulse test."

In 1922 the Lord Chancellor of England appointed a committee to consider and report upon what changes, if any, were desirable in the existing law, practice, and procedure relating to criminal trials in which the plea of insanity as a defense was raised. The committee approved of the M'Naghten Rules and held they should be maintained. It recommended an addition to the effect that "a person charged criminally with an offense is irresponsible for his act when the act is committed under an impulse which the prisoner was by mental disease in substance deprived of any power to resist." As indicated, the laws in some states of the United States exempt from criminal responsibility persons suffering from irresistible or uncontrollable impulse. To most psychiatrists, however, the word "impulse" is unsatisfactory for it covers only a small and very special group of those who are mentally ill. It suggests some sudden episode, yet in many cases the sufferer acts, not suddenly or impulsively, but coolly and with ingenious calculation. This is characteristic of many who suffer from paranoid schizophrenia or paranoid psychosis. Although courts have hung tenaciously to the M'Naghten "right and wrong test," it has been severely criticized, and increasingly, not only by psychiatrists but also by many eminent lawyers. In 1953 Justice Felix Frankfurter stated in testifying before the British Royal Commission on Capital Punishment: "The M'Naghten Rules were rules which the Judges, in response to questions by the House of Lords, formulated in the light of the then existing psychological knowledge. . . . I do not see why the rules of law should be arrested at the state of psychological knowledge at the time when they were formulated."

The above statement, quoting the opinion of one of the most eminent American jurists, reflects the view of an increasing number of lawyers.

In 1869, influenced by Dr. Isaac Ray, doubtless the most enlightened American psychiatrist in the medical jurisprudence of insanity, the Supreme Court of New Hampshire handed down an opinion sweeping aside the M'Naghten Rules. The court recognized simply that an accused person is not criminally responsible if his unlawful act was the result of mental defect. Under this decision, insanity is no longer defined as a matter of law; instead, it is made a question of fact to be determined by the jury like any other fact. This determination rests upon testimony of the psychiatric expert respecting the latest knowledge of human behavior and his interpretation of such knowledge in terms of his observations of the accused. If the accused has a mental disease and if the criminal act is the product of it, he is found not guilty by reason of insanity.

In 1954, in the case of Durham v. United States, the Court of Appeals for the District of Columbia Circuit handed down a decision adopting in substance the same rule as the New Hampshire one. This case involved a defendant, Durham, who had been convicted of housebreaking. He had previously been committed to a hospital for mental disease. At Durham's trial the issue of responsibility was raised. A psychiatrist testified that he thought Durham was of unsound mind but that he might give the correct answer if a question of right or wrong were put to him. The appeal court ruled that the trial court was in error in declaring Durham sane on an obsolete test of responsibility. The essence of the decision is contained in the following passage:

"We find that as an exclusive criterion the right-wrong test is inadequate in that (a) it does not take sufficient account of psychic realities and scientific knowledge, and (b) it is based upon one symptom and so cannot validly be applied to all circumstances. We find that the 'irresistible impulse' test is also inadequate in that it gives no recognition to mental illness characterized by brooding and reflection and so relegates acts caused by such illness to the application of the inadequate right-wrong test. We conclude that a broader test should be adopted. . . .

"The rule we now hold must be applied on the retrial of this case and in future cases is not unlike that followed by the New Hampshire court since 1870. It is simply that an accused is not criminally responsible if his unlawful act was the product of mental disease or mental defect."*

In 1957 the Vermont legislature adopted the following test of insanity when this is used as a defense in criminal cases:

"1. A person is not responsible for criminal conduct if at the time of such conduct as a result of mental disease or defect he lacks adequate capacity either to appreciate the criminality of his conduct or to conform his conduct to the requirements of law.

"2. The terms 'mental disease or defect' do not include an abnormality manifested only by repeated criminal or otherwise anti-social conduct. The terms 'mental disease or defect' shall include congenital and traumatic mental conditions as well as disease.

"3. The M'Naghten test of insanity in criminal cases is hereby abolished."

This statute seems to reflect the increasing dissatisfaction with the M'Naghten Rules as a test of criminal responsibility.

When testifying at a trial, the psychiatrist should remember that the determination of responsibility is a legal issue. The psychiatrist's function is to present the data; the application of the law to the facts is for the court and the jury. He will therefore not express any opinion as to whether or not the defendant can distinguish between right and wrong. Any testimony beyond professionally recognized medical data descriptive of the defendant's mental status, and informative to the court and jury, is therefore beyond the province of the psychiatric expert. All expert testimony should be free of moral and value statements. The psychiatrist will be wise not to attempt

to scale degrees of responsibility in terms of symptoms.

If a person charged with crime is found not guilty by reason of insanity, he may, in some states, at the discretion of the court be committed to a state hospital for mental diseases. In other states it is mandatory that he be committed. In some states the patient may, upon recovery, be discharged by the court that ordered his commitment; in other states, if regarded as no longer dangerous if allowed at large, he may be discharged by the governor. In one state the patient may be discharged only by act of legislature.

Patients are not tried or executed while insane. The issue in such a case is not the patient's ability, or lack of it, to distinguish between right and wrong, but his ability to confer with counsel and prepare his defense.

In one state, Massachusetts, the law (the so-called Briggs law) provides that a person who commits a capital offense or commits more than one felony, or who commits the same crime more than once, must be referred for examination by experts appointed by the State Department of Mental Health. The examinations are usually made at the jail where the defendant is being held. The psychiatrist's report is filed with the clerk of the court and is accessible to the court, to the district attorney, and to the counsel for the accused. If the examiner reports that the prisoner is suffering from mental disease, he is not directly asked to say whether the patient is able to distinguish between right and wrong, or whether he is able to refrain from doing wrong because of an irresistible impulse, but he is asked whether the patient suffers from a mental illness sufficiently severe to affect his responsibility and to require treatment in a mental hospital. It is apparently assumed that the examiner bases his opinion on the right-wrong test and the irresistible impulse test, but the reports submitted to the courts neither ask nor answer the question in these terms.

Under this law, juries have shown a commendable tendency to take the word

---

* Durham v. United States: 59 App. D. C. 144 (1929).

of the impartial examiner as against that of psychiatrists hired by either side. The "battle of experts" has become almost unknown in Massachusetts.

BIBLIOGRAPHY

Barrow, R. L., and Fabing, H. D.: Epilepsy and Law. New York, Paul B. Hoeber, 1956.

Davidson, H. A.: Forensic Psychiatry. New York, Ronald Press, 1952.

Diamond, B. L.: Isaac Ray and the trial of Daniel M'Naghten. Amer. J. Psychiat., *112*:651–656, 1956.

Donnelly, R. C., Goldstein, J., and Schwartz, R. D.: Criminal Law. New York, Free Press of Glencoe, Inc., 1962.

G. A. P. Report No. 26: Criminal Responsibility and Psychiatric Expert Testimony. Topeka, Kansas, 1954.

G. A. P. Report No. 45: Confidentiality and Privileged Communication in the Practice of Psychiatry. New York, 1960.

Group for the Advancement of Psychiatry: Report No. 61, Laws Governing Hospitalization of the Mentally Ill., 1966.

Guttmacher, M. S.: The Role of Psychiatry in Law. Springfield, Ill., Charles C Thomas, 1968.

Hall, J.: Mental disease and criminal responsibility —M'Naghten versus Durham and the American Law Institute's tentative draft. Indiana Law J., *33*:212–225, 1958.

Maclay, W. S.: The new Mental Health Act in England and Wales. Amer. J. Psychiat., *116*: 777–781, 1960.

Mental Health Act, 1959. London, Her Majesty's Stationery Office, 1961.

Meyers, D. W.: The Human Body and the Law., Chicago, Aldine, 1970. Reviewed in Science, *171*: 53, 1971, by W. J. Curran.

Rappaport, J. E. (ed.): The Clinical Evaluations of the Dangerousness of the Mentally Ill. Springfield, Ill., Charles C Thomas, 1967.

Ray, I.: A Treatise on the Medical Jurisprudence of Insanity. Boston, Charles C. Little & James Brown, 1838.

Rollin, H. R.: The Mentally Abnormal Offender and the Law. New York, Pergamon Press, 1969.

Tracey, J. E.: The Doctor as a Witness. Philadelphia, W. B. Saunders Company, 1957.

Usdin, G. L.: The physician and testamentary capacity. Amer. J. Psychiat., *114*:249–256, 1957.

Weihofen, H.: Guardianship and other protective services for the mentally incompetent. Amer. J. Psychiat., *121*:970–978, 1965.

Weihofen, H.: The Urge to Punish. New York, Farrar, Strauss & Cudahy, Inc., 1956.

Index

669